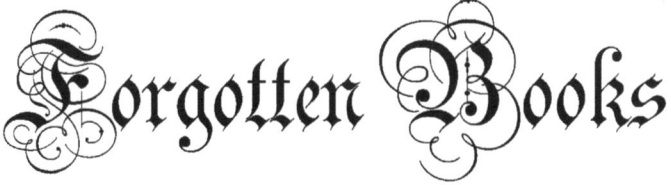
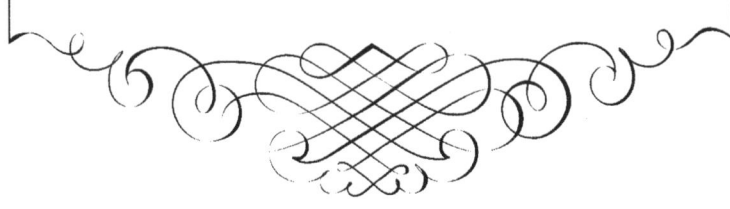

ISBN 978-1-5280-1093-1
PIBN 10940172

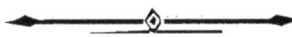

English
Français
Deutsche
Italiano
Español
Português

www.forgottenbooks.com

Mythology Photography **Fiction**
Fishing Christianity **Art** Cooking
Essays Buddhism Freemasonry
Medicine **Biology** Music **Ancient
Egypt** Evolution Carpentry Physics
Dance Geology **Mathematics** Fitness
Shakespeare **Folklore** Yoga Marketing
Confidence Immortality Biographies
Poetry **Psychology** Witchcraft
Electronics Chemistry History **Law**
Accounting **Philosophy** Anthropology
Alchemy Drama Quantum Mechanics
Atheism Sexual Health **Ancient History**
Entrepreneurship Languages Sport
Paleontology Needlework Islam
Metaphysics Investment Archaeology
Parenting Statistics Criminology
Motivational

PREFACE. ·

THE recognition of the value of this work of von Bergmann, vo
Brims, and von Mikulicz has been both prompt and widespread. It
appearance was immediately followed by translations into Spanisl
and Italian, and its first edition was in such demand that the earlie
volumes went out of print before the later ones could pass through th
press. The second edition, carefully revised and brought thoroughl
up to date in regard to literature and new matter, has been the basi
of the present translation. This work has been done by the collabo
rators with great fidelity and thoroughness, for which the editor desire
to express his warmest thanks. They have brought to their work no
only a keen enthusiasm and industrious effort, but also a wide surgica
experience, enabling them to add judicious references to methods o
practice, which are preferred by English or American surgeons
They have increased the number of illustrations by drawing on th
material found in recent German literature—a feature which, it i
believed, will enhance the value and add to the interest of the text.

This work is really encyclopedic in character. Many of its chapter
exceed in scope those of the text-book, or even special treatise. Al
have been written by men of acknowledged authority and large clinica
experience. While it is chiefly clinical in character, there are abundan
pathological data, details of original research and statistical facts
which render it the most important surgical work of the day. Th
editor feels justified in expressing the conviction that these volume
will be found of inestimable value to the student and the scientifi
surgeon, and at the same time a trustworthy guide to the best an
most recent methods of practice.

W. T. B.

New York, January, 1904.

CONTENTS.

INJURIES AND DISEASES OF THE SKULL AND ITS CONTENTS.

MALFORMATIONS, INJURIES, AND DISEASES OF THE EAR.

MALFORMATIONS, INJURIES, AND DISEASES OF THE FACE. PLASTIC OPERATIONS.

THE NEURALGIAS OF THE HEAD.

ANOMALIES, INJURIES, AND DISEASES OF THE SALIVARY GLANDS.

INJURIES AND DISEASES OF THE JAW.

MALFORMATIONS, INJURIES, AND SURGICAL DISEASES OF THE NOSE AND ITS ADJACENT TISSUES.

MALFORMATIONS, INJURIES, AND DISEASES OF THE MOUTH.

MALFORMATIONS, INJURIES, AND DISEASES OF THE PHARYNX.

INJURIES AND DISEASES OF THE SKULL AND ITS CONTENTS.

By Prof. Dr. E. von BERGMANN and Prof. Dr. R. U. KRÖNLEIN.

INJURIES AND DISEASES OF THE SOFT PARTS AND OF THE CRANIAL BONES.

By Prof. Dr. E. von BERGMANN.

CHAPTER I.

INJURIES OF THE HEAD BEFORE BIRTH AND DUR*I*NG LABOR.

INJURIES OF THE HEAD BEFORE BIRTH.

THE fœtus is so well protected in the uterus that it is affected only by extreme violence, such as penetrating wounds of the maternal pelvis. This protection is afforded by the liquor amnii and the position of the fœtus. The head is especially well shielded in the latter months of pregnancy, when it lies in the false pelvis immediately above the brim of the true pelvis.

The large majority of intrauterine injuries of the head, being fatal to the mother as well as to the child, are of little surgical interest. The losses of substance met with in the newborn have, however, a medico-legal significance, for they may result from attempts to expel the fœtus mechanically, especially when the wound is in the form of a slit and has sharply defined edges. Careful observation of the course of labor in cases in which mechanical interference was positively excluded shows that long-continued intrauterine pressure is capable of bringing about a condition of necrosis in the skin of the fœtus. In several such cases it was found that a process of granulation or even cicatrization had set in after the throwing off of the wound slough. Pressure against the sacral promontory undoubtedly can bring about circumscribed gangrene of the scalp.

It seems probable from numerous observations that a fall during pregnancy or a blow on the abdomen may project the fœtal head against the promontory and in this way bruise the skin. On the other hand, it is doubtful whether such a shock can break the cranial bones of the fœtus. In the few cases of fractured skull reported as occurring before birth, the injury might well have happened during birth.

INJURIES OF THE HEAD DURING LABOR.

All injuries of the head occurring during delivery have been simply classed together, whether caused by the parturient canal or by artificial means intended to assist the mother. There is no doubt that injuries of the soft parts or the bones of the head, or of both at the same time, may take place during normal labor. It is obvious that these injuries are of medicolegal interest, for when occurring in normally delivered children their cause might be sought for in a criminal act.

Erythemata and Excoriations.—Among the excoriations are placed those pressure-marks found on the scalp of the newborn. These are the result of long-continued pressure against the maternal pelvis, especially the promontory, or are produced by forceps. They appear as linear, spotted areas of erythema with ecchymoses, and on the cadaver as mummified areas. If the pressure has been of long duration the nutrition of the areas of skin involved may be impaired, leading to more or less superficial or deep necrosis, and these portions are thrown off by a process of granulation or suppuration. The pressure-marks produced by the promontory are either round red spots or lines extending from the parietal bones to the ear or even over the face. The pressure is applied to all the passing parts, being exerted continuously from the time the fœtal head engages in the pelvis.

In flat pelves pressure-marks are also seen. They are caused by the impact of the horizontal ramus of the pubis on the frontal bone at a point opposite the area on the parietal bone pressed on by the promontory. The pressure-marks left by the generally contracted pelvis are less typical. They are distributed irregularly over the head and are not very extensive, but their effect is more pronounced.

The pressure-marks produced by forceps correspond to the points of application of the blades. They are situated, therefore, on both cheeks in case the head is grasped symmetrically. If at the time the forceps were applied the head had assumed an oblique position in the pelvis, one blade would be in the region of an eye and the other in that of the opposite ear. It is a well-known fact that the facial nerve may be so severely pressed upon at its point of exit from the stylomastoid foramen as to produce complete paralysis. Fortunately, most of these palsies disappear during the first few days after birth.

Œdema, Ecchymoses, and Extravasations.—The so-called caput succedaneum is a circumscribed œdema of the scalp. After the escape of the liquor amnii the fœtal body is subjected to a uniform pressure, excepting the part that lies over the os uteri. At this point congestion, transudation, and even extravasation take place, the combined effect of which is to produce the caput succedaneum and extensive ecchymoses of the skin. As the membranes may rupture at the time of the complete dilatation of the os, or even after, the development of the caput may take place when the head is at the pelvic outlet. In these cases the soft parts of the pelvic floor or the parts surrounding the vulvar outlet exert the pressure. While the caput is generally hemispherical in form when produced by pressure of the os, in the latter case it is usually elliptical. In rare cases in which decided changes in the position of the head have taken place, two distinct swellings at different points of the cranium may appear. On account of the decided frequency of the first position (left occipitoposterior) the caput is generally on the posterior superior portion of the right parietal bone and extends from there to the posterior or lesser fontanelle. Only when the posterior fontanelle lies very low, does it extend wholly or in part over the occipital bone. In the second position (right occipitoposterior) it lies on a corresponding portion of the left side of the cranium. On the whole the position varies, of course, according to the engagement of the fœtal head. The size of this generally unimportant swelling is variable. The more powerful the pressure exerted by the uterine contractions or the more obstinate the resistance on the part of the os uteri, the larger will be the resulting caput. Its surface is darker than that of the surrounding parts, cyanotic, and mottled with purplish ecchymoses. After birth, with restored circulation, the smaller swellings rapidly disappear. The larger ones appear to change their position, as in the dorsal posture of the child the œdema sinks toward the occiput. Even the very largest capita generally disappear within three days and do not require treatment.

Cephalhæmatoma.—A peculiar extravasation on the head of the newborn is presented by the so-called cephalhæmatoma. It was first described and named by Nägele as a tumor-like collection of blood between the periosteum and bone of the cranium in the newborn. It is not rare, occurring in 0.5 per cent. or slightly less of all births. Termin and Scheglow have instituted careful anatomical investigations of the same in the foundling asylums of St. Petersburg and Moscow. Of 103 cases cited by them, 101 cephalhæmatomata were situated on the parietal bones, 45 on the right side, 47 on the left, 9 on both sides, and 1 each on the frontal and occipital bones. Three at one time were observed by Hennig, and 4 by Scheglow.

Etiology.—There are two causes of cephalhæmatoma: First, the condition that brings about caput succedaneum, namely, the circular pressure exerted by the maternal tissues. The fact alone that the cephalhæmatoma occurs at the same place that the caput does would point to a common etiology. Besides this, when the diagnosis of cephalhæmatoma is made early there will frequently be found over it the remains of the œdematous, hemorrhagic caput. Second, fissures and dents arising in the bones during labor cause effusions of blood between the intact pericranium and the broken or bent bone. Termin was the first to describe this type of cephalhæmatoma. The author has noted in a specimen, as also those of Scheglow showed, the external as well as the internal periosteum raised by an effusion of blood, while the bone separating the two collections was fissured.

The larger amount of blood in the tumor is effused at the time of birth, when, through separation of the pericranium, laceration of blood-vessels takes place. The hemorrhage continues for several days after birth, owing probably to the stasis caused by the act of respiration and the crying of the child. The swelling, therefore, continues to increase during the first period of extrauterine life, and may only be noticed after two or three days. It appears at that time as a flat, tense tumor, with a convex, smooth surface. At times it is only the size of a pigeon's egg, but occasionally it includes the entire extent of a parietal bone. It is bounded by the edges of the bone upon which it is situated, not extending beyond the sutures, owing to the fact that along these the periosteum is more firmly adherent. If a cephalhæmatoma continue for some time, say two weeks, there will appear a hard swelling at the point where the detached pericranium rises above the skull and surrounding the tumor at its base in the form of a ring, so that it feels on palpation as if there were a depression or even defect of the skull. This ring continues to increase in width, advancing from the periphery toward the centre, and finally covering the entire surface of the tumor. At the same time the elastic hard border becomes softer, markedly fluctuating, and less well defined.

The development of the ring and capsule about the tumor is the result of a bone formation produced by the detached periosteum. Beneath the

Fig. 1.

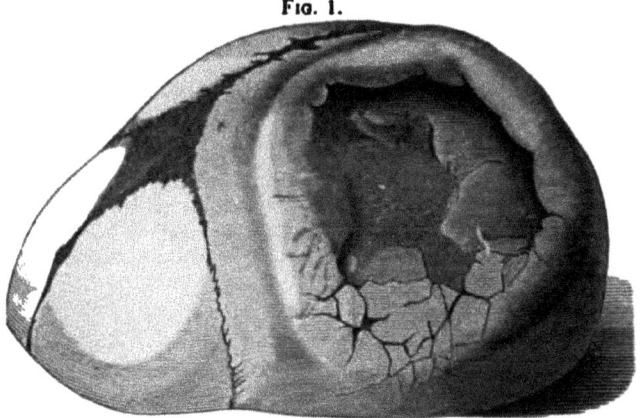

Cephalhæmatoma.

superficial connective-tissue layer of the periosteum there lies an equally thick and at times thicker layer of bone-forming tissue, consisting of layers of osteoblasts and numerous bloodvessels, and beyond this the true osseous tissue. It is in this osteoblastic layer that laceration of bloodvessels and blood effusion take place. The layer is split apart, some osteoblasts remaining adherent to the bone, the rest to the perios- teum. The osteoblasts on the internal surface of the detached periosteum develop disseminated plates and trabeculæ of bone. In all the specimens of the Moscow and St. Petersburg foundling asylums, which the author had the opportunity of observing through the kindness of Termin, the wall of bone is more thickly developed at the point where the raised membrane is attached to the bone itself and becomes thinner toward the centre. This is easy to account for, as at the angle of reflection more osteoblasts will be found than at a distance. As a rule, the formation of bone in the central portions takes place in the form of islands, the plates and scales of bone being separated from one another by non-calcareous connective tissue, and may, therefore, be compared to the Wormian bones. This relation is shown particularly well in the specimen of the Moscow foundling asylum, illustrated in Fig. 1.

If the bony shell surrounding the extravasation is completely closed a flattened boss at the site of the cephalhæmatoma simply remains after recovery. The bloody contents of the cephalhæmatoma may remain fluid for some time, perhaps more than four weeks following birth. The bony shell surrounding it is not always formed. Should the effused blood disappear within a few days, the raised periosteum returns to its former bed and no trace of the disturbance remains. In the majority of cases, however, the flattening, reabsorption, and formation of the bony shell require weeks or even months. During this period the child's general health is not impaired unless an abscess develops in the hæmatoma. This may be caused by abrasion of the swelling or by some external injury to the soft parts, such as incised or punctured wounds. The periosteum as well as the skin and connective tissue are involved in the process of suppuration. The result is usually simply a superficial necrosis of the cranial bone and destruction of the newly-formed bone-plates and tra-beculæ. As a rule, further danger is prevented by either early rupture or prompt incision. Cases have been reported, however, in which an abscess spread over the entire scalp, leading to total destruction of the exposed parietal bone and fatal meningitis.

Cases are recorded in which a cephalhæmatoma has been mistaken for a hernia, the bony ring at the base being mistaken for the margin of the hernial opening. However, cephaloceles do not occur at the sites of cephalhæmatomata.

Treatment.—The treatment of cephalhæmatoma by incision is un-necessary. Early incision might, in fact, be dangerous through loss of blood, as the effusion usually increases by slow oozing during the first few days after birth and the blood remains fluid. A very rapid increase in size is best treated by puncture and subsequent pressure. The same minor operative procedure might be considered in cases of delayed reso-lution. If, on the other hand, suppuration has set in and the skin is red and thinned and the outlines of the tumor lost in surrounding œdema, a large incision must be made, dividing the inflamed area, and the usual measures applied for limiting and bringing about a favorable termina-tion of a phlegmon.

Deformities.—The deformities of the child's skull present after birth are well known.

Etiology.—In its passage through the maternal pelvis the child's head is adapted to the existing relations by the cranial bones approaching and gliding over one another at the site of their articulations. The occipital and frontal bones are by this process pushed under the two parietal bones. The occipital bone, even under normal conditions, in the parturient canal,

on the contrary, they facilitate the process of labor. Within from twenty-four to forty-eight hours the bones return to their normal position. In case of marked overriding of the parietal bones there might result inter-meningeal hemorrhage from rupture of the veins leading to the superior longitudinal sinus or of the sinus itself.

In the same manner that the parturient canal changes the shape of the skull as a whole by the displacement of its bones, the shape of the individual bones may be changed and made more convex or more flattened. This change in form takes place in half of all cases of contracted pelvis. The pressure of the promontory against the parietal bone causes a decrease in its convexity, and is determined by the direction of the uterine axis tending to force the head against the posterior wall of the pelvis. The left parietal bone is more frequently flattened than the right one, owing to the fact that the first position occurs more than two and one-half times as often as the second. The pressure of the promontory may cause more than simple flattening of a cranial bone, occasionally producing more or less extensive depressions of two types—shallow, gutter-shaped and deeper, boat-shaped or funnel-shaped dents. The first type occurs almost exclusively along the coronary border of the parietal bone. Being caused by the promontory, they are found only in the posterior bone. The edge of the parietal bone projects somewhat along the coronary suture and falls away toward the depression which runs parallel with the suture. At the same time the portion of bone along the edge appears notched with several lines of fracture. A red pressure-mark will, as a rule, be found overlying the depression. In the shallow, gutter-shaped type the promontory has generally exerted pressure for some time; in the deeper, funnel-shaped type, on the other hand, for less time and with greater violence. The latter are consequently character-istic of labors that are terminated artificially, in which, either by forceps or by version, the head is rapidly drawn past the promontory. The blades of the forceps do not cause the denting; they are only the indirect means in so far as by forcible traction through the pelvis they cause the head to be pressed against the promontory. Of 32 cases collected by von Hoffmann, only 2 had been delivered without intervention on the part of the obstetrician. Of the 30 remaining, 23 had been delivered by forceps and in 7 version had been performed. The forceps are applied to the head in the transverse or longitudinal diameter, and accordingly either the frontal bone is depressed between the tuberosity and anterior fontanelle or the parietal bone between the parietal eminence and ante-rior fontanelle. In all cases of the after-coming head the depression was found in the parietal bone between the eminence and the ear or parallel with the coronary suture. Cases in which an exostosis or an ankylosed coccyx causes the depression are rare. The depressions are sometimes deep and extensive. As a rule, a cephalhæmatoma is found in the resulting bony fossa. Though most cases of deep depressions are combined with fissuring of bone, they do occur without the slightest loss in continuity of bone, as the author saw in Termin's collection in St. Petersburg.

Prognosis.—The gutter-shaped depressions have a decidedly better prognosis than the funnel-shaped dents. The former are generally not noticed until several days after birth, when the swelling of the soft parts has subsided. Schröder has reported, among 65 cases of the latter, 22 dead or stillborn children, 10 who died soon after as a result of the injury, and 33 who were in good health. Only a small number died as a result of intracranial hemorrhage, the majority of deaths being due to asphyxia, a consequence of protracted labor in cases of contracted pelvis. Most of the depressions are smoothed over in time, at times rapidly, often after months. There are, however, cases in which they continue through life. The counterpressure of the brain, the development of bone, the bony thickening taking place in the cephalhæmatomata generally found in the depression, all tend to restore the bone to its former level.

It is obvious that under certain circumstances depressions of the skull in the newborn child may have a medicolegal significance. They may be suspected to be the result of a criminal act after birth, or, on the contrary, similar depressions, as von Hoffmann has demonstrated experimentally, may be produced within the uterus. In such cases the cautious physician must consider the circumstances of delivery, especially the relative size of the child's head and the pelvis of the mother, besides the objective findings in the child.

Solution of Continuity of Bones.—It required some time to decide that real solution of continuity of the cranial bones in the newborn could take place as a result of pressure on the part of the parturient canal. As these fissures lead to fatal hemorrhage and brain lesions, they have frequently been the subject of legal investigations. It may be conceded that in rare cases the pressure of the forceps blades may cause fracture of the skull, particularly of the frontal bones. Generally, it is not the closure of the blades that is responsible for the fracture, but the violent pressure of the head against the promontory as it is forcibly dragged through the pelvis (Fritsch). As has been mentioned, there are found in connection with flattening of the parietal bones, as well as with gutter-shaped depressions of the same, fissures that radiate from the periphery toward the eminence. The depressions occurring in cases of the after-coming head are characterized by such fissures and even larger fractures. Moreover, it is characteristic of congenital fractures of the skull that they occur almost without exception in the parietal bones, extending from the sagittal suture to the centre of ossification or parallel with the sagittal suture. In the former case the fractures have sharp, smooth edges, as if the bone had split; in the latter it is irregularly serrated. These differences in appearance are due to the structure of bone in the newborn. Only about the centres of ossification (parietal eminence, frontal and occipital tuberosity) do we find the uniform structure of later life. Everywhere the bony tissue can be seen in the form of rays diverging toward the periphery. The line of fracture that extends in the direction of the latter is sharp and smooth; that which runs more or less obliquely to the rays is characterized by an irregular, notched border.

Besides these relations the physician must weigh the statements regarding the course of labor and the results of a pelvic examination before deciding or leaving undecided the questions as to whether in a given case the fissure was the result of pressure on the part of the parturient canal.

If extensive intracranial hemorrhages do not complicate fractures and if at the same time there is no danger of asphyxia, the child can live. Indeed, it seems as if newborn children could tolerate much in this respect, as the recovery from cephalhæmatoma shows, which so often covers fractured bones.

Fig. 2.

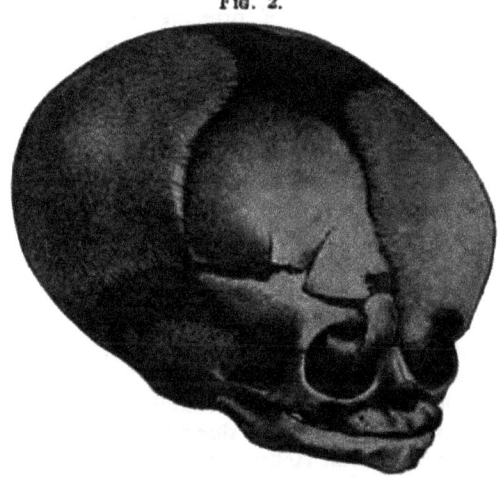

Fracture of right frontal bone in a newborn infant; fracture extending into orbit.   (Bruns.)

Rupture of the articulations has been observed along the line of the sagittal, coronal, and lambdoidal sutures. If one parietal bone is depressed to such a degree that the sagittal border of the other parietal bone projects sharply through the stretched soft parts, it is easy to understand how the membranous articulation may tear. The danger from this injury is due to the resulting rupture of bloodvessels, previously mentioned. The sinus itself may be torn without injury to the articular membrane, because its thinner wall does not bear the stretching which the ligamentous structures of the suture withstand (Olshausen). The intracranial hemorrhage resulting from a ruptured sinus is almost always fatal.

The separation of the condyloid from the squamous portion of the occipital bone is brought about in the extraction of the after-coming head either by forceps or the Prague method. The squamous portion is simply torn away from the articular portion or the squamous part is pressed against the articular and pushed off by the latter. Very often both mechanisms act together or in succession. Even this injury is not dangerous in itself, but on account of the accompanying hemorrhage and possible crushing of the medulla in the foramen magnum, which is narrowed by the displacement of the fractured articular portions.

Prognosis.—Fortunately, all mechanical injuries to the skull in fullterm children are seldom dangerous to life. The dead or stillborn children met with in cases of contracted pelves are asphyxiated, as the postmortem examination shows. The cranial injuries themselves are only dangerous to life in so far as they may cause cerebrospinal hemorrhage. These are more severe in cases of fracture and dislocation at the site of suture than in simple flexures and depressions. The prognosis is consequently more favorable in the latter. In the former the children are born with a vigorous cry. The extravasation increases rapidly, however, now that the skull is relieved of pressure, and constantly increasing symptoms of intracranial pressure are met with. Stupor, convulsions, and death follow each other closely.

Treatment.—The question has frequently come up in recent times whether surgical interference could be of any benefit. In asphyxiated children the indications for the obstetrician are clearly to employ artificial respiration and not to incise the skull. The only cases which seem to demand different treatment are those in which there is extensive and deep depression of the skull and paralysis of the opposite side, generally a paresis and not a paralysis. In these cases attempts have been made to elevate the depressed area by means of incision and the application of a bone-elevator, but the results have been doubtful. On the other hand, such cases have completely recovered without treatment.

Defects in Skull Not Due to Trauma.—Certain gaps and openings occurring quite frequently in the skull of newborn children were often mistaken for injuries received during labor or for fractures originating after birth, until von Hoffmann cleared up the whole matter by his investigations regarding physiological and pathological defects in ossification.

Diagnosis.—The differentiation of all these physiological cracks and fissures from real fractures is based on their constant location in the large majority of cases, their symmetrical distribution, the gradual thinning of their edges when observed by transmitted light, the absence of hemorrhage and ecchymosis, and, finally, on the firm adhesion found to exist between the periosteum and dura under the defect, as opposed to their separation and free mobility at the site of a true fracture.

Failure of or incomplete ossification is easily distinguished from fracture. In such cases the skull seems to be composed of numerous islandlike fragments of bone, which make it incapable of support and readily indented. At the same time such cases may show marked curvatures of the extremities and united fractures with and without callus.

CHAPTER II.

INJURIES OF THE COVERINGS OF THE SKULL.

A PLANE passing through the nasal process of the frontal bone and the root of each zygoma divides the cranium or skull proper from the face. The soft parts covering the skull, being of uniform thickness and conforming accurately to its shape, show its true size and form. From before backward we find the frontal, parietal, and occipital regions, constituting the middle zone of the skull, while that portion bounded above by the origin of the temporal muscle and falling away over each zygoma toward the face is known as the temporal region.

The soft parts consist, in the middle portion, of the occipitofrontalis muscle with its broad, flat tendon and the periosteum; laterally, the temporal muscles, with their aponeurotic covering, separate skin and periosteum. The connective tissue uniting the different layers is represented by the subcutaneous layer and the subaponeurotic layer. Only on the forehead is the skin thin and elastic; in youth smooth, in old age wrinkled and furrowed. The structure of the hairy scalp is exceedingly firm and the corium is rich in elastic fibres and muscular tissue. The fatty layer of the back of the neck and forehead is characterized by extraordinary rigidity; the fat-lobules in it are about the size of a pin's head and are embedded in a closely woven, dense connective-tissue framework. The skin is firmly attached to the aponeurosis and muscular portion of the occipitofrontalis and cannot be moved over the underlying parts nor raised in folds. The connective-tissue layer immediately beneath the occipitofrontalis muscle, however, is poor in adipose tissue and very delicate and elastic in structure, so that the entire extensive tendinous capsule is but loosely attached to the periosteum, enabling the scalp to be thrown into folds during muscular action and to be raised by extravasations and exudates.

INCISED, PUNCTURED, AND LACERATED WOUNDS.

Incised Wounds.—Incised wounds of the scalp are generally surgical incisions required in operations for covering bare bone or defects in rhinoplasty, and in the extirpation of tumors. Blows striking perpendicularly produce *simple* wounds; those obliquely, wounds with the formation of a *flap*, or, if an entire portion of skin is cut off, wounds with *loss of substance*. Incised wounds as well as those the result of blows generally divide the aponeurosis as well as the skin, owing to their intimate connection. Simple wounds of the hairy scalp do not, as a rule, e. The narrow muscles of the reticular layer of the skin are placed at right angles, so that the degree of contraction in the skin is the same in all directions. In the lateral portions of the skull vertical wounds will gape more than horizontal ones, as here the bundles of fibres run parallel with the median line, while horizontal wounds of the forehead will gape more than vertical ones for the same reason. If the aponeurosis is divided, the edges of the wound separate more or less, since the loose cellular tissue separating it from the periosteum allows free play of the contractile skin, while at the same time the aponeurosis is drawn in opposite directions by the action of its muscles. Where the occipito-frontalis aponeurosis is divided perpendicularly to the direction of its fibres, either in the frontal, temporal, or occipital region, the lower edge of the wound will be bowed out more than the upper. For this reason flap wounds, where the attached portion is directed toward the circumference of the hairy scalp, retract toward their base.

Prognosis.—The prognosis of incised wounds and those produced by blows is good, for the structure of the scalp favors primary union. The opposing wound-edges are of equal thickness, are situated on a firm bed, do not collapse nor curl up, and may be accurately placed according to their corresponding layers. If the precaution be taken that no blood-clot separates the edges of the wound, their coaptation will result in rapid union. The tendency is to primary union in those wounds that have not been caused in their entire extent by sharp instruments, but which are, to a certain degree, lacerated wounds. A blade may penetrate the soft parts in a vertical direction and by turning flat strip off a flap, and in this way tear into the skin at the angles of the wound. In this combination of incised and lacerated wound the torn portion will heal as well as the sharply cut.

Punctured Wounds.—Punctured wounds of the scalp, whether delivered in a perpendicular or oblique direction, produce short sinuses and generally involve the skull as well as the soft parts. The instrument causing the injury may glance off the bone and emerge from the skin at some distance, thus forming two wounds communicating by a subcutaneous, often tortuous canal. The only punctured wounds that attain any depth are those that penetrate beneath the zygoma from above. Against this bony edge knife-blades have broken off and remained fast.

Contusions.—Blows inflicted by blunt objects press the scalp against the bone beneath, contusing it. It is the same whether the blunt body strikes the head, or the latter while in motion meets with resistance from some other object, or in falling strikes the ground. If the violence be more severe, the underlying bone may be broken or the skin covering it divided, or both injuries may be brought about at the same time. Thus simple fractures are combined with contusions, while compound fractures are combined with contused wounds of the scalp, and only the mildest kind of contusions are limited to the soft parts. The injury affects the bloodvessels primarily. Hemorrhage takes place to a greater or less degree into and between the tissues, forming a swelling. According to the place of extravasation, we might distinguish between subcutaneous, subaponeurotic, and subperiosteal hæmatoma, were it not a rule for more than one connective-tissue layer to be infiltrated with blood. If the violence is inflicted in a perpendicular direction, hemorrhage takes place into the subcutaneous adipose tissue and is limited to a small surrounding area. Such a hæmatoma is sharply circumscribed and uniformly hard, as blood does not force the tissues apart, but simply infiltrates them. The skin can generally be moved with the swelling, showing it to be situated within the same. If the violence is directed in an oblique direction, the skin and the aponeurosis are both pushed over the periosteum, tearing the loose cellular tissue and wounding not only vessels, but also other portions of the soft tissues, and the hemorrhage takes place into the spaces formed in the delicate connective tissue and spread a considerable distance beyond the site of injury.

Circumscribed Hæmatoma.—Most of the circumscribed hæmatomata, or bruises, occur in childhood. A child too young to have learned to use its hands in preventing a fall, strikes its head or knocks it without much violence against an object, and this slight injury is the result. A weak blow or spent ball glancing off will cause a like bruise. After several hours the skin is discolored by the effused blood, and shows the familiar play of colors exhibited in the resolution of a contusion.

Treatment.—Absorption progresses without disturbance. No special treatment is indicated. In order to prevent unnecessary manipulation on the part of timid mothers or nurses, the physician may order applications of lead acetate or water with tincture of arnica.

Hæmatomata beneath the Aponeurosis.—Hæmatomata beneath the aponeurosis are more flattened and may spread over the whole cranial vault. The larger the hemorrhage the softer and more fluctuating is the hæmatoma. The softest part is at the centre, while the periphery is bounded by a hard belt of varying breadth, for the collection of free blood is bordered by a zone of simple infiltration of blood into the close meshes of the connective tissue. The resulting hard edge about the centre may be mistaken for an edge of bone, and lead to the idea that there is a depressed fracture. The mistake is particularly likely to occur if the violence causing the injury was considerable and at the same time cerebral symptoms are present. The wall-like edge of a bruise or hæmatoma rises from the general plane of the cranial vault, as opposed to the edge of a depressed fracture, and may be impressed or even made to disappear on pressure, while in the centre the uneven surface of displaced bone fragments is absent. If larger veins or arteries of the supra-aponeurotic tissue have been torn, the hæmatoma may be very extensive and cause considerable tension of the skin; they have been observed to extend from the frontal tuberosity to the superior curve of the occipital bone. However extensive the extravasation may be, absorption takes place.

Treatment.—Should the overlying skin be stretched by the hemorrhage until it is bloodless, puncture is to be preferred to incision. However, incision need not be feared with aseptic methods of operation and the avoidance of unnecessary digital exploration of the wound. It is difficult to locate the principal bleeding vessels, and extensive pressure may be required. For this reason, above the usual expectant treatment, which has been followed with happy results, is to be preferred. Should the cellular tissue be, and about extravasation, become infected through excoriations of the skin overlying a diffuse or circumscribed hæmatoma, the usual treatment for a phlegmon is demanded. The necessary incision should be made through the inflamed and œdematous scalp. In most cases several incisions and counteropenings at different points are necessary.

Hemorrhage of any extent beneath the pericranium following contusions is found usually in children, in whom the bone derives a rich vascular supply from its periosteum. These cephalhæmatomata of later life appear like the subaponeurotic hæmatomata, as flat or moderately curved swellings, soft, and with a distinctly raised border. Assuming the mechanism of their origin to be the same as that of the subaponeurotic hemorrhage, it is easy to imagine that by the displacement of the periosteum some of the branches derived from the emissary veins are torn against the sharp borders of their foramina. If the divided vessel is a large one, it may cause considerable hemorrhage with extensive separation of the periosteum. In this way many large fluctuating extravasations of blood may be explained that occur in connection with simple fractures.

Lacerated Wounds.—More frequent than all other injuries of the skull are the lacerated wounds produced by blunt instruments and objects of all kinds. They divide the soft parts at one or more places in a line or detach them in the form of a flap, tear or pull them into ribbons and shreds, or even pull off entire pieces, leaving losses of substance of greater or less degree.

Etiology.—Linear wounds are the result of bodies striking the head in a perpendicular direction, or they arise through the head striking or falling against angular objects. The scalp is thereby pressed against the bone beneath, contused and divided. It is not always bruised throughout the whole extent of the surface coming in contact with the object causing the injury, for on account of its dense structure it may burst at the moment of striking. If the force be then spent, there are presented one or more linear wounds; if it continue to act, the divided layer of tissue at the site of the first cut or tear is still further detached from the underlying parts, and in this way the usual undermining and formation of pockets takes place. If the blunt object penetrate the scalp with sufficient force, it may glance off the vaulted surface of the skull, catch the soft parts, and strip them off to a greater or less extent. In this manner angular wounds and three-cornered flaps are produced. The apex of the angle corresponds to the point of direct impact and the site of the greatest contusion, while the edges are produced by laceration. If the original direction of the force were oblique, the scalp may be extensively torn off and the flaps attain considerable size. This is the case where a blow is delivered with an angular piece of wood traversing the scalp from the parietal surface to the temple, or an irregular-shaped stone falling from above. A larger number of flap-wounds originate in another way, not at the point of impact, but at some distance. The scalp is pushed along its bed to such an extent that it can stretch no further and is torn. If the head be dragged forcibly over the ground for some distance or pushed along a rough surface, considerable portions of the scalp may be torn off. Likewise the same thing may happen if, in falling from a height, the head strikes a glancing blow and rubs against a hard object.

The character of contused and lacerated wounds varies with the manner of their origin. If the instrument causing the injury is relatively small and the force with which it was impelled considerable, the edges of the wounds may appear very much like those of the incised ones, and the surgeon must be careful about arriving at any conclusion regarding the shape and degree of sharpness of the instrument that caused them. The firm support offered by the skull and its smooth outline explain why clean-cut wounds can be produced by dull instruments. The vitality of the wound-flaps depends upon the extent of surface and the degree of violence with which the body strikes; the greater the former and the less the latter, the more evident are the signs of contusions on the edges of the wound. Lacerated wounds surrounding a torn-off flap may appear sharply cut. On closer observation, however, a more or less fine serration is rarely wanting, a condition that does not in the least impair their vitality. In other cases linear as well as flap wounds betray their origin through contusions and by the shreds and tabs of tissue. The points of skin at the angle of two wounds are always discolored and infiltrated with blood. The tissues in the immediate neighborhood and at some distance from the wound may show different degrees of contusion or form distinct swellings by larger extravasations of blood. The skin covering a dependent flap remains uninjured in case the latter was formed by an instrument penetrating the scalp and glancing off the bone, but is always extensively excoriated, scratched, and bruised when the tearing off is produced by abrasion against some hard object. The flaps formed in the latter accident consist of skin and aponeurosis, for the separation affects the subaponeurotic connective tissue, as in this alone can any extensive displacement of the two superficial layers take place. Of course, as a rule, in cases of extensive loss of scalp, some periosteum is stripped off at one or more places and remains adherent to the under surface of the scalp. In the same way the skull is deprived of periosteum to a greater or less degree in cases in which a wedge-shaped instrument is driven into the scalp and its edge penetrates the periosteum before glancing off.

The flaps vary in shape and size. Sometimes they are regular, crescent-shaped, or triangular, or they may be irregular, hacked, or torn at the edges. The attached portion, the base—whose ratio to the length as well as breadth of the flap is an important factor in determining its vitality—faces either the crest of the skull or its periphery. In the latter case the flap hangs over the face, neck, or ear, and if the latter be also torn off, it may reach the shoulder. As, on account of the spherical form of the skull, violence is more often directed in a slanting line than in a perpendicular one, it is easy to explain why flap-wounds are much more frequent than other kinds.

The severest lacerations are those tears, either diverging from one point or frequently intersecting, that result from explosions of gases or sudden considerable increase of air pressure, as the discharge of a blank cartridge from a gun held close to the head. Many gunshot-wounds hitherto explained in this way are, however, supposed to be due to an expansive action of the ball after penetrating the skull. Especially is this the case with modern small-calibre projectiles.

In a lacerated wound originating in any of the above-mentioned ways pieces of scalp may be lost and wounds with loss of substance result. This is most marked in so-called cases of scalping, the mechanism of which is peculiar in so far as the pulling of the hair causes a separation of the scalp. The first action of this pull, provided the hair be not torn out, is a laceration of subaponeurotic connective tissue. If the force be considerable and continuous, the scalp is torn into and pulled off entirely. The prognosis in such severe injuries is more favorable than would be expected, although several years may elapse before complete recovery takes place. The distortion of ears, eyebrows, and eyelids after spontaneous repair, with excessive cicatricial contraction, causes considerable deformity. For this reason early therapeutic intervention by Thiersch's method of skin-grafting is urgently indicated.

Prognosis.—The course of contused and lacerated wounds varies according to the changes that have taken place in the wound-edges and wound-flaps, and according to the methods of treatment applied. The experience of all surgeons has taught that primary union takes place very frequently, owing to the fact that the vitality of the edges of the wound is generally unimpaired. Perhaps only a part of the wound will heal by first intention, while the rest becomes infected, suppurates, and becomes neurotic, until finally repair takes place by granulation after the necrotic portions of the tissue have been thrown off.

In judging these cases, the appearance of fresh contused wounds may deceive. Many blue, bruised, and excoriated wound-edges, which look scratched and torn, recover within twenty-four hours and are capable of rapid union. As a matter of fact, we seldom see an extensive or even limited gangrene of the contused tissue. If the latter is thrown off and destroyed, the process is slow and unnoticeable. The vascular supply is very favorable for the nutrition of the scalp. An intricate arterial plexus, receiving supplies from all directions, is spread out over the entire cranial vault immediately beneath the skin, almost entirely preventing the cutting off of the blood-supply. This explains why the vitality may be preserved in flaps that have been extensively torn off and undermined. The arteries run for the most part above the aponeurotic capsule, and therefore remain within the flap when the subaponeurotic tissue is torn, whereas in other parts of the body the arteries run vertically upward from the deeper tissue-layers. As the arteries run from the periphery toward the crest of the skull, the chances of saving a flap are more favorable if the base is directed downward and the apex upward, notwithstanding which the author has seen rapid and complete primary union take place in a narrow, tongue-shaped flap, six and even twelve inches long, whose base was situated along the coronal suture. Even unfavorably situated flaps seldom become gangrenous to any extent unless the injuries are complicated at an early stage by infection of the skin and subcutaneous tissue.

The aponeurosis and the cellular tissue uniting it to the periosteum are more prone to necrosis. This destruction may result immediately upon a contusion or stretching, or it may follow œdema and purulent inflammation, with subsequent necrosis of the connective-tissue stratum, caused by pressure of the overlying tense aponeurosis. As this connective-tissue layer is usually the one to suffer most in the tearing off of the scalp, it is easy to see how more or less extensive abscesses may follow contused wounds. Extravasations of blood predispose to rapid extension of inflammation in this region as much as in other parts of the body. How much more the deeper layers suffer from contusions than the superficial ones is clearly shown by the fact that the cutaneous wound is often entirely healed, while the deeper-lying connective tissue is going through a process of suppuration. The products of inflammation thus dammed back are still another factor in determining the extension of the infective process and burrow into the tissue for some distance from the wound.

Diffuse cellulitis (phlegmon) is one of the most serious and unfortunately a very common complication of contused and lacerated wounds. The temperature accompanying it is high. The multiple abscesses resulting from it may be distributed over the entire cranial surface, at times very close to one another, or even above one another, separated only by periosteum. The greatest danger lies in further complications. The cellular connective tissue between the skull and aponeurosis blends insensibly with the periosteum. With the destruction of the former the latter may also become necrotic, exposing the bone, if it has not been laid bare by the original injury. This exposure of bone may lead to superficial or deep necrosis or an extensive osteomyelitis. This is more likely to be the result when an exposure is due to a secondary suppurative destruction of the periosteum than when it is torn off mechanically by the original violence. This process in the bone may be of great significance when involving the periosteum on the internal surface—the dura —or when causing a thrombosis of the vessels. The resulting changes in the skull contents and the danger to life will be referred to again in the chapters on Diseases and Injuries of Bones. The tension under which the products of inflammation exist in these affections of the soft parts of the scalp explains how the cranial contents may be involved in this inflammatory process without the presence of an intermediary bone lesion by a successive thrombosis of the vessels or by a progressive extension in the connective tissue surrounding the tracts of vessels. We are familiar with deep-seated cerebral abscesses that originated in a process transmitted through thrombosed veins.

Important, as determining what to do or not to do, is the experience that even the severest contusions may be inflicted without inflammation or suppuration of the wound-edges, while at times, through some specific infection, the severest and most obstinate cellulitis may result from a wound with the slightest degree of laceration. This complication, though rare at the present time, was seen quite often even in simple incised wounds in former days.

As in all wounds, *erysipelas* may complicate contused wounds at any stage. It is more to be feared here than elsewhere, as on account of the extensive injury to the connective tissue the infection, instead of being limited to the skin, has a tendency to invade the deeper layers and thus favor the frequent combination of cellulitis and erysipelas. Should erysipelas spread along the edge of a wound, with loss of substance, at the bottom of which there is bare bone, there is danger of bone necrosis and extension through the bone to the membrane of the brain, especially when it is combined with an extensive cellulitis. A simple cutaneous erysipelas has little tendency to invade the deeper tissues, but in combination with a cellulitis of the soft parts it may extend to the membrane of the brain.

Treatment of Wounds in the Soft Parts Covering the Skull.

The treatment of wounds, whether caused by dull or sharp instruments or objects, has so much in common that they may be discussed together. As a matter of fact, in the treatment of incised and punctured wounds and those caused by blows, the surgeon must be governed by the same circumstances as in contused wounds, for in every wound of the skull three things must be considered. In the first place, whether or not the *wound is infected;* secondly, whether the *flaps are viable;* and finally, what complications are liable to occur in the way of *brain* and *bone affections.* The last consideration is of more importance than the first two, and will receive special attention in the following chapters. Injuries of the scalp with or without primary cerebral affections are so frequent in the author's clinic that in his treatment a regular routine is followed. If more or less severe brain symptoms are present, as those referable to concussion or intracranial pressure, they are treated in the house division. The same is the case where there is evidence of fracture below the wound in the soft parts, or if there are present wounds with extensive areas of bare bone or with extensive loss of substance. All others are treated in the out-patient department.

The question whether or not a wound is infected at the time of injury cannot always be decided positively, but nevertheless may be determined with sufficient accuracy for all practical purposes. While it is possible that a clean incised wound may be infected by a knife-blade or the germs of infection be derived from the neighboring unclean skin, it is not necessary to consider these remote possibilities, as it will be sufficient for all therapeutic purposes to determine the probability of infection in a given wound. Wounds that contain dung and dust from the streets, garden loam, sand, mud, particles of masonry from walls against which the head may have glanced during a fall, also lime, mortar, coal, tree-bark, sawdust, machine oil, or portions of head-covering are considered probably primarily infectious. Wounds whose edges and immediate surroundings show evidence of severe contusions are also considered in the above class, as they are readily infected. In many cases the history of the injury and inspection of the instrument may lead us to suspect primary infection of a given wound, as in the case of a knife repeatedly used to slaughter animals or a pitchfork used to toss manure. Without question, all wounds are infected that show signs of inflammation on coming under observation. Surgical incisions during operation, sword-cuts and sabre-cuts, and sharply lacerated, simple, or flap-wounds, especially those in which the wounding instrument catching the scalp at some distance from the site of injury stretches and tears the scalp, are considered not probably infected.

The conditions governing the vitality of wound-flaps have been considered in discussing the mechanism of contused wounds, at the same time describing the appearance of the latter where their edges were in danger of becoming necrotic. The edges may be preserved in all sharply cut wounds produced by blows, also in most contused wounds produced by blunt objects. Both types have a tendency to primary union which the surgeon should attempt to obtain in all such cases.

The skin in the vicinity of every scalp-wound should be thoroughly cleansed and disinfected. The necessary procedure may be limited to the immediate neighborhood in cases of small and probably not infected wounds; but in the case of more extensive and very severe injuries, large flap-wounds, extensive contusion wounds with loss of substance, the entire scalp must be shaved. In many cases a surgeon has spared the hair only to have it destroyed by erysipelas a little later. Even the layman is well acquainted with the danger of injuries to the head, and if the surgeon insist upon it he can generally gain consent to removal of the hair. If the case be brought in several hours after injury, the hair will usually be found matted and glued together with dried blood, so that it will be necessary to soak and soften it before attempting to cut it. This is best accomplished by applications of sterile water with the assistance of an irrigator. After the hair has been removed by scissors the scalp should be shaved. The mechanical scouring thus produced effectively removes the pathogenic organisms vegetating in the scalp, among which *Staphylococcus albus* is most frequently present. During the process of scrubbing and shaving it is a good plan to fill the cavity of the wound with sterile gauze, thus preventing the entrance of soap and hair as well as dust scraped from the surrounding skin. Pressing in the tampons of fluff gauze will at the same time act as a temporary hæmostatic. A modern instrument called a "safety razor" or "razor-plane," is useful for removing the hair from the corners of the wounds and flaps of skin. Following the shaving, the head is thoroughly rubbed dry with a sterile towel and then cleansed with ether. The latter is an absolute necessity owing to the oily character of the skin. Before the skin is scrubbed with soap and warm water it should be washed with alcohol to dissolve the ether, as otherwise the water cannot reach the skin. The cleansing with soap and water is again followed by washing with alcohol, and finally with a solution of 1 : 1000 of corrosive sublimate.

Not until the wound is thus clearly presented can the surgeon judge its size and significance: the character of the wound-edges and the degree of contusion that the skin has suffered. If, in the inspection of a wound, foreign bodies, such as hair, sand, or particles of any kind are found, they should be removed with forceps or pieces of sterile gauze. A forcible stream of water from an elevated irrigator or dressing syringe should never be used for this purpose. A 0.6 per cent. salt solution is sufficient, allowing it to trickle gently over the surface of the wound by squeezing a gauze sponge wet with this solution. At the same time more firmly attached particles may be removed with a dry gauze sponge. With a well-disinfected finger all pockets and crevices of wounds should be explored for foreign bodies, fragments of bone, or depressed fractures, to determine whether the periosteum is preserved or detached and to discover any hairs that may be attached to the under surface of the flaps. All antiseptics are avoided in this cleansing process.

During the lengthy, tedious, but very necessary process of cleansing the surgeon must consider the question of hemorrhage. According to the experience of the author, the complete arrest of all hemorrhage is the most important part in the antiseptic treatment. Fluid or coagulated blood in a wound always causes a delay in its healing, and is at the same time a culture-ground for pyogenic organisms that would not multiply in the living tissue except for the pressure of the stagnant, decomposing blood-clots. Owing to the tense connective tissue in which the arteries run, it is not always easy to isolate and catch them for the purpose of applying a ligature. Hæmostatic forceps, provided with teeth and closed by a slide, will be found more suitable in these cases than the Pean artery-clamp. After catching the bleeding point with the forceps a sharply curved needle armed with a piece of catgut is passed through the tissues around the vessel near the clamp and tied. In cases in which the vessel slips from the surgeon's grasp or is torn off, it may be transfixed sub-cutaneously and ligated. Long, continuous compression by means of specially devised plaster straps is not to be recommended. The chief point is not to grow impatient in attempting to stop the bleeding. Many small vessels will usually quit bleeding if firm pressure be made over the bleeding points with a hard pad of gauze for three minutes. Dangerous hemorrhage from the vessels of the scalp, though uncommon, has occurred in the distribution of the temporal and occipital arteries. In extensive wounds of the head, however, the loss of blood is usually considerable. It is therefore important to control temporarily the hemorrhage by digital compression on the edges of the wound or flap. With the same object in view a thick, narrow rubber band may be passed from the forehead above the ear to the neck and back again on the opposite side, then drawn tight and clamped. The venous hemorrhage that follows this constriction is usually profuse. On the other hand, the elastic band prevents the more dangerous arterial hemorrhage. Ligation of the trunk of the occipital, temporal, and even the external carotid arteries has been performed in cases in which the local arrest of hemorrhage was despaired of. The occipital artery is best exposed where it emerges between the superior insertion of the trapezius and the splenius muscle, the temporal artery at a point half a centimetre in front of the tragus, where it crosses the zygoma and can be felt pulsating under the finger. Here the vessel is separated from the skin by only a sheath-like investment from the cranial aponeurosis.

Being satisfied as to the vitality of the wound-flaps and having completely controlled all hemorrhage, the probability of infection also having been excluded, the opposite edges of the wound should be brought together with fine silk that has been sterilized by steam or with fine catgut. Even in wounds that do not gape suturing will favor rapid union. In flap-wounds suturing is absolutely necessary. In these the sutures must hold the flaps in proper position to prevent their retracting toward the base. In case a flap is not straightened out, unfolded, and properly

FIG. 3.

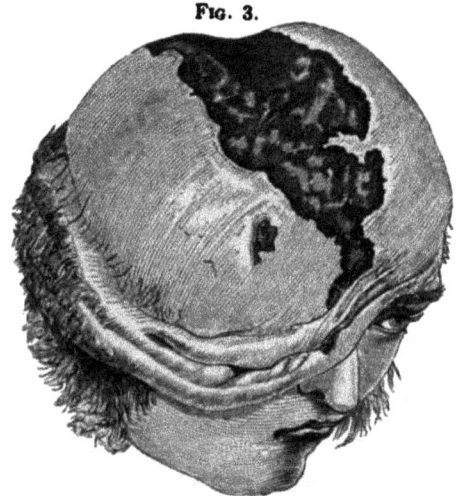

Result of faulty coaptation of flaps in wound of scalp.

coaptated, the result may be as shown in Fig. 3, taken from Hilton. When the case came to Hilton for treatment, more than six months after the time of injury, the skin was rolled up in a twisted, shapeless mass at the side of the skull, covered the eye and ear, while on the top of the skull large, necrotic portions had been thrown off by the exposed bone. The flaps should be sewed up, even in those cases in which there is apparently little chance of primary union. In such cases the connective-tissue layer of the flap may have sustained very little damage by contusions and be in a good state of preservation. Even if the wound-edges do not meet throughout their entire extent, a large part of the deep surface may become united to the underlying periosteum and bone, and thereby protect the skull, at the same time establishing for itself further source of nutrition. If primary union take place only here and there along the coaptated edges, these bridges of tissue will hold the flaps in place a great

leal better than any subsequent retention dressing can. It may often
ie of advantage to trim the lacerated edges in part, if not entirely, and
nake a cleaner-cut wound before suturing. There are cases, of course,
n which flaps have retracted so much toward their base that any further
rimming off would make it difficult to bring the edges of the wound
ogether without unduly stretching and distorting the flap. But even in
uch cases one should try to bring about their approximation by sutures,
s these alone can hold the connective-tissue layer of the flap firmly down
pon the underlying parts, insure healthy union, and re-establishment
f circulation and nutrition from below. In cases of large flaps with a
road base, one or more small incisions may be made along the line of
eflection to provide for drainage. Such incisions have been found
seful in cases that come under observation for the first time several
ays after injury, and where the attempt is made to freshen the edges.
Iere the so-called wound secretion is more profuse and the danger of its
tagnation is greater.

The bone exposed by the injury is best protected by freshening the
lap and suturing. No other means offer the same security from super-
cial necrosis. Drainage of all wound secretions is one of the chief
actors in obtaining rapid union and freedom from pus, and is the
est—indeed, the only—means of combating threatening infection. The
uthor, therefore, never sews up closely, as by continuous suture, any
round where he may expect oozing of blood, but leaves gaps here and
here between sutures to provide easy escape for accumulating wound
ecretions.

A wound which has probably been infected and which does not gape
nuch should not be sutured; in cases in which there is danger of a flap
illing down and where sutures are necessary to hold it in place, they
hould be wide apart and the edges of the wound between them be
llowed to gape, and in every instance a counteropening should be made
t the base of the flap.

In addition an attempt should be made to supplement the above by
ie manner of dressing these wounds. In the gaps and counteropenings
iat may have been made in wounds probably infected, strips of iodo-
)rm gauze should be laid, thereby maintaining the openings intended
)r drainage, and at the same time favoring removal of the fluids secreted
y the wound, through capillary absorption by the dry gauze, or, better
ill, by gauze impregnated with powdered iodoform. Strips of gauze
iould be inserted into the incisions at the base of flaps suspended by
itures and carried well up and under the same. For years the author
as substituted gauze for drainage-tubes in wounds of the head, as the
itter are difficult to hold in place in this situation, and troublesome to
:move and replace. When wounds become purulent iodoform gauze
innot be used for packing, as the secretion is too thick to be readily
bsorbed. The plug in the opening of the wound would block it up and
iuse an accumulation of pus in the bottom of the wound—just what is
iost to be avoided. Here extensive drainage is indicated, and for that
urpose the wound may have to be opened.

Besides the strips of iodoform gauze which the author inserts into wounds, and with which losses of substance are replaced or denuded bone covered, the protective dressing consists of layers of fluff gauze held in place firmly and with moderate pressure by turns of a bandage. If infection is probable, the bandage should be drawn less tight. The dressing should not press the flaps down on the skull or the edges of the wounds together, as was taught by Volkmann. Pressure should be just sufficient to cause absorption of all secretion from the wounds and to saturate the gauze. The author does not place layers of cotton over the gauze, as the absence of this covering favors evaporation of fluid, serum, blood, and pus, penetrating to the surface of the dressing. These dry much faster in gauze than in cotton dressings. Only in order to occlude securely the dressing, layers of cotton are placed about the neck, temple, and occiput, also the cheeks and chin. The dressing should then be securely, smoothly, and uniformly held by the well-known turns of a skullcap bandage, using a soft cotton or muslin bandage, the latter being covered by a few turns of a gauze bandage wet with corrosive sublimate to prevent slipping and displacement.

With this dressing everything is completed. The patient should be advised to refrain from all excesses and from severe or overheating work. No special régime is necessary, nor any device for cooling the head that will disarrange the dressing. If the dressing remain dry, it may be left in place from four to eight days. If much iodoform gauze has been packed into the cavities of wounds or into counteropenings, the dressing should be changed sooner. As soon as the dressing becomes saturated with secretion it should be replaced by a fresh one.

When a wound in a state of suppuration is presented the first time for treatment, the question comes up whether it is an active suppurative process or whether the active inflammation has subsided, and the surgeon is simply dealing with the·abundant secretion accompanying a .process of granulation. In the former case the treatment is that of an acute phlegmon; in the latter the only indications are proper drainage and appropriate dressing. As pus of the consistency of cream can never be completely absorbed by the materials used in dressings, the dressings should not remain too long in place. Whenever fresh dressings are applied, all crusts and inspissated pus attached to the hairs should be washed off with ether or hydrogen peroxide and growing hairs removed by the "safety razor," which can easily be sterilized by boiling. Of course, every abscess should be promptly opened; unhealthy, flabby, or necrotic granulations frequently be scraped off, and slowly healing areas be covered by Thiersch skin-grafts. The latter are found especially useful in cases with extensive loss of substance, such as those of scalping, and there will hardly be found a better place in which to apply Thiersch's method of skin-grafting. The whole extent of a large wound may be treated at one sitting, as first done with happy and permanent results by Socin. The cases treated in this way were granulating, and it was necessary to scrape off the superficial spongy layer. After bleeding had been controlled by moderate pressure with pieces of gauze soaked in normal salt solution, strips of epidermis 10 cm. to 20 cm. in length and 15 cm. in width, taken from the arms and legs of the patient, were spread over the surface of the wound until it was completely covered. Altermatt saw his patient a long time after the operation, and found the new scalp movable over the subjacent skull. The grafts can be made to grow on fresh muscles. They can be spread on the periosteum or the aponeurosis, or less satisfactorily on the bare bone, without waiting for the stage of granulation.

CHAPTER III.

DISEASES OF THE COVERINGS OF THE SKULL.

TUMORS OF THE COVERINGS OF THE SKULL.

Emphysema.—Emphysema of the soft parts covering the skull has frequently been observed. It follows traumatism, causing a subcutaneous opening into the air-sinuses of the cranial bones, most frequently after fracture of the frontal bone involving the frontal sinus, and quite rarely after fracture of the mastoid process. Usually it is limited to the immediate neighborhood of the injured anterior wall of the frontal sinus. A spreading of the emphysema from the frontal region over the face, the neck, the breasts, the arms, and the abdomen, and even the hand, appears to have occurred but once (Andral). However, this general emphysema disappeared within a few days, as it has in all other cases, without resulting in permanent damage. Emphysema does not always appear immediately after injury, sometimes only after several hours. In all cases it will increase if the patient be directed to breathe out, at the same time closing the mouth and nares. The site of injury may be detected by the course and direction of this increase. Voss observed the very rare occurrence of emphysema of the scalp in a case in which there was a fracture of the mastoid process. Here also emphysema had disappeared after three days.

Pneumatocele of the Head.—Opposed to the cases of diffuse emphysema of the skin, involving principally the subcutaneous areolar tissue, and recognized by a distinct crackling on palpation, are those tumor-like collections of air between periosteum and cranial bones, known as *pneumatocele cranii*, which have been observed to occur on the forehead and in the occipital region, especially near the mastoid process. Eighteen cases of occipital pneumatocele have been reported, and nine cases of frontal pneumatocele were collected by von Helly. The cases of pneumatocele that communicate with the frontal sinus do not occur before the tenth year for embryological reasons. They appear as irregular, hemispherical, tumors of variable size; they may be as large as a cherry or extend from the eyebrows to the occiput. The soft parts covering them may be more less elastic, but always have a uniform degree of tension.

The raised periosteum is more tense in cases of pneumatocele that recently or suddenly occurred than in those that are more gradual and have progressed for months or years. The tumors lie the scalp, which remains unaltered; there may be a thickened the periphery, and they may give a clear tympanitic note on The air contained in them may be forced by pressure into nus, and this act may be accompanied by a perceptible noise.

On breathing out, with the nose and mouth closed, the air-cyst suddenly swells. After a cyst has been emptied by pressure one may feel at times, though not in every case, some irregularity or defect in the anterior surface of the frontal bone. Some opening must exist in the anterior wall of the frontal sinus to account for the occurrence of the pneumatocele. Such defects are of three kinds: first, congenital; secondly, foramina, serving to conduct vessels; and thirdly, traumatic defects, inflammation, or suppuration of the anterior sinus-wall. In the latter case the anterior wall must have been destroyed by caries or necrosis.

Treatment.—In cases not resulting from an inflammatory process in the frontal sinus continuous pressure should be applied to the cyst. When an inflammatory process has been followed by partial necrosis, an incision should be made and all necrotic tissue and sequestra of bone be removed, with the hope that repair will be completed by granulation. If the opening in the frontal bone does not close of itself after this procedure, recurrence of the cyst may occur and necessitate a more complicated operation which will be given later.

Occipital Pneumatocele.—Occipital pneumatocele is similar in external appearance and clinical features to frontal pneumatocele, except in so far as its form is modified by the particular shape of the region of the skull in which it occurs. It generally originates in the region behind the ear, and separates the periosteum for a considerable distance.

Etiology.—The point of origin indicates the mastoid cells to be the source of air in the cyst. The outer wall of these cells is very thin, and may be broken through by trauma, carious process, or even spontaneously during violent exertion, thus allowing air to escape. In the skulls of very old individuals the outer lamella of the mastoid process may be so thin as to be broken through by strong pressure with the finger, like an egg-shell. Besides the acquired losses of continuity of bone in the mastoid process, there are cases in which foramina of vessels communicating with the air cells may provide a means of exit for the contained air, as in the case of the frontal bone. From Flesch's investigations it is known that in such cases a process of absorption in the superficial layers of the bone takes place. At all events, many more spontaneous than traumatic pneumatocele have been seen in which, as in Sonnenburg's case, after opening the tumor the communication with the mastoid cells could not be discovered. Similarly the not infrequent persistence of the mastoid-squamous fissure may play a part in the etiology of occipital pneumatocele.

The raised periosteum confines the air in a circumscribed swelling. By pressure it may be diminished in size and the air forced through the middle ear and Eustachian tube into the pharynx, while the swelling will increase in size and become more tense if the middle ear be inflated by Politzer's method. The tumor may continue for a long time and demand active surgical interference to accomplish its removal. Anatomical examination shows irregularities such as erosions with a smooth floor, or trabeculæ and ridges on the surface of the bone, and in addition a low bony wall where the raised periosteum is reflected.

Treatment.—If pressure, bandages, and puncture are not successful an operation will be necessary. Simple incision, with iodoform packing, may be tried. As in most cases only minute openings exist, it may be assumed that they will close by the formation of granulation tissue. This happened in Sonnenburg's case. Kramer found it necessary to do more, as in spite of two successive operations the tumor recurred. In this case there was a visible space of communication—namely, a cleft in the occipital bone—this was covered by a König-Müller osteoplastic flap. This operation was followed by recovery.

NEOPLASMS OF THE COVERINGS OF THE SKULL.

Lipoma.—Lipoma of the hairy scalp and forehead is rare. In 685 cases of single lipoma Grosch found only 13 in the scalp and forehead—less than 2 per cent. Stoll found somewhat more; 45 per cent. in 133 cases from the clinic of Tübingen. Chipault collected from the literature on the subject 54 solitary, 2 symmetrical (located in two places on the head), and 10 multiple lipomata (appearing in combination with numerous fatty tumors in other parts of the body). Diffuse lipomata of the back of the neck extend to the occipital region, and of the front of the neck laterally over the mastoid process. The favorite situation for lipoma is the forehead, which was the site in 37 out of Chipault's 54 cases, though the forehead represents only one-fourth of the entire cranial surface. On this relation of frequeney Grosch based his theory of the antagonism between the hairy parts of the body and the occurrence of lipoma, referring principally to the large number of sebaceous glands and their action in preventing the development of these tumors. In the parietal region lipomata occurred four times, in the temporal region five times, and in the occipital region eight times.

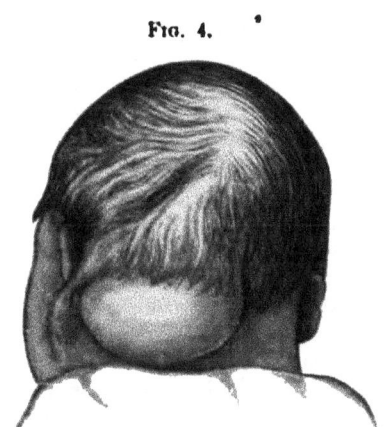

Fig. 4.

Deep-seated lipoma of scalp of infant. Tumor differentiated clinically from cephalocele by Röntgen ray. Microscopic examination after removal showed large fat cells with a connective-tissue stroma rich in cells.

Lipoma of the frontal region is always situated in the delicate, elastic connective tissue beneath the occipitofrontalis muscle, where there is absence of all adipose tissue. There is usually a wall around the base of the tumor rising above the level of the cranial bones, feeling very much like a bony ridge, and giving the impression that the growth is situated in a depression of the bone. In most cases, however, this is due to a simple, hard infiltration of the pericranium, like that felt in the case of hæmatoma. In only one case did the author find a frontal congenital lipoma in a shallow fossa of the bone, a condition similar to that found in congenital dermoid of the scalp. Somewhat the same condition was observed by Lannelongue in 1 case and by Chipault in 2 cases of congenital frontal lipomata.

Lipoma of the head usually appears as a rounded, dome-like swelling, or flattened tumor, generally attached by a broad base, and only rarely in cases of excessive growth becoming pedunculated and pendulous. An enormous lipoma in a negress was described by Roger and reproduced by V. von Bruns in his *Atlas*. It had been growing since the unhappy possessor was two years old, and attained a length of more than three feet, reaching the woman's knees. Lipomata are generally of slow growth, the increase involving all parts of the tumor uniformly. The skin over a lipoma is unaltered, freely movable, and in case of the frontal region may be raised in folds. The surface is not always lobulated, but smooth and homogeneous, because in the structure of the lipoma the connective tissue—that is, the element which forms the septa of the lobes—is less developed than the purely adipose tissue. Lipomata are therefore not always tense and elastic, but often quite soft, as if fluctuating. They have frequently been mistaken for sebaceous cysts of the scalp; but a sebaceous cyst is always movable with the skin, no matter how deeply its sac reaches into the subcutaneous tissue, while a lipoma is not. The mobility of the latter over the underlying parts may be very slight, owing to its frequent attachment to the periosteum.

Diagnosis.—A lipoma is differentiated from dermoids by the position of the latter in certain definite places on the skull, and by the occurrence of dermoids at birth, while lipoma usually occurs in later life. Cephalocele would be excluded by the constant site of its occurrence. The relations of lipoma to these congenital tumors will be referred to below. Lipoma may be mistaken for chronic tuberculous osteomyelitis occurring frequently in the frontal bone; this is rarely solitary and generally of irregular outline. In addition there are usually found other tuberculous lesions in different parts of the body, and the child is apt to be ailing and anæmic. Syphilitic gumma is recognized by its multiple occurrence, manner of growth, and other symptoms accompanying the tertiary period.

Treatment.—As lipoma of the head is hardly a serious matter, the surgeon is usually consulted for cosmetic reasons, and his scalpel can readily effect its removal. The excision of unusually large and pendulons tumors may be troublesome on account of excessive hemorrhage, but even in these cases operation is not contraindicated.

Fibroma.—Whether hard, lobulated, fibrous-tissue growths occur in the soft parts covering the skull is questionable. A papillomatous form of fibroma has been described, appearing like soft, ulcerating warts, but the author's knowledge of them is too imperfect to distinguish them from sarcomatous warts or from neuropathic papillomata of similar form. On the other hand, soft circumscribed or diffuse connective-tissue growths are of great pathological and surgical interest, especially since von Recklinghausen has taught their relations to the peripheral nervous system. Four types may be distinguished: (1) soft multiple fibromata, fibromata mollusca, which originate in the sheaths of cutaneous nerves; (2) the pigmented "neuronævus," in which regular minute fibromata are attached to the finest terminal twigs of the cutaneous nerves; (3) the "racemose neuroma" of P. Bruns, in which coils of thickened nerve-fibres, cylindrical or spindle-shaped, are twisted and intertwined like grape-vines; and (4) elephantiasis of neuropathic origin or "elephantiasis neuromatosa congenita." The four types may exist in combination with each other much more frequently than formerly was supposed.

A case of elephantiasis of the skin is shown in Fig. 5, in which the appearance of the twenty-year-old male patient was grotesquely changed. The growth looked like a cap of dough placed upon the top of the head and over the occiput. This thick tab of skin could be grasped by the hand and thrown from one side of the head to the other, covering either ear. Over the rest of the body were numerous fibromata, soft and of different sizes, some so small that they could be felt like mere papules, while others were of considerable dimensions. Some had a faint brownish surface, others were more intensely pigmented. Between the soft fibromata were many pigmented spots. In some of the latter, which were removed, the microscopical examination after osmium staining showed rows of minute fibromata, many of them made up of coiled and twisted nerve-fibres like microscopical racemose neuromata. · Besides a large number of the soft fibromata, the author dissected off the cap-like tumor of the head. The resulting wound could not be completely closed, so that skin-grafting by Thiersch's method was found necessary.

The large, folded, tab-like cutaneous tumor, which showed numerous pigmented areas on its surface, besides abundant hairs, was found to consist of soft, rich, connective tissue, representing an extraordinary degree of proliferation in the subcutaneous connective tissue, like the

Fig. 5.

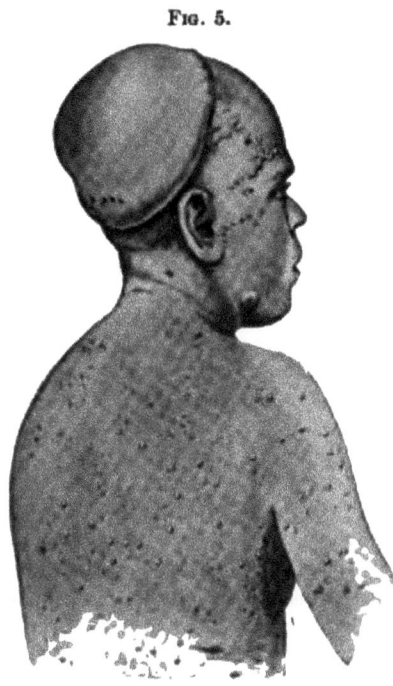

Elephantiasis of the scalp.

involve the skin in these forms to a slight degree only, as they do also in some forms of cephalocele.

Simple angiomata are congenital, but they are mostly smaller immediately after birth than four or five weeks later. They seldom originate in later life, and in such cases are limited to scars and contused wounds. The racemose, arterial angioma, on the other hand, has been definitely shown to originate in later life as a direct result of traumatism.

The extensive flat telangiectasis, of a uniform pale-red color, not raised above the level of the general surface, usually disappear of themselves after a time. In one family the author observed that each child was born with one of these large bright spots on the occiput, yet in each case it disappeared within two years. The growth of the hair was not in the least affected. Even the purplish spots with a raised undulating or irregular surface may disappear spontaneously, especially if they are small, and the white retracted streaks on their surface are numerous or predominate. However, their disappearance usually requires a long time, and there may always remain glistening white areas marked by fine bluish veins and characterized by absence of hair. Cases in which the growth has spread out under the skin have been seen to recede by a kind of spontaneous atrophy. Quite frequently the entire growth has become cicatrized and contracted following a process of inflammation and ulceration.

TREATMENT.—The same result is aimed at in the surgical treatment of these tumors, and this end is probably reached better by means of caustics than with the knife. The superficial slough resulting from the application of caustic, preferably fuming nitric acid, is slowly thrown off, leaving at first a purplish scar, which gradually pales until it becomes white.

The use of caustics, even if repeated application is required, will not affect a child, while in excision the surgeon has to face not only troublesome hemorrhage, but also the possibility of subsequent infection of the wound, which makes the latter method less applicable in spite of all precaution, especially in the treatment of cases in out-patients' departments. The purplish racemose nævi of the forehead, either those that are prominent and projecting, or those that have spread beneath the skin, are an exception to this method of treatment. They should be cut out; a fine white linear scar is left which is hardly noticeable in the course of time. Thick, projecting masses of spongy tissue, either above or beneath the kin, should also be excised. The operation may be made bloodless by means of a ring of rubber surrounding the growth and pressed down firmly upon the underlying bone. Some of the fine red lines of vascular tissue may be difficult to dissect out, in which case they should be scraped off with a sharp spoon. It is often surprising to find how little bleeding accompanies the radical removal of these growths, and the moderate hemorrhage that does occur is usually easily controlled by clamping and tying a few of the larger vessels as soon as the rubber ring is removed. In spite of the looseness of the surrounding tissues, it is difficult to cover the denuded surface and to bring the edges of the wound together in the cases in which it has been found necessary to remove much skin. In young children the dressing is held in place by rubber tissue strips sewed to a butterfly-shaped piece of adhesive plaster according to Thiersch's method, and this is changed whenever it becomes moist.

Special precaution must be observed in operating on cases of angioma situated over the anterior fontanelle, as the growth is seldom shallow or superficial, but generally extends down to the longitudinal sinus. In these cases repeated cauterization is preferable to dissection, or, as Thiersch has recommended for similar growths on the lips and cheeks, multiple puncture with a fine needle-like thermocautery.

Therapeutic interference is positively indicated in these cases on account of the liability of hemorrhage, and also because of the tendency to further proliferation. They usually grow superficially; the neighboring bloodvessels, especially the veins, become dilated, lengthened, and convoluted, and along these the tumor progresses. They may also invade the deeper tissue layers, reaching and even penetrating the bone. Under these circumstances they cannot be distinguished from diffuse cavernous angiomata, or they represent that form of new growth known as hypertrophic simple angioma (hæmangioma simplex hypertrophicum). They are characterized by being composed chiefly of sinuses filled with

FIG. 6.

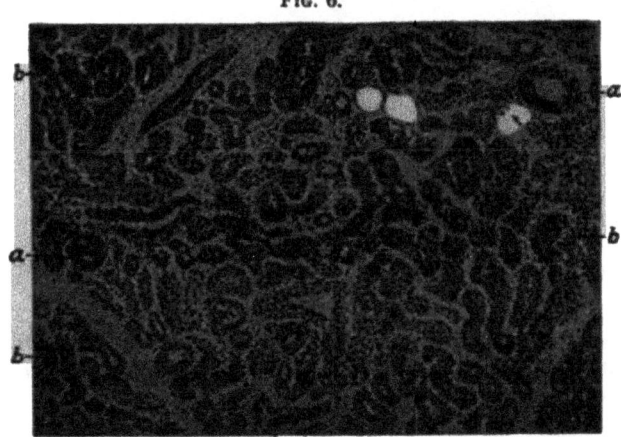

Hypertrophic simple angioma.   *a.* Bloodvessels filled with blood.   *b.* Empty collapsed blood-vessels with thick walls.   (Ziegler.)

blood. But besides these there are strands of endothelial cells intersecting the vascular network. Ziegler gives a microscopical section of such a tumor taken from the top of the head, in which may be noted the similarity in structure of the illustrated angioma with that of an endothelial tumor called endothelioma vasculosum or telangiectodes. (Fig. 6.)

√ **Cavernous angioma** (*hæmangioma cavernosum*) is not composed of dilated and intertwined vessels, but consists of a spongy mass of blood-filled sinuses, like the corpus cavernosum of the penis. On the cranium it occurs generally as a diffuse variety, whose similarity with the progressive subcutaneous form of simple angioma has been referred to above. The transition from simple vascular nævus or angioma to cavernous angioma may be frequently observed. The bright-scarlet patch becomes a prominent nævus, its surface becomes irregularly lobulated, and the growth increases laterally and in depth. Certain forms of cavernoma, appearing shortly after birth and increasing rapidly in extent of surface and depth, are of special interest on account of their relation to the cranial bones and the contents of the skull. They burrow through the bones and establish a connection with the intracranial vascular system. Lannelongue collected 12 cases of congenital angioma that showed this connection with the longitudinal sinus after traversing the cranial bones. They were either superficial or subcutaneous; some simple,

Fig. 7.

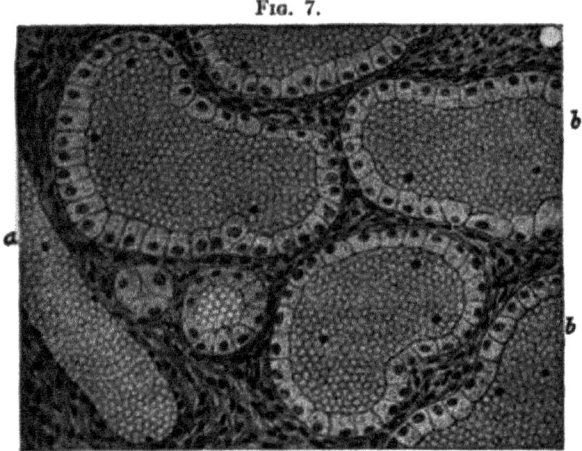

Cavernous angioma of scalp. × 390. a. Spaces lined with flat epithelia. b. Spaces lined with cylindrical epithelia. (Ziegler.)

others cavernous, most of them running out in many branched venous ramifications. The emissary veins as well as those of the scalp were dilated, and the bones retarded in their development, as a result of the new growth in its proliferation having extensively invaded the skull.

TREATMENT.—While it is obvious that careful operation is indicated in the case of simple or cavernous angioma growing rapidly toward the deeper tissues, at the same time, if it has been determined that the growth has penetrated to the cavity of the skull, it is much the safer plan to use multiple puncture with the thermocautery. This method has the advantage of producing less reaction in the tissues bordering on the slough. If the cauterized area be then covered with several thicknesses of iodoform gauze, and these are held firmly in place by strips of bandage saturated with photoxylin, the slough is thrown off without any suppuration. After a short time the cauterization by puncture may be repeated.

Racemose arterial angioma (*angioma arteriale racemosum*), called by
Virchow "Rankenangiom," occurs more frequently in the arteries of
the head than in those of the hands and feet, and is characterized by
a dilatation, convolution, and thickening of a number of neighboring
arteries, the change involving not only the trunks of the vessels, but
their branches as well.

According to the description of the majority of cases reported, this
neoplasm occurs principally on the head, and an excellent specimen from
von Brun's clinic is shown by Müller and Ziegler. (Fig. 8.) The authorities name two causes: first, developing from congenital angioma, and,
secondly, traumatism. The development of phlebectasis at the periphery

FIG. 8.

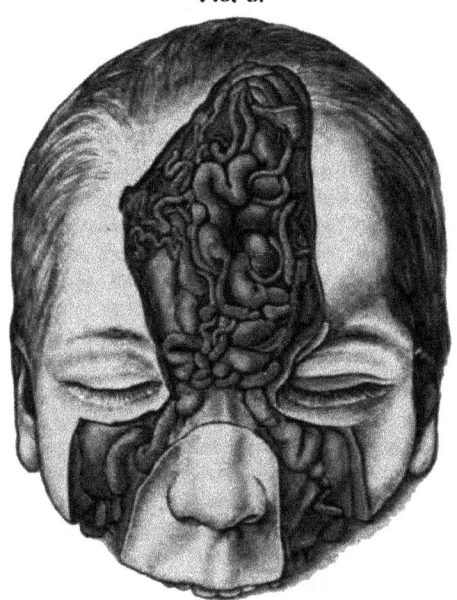

Racemose arterial angioma. (Ziegler.)

of superficial angioma has been mentioned above; in the same way it
has been observed that dilatation of the afferent arteries takes place
first in the smaller branches, later in the larger trunks, the capillaries
developing, as the proliferation of the growth goes on, into a higher order
of vessels. In regard to their mechanical or traumatic origin, these
tumors sometimes follow severe contusions, rarely contused wounds.
After the wound heals a pulsation gradually becomes noticeable at the
site of the contusion or scar. In some instances where a good-sized
artery has been injured a small, circumscribed aneurysm appears at
the seat of the injury. Later there is a widening of the affected artery.
This is followed by similar changes in the anastomosing branches and
finally of their respective trunks.

König observed the development of a racemose angioma on the ear of a boy who had the habit of constantly pulling at the lobe of his ear. Seventy-four cases of racemose angioma of the scalp were collected by Heine and Körte, and quite a number have been reported since then: 20 were located in the region of the ear, 18 on the forehead, 4 on the lateral half of the skull, and 1 in the region under the ear, while in the rest the site of the growth was not mentioned. The clinical features are well marked. At the periphery of the growth dilated arteries are visible and can be distinctly felt. The frontal and superficial temporal arteries are more frequently involved than the occipital and auricular. The growth may be resolved into a number of anastomosing branches communicating with each other in a complex system or network, and seems to be made up of a number of pulsating strands, feeling like a bundle of earthworms. Ferrier has given the name "cirsoid aneurysm" to those growths in which dilatation was limited to one of the external arteries, distinguishing these from all other varieties of racemose angioma; but there seems to be no sufficient reason for this, as the changes in the wall of the one vessel are exactly the same as those found when two or more are involved. The increase in length as well as in transverse diameter of the arteries is a very active process and the forerunner of the tumor formation. This process is combined with the formation of small saccular aneurysms and fatty degeneration of the elements of the vessel-wall. These changes occur at intervals in the course of the vessel, and, since the process advances toward the centre from the periphery, can be traced to the carotid artery. Usually a quarter, if not half, of the entire surface of the skull is occupied by this vascular network. The skin covering the enormous collection of anastomosing arteries may be thin and smooth, or thick and warty. There is always a blue tint shining through; but the skin may be of a deep purplish color and appear cyanotic. The tumor is flattened and not raised markedly above the general surface. The most striking feature is the pulsation, which not only can be felt, but is also distinctly visible throughout the extent of the tumor. Compression of one afferent vessel does not stop the pulsation, on account of the very extensive anastomosis, except where the growth is limited to the region of one terminal artery and no other vessel can furnish a blood-supply to the tumor. On applying the ear or stethoscope a whirring, blowing noise is heard where smaller vessels empty into larger ones; or, conversely, larger ones empty into smaller ones. The sound is synchronous with the pulse. The pulsation and murmurs may prove very annoying to the patient.

Racemose angioma grows rapidly at first, but later becomes quiescent and remains stationary. Periods of growth may alternate with stationary periods, especially during pregnancy.

There is always danger of rupture of the skin at any time, and the resulting hemorrhage, whether preceded by inflammation and ulceration or not, is the cause of death in many of these cases. This danger, as well as the liability to external injury, justifies surgical interference, even if this requires radical and even doubtful methods.

DIAGNOSIS.—From what has been stated above, the diagnosis of racemose angioma offers no difficulty. However, it is important to remember in every case of pulsating tumor of the skull that there is no part of the body where so many different kinds of pulsating tumors are to be found. We meet with these pulsating tumors, according to Stierlin's classification: in racemose arterial angioma, mentioned above; in arteriovenous aneurysm (to be mentioned later); in aneurysm of cranial arteries; further, in subperiosteal varix communicating with the longitudinal sinus; in cephalocele; sarcoma perforating the dura mater; in dermoids situated in cranial bone-clefts and resting directly on the dura mater; in pulsating osteosarcoma; and, finally, in pulsating sarcoma of soft parts, first described by Stierlin.

Racemose angioma may be distinguished easily from solid, smooth, pulsating tumors, especially those cases of sarcoma referred to above, by the peculiar feeling of the separate elastic tubes filled with blood. The differentiation from arterial aneurysm and arteriovenous aneurysm will be discussed at length below.

TREATMENT.—The different methods of treating racemose arterial aneurysm have been very thoroughly discussed by Siegmund. Heine, to whom we are indebted for the first monograph written on these new growths, divides the methods of treatment into three classes: First, those methods which by limiting the blood-supply bring about obliteration, shrinking, and atrophy of the dilated bloodvessels. Among this class are: long-continued pressure, applied at intervals, on the afferent vessels (discarded because ineffectual); ligation of each afferent vessel (doubtful benefit), and the ligation of the larger vessels of the neck, the direct effect of which is to inhibit the pulsation of the tumor without producing any permanent results so far as can be observed.

Several times surgeons have been rash enough to tie at the same time both common carotids, with only partially good results.

This method seems a very unsatisfactory one when one considers that in tying the carotids the nutrition of the brain and of the face also is seriously imperilled and that the operation has been successful in only 3 of 52 cases of ligation of the carotids, according to Heine's enumeration. Consequently physicians have turned to the second class of methods, which attempt to bring about obstruction of the bloodvessels and their subsequent destruction. In these methods the injection of coagulating fluids, principally ferric chloride and absolute alcohol, play an important part. Körte reports 7 cases in which this method was used. But this procedure is dangerous, as experience has shown. The resulting thrombosis may extend to the bloodvessels of the dura, or even to the heart, and so directly imperil life.

During the injection temporary pressure is made to prevent the entrance of the injecting fluid into the larger vessels, and to prevent its being carried through them; but this means of protection is as unreliable as the thrombus that we endeavor to produce. Nevertheless, this method has shown some good results, more, at any rate, than electropuncture and electrolysis. The alcohol should be injected as much as possible between the arteries in order to produce an inflammatory reaction in the connective tissue, subsequent contraction of which may produce sufficient pressure on the vessels to close them. Two cases have been reported cured by this method.

The last group of methods in Heine's classification includes all those which aim at the direct destruction and removal of the diseased vessels. The destruction by potential cauterization has shown itself to be as dangerous as destruction by the actual cautery. Fatal hemorrhage has followed removal of the slough following cauterization by acids and burning. The most effective of the methods belonging to this class is dissection with the knife, and is recommended by Heine as well as Siegmund, having given positive results in 9 cases. One must not forget, however, that in only a few cases of racemose angioma have these good results been obtained, while in a large number fatal hemorrhage has resulted from the operation. A heavy rubber ring encircling the vault of the skull in the plane of its base makes the operation much easier. Heine secured some advantage in his operations by tying the external carotid as a preliminary step. From the preceding we would deduce the following: that in the case of small racemose angioma it is advisable to excise the growth with the assistance of a constricting rubber band, and the ligation of the external carotid immediately before the operation; in the case of larger growths in older people it is best to leave them alone and to protect them from external violence by suitable caps. In younger people they should be injected with ferric chloride, while at the same time constriction is made about the forehead and occiput, or pressure with a rubber ring about the region which is to be injected, in order that the circulation may be temporarily suspended in these parts. Kötschau reports successful extirpation of a very extensive growth which had led to a very exhausting hemorrhage, and was gratified with the condition of his patient eight months later.

Aneurysms.—Simple aneurysm of the arteries supplying the scalp is almost always caused by some injury of the vessel. The superficial temporal, on account of its extensive distribution and its course along the surface, is the one most exposed to violence and the one most frequently the site of aneurysm. The author has had the opportunity of operating in 3 such cases, in each of which the aneurysm was small. Cases have been reported, however, in which they were the size of a goose's egg, which would probably have ruptured under the thin skin of the temple in a short time. These aneurysms may be sacculated or spindle-shaped. It was mentioned above that occasionally such aneurysms may be combined with the dilatation of an artery throughout its entire trunk and all its branches, thus forming a transition to the racemose arterial angioma. The diagnosis is as a rule simple.

Treatment.—The treatment of aneurysm in all cases consists in extirpation of the sac. De Sauti collected histories in 40 such cases.

Arteriovenous aneurysm, for which the author operated in only one case, occurs likewise most frequently in the region of the superficial temporal artery, and is brought about in this vessel by punctured or incised wounds. The dilatation of the superficial veins is the most conspicuous symptom; in addition, all the symptoms of arteriovenous aneurysm as described by von Bramann. The peculiar whirring sound is heard louder at the point of communication between artery and vein. In most cases there is a direct connection between the vein and artery as in aneurysmal varix. Pressure with the tip of the finger on the point of communication causes all pulsation to cease.

DIAGNOSIS.—Keeping in mind their traumatic origin, the diagnosis is not difficult.

TREATMENT.—The treatment consists in searching for the communicating portion and excising it after double ligature of both artery and vein.

Sinus Pericranii.—There is a peculiar cyst-like growth filled with fluid blood, best known under the name "sinus pericranii," given it by Stromeyer. It is situated beneath the cranial periosteum, and is connected with the longitudinal sinus by a wide emissary vessel. Its traumatic origin has been mentioned. The forms of congenital subcutaneous or cavernous angioma, put in the above class by Lannelongue, have been previously mentioned, as their external appearance distinguishes them decidedly from the sinus pericranii of Stromeyer. The latter is probably always traumatic in origin and situated in the middle line of the skull, on the forehead, or on the occiput. Lannelongue collected observations in 7 such cases. The tumors are covered with normal or thinned and at the same time bluish skin, and are rarely larger than a walnut. Soft and elastic, they impart a distinct sense of fluctuation, and may be forced into the hollow of the skull, where a cleft may be felt in the bone or a bony ring about the base of the tumor. Slight pulsation has occasionally been noticed, but what is most noticeable is the fact that in throwing the head back, or allowing it to fall forward, the growth swells and grows tense. The same thing takes place in coughing and on exertion, sometimes even on simple expiration. Continuous pressure is probably the only therapeutic method that has been applied to these cases. In threatened rupture of the sac, with danger of hemorrhage, tamponing with iodoform gauze is indicated to arrest bleeding, as in all other cases of hemorrhage from a sinus. There may also arise the question of closing the opening in the skull by some osteoplastic operation.

Sarcoma.—Sarcomata of the soft parts of the skull occur either as sarcomata of the skin or sarcomata of the fascia. The first originate primarily in the intact connective tissue of the skin or subcutaneous tissue, or they develop secondarily to some disturbance in the normal structure of the tissue, as from keloids, warts, or pigmented moles. They occur at any period of life and in any region of the skull, though as a matter of fact the warty forms of sarcomata (flesh warts, bleeding easily) belong to old age, and the fascial sarcomata occur principally in the temporal region.

The forms of sarcomata which will here be considered are rather rare tumors, and do not differ in anatomical structure or in clinical aspect from sarcomata ..... in other parts of the body. There are two ..... soft nodular tumors and warty growths. The former may be ..... considerably above the level of the skin and have overhanging ..... -like edges. In other cases in which the growth has extended into the deeper parts, the skin covering it is very slightly raised. The nodular sarcoma offers a very bad prognosis, as it invades not only the neighboring tissues in the form of secondary nodes, but also gives rise to metastatic growths in the lymph-nodes of the head and neck. This fact might lead to their being mistaken for carcinomata, but in the case of sarcomata the skin is altered in an unmistakable manner before the growth invades the deeper tissues, while in sarcoma the skin covering the tumor remains intact.

When ulcerations occur in sarcomata they are flat and smooth, while those of carcinomata are undermined, irregular, and crater-like. Sarcoma is disseminated over the neck, face, and back at a very early stage, and at the same time metastasis forms in the internal organs.

The endothelial sarcomata developing secondarily in small pigmented nodes or warts have a particularly malignant character. They develop in diffuse nodular growths, or in the form of numerous hard knots, distributed over the face, neck, and chest, and having a tendency to form early metastases in the internal organs. Their structure is for the most part that of alveolar sarcomata. The pigment particles prefer the cells lying deeply in the connective-tissue stroma, and are found everywhere in the growth.

In sarcomatous warts, on the other hand, the prognosis is more favorable, whether they occur primarily as such or whether they develop secondarily in fibrous papillomata, and the patient is led to seek surgical aid on account of the hemorrhage which is often brought about by scratching the soft, cockscomb-like excrescences. These growths must be removed by wide excision through sound tissue in order that they may not recur.

A growth occurring in a case described by Mulert had existed on the scalp for fourteen years before it began to increase in size. It became ulcerated on the surface, and caused the development throughout the entire surrounding scalp of numerous new growths of similar anatomical structure. Mulert pointed this out as an example of multiple endotheliomata of the scalp. The tumors that at the present time are called endotheliomata originate from the same kind of cells as the sarcomata, but they are distinguished from the latter by the fact that in them the newly proliferated cells are arranged after the structure of lymphatics, and their similarity to lymph-channels can still be recognized. The case of ..... had all the clinical features of warty sarcomata of the skin.

A sarcoma of the soft parts of the skull is described by ..... It involved the fascia in the temporal region, and was composed of ..... cells enclosed in a fine meshwork of capillaries. In all ..... the endothelial and perithelial cells of the excessively hypertrophied ..... cells were the starting point of the sarcoma, and in this ..... much like those cases of subcutaneous hypertrophic angioma and of endothelioma from the author's clinic, reported by Nasse. The striking feature in these tumors was the pulsation, which was not transmitted, but existed in the growth itself.

Sebaceous Cysts.—The scalp is the favorite site for the development of sebaceous cysts (wens). These cysts of the scalp seem to be more frequent in women than in men. According to Chiari, they do not occur before the fifteenth year. The statistics of the author's polyclinic show that multiple cysts are about as frequent as single ones. These figures may be inaccurate, as, in the case of a large, striking cyst, smaller ones occurring at the same time are liable to be disregarded. Poncet operated at one sitting on 22 sebaceous cysts in one patient.

The growths are not different, either in their anatomical structure or clinical features, from sebaceous cysts in any other part of the body. In several cases the etiology was referred to recurrent attacks of erysipelas of the scalp. Probably the excessive desquamation of epidermis scales occurring so commonly in many people is a more important factor in their origin. Occurrence of sebaceous cysts in several succeeding generations of the same family has repeatedly been observed. They are true retention-cysts of hair-follicles and sebaceous glands, and as such always occur in the skin of the scalp, but in the course of development may invade the subcutaneous tissue. According to Chiari, sebaceous cysts may be entirely separated from the elongated hair-follicles; they are, however, never found beneath the pericranium like the dermoid cysts. By their shape sebaceous cysts of the scalp differ from those found in other parts of the body in that they may be less prominent and less dome-shaped, owing to the fact that the tense scalp flattens them out by pressing them down on the underlying bone. At other times, apparently when superficially placed, they are elevated considerably above the level of the skin, and by drawing out the latter become pedunculated (atheroma pendulum). The usual site of this variety is in the lower portions of the occipital region. The resistance offered by the cranial bones brings about another characteristic feature, the loss of hair over extensive cysts, which is caused by the progressive thinning of the skin covering the tumor and subsequent atrophy of the hair-papillæ. In this way occurs the disfigurement seen so often in older men and women, when the skull is studded with numerous bald protuberances. (Fig. 9.)

Sebaceous cysts vary in size from that of a hemp-seed or lentil to that of a man's fist, or even larger. Small cysts are always hard; large ones always soft. In the latter case the feeling varies according to the consistency of the contained fluid. It is like that of moulding clay or distinctly fluctuating. The elastic tension is always uniform no matter what the degree, and the surface of the tumor is smooth. At times sebaceous cysts present a transverse groove, or they may consist of several prominences, probably owing to the confluence of several separate cysts, which is very possible when their multiplicity is considered. The thinned skin appears very pale as compared with that of the neighboring parts. Very often the summit of the tumor shows pitted hair-follicles destitute of hair, or it may be the seat of a comedo. At other times sebaceous cysts appear livid and blue, due to congestion of the stretched skin. Chiari and Fritz König have explained many details of their histological structure. According to these observers, they are caused by cystic dilatation of the hair-follicles, as well as sebaceous glands, by the occlusion of their excretory ducts with necrotic epithelial cells, fat, and sebaceous materials. The wall of the follicle in both cases is composed of fibrous connective tissue with few nuclei, lined with epithelium composed of stratified squamous cells without the basal, cylindrical cells found in the Malpighian layer of the epidermis. The contents of the cyst are composed of the decomposing horny scales of epithelium and the secretion of the sebaceous glands. In the case of sebaceous cysts arising from hair-follicles, stumps of hairs are also found.

FIG. 9.

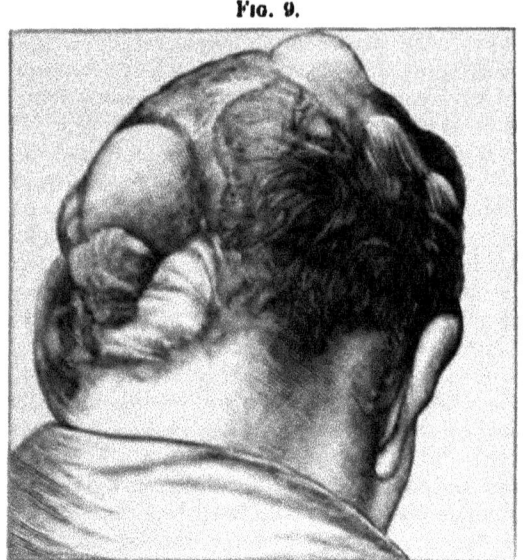

Sebaceous cysts of scalp. One on the left has undergone a carcinomatous change, the surface showing a characteristic ulcer about the size of a twenty-five-cent piece.

Sebaceous cysts of the scalp may undergo a variety of secondary changes. Fistulous sebaceous cysts may be produced by spontaneous rupture or by manipulations on the part of the patient in attempting to remove or empty them. These may continuously secrete their contents, or by temporary occlusion intermittently swell and subside. Should pyogenic micro-organisms find entrance to a cyst, either through a fistula or the still patent duct of a follicle, they may set up a purulent inflammation causing liquefaction of the contents and destruction of the sac, or the purulent process may dissect around the sac and lead to the throwing off of the entire cyst. Further, sebaceous cysts may become calcified or even produce real bone in their walls. In such cases, instead of the uniformly soft walls, hard particles or granules, producing crepitation, are felt as they are rubbed against each other. Malignant degeneration of the epithelial lining of the cyst may lead to the development of a carcinomatous growth, as will be discussed below. (Fig. 9.)

Diagnosis.—The features of diagnosis, especially the differentiation from dermoids and lipoma of the head, have been dwelt upon in the description of the latter class of tumors. As a matter of fact there is no difficulty in recognizing them, except in cases in which sebaceous cysts have become entirely separated from the skin, or in which a cyst has broken down and secondary changes, such as suppuration, have set in. The diagnosis can usually be based on the fact alone that the growth is situated within the skin.

Treatment.—As in a few cases only, sebaceous cysts get well spoutaneously by the emptying of their contents, and as no danger whatever is involved in their removal under aseptic methods and the appropriate treatment of wounds, the patient ought always be advised to get rid of such annoying and disfiguring growths. Thorough disinfection of the surrounding skin should precede the operation, even if this involves the sacrifice of hair. The hair over the entire surface of the tumor and over a fairly wide zone about its base should be shaved. Thorough scrubbing of the scalp at some distance from the cyst is sufficient. The scalp near the tumor having been shaved and scrubbed, should always be washed with ether, etc. For local anæsthesia Braun's modification of the Schleich infiltration method should be employed. The unnecessary preliminary freezing is omitted and eucaine-B substituted for cocaine. The first injection is made at the base of the tumor, from which point the resulting wheal spreads to its summit. Dissection is carried out with the knife; an incisiou is made in a line over the summit of the tumor and the skin dissected back on either side, or, better still, especially where the skin is thinned or necrotic, an elliptical or spindle-shaped incision is made over the top of the tumor. This flap of skin is allowed to remain attached to the growth, and not only prevents the cyst from bursting, but also forms a convenient means of holding the sac in dissecting it out. Frequently in spite of all precaution the sac may be injured during the first incision, and then should be quickly grasped and held by an artery clamp during its further dissection. Care must be taken not to mistake the outermost layers of the cyst contents, which may often be quite tense, for the sac itself. If upon completion of the dissection too much skin has been left to cover the wound evenly, the redundant portion should be trimmed off, as it is important that the skin-flaps should lie smoothly and without folds or wrinkles. The author never employs sutures. Hemorrhage should be controlled by ligature or compression for one minute with gauze sponges, the edges of the wound are carefully placed, leaving a small crevice between them, and the dressing completed by a compress of fluff gauze held firmly in place by several snug turns of a bandage. In this way all retention of wound secretion is prevented. All gluing with collodion, etc., produces occlusion of the wound and increases the danger of erysipelas and inflammations of the tissues surrounding the wound. It must be borne in mind that pyogenic organisms may find their way into the cavity of the wound from the neighboring scalp, and if these are sealed up they exercise their destructive tendency, while if they are constantly removed by the flow of exudate into the dry gauze of the dressing they become desiccated and do no harm.

Λ Dermoid Cysts.—Dermoid cysts occur on the head, as they do on other parts of the body, before the second or third year, at the very latest about the time of puberty. In this respect they differ from sebaceous cysts, which do not as a rule appear before the fifteenth year.

According to Roux, von Beneden, Lannelongue, and von Bramann, dermoids are probably formed by a folding in of the ectoderm after the manner of formation of the crystalline lens, and their origin must be referred to a very early embryological period. The fact that they occur almost without exception on the head, face, and neck can be explained by the different relation the amnion bears to the head and to the rest of the body.

Dermoid cysts of the soft parts of the skull are always congenital. They may, however, be so small at the time of birth as to escape notice. They occur almost without exception singly and present a prominent hemispherical form. The skin covering them is unaltered and movable. They are found not beneath the skin merely, but also deep down below the aponeurosis and occipitofrontalis muscle, generally in saucer-shaped depression of bone, the latter not being the result of atrophy following pressure, but due to lack of development of bone owing to the intimate attachment between pericranium and cyst. The connection between the latter and the periosteum is so close at times that portions of it must be dissected away in removing a dermoid cyst. The growth of bone may be so much interfered with by the influence of a dermoid cyst that at the bottom of the hollow in which it is placed bone may be entirely absent and the dura mater be directly exposed.

Diagnosis.—Dermoids are distinguished from other cystic and solid tumors of the head not alone by their deep situation, but also by their constant location. They are found in the neighborhood of the anterior fontanelle, the posterior fontanelle, and over the mastoid process, but most frequently at the outer edge of the supraorbital margin and the neighboring temporal region, further at the inner angle of the eye, over the glabella and the root of the nose. This typical location of these growths is the result of the folding in of ectoderm during foetal life, as explained above. The dermal inclusions correspond with the points of union of their respective embryonal clefts. In adult life dermoid cysts may not be found exactly over the lines of union, as such cysts in the course of bone development being adherent to bone and periosteum, recede from their original site more and more away from the margin of the cleft. Dermoids of the orbital ridge and intraorbital dermoids are especially interesting on account of their relations to the bone. It is very probable that they have some etiological connection with the formation of the primitive crystalline lens through a folding in of ectoderm, just as the dermoids of the ear arise through a closure of the primitive labyrinth. It occasionally happens that one portion of a dermoid is placed within the orbital cavity, deep in the retrobulbar tissue, while the other is found in the temporal fossa. Both divisions are connected by a middle portion or isthmus, traversing a defect in the outer orbital wall (twin-sac dermoid).

The origin of dermoids through the inclusion of portions of epidermis is corroborated by the histological structure of these cysts. The wall is generally considerably thicker than that of sebaceous cysts, and consists of tissue having the character of normal skin and possessing papillæ, hair-follicles, and hairs, even sebaceous and sweat-glands. After washing out the contents, superficial examination will disclose this cutaneous lining as a continuous layer of whitish appearance. In most cases this lining exists throughout the entire extent of the cyst-cavity, more rarely only in part, as according to König the covering portion may be broken down and defective, and skin, hair-follicles, and sebaceous glands are absent. In their place a very soft connective tissue is found, characterized by a close meshwork, in which large polynuclear giant cells are embedded. This may be recognized as a circular brown spot. The contents of dermoids are very much like those of sebaceous cysts, but occasionally may be of an oily character, as noted in a case each by Reinhold and Le Dentu. The contents may be mixed with blood or blood-pigments as a result of hemorrhage into the cavity of a cyst, and then appears of a brown or maroon color. Finally, the contents may be serous or watery, which has at times led to a dermoid cyst being mistaken for meningocele, especially where there was absence of bone under the dermoid, and the pulsations of the brain were transmitted to it. This mistake may also be made when the edges of the bony depression in which it is lodged are very sharply defined, or the bony ridge surrounding the base of the tumor feels like a hernial opening. The differential diagnosis of dermoid and cephalocele will be taken up more fully in the section bearing on the description of the latter. The most important point in the diagnosis of the first is their constant occurrence in certain localities, as cephalocele never occurs over the anterior fontanelle or mastoid process. There might be a possibility of confusion in the case of a dermoid of the inner angle of the eye or glabella. Dermoids of the scalp are liable to the same secondary changes as sebaceous cysts, with this difference, that inflammation and suppuration take place only as the result of some injury opening the cyst and giving entrance thereby to pyogenic cocci and their further cultivation. Pressure does not bring about a diminution in size in every case of cephalocele; at the same time, however, this phenomenon is naturally never observed in dermoids, nor are cerebral symptoms excited by this compression. Orbital dermoids present more difficulties in diagnosis than do dermoids of the anterior fontanelle, sagittal suture, or mastoid process. The exophthalmos produced by them may be the result of other orbital tumors.

Treatment.—In children there is no question about the positive indications for removal of dermoids, as the bone beneath the tumor cannot attain its normal thickness and firmness as long as such an interference with its development and growth is present. Should the dura be exposed in the course of dissection, care must be exercised not to open it; the sac of the cyst can usually be separated without any difficulty. The enucleation of orbital dermoids requires osteoplastic section of the outer wall of the orbit, which should include the entire outer edge (zygomatic process of the frontal bone, frontal process of the malar bone, and those portions of the outer wall lying between this margin and the orbital fissure). The bone incisions should be made with a chisel and planned in such a manner as not to destroy the natural attachment of the bone fragment with the temporal fascia, the fibres of the temporal muscle, and the skin covering them. The flap of bone having been cut out by the chisel and loosened is turned outward, together with the flap consisting of muscle, fascia, and skin of the temporal region, thereby giving access to the lateral portion of the orbital cavity.

Carcinoma.—Carcinoma of the soft parts covering the skull can proceed only from the epithelium of the skin and the epithelial cells of the hair-follicles and sebaceous glands. In this region, as in every other, may be distinguished flat or superficial, deeply growing, and fungus-like or papillomatous forms. The flat forms are found most frequently in the temporal region. Those cases of nodules growing deeply and beneath the surface are usually found in the occipital region. All of them, and the papillomatous forms in particular, have little tendency to reach as far as the bone, or invade it and spread through it. In regard to their frequency of occurrence, the author has observed in 675 cases of skin carcinoma (epithelioma) 36 in the temporal region (temple, forehead, and ear)—that is, about 5.3 per cent. Almost all attacked old people; in one case only the subject was an eighteen-year-old girl.

The flat or superficial form of carcinoma is characterized by slow growth, especially in the beginning of its existence. After considerable time a stage of rapid proliferation is reached, extending over the surface and to the deeper tissues, and in such cases a change into the deeply penetrating nodular form has been observed. A peculiar form of carcinoma is found especially in the temporal region ("lupus-like carcinoma, *das Lupus ähnliche Carcinoma*"). It begins in the form of small nodules whose surface scales off and becomes shrivelled up. Surrounding these fresh eruptions occur, while at the same time the part first affected becomes changed to a smooth, glistening, hairless scar. In this manner it proceeds, the small nodules uniting to form a wall, serpiginous in outline, or curved, with the convexity outward, from the temple to the hairy scalp and forehead, posteriorly toward the ear and down over the cheek, while the central scar follows close behind, growing continually larger. Only the low surrounding wall, which indicates by its notched edge the origin from separate tubercles, shows the microscopical character of carcinoma—small collection of epithelial cells in a framework of broad bands of connective tissue. Following the fatty degeneration of the epithelial cells the connective-tissue stroma undergoes cicatricial contraction. The central scar is destitute of hair and is without sebaceous glands. It grows very slowly.

The author had the opportunity of presenting such a case in his clinic at the time the treatment of lupus by injection with tuberculin was being developed. While the injection of tuberculin was always followed by some reaction in the way of inflammatory symptoms in the case of a skin area affected by lupus, in this case the largest doses gave not the slightest result. There was no trace of a reaction; neither the central scar nor the growing peripheral portions of the affected temporal region showed any reddening.

During the last few years the question regarding the relations between carcinoma and adenoma of the sebaceous glands has arisen with respect to these new growths in the scalp. Adenoma of the sebaceous glands usually follows a preceding circumscribed seborrhœa of the skin of long standing. The area affected is covered with crusts of horny epithelium, which peel off or are washed off, leaving a somewhat thickened skin slightly reddened or bleeding slightly here and there. Sometimes adenoma of the sebaceous glands follows this obstinate condition; but again the immediate consequence may be a carcinoma. If the surface becomes ulcerated, the appearance is so like that of an ulcerating epithelioma that only microscopical examination of large and extensive sections can determine their true character. During the last two years five or six cases of adenoma of the sebaceous glands of the head and face have been so determined by such examination at the author's polyclinic. These were non-ulcerating, however.

The multiple occurrence of these cases of adenoma would lead one to suspect that he is not dealing with carcinoma, for the author has shown a case in which two ulcerating adenomata were situated side by side on the forehead and at the same time there was one on the cheek of the patient.

Three cases from the clinic of the author were recognized by Nasse as epithelial growths. They were spherical or lobulated, generally hard, and in each case covered with unaltered skin. Although they were multiple and in their course appeared for some time to be of a harmless character, they showed an alveolar framework of connective tissue, the spaces of which were filled with cells of epidermal type and numerous horny concretions or epithelial pearls. They appear similar to the calcareous endotheliomata described by Perthes, which are found very frequently on the head. They are also very much like Lejar's "polymorphous epithelioma" (*polymorphes epitheliom*). A rare case, reported by Nasse, in which there was no capsule, while the neighboring hair-follicles showed an irregularity of structure—a sign of transition into epithelioma —is closely related to one observed by Poncet in which similar but ulcerating growths (épitheliomes alvéolaires avec envahissement myxomateux) of thirty-two years' duration had developed from sebaceous glands. In several cases, after existing for years and decades, these adenomata have been positively known to undergo a carcinomatous change (Shattock).

The development of carcinoma in existing sebaceous cysts has been mentioned in the clinical description of the latter. Either the easily recognized new growth springs up in the cleft of an ulcerating or sup-

growing sebaceous cyst, or on the inner wall of the closed cyst appear soft branching papillomata, which break through the cyst-wall and appear on the surface as papillomatous carcinoma. The inner surface of these dermoid cysts has been known to produce cauliflower malignant growths, but true carcinoma was not observed until Wolff reported such a case. This carcinoma of the wall of the cyst arose from the deepest layers of the rete Malpighii, and was similar to the superficial adeno-epithelioma described by Krompecher. The development of carcinoma has been observed to take place in the cicatrix of lupus or the ulcerating nodule of lupus in the temporal region.

Melanocarcinoma (pigment carcinome) occurs less frequently on the scalp than does melanosarcoma.

Skin carcinoma (epithelioma) may spread extensively over the surface or penetrate to considerable depth. The nearest lymph-nodes to be affected are those of the retromaxillary fossa, the posterior auricular and lateral cervical regions.

Treatment.—The treatment of carcinoma consists in thorough removal by dissection. As long as the malignant new growth is movable with the skin, only the soft parts need be involved in the excision. As, however, they frequently invade periosteum and bone before coming under the observation of a surgeon, their removal often requires quite extensive resection of cranial bones. It has been demonstrated that quite extensive losses of continuity of the cranial bones can be borne without injury. At the present day surgeons are enabled to close such extensive defects of the skull with bone by means of the König-Müller method. The plastic operation may be performed immediately; or, in case the primary operation has exhausted the patient, may be deferred until some time after the extirpation of the growth. In the frontal and occipital regions we need have no fear of going beyond the dura and removing portions of the cerebral cortex.

INFLAMMATIONS OF THE COVERINGS OF THE SKULL.

Erysipelas.—The etiology and clinical features of erysipelas on the scalp are the same as in all other parts of the body. It is always a disease caused by wound infection, and is dependent on the cultivation and propagation of Streptococcus erysipelatis in the lymph-spaces of the skin. It has been shown by observation and experiment that erysipelas may be produced in the human being by cutaneous inoculation with strepto-cocci cultivated from deep-seated collections of pus. This fact explains why erysipelas may follow an existing purulent inflammation caused by streptococci. In every case in which such cocci are found in connection with any purulent inflammation of a wound on the head there is danger of erysipelas setting in. Besides the location and manner of infection, the virulence of the invading streptococci determines how far the disease will spread in the skin and subcutaneous tissue. It is remarkable how variable may be the degree of virulence. Considering the fact that the bacteriological flora of the scalp include this streptococcus, w

see how important thorough disinfection of the scalp is in
erysipelas and abscess of the scalp, so much dreaded former
    Erysipelas either originates in the scalp or extends to it fro
or neck. Occasionally it arises from the external auditory
cases in which a streptococcus angina has travelled through t
chian) tube to the middle ear. Whenever erysipelas occurs
on the scalp, it is usually in connection with virulently infect
purating wounds. Notwithstanding this, its early appearan
overlooked, as erysipelas of the scalp compared with that of
of a very pale rose color. One should look for the doughy
the neighborhood of the wound, which is usually well mar
sharply defined red border is first recognized about the for
ears, which are always markedly swollen. The discovery of s
beneath the scales of epidermis and in the hair-follicles of a
explains the occurrence of erysipelas in connection with
wounds, especially small scratches. The formation of bleb
usually occur on the head, while it is the rule on the forehead
of ear. Erysipelas runs a shorter average course on the head t
on the trunk and extremities, generally from seven to nine c
extension of erysipelas usually stops at the hair-line of the nec
is not the case with respect to the face. It occurs, how
frequently here than anywhere else. Von Bardeleben has calc
there are 20 cases of erysipelas of the head to 1 in other parts o
He includes in the above enumeration erysipelas of the face.
    The temperature in erysipelas of the scalp is constantly high
ing for the delirium, semistupor, and the muscular twitching
referred to a complicating meningitis. Meningitis in conne
erysipelas of the scalp occurs only through a streptococcus pu
which extends to the cranial cavity through the site of a frac
means of an osteomyelitis traversing the bone, or also by an
of a thrombosis of the cutaneous veins through the emissa
longitudinal sinus.
    As sequelæ abscesses of the scalp have been frequently obs

the absence of any other direct specific therapeutic measure Landouzy recommends the injection of antistreptococcus serum.

Phlegmons.—Phlegmons of the scalp may be either circumscribed or diffuse. The circumscribed form, as furuncle and carbuncle, is always caused by a staphylococcus infection, and occurs commonly in the region of the back of the neck, but may extend to the occiput. The diffuse phlegmons (cellulitis purulenta), on the other hand, are generally caused by a streptococcus infection rather than by one with staphylococci. They extend over some surface in the connective-tissue layers of the scalp, very often in combination with an erysipelas of the skin. As they lie above and below the aponeurosis, they cause the destruction of the latter, and in the later stages of the process large shreds of necrotic tissue can be pulled out. Total destruction of the connective tissue exposes the bone and leads to its superficial necrosis, if not to a more extensive and deep destruction. Besides occurring after wounds of the scalp, abscesses may develop in connection with osteomyelitis of the cranial bones, also as the result of extension of an abscess in the pterygopalatine fossa and the parotid region to the temple. The danger of these abscesses lies in their extension to the covering of the brain, and the extension of thrombosis to the venous sinuses of the dura mater. The destruction of thrombi and the subsequent emboli bring about a fatal condition of pyæmia. The tension under which the products of inflammation exist in the soft tissues of the scalp accounts for the tendency to spread to the deeper tissues. Abscesses following punctured wounds are considered very serious, as they occur first beneath the aponeurosis and are subjected to considerable pressure by the stretched membrane. The increasing swelling in the neighborhood of such slight wounds, the induration, temperature, the pains extending throughout the head, and the beginning enlargement of the post-auricular lymph-nodes and those of the occipital region, all call attention to the disease at its onset.

Treatment.—It is important to recognize this onset, as we can accomplish much in the treatment of these abscesses by early, extensive, and deep incisions through aponeurosis and periosteum to the bone. Fortunately the aseptic and antiseptic method of treating recent wounds allows little opportunity to test the efficiency of these incisions. We do not inject or irrigate with corrosive sublimate or carbolic acid solutions in these incisions, but simply keep them open by laying in iodoform gauze or drainage-tubes. While Landouzy is loud in praising the efficiency of antistreptococcus serum in all cases of abscess, Petruschky acknowledges that it has had no effect whatever.

On the head, as everywhere else, incisions should be so planned as to secure the best drainage, while the further treatment should aim to bring about the same result by means of absorbing dressings. Packing the wound-cavity with absorbent sterile gauze is only necessary as long as there is liability to hemorrhage. After the first dressing strips of gauze or rubber drains should be laid in the wound for the purpose of keeping its edges apart and to insure complete evacuation of pus.

CHAPTER IV.

INJURIES OF THE BONES OF THE SKULL.

FRACTURES OF THE SKULL.

Occurrence.—According to Gurlt's statistics of the relative frequency of fractures, 757, or 1.45 per cent., of 51,938 cases of fracture treated at the London Hospital were fractures of the skull; this includes the cases that were received into the hospital and those treated as out-patients. In the tabulated calculations of v. Bruns there were 292 out of 8560 fractures, or 3.4 per cent.; these tables were taken from reports of several hospitals. Recently, Chudovsky compared the above figures with those he had taken from observation on 2366 cases of fracture, from the second surgical clinic of Buda-Pesth, in which 90 were fractures of the skull, or 3.8 per cent. Sixty per cent. of all fractures of the skull occur between the ages of twenty and forty years, and nine times more frequently in men than in women. Fifty per cent. of the cases were caused by falls, 35.5 per cent. by blows or kicks, and 9.2 per cent. by being run over; 52.2 per cent. were fractures of the vault of the cranium, and 47.7 per cent. fractures of the base. Fractures of the vault were simple in 32.6 per cent. and compound in 67.3 per cent. of the cases. The fractures of the vault were located in the frontal bone in 44 per cent., in the parietal in 40 per cent., in the temporal in 40 per cent., and in the occipital bone in 2 per cent.

In war records the relative frequency of fractures of the skull as compared with those of the rest of the body differs from the above figures. Of course, those cases of dead and wounded in which the location of the injury is not reported should be excluded. All information regarding the wounded during the Franco-Prussian War of 1870 and 1871 shows the great danger in gunshot-wounds of the skull; fully one-half of those left on the field were head injuries.

According to Table III., vol. iii., sec. 1, p. 3, *Sanitary Reports of the German Army,* during the war against France, 1870-'71, 12.7 out of 100 wounded in the hospitals had been struck in the head. The wounds of the head exceed those of the back and chest (11.2 out of 100), and still more those of the neck (1.6 out of 100). Of 10,013 Germans wounded, there are exact accounts of 6011; 64.6 per cent. had received injuries of the skull and 35.4 per cent. injuries of the face. Of the former, 2090 were put down as injuries of the soft parts, and 993 as gunshot-wounds of the bones, with accurate description of the injury. Here also the frontal bone had been most frequently injured.

Prognosis.—Considering at this point the prognosis of injuries of the skull in war and in civil life, it must be borne in mind, above all else,

that fractures of the skull as such have no peculiar or special significance
in themselves, and that they are of importance only on account of their
relation to the brain. The prognosis depends very little on the
extent at the time, but entirely on their relation to the brain, the complicating injuries to its substance and vessels, and the disturbance in its
circulation, and some such complicating injury takes place in about 46
per cent. of the fractures of the vault and 64 per cent. of the fractures
of the base.

Beneath the vault are portions of brain injury of which can be borne
without marked disturbance of function, while at the base are situated
the medulla, the crura, and the pons. This would explain the difference
in mortality-rate; but further than this, it may be assumed that a more
general deformity of the skull as a whole is produced in connection with
fracture of the base, while in fractures of the vault the inflicting violence
is limited more to the site of injury. The mortality-rate of gunshot fractures in the Franco-Prussian War was 51.3 per cent., while in six wars
during the second half of the last century the rate was 60.2 per cent.

Forms.—The different forms under which solution of continuity of
the cranial bones takes place may be arranged in the following order:

1. FISSURED FRACTURES traverse the bone, as their name would indicate, in the form of linear cracks or splits. They occur as the result of a
bursting or bending of the skull, and will be discussed at greater length
in the chapter on the Mechanism of Fractures of the Skull. They generally involve all three layers of the cranial bones, seldom only one table.
The large majority of them do not gape through any great part of their
extent; at the same time it is not rare for the edges to be separated a
little and not in actual contact, but as they are sharply defined and
smooth and opposite to one another without deformity or displacement,
they may be classed as fissures in the strict sense of the word. At times
fissures may be so fine that they are not noticeable on autopsy after
stripping off periosteum, and are only discovered after maceration of the
bone. Fissures are single or multiple; they may be simple or forked, or
dividing into many branches. Sometimes their branches after diverging
for some time become joined again, circumscribing larger or smaller
areas of the base or vault. They may be long or short, straight or curved,
limited to one bone or running through many. Only rarely are they
confined to the lines of suture, but generally continue across them. A
fissure reaching a suture, either by changing its direction or not, may
follow the course of the same, tearing it open, and, having continued
thus for some time, diverge again and start off in another direction.
Fissured fractures may occur alone or in combination with penetrating,
gunshot, or lacerated wounds with splintered, comminuted fractures, or
fractures with fragments and loss of substance. In such cases it is very
characteristic of them to run in curves or closed circles surrounding a
defect or depressed area of fracture.

2. FRAGMENTED, COMMINUTED, AND SPLINTERED FRACTURES (French:
comminutivæ, assulares).—In fragmented fractures there is only one
line of fracture which encircles an area of skull in a curve, or an angular

broken line cutting off its connection with the rest of the skull. They represent the fractures by bending. In splintered or comminuted fractures a greater or less portion of the skull has been broken into a large or small number of pieces. The splinters of bone may be entirely detached or they may still have more or less connection with the neighboring bones and soft parts. Both forms differ very much according to whether they are limited to a comparatively small area of the skull or whether they involve a large portion or even the entire vault and base. The comminuted portion of the fracture consists either of irregular splinters, needles, disks, or wedges. At other times the fragments present more regularity of outline, radiating from a central point, in which case the term *stellate fracture* is applied.

As the distinction in degree and extent of a fracture of the vault is of significance in the prognosis and therapeutics, so also a distinction according to the displacement of the fragments is to be made, especially the depression into the cavity of the skull. and against the dura, on account of the relations to the skull contents. We distinguish between fractures *with* and fractures *without depression*. The entire fragment circumscribed by the line of fracture may be depressed (*peripheral depression*) or the periphery remains attached and in place while the remaining portion slopes gradually toward the centre, which is the deepest part of the depression, like a funnel (*central depression*). (Fig. 10.) In this case the external table of the depressed centre is usually fissured, while the inner table, still more depressed, is always more extensively separated. The accompanying illustration (Fig. 11) is taken from the case of a man who apparently fell, striking his head on a pointed stone, and died two weeks later. The encircling crack (a) involves only the outer table, as the illustration showing the inner table (Fig. 12) clearly indicates. The form thus figured is characteristic of fractures produced by striking against an angular object, by pitchers and tankards thrown at the heads of fellow-drinkers, also by hammer blows.

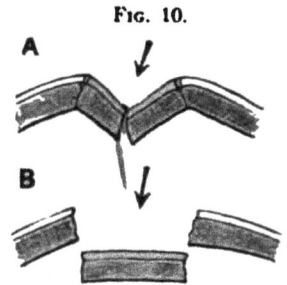

FIG. 10.

A

B

A. Central depression. B. Peripheral depression.

In other cases the depressed disk of bone is either broken into many fragments or only slightly cracked. In the latter class it frequently happens that only the centre of the depressed fragment is entirely broken through, while the peripheral portion is bent, though still attached, so that the broken portions of bone hang down into the cranial cavity like a trap-door. Viewed from within, the penetrating projection looks either like the ridge of a sloping roof or a many-sided pyramid. At times the edges of the fractured surfaces are in such close apposition that even after maceration, if the skull be filled with water, it trickles very slowly through the site of fracture. It is obvious that depressions of this character, by virtue of such firm fixation and apposition, offer the best chances for restoring broken and lacerated channels of nutrition. The same holds good for all gutter-shaped depressions, and even cup-shaped ones if they

FIG. 11.

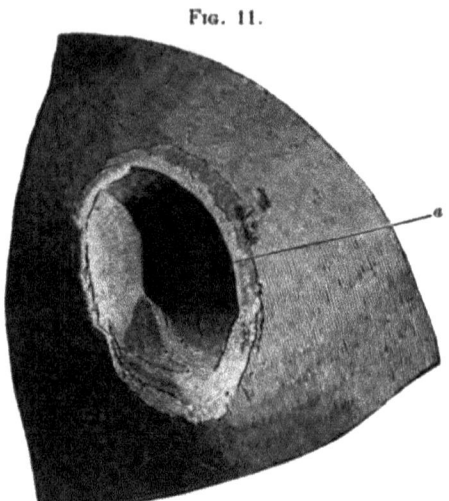

Fracture of the outer table of the skull.

be not deep. On the other hand, the conditions for nutrition are much less favorable in that class of fractures in which the depressed portion of

FIG. 12.

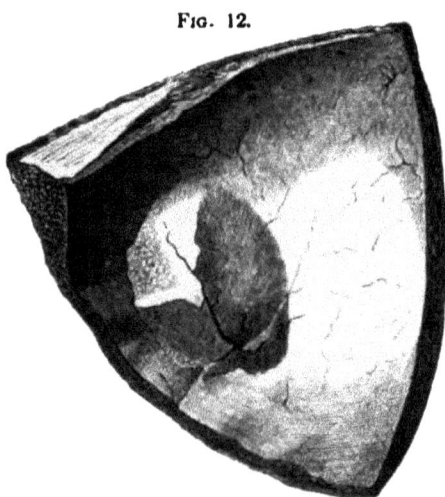

The same fracture seen from within.

bone is broken into many fragments of greater or less size. The number of these is greater than one would expect when, as is quite commonly the case, the individual splinters are themselves broken transversely. They are usually pushed over one another or under the adjacent edge of fracture, between bone and dura, or displaced laterally. They may penetrate the dura in a perpendicular direction, and become embedded in it and in the brain. If they have sharp edges or are pointed, they are capable of penetrating deeply and becoming firmly wedged. On account of this danger to the brain membranes and to the brain itself these localized fractures with shattering into sharp lamellæ and needles are of more serious import than simple depressed fractures of the same locality and size. The important point is that all fractures with distinct and circumscribed areas of depression are strictly and definitely limited. It will be shown below that these depressed fractures are caused through violence by blunt objects, but that this is of such a character as to be limited to the site of injury.

3. PERFORATED FRACTURES AND FRACTURES WITH LOSS OF SUBSTANCE.—To this class belong, first, perforating gunshot-wounds of the skull; further, fractures caused by penetrating hooks or falling spikes and bolts. The outline of the perforation in gunshot-wounds depends so much on the manner of occurrence that the forms and mechanism of gunshot-wounds will be discussed under another heading. Extensive losses of substances are produced by glancing fragments of shells. In comminuted fractures in which the skull is broken into many pieces, some of the fragments may become entirely loosened, and according to the direction of the blows be knocked out entirely, leaving extensive openings in the vault of the skull.

The different forms of fractures involve either both tables to the same extent, the inner table more than the outer table, as is usually the case, or finally only one table. Under the latter circumstances it may be either the outer or the inner table. Fracture of the "vitreous" (inner) table alone is not so rare as formerly supposed.

The greater involvement of the inner table occurs in fissured as well as splintered fractures, but in the latter rather more frequently than in the former. The fissures and cracks of the internal table may often be more extensive and more complex than those of the external. Very often they traverse the skull in an oblique direction, in which case the fissures do not always correspond on both surfaces.

In connection with these cases may be mentioned those so-called *isolated fractures of the vitreous* or *inner table*. Either there is only an involvement of the inner table so that the outer table remains absolutely intact, or the outer table is just superficially injured, appears slightly dented, or shows a fine, hair-like fissure. The inner table is generally splintered into many separate fragments, and depressed into the cavity of the cranium in the shape of a cone, only very rarely it may be divided by a single, simple crack.

Solution of continuity of the outer table alone is described by surgeons as occurring frequently. The author is in possession of the skullcap of an officer wounded at Plewna, in which a large portion of the external table had been pried off by a bayonet-thrust. It is a fact that gunshot-wounds diagnosticated as simple injuries of the external table offer a comparatively favorable prognosis. In the German military hospitals during 1870-'71, of 226 gunshot injuries assumed to be of the outer table alone, occurring both in Germans and French, only 23 cases were definitely reported as fatal. The excellent results do not prove by any means that the injury was really limited to the external table. In the case of the external table alone being depressed there may be very limited denting in, perhaps only a few millimetres deep. If the depression has a circumference greater than a finger-nail, or if it has a circumference about the size of a mark piece, as in the case in a depression following a blow by a hammer, one can be sure of finding a fracture of both tables, and as a matter of fact the inner table more extensively broken than the outer. The assumption that projectiles striking in a tangential direction tear away only the outer table is rarely if at all applicable to modern small firearms. When the projectile of the latter strikes the skull in the above-mentioned direction, it seldom produces simple contusions, but much oftener fracture of the inner table or of both tables. The lateral action of these projectiles is considerable, and involves the whole thickness of the skull in all cases in which there is actual tearing away of bone-substance. Where the diploë exist in more massive layers, as in the mastoid process, the external angular process of the frontal bone, and possibly also the external occipital protuberance, of which 23 cases bear evidence, reported by v. Beck in the war of 1870-'71, the rule does not hold good.

The Mechanical Processes Involved in Fracture of the Skull.—Two things determine the elasticity and rigidity of the skull: the character of the material (the bony tissues entering into its construction) and its shape. The elasticity of the bony tissues is that quality by virtue of which these tissues resume their original form when distorted by stress and strain. This quality has been carefully determined by Rauber, as well as the rigidity of the bony tissues. Considering in the usual way as the modulus of elasticity the weight which would elongate a body of a transverse section equal to a given unit to double, or compress it to half of its own length within the limits of its elasticity, then the modulus of rigidity is the force which would break a body of a transverse section equal to a given unit—that is, either tear it apart by traction or crack it by pressure. Bone, like ivory, is very elastic, and has a modulus of elasticity of 1800 to 2000 compared to that of bronze or brass, which is 6900 or 6400. The tensile strength of bone is less than its resistance to pressure in about the ratio of 9 to 12.

The determination of the elasticity of the skull as a whole, a spherical body constructed of elastic material, is still more important. One can convince one's self of this elastic quality by allowing a skull to fall on an inelastic floor; it does not remain at rest, but makes several bounds like a ball or ivory sphere: an inelastic body would remain motionless after being thrown.

The distortion produced by violence caused by a broad smooth surface is not limited to a circumscribed portion, but produces a change in form of the entire skull. If in falling the summit of the skull strikes, or the same is struck by a blow from a broad surface, the vertical diameter is shortened, while at the same time the occipitofrontal and biparietal diameters are increased. The particles of the skull in the direction of the increased diameters are drawn apart, and those in the diminished diameters are pressed together until at last the skull breaks or, more properly speaking, bursts.

As the skull is elastic, the lines of fracture must gape when the skull is burst or fractured, but as soon as the violence ceases to act they return to their original position and become closed. This explains how orbital fat is caught in fissures of the orbital roof, also dura mater; even the basilar artery may be included in clefts of bone, and especially hairs, which may be so tightly fastened as to persist in the dried skull. Neudörfer found in the skull of a wounded hussar, beneath a fissure as fine as a hair, a piece of felt hat that had been caught in the skull. An important point in regard to the opening and shutting of fractured and depressed fragments of skull is the fact that even large pieces of projectiles may penetrate without the aperture through which they entered the skull being visible. The author is in possession of a very instructive specimen of this kind. The external surface of the skull shows a moderate gouging out of the external table, but not the slightest opening is visible even when the macerated skull is held up to the light, and the site of injury illuminated, and yet it was penetrated by a fragment of a bullet almost half the size of a Snider projectile, for the latter was embedded in the medulla of the hemisphere.

V. Wahl, considering the elasticity of the skull, has divided all fractures of the skull into two fundamental forms: bending and bursting fractures. Under these and their combinations with each other all fractures of the vault and base may be classed, even such different varieties as fissure, comminuted and perforating fractures. The mechanism of bending fractures is more clearly carried out in those fractures produced by injuries with objects and instruments of relatively small surface, while that of bursting fractures in those produced by violence caused by extensive surfaces.

Since v. Bruns' experiments it is known that whenever the skull is compressed in any given diameter there is a shortening in the direction of pressure, while the diameters of the circles perpendicular to this line of compression are increased. The form of the skull is changed in these directions by every violence whether acting on a limited and circumscribed area or more extensively. Analyzing the first case, and assuming that a bolt of from 2 cm. to 4 cm. in diameter falls and delivers a blow on the skull: immediately two forces are at work—first the entire form of the skull is changed, and then the particular locality in a special manner. According to the extent of the surface possessed by the striking body, an area of skull is flattened, then depressed and bent in. If the action be momentary, as in the case of a blow, and its force exhausted by the elasticity of the depressed portion of skull before its limit of elasticity has been reached, it rebounds to its former position and no

permanent change in form results. The bending in, however, results in
fracture when the molecules of the skull have reached a degree of separation in which the force of cohesion no longer suffices. This takes place
first in the inner table, the fracture of which alone has always attracted
the attention of surgeons. Originally the great brittleness of the inner
table (called on this account the vitreous table) was made answerable
for these fractures. Teevan first explained it correctly as being due to
the small tensile strength of the bone-tissues as compared with the resistance to pressure. The usual direction of the inflicting violence from
without inward explains why the internal table alone is broken, or why
in combination with the external table it sustains more extensive fracture.
As mentioned above, the circumscribed solution of continuity of a limited
and small area of the skull is the result of a bending in of the skull beyond
the limits of its elasticity, and must therefore always begin in the inner
table.

In attempting to break a stick by bending, it always begins to break
on the convex, stretched side, and not on the concave, compressed side;
for the resistance offered by the molecules against being torn apart is less
than that offered against compression, as Rauber has demonstrated. In
breaking a stick by bending over a knee the fracture never begins at the
point which is held in contact with the knee, but always at a point
directly opposite. In the accompanying illustration (Fig. 13), taken from

FIG. 13.

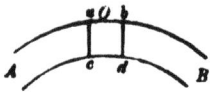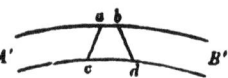

Teevan, let *A B* represent the arch of the skull, and *O* the point of impulse
of a nearly spent ball. By the impact of the same the neighboring portion
of the skull becomes flattened out, making *A' B'*. Take two parallel lines,
a c and *b d*, placed vertically on either side of the point of impact. When
the flattening *A' B'* takes place, the parallel lines *a c* and *b d* will diverge,
the points *a* and *b* will approach each other, and the points *c* and *d* will
be at a greater distance from each other. From this it follows that in
the presence of such flattening of the arch of the skull the external table
is pressed together and the internal table is stretched. Precisely as in
the case of the bent stick the fracture commences at the side of extension.
If the acting force be exhausted at this moment by the power of resistance
on the part of the cranial bones, the solution of continuity may be limited
to the inner table, and the only remaining trace of the above-described
flattening will be the isolated fracture of the vitreous table. If the usual
direction of bullets striking and penetrating the skull were in an opposite
direction, so that the inner table would be the one to receive the impact,
the outer table would be the one more seriously affected, for the reason
explained above. Teevan attempted to prove this by blows delivered

with dull instruments, against the concave surface of the skull, and besides the results obtained in his experiments was able to prove the correctness of his theory by a specimen in Guy's Hospital Museum. This specimen was the skull of a suicide who had shot himself in the right temporal region. The bullet had traversed the entire brain, reaching the inner surface of the frontal bone at a point obliquely opposite on the left side, where a discoloration by the lead showed that it had struck. The inner table was uninjured, but the outer table showed a decided cleft. A second specimen equally instructive was given to the author by Thiersch. The shot of the suicide had been directed into the mouth, penetrated the hard palate and body of the sphenoid bone, and the ball travelled to the inner surface of the posterior portion of the left parietal bone, where it lacerated the dura and remained embedded. The inner table is entirely uninjured, but the outer table is fissured. A hæmatoma had formed over the fissures beneath the pericranium. It is clear that such results contradict any assumption that the inner table is more brittle than the outer one, but is satisfactorily explained by the fact that in the process of bending in solution of continuity takes place first at the point of tension.

The funnel-shaped depressions, of which there is an illustration in Figs. 11 and 12, taken from a comminuted fracture, are the result of an injury by an object with a small surface. Only the centre of the fragment receives the force of the impact, and becomes flattened. The pressure is continued beyond the region receiving the blow. If the force of impact against the centre of the fragment does not cease, so that the fragment is pressed inward, the elasticity of the surrounding structure may produce a contraction of the base of the inverted hollow cone and prevent its springing to its former position. However, in such cases, as experience teaches, the elasticity of the bony skull is always (with an exception soon to be mentioned) carried beyond its limit and the portion pressed inward is broken to pieces. For this reason indentations of the skull are always combined with fractures and fissures. The walls of the skull are less elastic and less ductile than the skull of a hollow metal sphere, which may be deeply dented without necessarily producing fractures. At the site of a dent in the skull there are always found splits and fissures, and in the majority of cases comminution and splintering. Where a blow is delivered against the skull, the flattened or dented portion either rebounds at once to its normal shape or immediately sustains fracture. The exception referred to above occurs in the skull of the fœtus and in that of young children. V. Hoffmann decided in a case in which there was a deep, spoon-shaped depression in the skull of a newborn child that the child had been in all probability murdered by its mother. He demonstrated that not only the long-continued pressure of the sacral promontory, acting on the head of the child, wedged in the brim of the pelvis could produce such a smooth, seamless depression, but also that forcible pressure with the finger against the parietal bone of the newborn child could produce the same result and bring about a spoon-shaped depression without fissure.

The process just described of stretching and bending in of the cranial arch at the point of impact, and the resulting elastic extension of the part surrounding the indented cone, explain the formation of fissures in the neighborhood of the depressed or non-depressed comminuted fracture, and around the majority of perforated fractures. Imagine a spheroid of the skull to have two poles, according to v. Wahls' description, one pole corresponding to the point of impact, the other diametrically opposite. The meridians or horizontal circles extend through the poles, while the equatorial or vertical circles are circumscribed about the poles. Through the flattening of the skull the latter are stretched. If this stretching occurs only throughout a limited area and rapidly exceeds the limits of elasticity, the bone within the circle surrounding the pole of impact is broken from without inward, so that the depressed portion is surrounded by a fissure, as in Fig. 11. Such a fracture is called an "indented, punctured, or bending fracture." These circular fissures surrounding the point of impact are also characteristic of perforated fractures, as in Fig. 42, illustrating a penetrating gunshot-wound of the skull. In the latter it is usual to find several concentric fissures surrounding the site of perforation.

Every violence acting on the skull that is sufficiently great to make it weak, no matter how limited its surface of contact, does not merely change its shape at the site of impact and immediate surroundings, but also causes momentarily a change in form of the entire skull within the limits of its elasticity if it remained intact, and beyond this point if it breaks. A like act of violence diminishes the diameter between the two poles and lengthens the meridional circles passing through the poles. Such a blow does not merely stretch the equatorial circles circumscribed about the point of impact, but also the meridional circles passing through the point of impact by the shortening of the skull as a whole. The meridional circles are forcibly stretched from within outward, separated from one another, torn apart, and burst asunder. Fractures in the direction of these circles are called bursting fractures.

The "bending fractures" are the result of violence immediately at the site of impact. Bursting fractures are the result of change in form of the entire skull. The smaller the surface of the inflicting instrument, and at the same time the area of contact on the skull, the more probable is a bending fracture. The greater the extent of surface of the inflicting object, the more probable is a bursting fracture. By the combination of bending and bursting fractures those lines of fracture are explained that surround extensive comminuted fractures and radiate from the same in all directions or in only one. V. Bruns writes: "If the skull were equally thick and elastic in all parts, and were its form that of a true sphere, the lines of fracture could be calculated mathematically." The paths of these lines would then be entirely dependent on the size of the body inflicting the violence and its direction. But the skull does not present the shape of a regular ovoid, nor does it offer the uniform resistance of a homogeneous body. The base is not only more flat than convex, but at the temporal and frontal portions is also sharply bent in at an angle. The irregularities, fossæ, and foramina, the large cavities and small fissures, forbid the idea of considering uniform resistance possible. In addition there are thin, translucent fossæ, without diploë, and firmer edges, buttresses, and supports. The base therefore offers proportionally less resistance than does the vault. That is the reason why bursting fractures have their points of origin in the base, and are prolonged from there forward, laterally, or posteriorly, according to the meridional circle affected.

The occurrence of hursting fractures, and their combination with bending fractures, are best studied at the base. The greatest degree of tension sustained by the flattened meridian circles is at their mid-point, where they cross the equator of the sphere. At this place bursting ought to

Fig. 14.

Fig. 15.

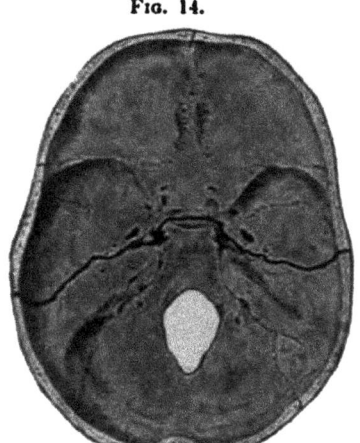
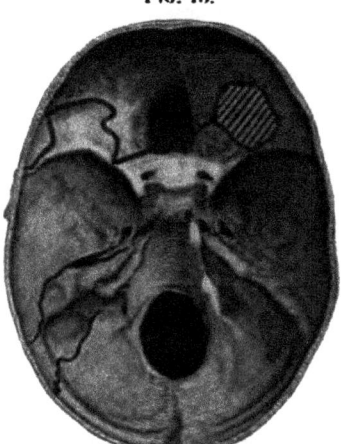

Bursting fracture.

Fracture of base from a fall down stairs; death in two hours from lesion of the cerebellum.

begin in each case; as, however, the base of the skull possesses less rigidity than its convexity, the bursting almost always takes place in the basal portion of the meridian. Whether the point of origin is placed in the middle, anteriorly, posteriorly, or laterally depends largely on the course of the flattened meridian through the base, and the relative thickness of the portions it traverses. Compression from side to side produces the greatest degree of deformity, causing the skull to burst and bringing about the results best calculated for study. This may be demonstrated by an experiment: when the skull is suspended freely, it is not broken by blows with a hammer directed against its sides, but when the skull rests on a firm support the same degree of violence produces solution of continuity. A fracture of the base, produced by pressure on both sides of the skull, connects the two poles of impact by a line running through the base—that is, in the line of a meridian intersecting the axis of pressure. The above result has been demonstrated not only in the given experiments, but also by observations in life, where the points of impact were carefully noted and the results corroborated by autopsy. The above fracture is shown in Fig. 14. It is taken from a specimen in the author's collection, and belonged to an individual who was run over. Lateral pressure is found to occur in practice most frequently in those cases in which a wagon-wheel passes over the side of the skull lying on the ground, or a large piece of wood strikes the temple of a person lying asleep on a bench or bed. Those are the cases in which symmetrical transverse fractures of the middle fossa of the skull are produced, typical bursting fractures often combined with bending fractures on that side of the skull receiving the impact.

In general two lines may be distinguished in these transverse fractures. One runs parallel with the longitudinal axis of the petrous portion of the

Fig. 16.   Fig. 17.

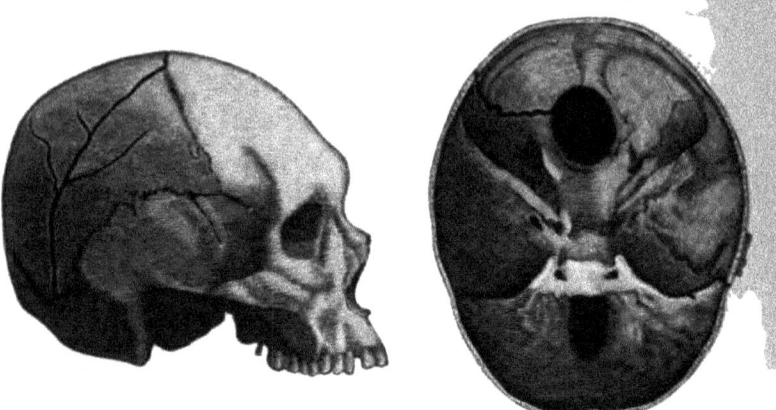

Fracture of right parietal and diastasis of coronal and lambdoidal suture.

temporal bone, the other runs farther forward in the greater wing of the sphenoid. If the line passes through the jugular process (apparently the favorite route) it remains pretty well within the pars tympanica in about the direction of the anterior inferior border of the petrous portion, the bone being very thin in the situation, or it passes a little higher, opening into the middle ear and labyrinth. In a few cases the line of fracture passes still nearer the superior border, and such are the cases in which the line traverses the porus acusticus externus. The second line of frac- ture in the middle fossa, which passes through the wings of the sphenoid, is as a rule combined with fracture of the zygomatic process or separation of its suture. At times the direction of the force exerted and the position of the skull that is struck determine the course of the fracture of the base.

In a certain sense compression of both sides of the skull takes place in falls in which the head is struck. In this case not only does the skull strike the ground, but the spinal column following after also presses on the condyloid processes of the occipital bone with the weight of the entire body and the velocity attained in rapid descent. The atlas striking vio- lently against a circumscribed area of the skull (the condyloid processes) brings about the lateral circles of a bent-in fracture. The fractures at the base brought about by impact of the spinal column are called *ring frac-tures*, for frequently the entire periphery of the foramen, against whose side force is exerted, is surrounded by a circular line of fracture in such a manner that the whole of the outlined boue-fragment is broken loose and displaced into the cranial cavity. The fracture begins symmetrically on the right and left sides, behind the condyloid process of the occipital bone, surrounds these, and proceeds on each side toward the jugular foramen, forming an arc whose concavity is directed toward the median line. From the jugular foramen the fissure proceeds to the carotid fora-men, stopping before it reaches the sella turcica, and, turning transversely, joins the fissure of the opposite side, that has followed a similar course.

Fig. 18 shows a specimen taken from the cadaver of an individual who died recently in the author's clinic. The man had fallen from a consid-

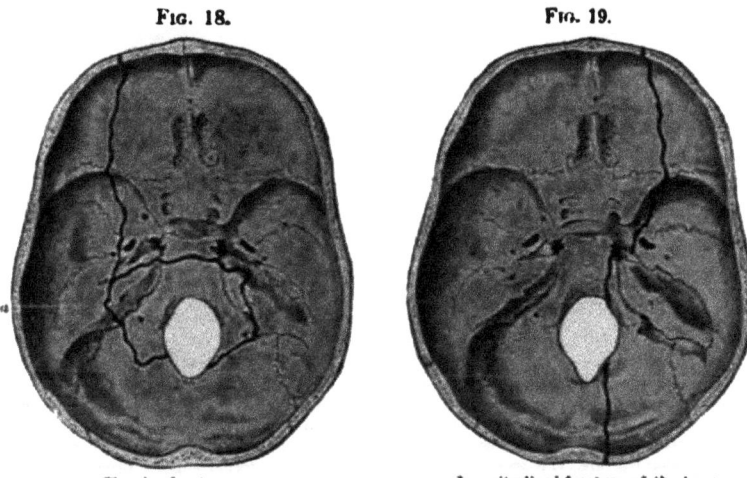

FIG. 18.　　　　　FIG. 19.

Circular fracture.　　　　Longitudinal fracture of the base.

crable height, striking on the left side in the anterior portion of the temple, as was shown by a wound of the soft parts at this site. The circular fracture began on both sides, in the posterior portion of the foramen magnum, proceeded forward and outward, around the condy-loid process, broke off the extreme tip of the petrous portion of the tem-poral bone, and broke the attachment of the latter to the basilar process of the occipital as far as the anterior lacerated foramen; from this point it is united with the fracture of the opposite side, that has followed a similar course. With the left side of this circular fracture is combined a fissure extending to the frontal bone, a bursting fracture which joins the bending fracture at *a*. By falling and striking the occiput the longi-tudinal fracture of the base illustrated in Fig. 19 was produced. Com-binations of bursting and bending fractures of the base, as well as the vault, are shown in numerous illustrations; also one of the author, illus-trated in Fig. 20.

Certain differences exist between fractures caused by pressure on two points more or less opposite to each other and those caused by pressure on only one side. These differences are probably due to certain slipping aside and yielding of the skull when it is not firmly held. While in bilateral compression the bursting begins at the mid-point of the meridian intersecting the poles of impact—that is, at some distance from the point of impact—in unilateral compression the bursting fractures begin

FIG. 20.

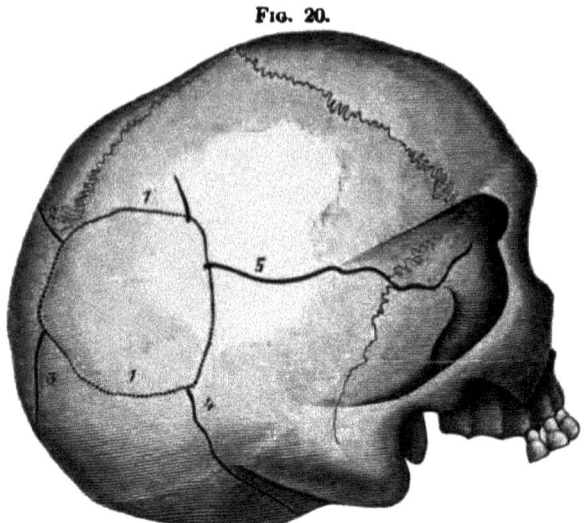

Bending and bursting fracture. Bending fracture outlined by dotted line; bursting fracture by continuous line. Fracture caused by bilateral compression; point of impact the occipital region. Poles connected by bursting fracture (1), which begins on the vault at the bending fracture and passes through the posterior fossa, then through the clivus, sella turcica, and roof of the orbit. The bursting fracture (2) passes over the left parietal to the external angular process of frontal; the fissure (3) has a short course, while (5) passes over the right parietal to the great ring of the sphenoid and ends in the sphenotemporal suture.

at the pole of impact. The fissures are widest at this point, becoming narrower toward the base and terminating in fine, often microscopical branches. While fissures of the base that are the result of bilateral compression extend through more than one fossa, when in a longitudinal direction generally through all three, those resulting from unilateral compression usually reach only as far as the middle of the base.

Knowing the direction of the acting force and the point of impact, the latter being usually indicated by the wounds and contusions of the soft parts, the surgeon is enabled to determine the course of a fissure through the base. Conversely the surgeon, judging from the course of the fissure found at autopsy, can determine the probable direction of violence and the site of impact, whether it was on the parietal, temporal, frontal, or occipital regions. If a fissure extends through all three fossæ of the skull or extends symmetrically right and left through both middle ones, the head of the deceased must have been resting on the ground or other hard surface when the compression was exerted. Ring fractures of the base indicate falling from a height.

Isolated short fractures of the base are incomplete bursting fractures. These are most frequently seen in the orbital plates, and usually on both sides at the same time, as was shown in the autopsy of President Lincoln. The author has several specimens taken from cases of gunshot fractures of the parietal and occipital regions, and considers them incomplete bursting fractures beginning at the weakest point of the base, especially when, as in his cases, the force of impact was directed against the occiput. Transverse fracture of the sella turcica may be conceived of as an incomplete ring fracture caused by the impulse of the after-coming spinal column.

Fig. 21.   Fig. 22

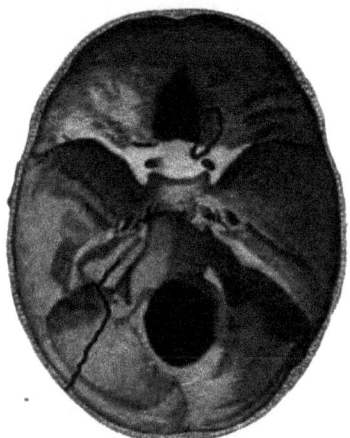 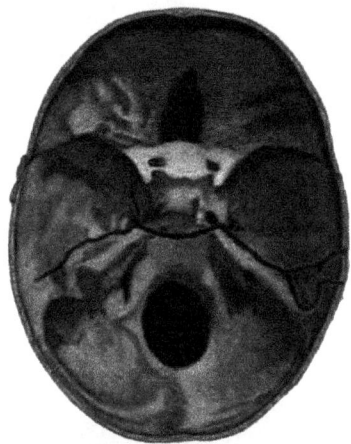

Fracture of occipital bone with small fracture of right orbital process of frontal bone from kick of horse.   Fracture of base, from fall from scaffolding. Hemorrhage from right ear and nose. Death from meningitis.

Bending fractures about a gunshot fracture are important factors in determining the direction of the projectile. This will be discussed fully when considering gunshot-wounds of the skull. The outline of the depression, the splitting of the cranial vault, the greater or less splintering of the inner table or outer table, all enable one to determine the character of the inflicting object with quite a degree of certainty. With this object in view, Paltauf made experiments on the cadaver. When caused by blows with a rounded hammer, the concentric circles about the site of impact were numerous and distinctly marked, while in those caused by an angular one the fissures extended radially at angles to one another. As a result of blows from a hammer there were extensive splitting, loosening, and breaking off of the inner table without any impression having been made on the surface. Perforated fractures that give the outline of the inflicting object may be called, according to Puppe, *moulded frac-*

tures. In determining the character of the inflicting instrument it is also necessary to examine critically the lesion of the skin, and even to observe

FIG 23.

FIG. 24.

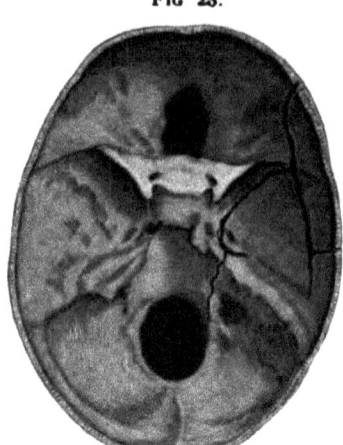
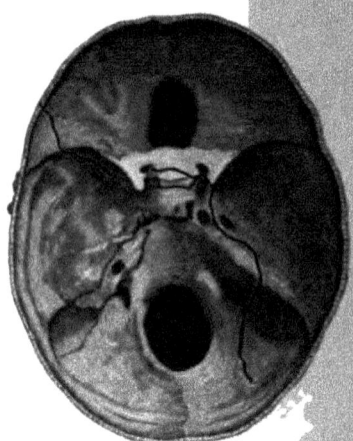

Fracture of base from blow with a boot.   Fracture of base from fall from train.
Death from meningitis.   Death from meningitis.

the hair. The course of the fissure at the base not only indicates the site of injury, but also the degree of violence. By taking into account the above relations, one can differentiate between a fall and a blow as the cause of death. This is often of great medicolegal importance.

FIG. 25.

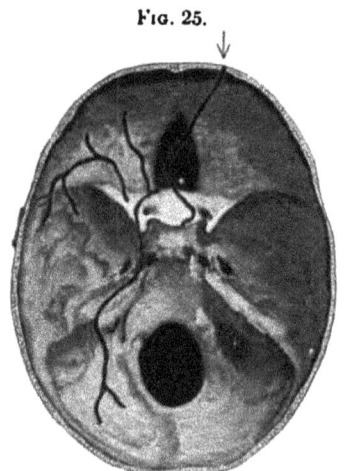

Bursting fracture. Patient slipped, striking head on a stone. Direction of force indicated by arrow.

Besides bending and bursting, expansion must be mentioned as a factor in the production of fracture of the skull, which will be discussed more fully in connection with gunshot-fractures, also the action of wedges. Bohl found on driving a chisel into a bone that the bone was split, a fissure beginning at the apex of the chisel and following the direction of its edge. As the chisel was driven in further the fissure was opened wider, and on the chisel being withdrawn the fissure snapped together again, the action being exactly the same as when the skull is split by the blows of an axe. This true wedge action is carried out when a bolt or projectile with conical head penetrates the skull or whether a blow is struck by an instrument intended for such purposes.

The short, radial fissures present in perforated fractures may be referred to this wedge action. As at the same time that these radial fissures are produced concentric bending fractures are caused surrounding the defect, the two intersect each other. The portion of the skull immediately struck by the entering wedge is finely splintered, while the surrounding portion, by the intersection of the radial and concentric lines of fracture, is broken or splits into fragments.

Diagnosis.—The diagnosis of fractures of the skull requires evidence of solution of continuity, which may be obtained directly in fracture of the vault and indirectly in fracture of the base.

Though important as regards prognosis, cerebral manifestations usually accompanying fractures are of little assistance in making a diagnosis. They are merely the results of brain lesions, and have no connection whatever with fractures themselves. It is easy to understand that knowledge regarding a fracture can be more easily obtained if it be easy of access; consequently the diagnosis is less difficult in compound than in simple fractures.

FIG. 26.   FIG. 27.

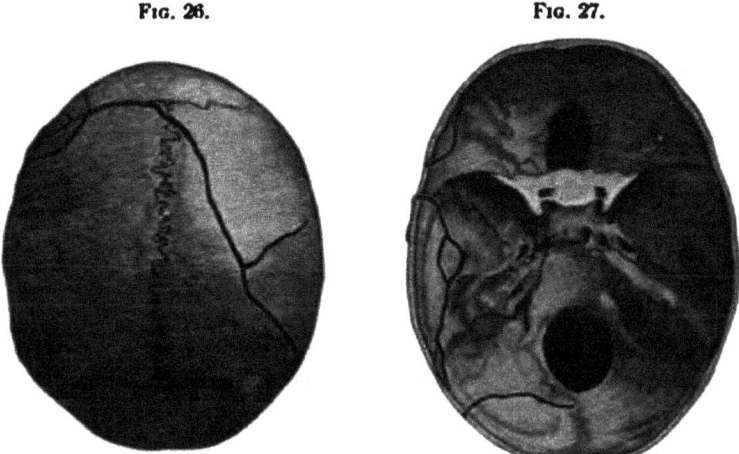

Fracture of vault and base, due to fall from window.

In *simple fractures* only palpation of the surface of the skull is of aid in discovering a fissure, the edge of a fracture, or an area of depression. By the sense of touch deformity can be appreciated only when the latter is of considerable depth and breadth; if of mild degree, it may be masked by the thickness and density of the soft parts. Detached and freely movable fragments can generally be detected on careful palpation. The more extensive the comminution of bone, the easier it can be determined.

When a depression is felt under the examining finger, it cannot be referred to recent violence unless one is satisfied that it did not exist before the injury. In this connection must be excluded: 1. Depressions produced in the course of parturition and by previous injuries. 2. Senile atrophy of the skull, which progresses from without inward, producing usually only shallow depressions, but which may occasionally bring about deep, sharply defined grooves easily felt on external manipulation. 3. The hollows found in the skull of syphilitic patients, which often present depressions beneath the scalp, due to the breaking down of gummatous ostitis. The burrowed-out hollow may appear even deeper than usual in these cases, as the central necrosis is surrounded by a reactionary hypertrophy of bone. 4. The natural prominences and irregularities that are the result of peculiar cranial development, such as an occasional higher or lower position of the apex of the occipital bone opposite the adjoining parietals. The history, the absence of injury to the soft parts, or the presence of an old scar over the supposed depression, and the occurrence of other syphilitic manifestations, also the symmetrical occurrence of involution fossæ, are all of value in preventing error.

Difficulty in examination arises frequently in connection with contusions of the soft parts which may lead to the assumption that the bone has been depressed where no fracture exists. While it rarely happens that any of the above forms of depression cause the surgeon to have any doubts, a flat hæmatoma with a hard, firm base has often led to error. The method of palpation was mentioned in the description of subcutaneous hemorrhages of the scalp, by which may be ascertained whether that portion of the skull in the centre of the hæmatoma is really deeper than the rest of the bony surface in case a depression is suspected.

Phlegmonous swelling, like extravasations, may simulate depressions. The tumor, which at first is uniform in consistence, softens when suppuration takes place, presenting a deep centre surrounded by a harder peripheral portion.

The subjective symptoms are not of much help in making the diagnosis. The patient who has been struck on the head and lost consciousness, or, at any rate, sight and hearing, is in no condition to answer questions. The half-conscious patient, by stretching his hand toward the painful spot on the skull, has little intention of hinting to the physician that this is the site of injury. The pain at the site of fracture is not more fixed than that of common bruises or wounds of the skin. It is true that in fracture of the skull the signs of concussion of the brain are rarely absent; but it is equally true that concussion of the brain is just as frequently, if not more frequently, present without fracture of the skull.

The diagnosis of subcutaneous fractures can be made with certainty only in those cases in which there is displacement toward the cranial cavity or in which fragments have been broken loose. It may happen that depressed pieces of bone are hidden beneath the temporal muscle or beneath even moderate extravasations of blood. Consequently many such fractures of the cranial vault, perhaps the majority of them, remain undiscovered. Should patients die as a result of the accompanying injuries of the brain or of some intercurrent disease, one may be surprised at discovering very extensive fractures. This is of such frequent occurrence that enumeration of cases can safely be omitted. The author is fully convinced that the apparently infrequent occurrence of fissures in the skull of children can be explained only by the mild degree of disturbance that they occasion, and by the fact that they are rapidly followed by complete recovery.

Fortunately the welfare of the patient is seldom dependent on the positive or accurate diagnosis of subcutaneous fractures. The treatment required is only that of the accompanying contusions. These therapeutic principles are the natural outcome of the present opinion regarding the relations of open and subcutaneous injuries and the former experience regarding the different course followed by simple and compound fractures. Formerly when the treatment of fractures of the skull was believed to require specific measures, the physician was obliged to do everything toward arriving at a positive diagnosis. For that reason it was considered imperative to make incisions into the soft parts and expose the bone in order to be sure that no fissure would remain undiscovered. Although A. Cooper severely criticised those surgeons who, for the sake of diagnosis, were willing to change a simple fracture into a compound, the rule of making an incision at the site of suspected fracture remained in force as long as surgeons were convinced that subcutaneous fractures of the skull demanded more or other interference than contusions of the soft parts. At the present time these ideas have been entirely dispelled, and one is satisfied to act for the welfare of the patient, no attempts at establishing the diagnosis being made. In the case of subcutaneous fracture of the skull, operative interference is necessary only on account of an accompanying lesion of the brain, and not because of the fracture itself, as will be discussed in the succeeding section.

A peculiar condition following subcutaneous fracture which has been observed only in children is the development of a more or less circumscribed swelling filled with fluid and situated beneath the scalp. It was first observed and reported by Haward; later it was described as meningocele spuria (traumatica) by Billroth, and at the present time is called cephalohydrocele traumatica. It is characterized by a slit-like ovoid or round defect of bone in the skull of children. There is at the same time a defect of the dura beneath the bone, so that the cerebrospinal fluid can flow through a sinus in the pia mater and extend beneath the scalp. The cleft in the skull does not close; the edges become sharpened and the fluctuating swelling pulsates synchronously with the cardiac beat and the movements of respiration, as do the rest of the skull contents. In all cases that have been operated upon or dissected post mortem the cyst continued on through the membranes of the brain, generally communicating with one of the lateral ventricles. On account of this relation these tumors are very interesting, for, besides violence during or just after birth, there is a second etiological factor. It seems to the author that some disturbance in the normal development of the brain must be responsible for their origin. In his opinion porocephalon may be distinguished as with or without defect of skull; among the latter class must be placed cases of meningocele spuria (traumatica).

Should fracture of the vault of the skull be suspected in connection with wounds of the soft parts, no special methods of diagnosis are required in such doubtful cases, for they should be treated as other contused wounds of the skin and aponeurosis that are not complicated by fissure of bone. The circumstances are different, however, when the site of fracture is exposed. What the finger feels may be controlled and completed by the sense of sight. It is easy to determine the presence of solution of continuity at the surface of the bone, but it is not always easy to appreciate the true nature of the fracture. Great difficulty is frequently met with in the case of hair-like fissures, as these may be mistaken for lines of sutures, a groove for a bloodvessel or an adherent hair. As far as the sutures are concerned, the knowledge of their situation and their notched borders prevent the possibility of error. It must be borne in mind, however, that before the third year the notches have not developed along the lines of suture, and that, on account of Wormian bones, sutures may develop at unusual situations. Special diagnostic manœuvres formerly much practised are not only unnecessary, but absolutely wrong. In recent cases blood oozes from a fissure, which enables one to recognize it as soon as the blood has been wiped from the surrounding surface. If, notwithstanding all this, it should remain undiscovered, it is of little importance either from the point of view of diagnosis or of treatment. Further, in making the diagnosis, the surgeon must distinguish between fractures of the outer table alone and those involving the entire thickness of bone. This question may not be definitely settled in a given case; one takes into consideration the depth of the depression and keeps in mind that as a rule the inner table is more extensively fractured than the outer table in strictly localized fractures. The chances of fracture of the outer table alone are greater in the parts of the skull in which the diploë are excessively developed, as was mentioned in a previous section.

It was formerly the custom to determine the degree of splintering of the inner table by passing fine probes or sounds through the fissures in the outer table in order to determine the mobility of the layers they encountered. This procedure is uncertain and too questionable to be imitated. The surgeon should bear in mind that the diagnosis on the living person is made only for the purpose of treatment, and that much probing is not only useless, but also may easily do much harm. The more localized the acting violence and the more limited consequently the extent of fracture, the more probable—in fact, certain—is it that the internal table is more comminuted and splintered than the appearance of the surface would indicate. If in addition there is a rather deep peripheral or central depression of comparatively small area, the internal table is undoubtedly considerably shattered and broken up. The important and relevant feature of diagnosis is therefore to determine whether in a given case there is a circumscribed fracture limited to a small area of the skull, or whether there is extensive fragmentation with far-reaching and branching fissures.

The diagnosis of isolated fractures of the inner table is absolutely uncertain. One can only assume the presence of detached fragments by their influences, for if they penetrate the central convolutions of the brain there may result monospasm and monoplegia.

For therapeutic reasons it is desirable to recognize displacements, depression, and mobility of fragments. The removal of sharp-pointed splinters may be necessary if they are directed against the brain. For that reason digital examination is indicated. The purpose of this is to determine only the gross relations at the site of fracture, as these determine the nature of the therapeutic intervention. Sufficient information can be obtained by passing the tip of the finger gently over the area of fracture. It is not necessary to incur the risk of forcing splinters in further, or stripping the dura more extensively than has taken place already by penetrating to any degree with the finger. The investigation in regard to the relation of fragments must never be carried too far. It is an error when, for the purpose of diagnosis, excessively minute accuracy is attempted.

Losses of substance within the area of fracture, as well as open clefts or detached fragments, make themselves known by the pulsating blood that collects in the wound.

The uninjured condition of the dura mater is important from the point of view of prognosis. In case of considerable loss of substance, its integrity may be determined by inspection. In other cases the prolapse of brain-substance is a positive sign of its having been injured. Flow of cerebrospinal fluid does not take place often in fractures of the vault.

The most important feature of diagnosis in fracture of the skull is the accompanying disturbance of the cranial contents, and belongs therefore to the section on the injuries of the brain and its adnexa.

The symptoms of fracture of the base are as indirect as those of the vault are direct. By the knowledge obtained in regard to the process of occurrence by the history and observation of the site of external injury, the surgeon is enabled to determine not only the presence of a fracture of the base, but its course and extent as well. The points in their diagnosis are as follows:

1. The spreading of hemorrhages from the site of fracture to certain points under the skin, where they appear as ecchymoses.

2. The flow of brain-tissue, blood, and serous fluid from those cavities immediately adjoining the base.

3. The disturbance in function of those nerves situated at the inferior surface.

Where the skin and mucous membrane are attached to the base of the skull by loose connective tissue, blood extravasations appear. The skin of the eyelids and the connective tissue of the eye, the mucous membrane lining the pharynx, the region of the mastoid process, and the sides of the neck are situations where in case of fracture of the roof of the orbit or of the middle fossa of the skull ecchymoses appear. Their appearance here is, however, positive evidence of fracture only when there is no question that the injury was inflicted at some point at a distance, and it is certain that they are not the result of contusions of the soft parts at that particular locality. Their late appearance is also characteristic, for they do not immediately follow the injury, but develop some hours or even days after, corresponding to the distance they must travel from the source of hemorrhage—i. e., the site of fracture—to the subcutaneous areolar tissue.

The so-called "black eye" is such a frequent accompaniment of persons who are exposed to violence that one must be especially warned against making a diagnosis on that one symptom alone. At the same time the appearance of ecchymoses at a certain time and at a certain place is of inestimable value when it occurs under positively fixed circumstances. It is of great practical significance that in all observations of such cases Berlin found hemorrhage from fissures and fragments in fracture of the roof of the orbit into the adipose tissue of the orbital cavity. Only the very finest fissures bleed little or not at all; all others produce hemorrhage into the orbit, as the periosteum is always torn at the same time that the bone is broken. Berlin refers to a series of autopsies the results of which were placed at his disposal by Hölder. Hölder examined the orbital fat for the presence of hemorrhage in cases of bursting fracture of the orbital roof. He found orbital hemorrhages in 69 of 79 cases, and in only 6 was there hemorrhage into the orbital fat without solution of continuity of the wall of the orbit. Taking into consideration the additional fact that blows with the fist on the eye or on the frontal region rarely produce orbital hemorrhage, it is safe to conclude the existence of fracture of the orbital roof in the presence of retrobulbar hemorrhage. The above-mentioned hemorrhage takes place in three ways: (1) extravasation of blood into the eyelids; (2) hemorrhage into the connective tissue of the eyeball; and (3) protrusion of the eyeball—exophthalmos. In regard to the first two forms, it is well to know that they occur with and without injuries of the skull. They are usually the result of contusions of the eye, blows with the fist and from other sources, or blood trickling from wounds in the neighboring regions of the face and head. In nearly every operation on the forehead both eyelids are found suffused with blood at the time of the first dressing, appearing of a purplish color or presenting the play of colors found in extravasations undergoing absorption. In order to make deductions from the effusion of blood into the conjunctiva, the site of injury must not be the eye, forehead, or the adjacent portions of the face. Even when it is known that the occiput has suffered violence it must be positively excluded that the patient did not strike his face in falling.

Similar limitations must be placed on the significance of ecchymoses of the bulbar conjunctiva and those of the eyelids. Even moderate concussion transmitted from distant portions of the body may bring about rupture of the delicate conjunctival vessels. The extravasations of blood in the sclerotic in children suffering from whooping-cough are well known. All macular extravasations of the connective tissue occurring immediately after injury are therefore without significance. If a suffusion into connective tissue is to be accepted as a sign of fracture of the orbital roof, it cannot have appeared a short time after injury, but must be delayed in its occurrence hours or even days. If the extravasating

blood originates in the orbital fat, the ecchymoses of the bulbar conjunctiva will appear before that of the lids. The outer skin and cellular tissue
of the eyelid are separated from the conjunctiva, and the areolar tissue
of the orbit by the tarso-orbital fascia, which extends from the supraorbital and infra-orbital ridges to the corresponding tarsal edges like a
thick, dense partition-wall. For that reason blood coming from the
deeper tissues collects around the bulb first and appear sooner under the
conjunctival mucous membrane than under the integument of the eyelid.
If the surgeon is able to prove that the posterior portion of the skull or
the parietal region was the region directl exposed to violence, and that
some time later the bulbar conjunctivayand subsequently the eyelids
had become suffused with blood, he may with a degree of certainty
make the diagnosis of fracture of the base, probably of the middle,
though possibly of the posterior fossa of the skull and extending to the
roof of the orbit. No matter how important, even with its limitations,
the above symptom may be, one cannot exclude fracture of the orbital
roof on account of its absence.

Exophthalmos occurring immediately or soon after violence, followed
by ecchymoses of the conjunctiva and eyelids, is an undubitable sign of
orbital hemorrhage, and, on account of the relation of the latter to fracture of the orbital roof, a sign of fracture of the base.

Ecchymoses into the mucous membrane of the pharynx are rarely
observed, not only because the region of the pharynx is not apt to be
inspected, but also probably owing to the rare occurrence of fissures in
the basilar portion of the occipital bone. The dense connective tissue
of the upper part of the nasopharynx does not favor the extension of
extravasations.

Moderate ecchymoses in the region of the mastoid process parallel with
the posterior wall of the ear and extending along the sternomastoid
muscle have been frequently observed, together with hemorrhage from
the ear. A fracture extending through the squamous portion of the
temporal bone may produce this as well as fracture of the mastoid portion. In case of fracture of the posterior fossa hemorrhage may find
its way through the thick muscles of the neck to the skin. In a few
days the easily recognized discoloration may appear under the skin of
the neck. Blood from the region of the lambdoidal suture and occipital
bone may, however, infiltrate the same region of the neck. These various
sources of origin of hemorrhage explain why this symptom can be an aid
to diagnosis only under positively determined circumstances, such as are
rarely met with. If, for example, the surgeon has made the diagnosis
of fracture of the petrous portion of the right temporal bone and finds
ecchymoses two or three days later in the region of the left mastoid
process, it is probable that there has been a fracture crossing both
middle fossæ of the skull symmetrically.

The *flow of brain-tissue* from clefts of bone produced by fracture
through the divided soft parts is a positive sign of fracture of the base
and at the same time of injury to the brain membranes. This has been
observed in the external auditory canal and the nose.

The brain-substance reaches the external auditory canal through fissures opening on its superior wall. Even small fractures at this site favor prolapse. Holmes shows in an illustration taken from a specimen this projection of the brain into the external auditory meatus through such a cleft produced by fracture. Rarefaction and thinning of the tegmen tympani, which are quite common, cause a tendency to more extensive fissuring and fracture with loss of substance.

The *flow of brain-substance from the nose* has been reported; it is very uncommon. Prolapse into the pharynx does not appear to have been observed. The reverse was seen by Hewitt, who observed the contents of the pharynx reach the interior of the cranial cavity through the cleft of a fracture.

The *hemorrhages from cavities and canals* that adjoin the base take place from the external auditory meatus, the nose, and the pharynx. Those from the external auditory meatus are the most important from the point of view of diagnosis. The petrous portion of the temporal bone is traversed by numerous canals which are torn at the time the fracture takes place, and which are the source of hemorrhage; or the latter may occur from the cerebral bloodvessels and those of the membranes and find its way out through the fissures in bone. Immediately adjoining the posterior wall of the tympanic cavity lies the transverse sinus; while the inferior wall, a thin leaf of bone perforated by a nerve and arterial canal, separates it from the internal jugular. Above the roof of the cavity lies the middle meningeal artery, and along the upper bony portion of the Eustachian tube, really a part of the tympanic cavity, runs the carotid artery. Arteries are not easily torn in connection with fractures of the petrous portion. The carotid is particularly capable of resistance, as it presents an elastic tube not adherent to the wall of the foramen through which it enters the cavity of the skull. The sinuses, however, are closely attached to the sides of the bony grooves in which they lie, and are wanting in that degree of elasticity possessed by arteries.

Hemorrhage from the ear accompanying injuries of the head may be from various sources: (1) bursting and laceration of the ear-drum; (2) fracture of the anterior wall of the external auditory meatus; (3) violent separation of the cartilaginous and bony portions of the auditory canal; (4) a fracture involving the cells of the mastoid process and the posterior wall of the auditory canal; (5) fissures and fractures of the base of the skull. In every case of hemorrhage from the ear it must be ascertained that the blood does not reach the ear from without by the result of a wound of the walls fine or external ear.

The wounds of the drum membrane and the parts contained in the tympanic cavity are numerous, but small and insignificant. Any considerable amount of hemorrhage is probably not due to rupture of the membrane (tympani) or laceration of the lining of the tympanic cavity, but to a much deeper seated lesion. If in connection with a moderate amount of hemorrhage examination with the speculum shows a rupture of the membrane, the source of blood is immediately accounted for. At the same time the amount of hemorrhage occasionally met with a rupture of the drum membrane has been more excessive than would be expected.

Fractures of the anterior wall cause considerable hemorrhage into the external auditory canal, as does also tearing off of the external ear or its displacement at the side of the head. There are cases in which a fissure originating at the summit of the skull extends to the mastoid process without involving the petrous portion, yet, nevertheless, causing considerable hemorrhage from the ear.

Not in every fracture of the petrous portion does hemorrhage find its way out through the external auditory canal. If hemorrhage originates in fissures of the roof of the anditory canal and the integument lining it is torn at the same time, the blood follows the shortest course and appears externally. The drum membrane may remain uninjured in this case, as has been shown in numerous instances. Hemorrhages from fissures involving the porus acusticus internus, the labyrinth, and the tympanic cavity appear externally as soon as the drum membrane is ruptured. In all cases the hemorrhage is characterized by its large amount, dropping continuously or flowing in a constant stream. It is usually of some duration, continuing for days, and it is difficult to control. When the blood wells up or spurts, large venous sinuses or the carotid artery itself have probably been injured. In spite of these circumstances the diagnosis of fracture of the base cannot be made on the symptom of hemorrhage alone, no matter how excessive it may be.

If the fissure be limited in its course to the middle or internal ear and the drum membrane be not ruptured, there may be entire absence of external hemorrhage. In such a case the tympanic cavity may be filled with blood which is shut in by the drum membrane. Naturally in such cases hemorrhage would reach the pharynx through the Eustachian tube and be swallowed or ejected, or the bleeding from the nose would attract attention. The flow of blood through the tube would probably take place sooner than rupture of the membrane as a result of increased pressure. In 15 of 32 cases of fracture of the middle fossa of the skull carefully investigated by Prescott Hewitt there was hemorrhage from the ear continning for some time, and in every one of them the post-mortem examination bore out the diagnosis made on the living subject. In 12 of the remaining 17 cases the fracture was limited to the tip of the petrous portion, so that the tympanic cavity escaped; in 5 cases the latter was involved without, however, producing rupture of the drum membrane.

It must be borne in mind that extravasations of blood showing through the uninjured drum membrane do not in themselves indicate the presence of fracture. They may occur independently as the sole result of shock or concussion sustained by the head in any injury. It has been more frequently demonstrated that laceration of bloodvessels can take place in this region without fracture than in the case of the orbital adipose tissue.

Hemorrhages from the nose have been undoubtedly caused in many cases by fracture of the horizontal plate of the ethmoid; in other cases the nasal hemorrhage is from the Eustachian tube, the result of fissures of the petrous portion of the temporal. Bloody expectoration and vomiting of blood is a frequent occurrence in fracture of the base. According to Prescott Hewitt's investigations, 14 of 32 patients bled from the nose or mouth. Autopsy showed fissures of the ethmoid bone in 4 cases, fracture of the body of the sphenoid in 3 cases, of the basilar portion of the occipital bone once, and fracture of both ethmoid and sphenoid 5 times.

The flow of serous fluid from the ears in cases of injury to the base of the skull is a result of and a symptom of fracture of the petrous portion. The subarachnoid spaces are the sources of this fluid. The dura and arachnoid membrane are torn in every case of fracture, thus opening up these spaces. The drum membrane must be torn in the same way that the subarachnoid space is opened up, as otherwise there would be no communication between the outer and middle ear. The fluid flows from the subarachnoid spaces through the tear in the brain membranes and the fissure in the bony wall of the inner ear, particularly the thin bony plate separating the antrum from the internal ear, enters the labyrinth and flows from this through the broken bony wall or the ruptured membrane of the foramen ovale. The middle and inner ear are more frequently involved in transverse or oblique fractures due to violence against the occiput than in longitudinal fractures. In a certain number of cases of the latter, though by no means in a large number, the external auditory canal is affected. It is of interest, therefore, that Roser observed the flow of serous fluid in a case with uninjured drum membrane, and apparently coming from the roof of the auditory canal. Von Troltsch considered it possible that in fractures of the roof of the bony auditory canal or of the tegmen tympani, with laceration of the soft parts on either side, serous fluid would flow from the ear. Luschka was opposed to this view, as he considered the subarachnoid space of the adjacent temporosphenoidal lobe too shallow. At the present time, when it has been shown that all the subarachnoid spaces communicate with one another and the flow of fluid has been observed to take place from compound fractures of the vault, in which situation the pia is just as tensely stretched, this route does not seem at all unusual.

The time at which the flow takes place is often immediately after the injury, so that a few hours later all the fluid may have trickled away. In other cases the flow from the ear takes place twenty-four hours or more after the injury. The late occurrence seems to prevail in the majority of cases. The quantity of the fluid is always considerable. In the usual position of the head resting on the injured side, it flows in rapidly succeeding drops. The flow is temporarily increased by snuffling, sneezing, coughing, and especially by vomiting. The fluid collected amounts usually to a small tablespoonful in fifteen minutes, or from 150 to 200 grams in twenty-four hours; occasionally the amount is a great deal more. The quantity is not surprising, as experiments on animals have shown that the cerebrospinal fluid is very rapidly resupplied. In addition the flow is favored by the diminished intracranial space as a result of collections of blood.

Chemical analysis shows the fluid flowing out to be identical in nature with that of the cerebrospinal fluid. It is at first colored red by being mixed with blood; later, however, it becomes entirely clear, flows like water, and is not at all mucoid in character. It is alkaline in reaction, contains only a trace of albumin, scarcely becoming cloudy on boiling. On the other hand, it is very rich in sodium chloride. If sufficient of the fluid be collected to make the boiling test and a second specimen be tested with a solution of silver nitrate, the first remaining clear, while in the second an abundant precipitate is formed, the diagnosis is certain.

When in case of fracture of the petrous portion the drum membrane remains intact and the subarachnoid space is opened up as far as the tympanic cavity, the fluid may flow through the tube into the nares. This is probably the only explanation for the rather interesting phenomenon of the fluid flowing from the nose. The first case of this kind properly explained was reported by Robert. The flow is generally observed to take place from one nostril, and is characterized by its amount and the fact that if the head be placed in a position to direct the flow from the injured side it will at once be considerably increased, or it may flow from the ear and nose at the same time. Besides coming through the tube the fluid may originate in fractures of the anterior fossa, the communication with the nasal passages being established through the cribriform plate of the ethmoid. Such cases have been reported. Anna Heer described the flow of cerebrospinal fluid in 4 out of her 58 cases, in 27 of which it took place from the ear and in 2 from the nose.

Traumatic *emphysema* in connection with fractures of the mastoid process has already been discussed. This symptom is a positive sign of such fracture, but is rarely observed.

Paralyses of single cranial nerves are produced by fracture of the base when the line of fracture traverses the canal or foramen through which the nerve emerges from the skull. Either the nerve is lacerated, or divided, or compressed, or bruised by a detached fragment. The result of this injury is immediate loss of function—that is, paralysis of the region supplied by it. The same paralysis may, however, be produced without fracture; either the nerve alone is torn against the edge of its foramen, or its central origin in the brain sustains some injury, or it is pressed upon by some exudate or extravasation within the cranial cavity, or in the bony canal through which it passes. Besides those paralyses of cranial nerves following immediately or soon after injury, there is a second form of paralysis which sets in during the course of disease and depends on an inflammation extending along the nerve-trunk. This neuritis is generally of an ascending form and not without danger, as pyogenic organisms may travel along the nerve and reach the pial membrane at the base of the brain.

The facial nerve is most frequently paralyzed. Anna Heer found paralysis of the facial nerve 10 times in 11 cases of injury to the cranial nerves out of 58 cases of fracture of the base. In 4 cases there was paralysis immediately following injuries of the head and remaining permanent. It is unquestionable that in these cases there was complete solution of continuity òr contusion of the nerves. In the remaining cases only pareses were present. Köhler observed paralysis of the facial nerve 22 times in 48 cases of fracture of the base. The character of the facial nerve paralysis and its combination with that of the aeustic and abducens nerves enable the surgeon frequently to determine the course of fracture through the petrous portion.

There are two cases to be added to the examples given of head injuries. One taken from the investigations of Anna Heer is a fracture of the base

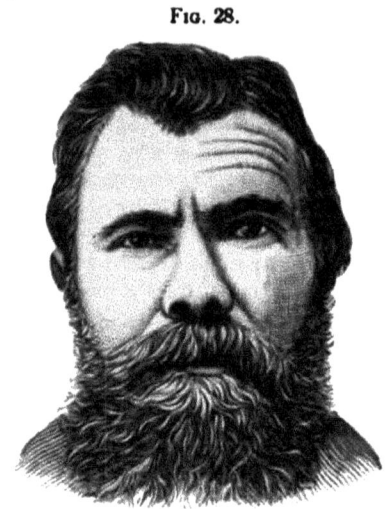

Fio. 28.

in a twenty-year-old miner. As there was paresis of the right facial nerve and absence of the sense of taste in the right half of the tongue, while the soft palate was symmetrical, the line of fracture must have crossed the facial nerve between the geniculate ganglion and the giving-off of the chorda tympani nerve. Another case is taken from L. Bruns' lecture before the neurological section of the "Naturforscherversammlung" at Cologne, 1888. In this there was paralysis of numerous cranial nerves following a fracture of the base caused by falling and striking the left side of the skull, resulting in complete evulsion of the left ear and accom-panied by hemorrhage from the right ear. On the left side there was paralysis of branches of the oculomotor nerve (ptosis and my-

Paralysis of facial nerve following fracture of base, right side. Patient fell from ladder, striking head on stone floor. Escape of cerebrospinal fluid from right ear. Photograph two years after injury.

driasis), the trochlear, the abducens, the entire trigeminal, including com-plete paralysis of its motor division, on the right side total peripheral loss of function of the facial; the soft palate, however, was raised symmetrically during phonation. On the right side no other nerve was affected, but there was absence of sense of taste on the right side, while it was well preserved on the left side. According to this, one is enabled to judge in regard to the course of fracture that it runs transversely through both middle fossæ of the skull, on the left side it follows close to and parallel with the infe-rior anterior border of the petrous portion in course of which the oculo-motor, trochlear, trigeminal, and abducens nerves were injured. From here the fissure ran through the sella turcica, turned backward in trav-ersing the right middle fossa, approaching the superior border of the petrous portion, and opened up the auditory cavities, thus accounting for the hemorrhage from the ear. As the functions of the soft palate were maintained, the facial nerve must have been injured in the aquæ-ductus Fallopii below the geniculate ganglion. This would explain the

loss of sense of taste in the anterior portion o
the lingual.

Anna Heer found paralysis of the acustic ne
following an injury capable of producing fractu
an unreliable symptom. Only in cases in whic
with flow of cerebrospinal fluid and facial paral

Fig. 29.

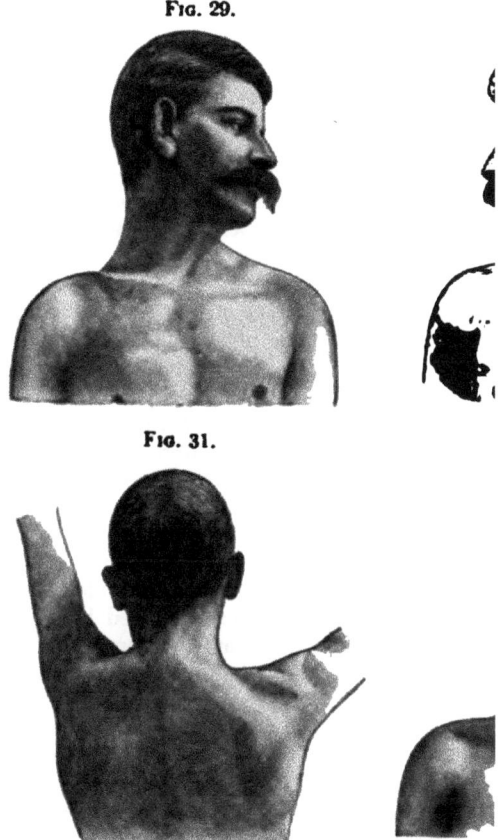

Fig. 31.

Paralysis of hypoglossal (tongue deviates toward left when p
(trapezius and sternomastoid on right side) following fracture o
down stairs. Hemorrhage from nose and right ear.

immediately following injury, is it justifiable tc
petrous portion extending from the internal ea
and tympanic cavity, and even further still to
canal. Disturbances of bearing may be bro
directed against the skull that does not neces
either through hemorrhage into the labyrinth

also by injury to the fibre tracts leading from the centre to the periphery. The various causes of deafness after falls and blows are fully discussed by Kaufmann.

After the facial the abducens nerve is most frequently affected by fractures of the base. Schröder collected 58 cases of abducens paralysis complicating fractures of the base. Forty-eight of these immediately followed the injury, which was not at the base in every case, being frequently of cerebral origin (nuclear, fascicular, and cortical) no doubt, as they complicated other brain and nerve lesions; in only 12 unilateral and 8 bilateral cases was the paralysis strictly isolated.

Although the injuries of the cranial nerves at the base are of diagnostic importance, they are not so important as those facts and circumstances that inform us of the site of impact of the pressure, knock, or blow that produced the solution of continuity of the skull. Being informed of the degree, manner, and direction of the violence, and one of the above symptoms by its presence, leading the surgeon to assume a fracture of the base, he is enabled to judge of its course, whether there is a longitudinal fracture from the ethmoid to the foramen magnum, a transverse fracture through the middle fossa of the skull from one ear to the other, or one running obliquely from the roof of one orbit diagonally across to the posterior fossa on the opposite side. If at the time of injury the head was supported (the injured patient lying with the back of his head on the ground, as he was struck on the forehead), one is justified in assuming that the line of fracture extends through all three fossæ of the skull; while, on the other hand, if a standing fencer is struck on the forehead, the fracture will probably not extend beyond the anterior fossa. If the patient should have fallen from a high place, striking the top of his skull, the surgeon may expect to find numerous lines of fracture at the base, the combination of bursting fracture involving the middle fossa and bending fracture of the condyloid processes produced by the violent impulses of the after-coming vertebral column. Inspection of an open compound fracture situated at the vault may at times disclose fissures that are prolonged through the base.

Course.—No fracture of the skull is in itself dangerous to life. Its seriousness is dependent on two rather frequent complications. One of these is the accompanying injury of the brain and its appendages; the other complication is a subsequent wound infection. The dangers of concussion of the brain, cerebral pressure, contusions, wounds, and rupture of the brain are common to all classes of fracture of the skull; the dangers of purulent cellulitis and osteomyelitis, of meningitis, cerebral abscess, and thrombosis of sinuses, are peculiar to compound fractures with division of the soft parts as far as the bone.

Therapeutic measures to be applied depend on whether the skull contents are involved in the injury. What may be accomplished in these cases by primary operative interference will be fully discussed in the chapter on injuries to the brain. At this point only those measures are considered which are demanded in the proper treatment of fractures themselves.

Prognosis.—The opinion generally expressed that the prognosis is more unfavorable in fractures of the base than in those of the vault is founded on facts; however, the solution of continuity of bone itself does not produce an unfavorable course, but the accompanying brain lesion, which is more extensive, deeper, and more severe than in circumscribed fractures of the vault, because in the production of the former a greater degree of violence and change in form of the bursting skull is necessary. To what extent and in what vital centres and to what degree the brain has been injured remain the governing and deciding factors in the prognosis and therapeutics of fractures of the skull. The obscure and contradictory statements of older and later writers are to blame for the fact that a sufficiently clear distinction was never made in former times, nor is always made at the present time, between the effects of brain lesions and what is the result of bone injuries. It is a well-known fact that until the beginning of the last century the finest fissure of bone was considered an indication for trephining, and that it took some time to arrive at the conclusion that by trephining the original form of fracture present in a given case was simply transformed into one with loss of substance. To this was added the prejudice against allowing fractures of the skull to be repaired, as other fractures are, by the formation of new bone, demanding that they should be kept open and remain ununited.

The so-called provisional callus or primary diffuse, hard swelling, present in fractures, is absent in fractures of the skull, and the permanent callus, though always present, is never so extensive as in fractures of the extremities or even those of flat bones elsewhere, as, for example, the scapula and ilium. This is surprising, for it is wrong to suppose that the cranial bones and the periosteum covering them show little tendency to form new bone. This is shown to be quite the reverse in observing the production of bone in exostoses and hyperostoses, in the osteophytes of pregnant and puerperal women, in diffuse osteosclerosis, and in the complete repair of defects produced by necrosis.

There are two causes that determine the delayed and incomplete repair of cranial bones after injury: first, the destruction and actual loss of the osteoplastic layer of outer and inner periosteum at the site of a localized fracture, especially where it is combined with splintering and displacement of fragments; second, the impaction and immobility of fragments occurring particularly in bursting fractures. The displacement of fragments caused by every voluntary and involuntary muscular action is commonly known to be the factor that stimulates the formation of new bone on the part of the soft tissues and causes its extension far beyond the site of fracture. This irritation is absent in case of the skull. The surfaces of the fracture remain from the beginning to the end of the process of repair in the position in which they were placed by the act of violence, and for that reason no provisional callus is formed. In addition there is present in many cases the inhibiting influence produced by collections of blood beneath the raised periosteum and above the depressed dura. The formation of callus in case of fractures of the skull is usually confined within the limits of periosteum. Spicules, knobs, and lumps have been rarely observed to extend beyond the connective tissue into the aponeurosis or projecting between the fasciculæ of the temporal muscle. Osteophytes on the inner surface of the skull are a rare and exceptional occurrence. An interesting specimen of this kind from the collection at Leipzig has been illustrated, and the author found several others on autopsy in which death took place shortly after injury, consisting of a velvety, sandy deposit between dura and bone. A more extensive participation of the internal periosteum shows itself later by the fact that the fissures, when viewed from within, appear more completely filled with bone than when viewed from without. The final result of the callus formation is the closure with bone of gaps and fissures, although a complete smoothing over generally requires more time than in the case of fractures elsewhere. While in some cases autopsy showed only incomplete repair after more than a year, in others the fissure was completely filled with bone after from two to four months. Suppuration, severe intercurrent diseases or complicating affections of the brain and brain membranes are factors in making the time required for repair a variable one.

Short fissures and shallow depressions may be so completely filled with new bone-tissue that all traces of them are covered up. In these cases, however, a measurable increase in thickness at the site of previous injury indicates that there has been a deposit of bone in excess of that required to fill the defect. In the case of more extensive and more gaping fissures the bone deposit fills only the deeper parts of the defect. This cementing is always more complete at the inner than at the outer surface, so that when viewed from within all traces of the injury may have disappeared. Generally the callus is traversed by small foramina for the transmission of bloodvessels which unite at intervals to form small cavities. The longitudinal diameter of the latter corresponds to the line of fissure. The grooves and hollows remain as traces of fracture for a long time or even for life, and are characterized by smooth, soft, rounded borders. Fissures at the base behave exactly as do those of the vault, as v. Bruns demonstrated in an extensive collection of cases.

The greater degree of vitality of the inner table is shown by the more complete process of repair and the development of osteophytes on the inner surface, and this characteristic quality is again shown by the fact that broken-off fragments may become completely united. It has been confirmed by repeated observations that fragments from the inner table that have lost all connection have re-established channels of nutrition and become completely and firmly attached. It is obvious how important these observations are in determining and treating isolated fractures of the inner table. The splinters of bone become united as a rule, unless the wound is infected. Their occurrence is no indication for opening the skull, provided they do not cause irritation of the cranial contents.

Process of repair in fractures with loss of substance rarely goes on to a complete filling in with callus. As a rule some defect remains which is closed by dense, glistening, fibrous connective tissue.

It is a very exceptional occurrence for a defect as large as the one produced by Küster in removing a sequestrum from the frontal region to be so completely filled in by bone as the same author found it twenty years after. A certain attempt at bone formation and partial closure takes place in case of most defects, although it is a fact that complete bony repair of larger defects is a rare occurrence, and cannot be expected in the case of defects of more than 6 to 8 cm. in diameter.

Treatment.—The treatment of fractures of the skull is necessarily different in simple solutions of continuity covered by unbroken skin than in compound fractures in which the soft parts are involved as well. The relations of the fracture beneath the skin, where the latter is bruised but not lacerated, are not easily determined, except that localized fracture of the vault may be suspected on account of the degree of violence and possible cerebral symptoms. At times there will be not the slightest ground to suspect that there is a fissure in the bone beneath a bruise on the forehead of a child who has recently fallen out of bed, and yet fracture may be present. There are rare cases in which a greater or less portion of the skull may be felt to be broken into numerous fragments beneath the uninjured skin. The author has shown such cases in his clinic, and in them complete recovery took place. To make an incision in case of completely detached fragments is only indicated when they are partially tilted and depressed, so that an edge or border either lacerates or irritates the dura—an irritation that is usually produced in circumscribed depressed fractures. When in the case of limited funnel-shaped fractures with depression this irritation remains constant or causes repeated injury of the pulsating brain, or when on account of the clinical symptoms such seems probable, it will be necessary to incise and remove the cone-shaped fragment of bone, although in doing so a simple fracture is transformed into a compound one. As a matter of fact the author has never seen, nor have other observers, a funnel-shaped depressed fracture occur without a wound of the soft parts, which is easily explained by the mechanism of this form of fracture as described above. A blow with a more or less pointed or angular object, by which they are brought about, will also divide the skin overlying the depressed fragment of skull. Special considerations regarding the treatment of depressed fractures will, therefore, be discussed under the head of compound fractures of the skull.

Compound fractures of the vault of the skull are an important as well as gratifying field for the art of surgery. Since the introduction of antiseptic methods their treatment has been most fortunate, with excellent results, and has shown great progress. A series of collective statistical reports regarding the past and present have placed them in a very favorable light. Reference will only be made to the reports of Socin, Estlander, Köhler (in the *Charité-Annalen*), Kramer, Leydal, Wagner, Lubeck, Leser, Burkhard, Sick, Broca and Maubrac, MacEwen, and others. Of 43 cases of fracture of the vault in the report of Burkhard from the "Nürnberger Stadtkrankenhause," in which there was no evidence of complications on the part of the skull contents, 42 recovered

from the injury, and of 83 cases of recent compound fractures of th
skull treated by Wagner, only 2 died. In the treatment of compoun
fracture there are two indications: to transform an unfavorable form o
position into one that favors union, and to prevent the infection o
wounds, just as in compound fractures elsewhere.

The first indication need only be considered in case of completel
detached splinters of bone and depressed fragments that have bee
driven deeply into the cavity of the skull, for slight displacements of th
edge of fissures are of no significance. At all times depressed fractun
have been the ones in regard to which the question of primary trephinin
has come up and been discussed. Narrowly limited depressions nev
cause symptoms of compression of the brain, no matter how deep the
may be, for the diminution of intracranial space brought about by th
projecting cone-shaped fragment of bone is never sufficient to distur
the circulation of the brain and its membranes. For this to be produce
reqnires rapidly developing hemorrhage into the cranium, which woul
indicate opening the skull even in those cases in which there was n
depressed fragment of bone. As the symptoms of intracranial pressui
are not produced by depression, its removal will not relieve them. It
probable, however, and often has been demonstrated that a cone-shape
collection of bone splinters, or even one splinter from the inner table
the skull, may pierce the dura and injure an underlying convolutio
Such a condition can only be recognized as a rule when the site of depre
sion lies over the motor area of the cerebral cortex, in which case mon
spasms and monoplegias disclose the seat of the brain lesion. In near
every other region limited and slight changes of the gray matter of th
cerebral cortex produce no symptoms and remain undiscovered. Whei
ever a narrowly limited depressed fracture is combined with localize
brain symptoms, the depressed, splintered, cone-shaped fragment of bo
must be removed, whether in case of a simple or a compound fractur
When a fragment of bone has been pushed under the adjacent edge
the skull, the latter may be chiselled away and the depressed fragmei
raised to its proper level.

Depressions limited to a small area have been held responsible for
subsequent epilepsy, and to remove or elevate depressed areas of bor
in every case has been considered positively indicated. As a matter
fact, epilepsy occurs as frequently in connection with head injuries
which no fracture exists. Depression is no more a factor in the etiolog
of this disease than any other scar of the brain or external soft par
that has become adherent to the skull. At present it is known th
even-when an act of violence not exceeding the limits of elasticity
the skull flattens or bends in the latter without producing fracture, tl
portion of brain underlying the site of impact may be contused. Tl
depressed segment of skull, being elastic, springs back into its form
position, but the portion of brain injured at the moment of depressio
undergoes a sclerotic degeneration from which may originate an attac
of Jacksonian epilepsy; the same may take place as the result of damag
to the cerebral cortex following depressed fracture. The author do

not consider it justifiable to elevate every depressed fracture on account of the possibility of a subsequent epilepsy.

While depressed fractures may be considered unfavorable for recovery only within certain limits, there are two other types of compound fractures of the vault that stand in a more unfavorable light. These are compound comminuting and perforating fractures that penetrate to the brain. A depression with little splintering and only slight disarrangement of fragments requires no more interference than a simple fissure. But small detached splinters lying free in the cavity of a wound should be removed and a sharp edge or border should be trimmed. The case is quite otherwise in localized comminuted and shattered fractures of the vault. These are usually accompanied by serious injury of the underlying portions of the brain. Under such circumstances a variety of methods may be applied to improve the conditions of the fracture and the wound of the soft parts. Such are the removal of foreign bodies that have penetrated or are still embedded in fragments, and which is best accomplished by chiselling them out, instead of pulling them out with sequestrum forceps. Also the removal of completely detached splinters of bone and those that have penetrated the brain and dura. These would be a constant source of irritation to the brain, and their subsequent· necrosis would lead to long-continued suppuration. Finally the parts are cleansed, hemorrhage is arrested, and absorbing dressings are applied. In these cases the opening of the wound is indicated to determine what lies at the bottom of a wound which may be filled with blood-clots, hair, or other foreign bodies, bone fragments, shreds of contused soft parts, and fragments of prolapsed brain. The conditions found in perforating fractures and pre-eminently gunshot fracture, are similar to those found in the class of severe comminuted fractures just mentioned.

Socin, Wagner, and Lübeck considered primary disinfection of the wound the principal object in exposing and trimming off the area of fracture. The primary disinfection of wounds should be the indication for surgical interference, not the fear of any unfavorable results in consequence of depressed fragments. The removal of splinters, the trimming of the edges of a perforating fracture, even the chiselling of the edges of a fissure, should be carried out in any case in which it may be assumed infectious materials or organisms have entered the cleft of a fracture. The removal of bone should be considered only as part of a thorough primary wound disinfection. This should be the principal purpose of the surgical treatment. "It must be emphasized again that the so-called primary disinfection of all kinds of open injuries is the nucleus of the entire modern treatment of wounds, and will always remain so."

In describing the treatment of contused wounds of the scalp the author has expressed his views regarding the primary disinfection of wounds. Here, as there, he considers it necessary that the wounds be thoroughly cleansed of all dirt—large and small foreign bodies of all kinds, hair, portions of head-covering, pieces of skin, entirely or partially detached shreds of fascia and connective tissue, fragments of brain, etc. In severe cases pulling apart the edges of fracture will not be sufficient; in most cases considerable incision and chiselling will be required. The process of cleansing may be carried out with the assistance of forceps and scissors, as well as digital exploration, while the wound is constantly being wiped out with pieces of dry sterile gauze. It may be necessary to cut off contused portions of skin, to scrape the soiled edge of a wound or bone-fissure with a sharp spoon, or to trim off or pinch off the edge of a fracture or splinter of bone with a gouge or Luer's forceps, and to widen a fissure with a few blows of a chisel in order to remove hairs that may have become caught in it. The author never permits the application of disinfecting solutions of any kind to the wound; neither carbolic acid, nor sublimate, nor zinc solutions; neither thymol nor lysol—not a single antiseptic. In order to obtain a smooth, clean wound leading to the brain it may be necessary at times to remove the entire portion of the skull that has been splintered and comminuted; in one sense of the word, to trephine—that is, to remove the injured bone with chisel, Collins', Luer's, or Lane's bone-forceps. It is not necessary to state that the head should be completely shaved, including the region of the neck, and washed with ether, alcohol and water, again with alcohol, and finally with corrosive sublimate solution, as was described in the treatment of contused wounds of the soft parts. Disinfection should be followed by thorough arrest of all hemorrhage. The wound should be absolutely dry before it is closed, or, if not closed, before it is protected by dressings; blood should not be allowed to collect at the bottom or in any corner or pocket, and to avoid this counteropenings should be freely made.

The above process should be carried out in every case, even if the in-jured person be exhausted or appear in a dying condition when presented for treatment. Whether the surgeon stops at this point depends on the general condition of the patient, especially the degree of cerebral disturb-ance. If the pulse is strong and syncope and collapse do not appear to be imminent, the author considers it proper to cover the site of a recent fracture where there is absence of soft parts with a flap from the neighbor-ing sound scalp. Drawing together the edges of the wound may accom-plish this. If, however, the scalp over a comminuted or perforated frac-ture is severely and extensively contused and consequently destroyed, or if, in preparing the wound for dressing, so much has had to be trimmed off that even after undermining and with appropriately placed counter-openings, the soft parts cannot be sufficiently approximated to cover the exposed site of fracture, the latter should be covered by a plastic opera-tion. The author pleaded this point in presenting a case before the "Congress deutscher Chirurgie" of 1882, and has since then frequently used this method with very good results. Large flaps with broad ped-icles for nutrition, adjacent to the loss of substance, as Schwimmelbusch suggested for rhinoplasty, are easily formed from the soft parts. The precaution should always be taken to make wide counteropenings, or to allow part of the loss of substance caused by the inflicting violence to remain open no matter what method is used to cover the site of fracture but might frequently be applied as a secondary operation to close defects resulting from the removal of comminuted fragments of the skull. Leydel used this method to close defects after only eight days—that is, at a time when the process of repair had not been completed. Others, however, have waited longer, until after the wounds have healed.

There are several methods that may be employed to close defects of the skull after they have become covered with skin. The author prefers that of König and Müller to all others. Overlying the defect in the bone, a flap with a pedicle is outlined by making an incision on three sides. In the immediate neighborhood a second flap is outlined, 0.5 cm. more in diameter, with its pedicle in the opposite direction, so that a spur-shaped bridge of skin remains between them. The second flap consists of skin, periosteum, and the upper layers of bone, and is lifted up by means of a chisel held horizontally. Both flaps are twisted about their pedicles, consisting only of skin, aponeurosis, and periosteum, and made completely to exchange their position. They are held in place by sutures. The method is not simple, and in cases of large defects requires considerable interference. Further, it is not applicable to the skull of children, where, on account of the lack of development of the diploë, the skull is too thin to be split longitudinally, and for the same reason cannot be carried out in the temporal region. One would naturally seek other means to secure firm bony closure of defects. Since it was observed and experimentally demonstrated that absolutely detached fragments of bone could become reattached, extensive efforts have been made to apply Wolff's method of attempting to reinsert buttons of bone removed by trephining and allowing them to grow on. Not only the fragments of bone removed in caring for a compound fracture were placed in the gap, but larger pieces of bone recently removed from other portions of the body—as the tibia, for example (Seydel)—were used to fill up the defect. According to Barth's investigations, which were later corroborated by Marchand, these fragments of bone always lost their vitality when transplanted. They only act as foreign bodies, stimulating the living tissues about them to produce new bone, the latter holding them fast and finally growing through them. As the fragments of bone placed in a defect simply play the part of a passive foreign body, the question arises as to which kind of foreign bodies will be more likely to produce sufficient formation of new bone to bring about the firm closure of the defect. Fränkel and v. Eiselberg have reported the successful use of celluloid plates, and Senn has used pieces of decalcified bone. This question was decided earlier by Barth, but more definitely by Grekow. According to these, the best material to produce sufficient growth of new bone to fill even large defects is a disk of spongy, thoroughly calcined bone. The grafting of a defect must be preceded by the removal of all scar-tissue and the freshening of the thinned edges of bone, either by scraping with a spoon or cutting it with the Luer forceps, so that in every case the implanted disk of bone shall be in immediate contact with the marrow within in the diploë of the edges of fracture to which it must be accurately fitted. The inserted fragment should be entirely covered

tured area of bone, it may be brought to a stop by the free drainage of
the products of inflammation with which the tissues are saturated. Early
abscesses of the cerebral cortex lying immediately beneath a circumscribed compound fracture of the vault are the result of pus retained in
wound-pockets and beneath occluding fragments of bone. In the absence of spreading purulent inflammation of the soft parts surrounding
the site of fracture, they are revealed by the coating covering the granulations that have begun to grow at the bottom of the wound. The red
field has become changed to a yellow mass, with here and there an opening through which a drop of pus exudes. An acute traumatic abscess
is recognised more easily by the changed appearance of the hitherto
healthy wound and the onset of rise of temperature than by the cerebral
symptoms. In many cases it cannot be distinguished from a beginning
meningitis of the vault. That is no reason, however, why a purulent
and inflamed wound at the site of fracture should be disregarded. Incision and drainage are, moreover, the only method, and in many cases
an effective method with which to treat the symptoms of meningitis.

As in other compound fractures, an infection, especially with staphylococci, may result in an acute traumatic osteomyelitis in connection with
fracture of the skull, and it is this complication which predisposes to the
further danger of purulent leptomeningitis, thrombophlebitis, and meta-
. tatic or pyæmic abscesses. If recognized early and met by energetic
interference, recovery may take place.

Fractures of the base require special consideration, among other
reasons, because their presence is not so easily determined as in the
case of the vault. A large majority of them never come under treatment, as the accompanying injury of the most important parts of the
brain lying at the base results in instant death of the injured individual. The great degrees of violence that are required to produce this
class of fractures, together with the great deformity of the skull resulting, cause the most extensive injuries of the brain that are beyond all
surgical help. Patients suffering from fracture of the base who are not
killed instantly are in the greatest degree of danger during the first
twenty-four to forty-eight hours. Of 23 cases of fracture of the base that
survived this period, Wagner met with not a single death. If the fissures,
running longitudinally, transversely, or diagonally through the fossae of
the skull, were always subcutaneous, one might conclude from the circumstances that fractures of the base were not dangerous in themselves,
but that the cause of death lay in the accompanying cerebral lesion. As
a matter of fact, however, the fractures of the base are only rarely subcutaneous throughout their whole extent, and generally reach the surface
at definite localities at the site of cavities let into the floor of the skull
that communicate with the outside, the frontal and sphenoid sinuses,
the cells of the ethmoid, and the nasal passages, the pharynx, and especially the tympanic cavity, Eustachian tube, and the external auditory
canal. These cavities are particularly liable to cause infection, owing to
the invasion of microörganisms that find their habitat in them. Some
time ago an officer who had been thrown from his horse was brought to

the author for treatment suffering from a fracture of the base. He died during the second week, and an autopsy showed a collection of pus above and below the lacerated dura immediately overlying the horizontal plate of the ethmoid. A. Fränkel showed conclusively that infection of the pia mater in a case had resulted from pyogenic organisms that had found their way from the nose through a fissure in the bone and advanced anteriorly. In this case there was a meningitis caused by *Diplococcus pneumoniæ*, ending fatally on the twenty-sixth day after a fracture of the base involving the orbital roof had been sustained. Microscopical examination showed the same cocci to be present in the nasal mucous membrane that were found in the meningeal exudate. As these are frequently found physiologically in the nasal passages, there can be no question that the infection of the wound at the base of the skull was brought about by the *Diplococcus pneumoniæ*. Other closed cavities at the base of the skull may be infected by organisms that are naturally found in these cavities, as, for example, the tympanic cavity which communicates with the superior nasopharynx through the Eustachian tube. This is particularly liable to take place from the external auditory canal, regarding whose rich microscopical flora bacteriological examinations of aurists have testified. The cause of infection finds entrance through a laceration of the drum membrane or through a penetrating wound of the roof of the auditory canal that communicates with the fracture in the bone. Unquestionably infection of fractures of the base can take place in this way, even if the fracture communicates with the outer world through a hidden and minute wound of the mucous membrane. It is probable that the abundant early hemorrhage affords some protection against the invasion of infectious organisms by washing them out of the nose and mouth.

V. Volkmann was the first to attempt by antiseptic means to prevent the infection of fractures of the base. Some years ago the author gave up entirely the use of antiseptics for irrigating the auditory canal. By this method thorough disinfection of the auditory canal or the tympanic cavity can never be carried out. It may only result in carrying infectious materials, wax, and shreds of epidermis to the site of fracture. The auditory canal should be wiped out; and if, as is usually the case, hemorrhage continues, it should be filled with a tampon of gauze. This should he removed frequently during the first day whenever it has become saturated with blood, while a light sterile dressing holds it in contact with the external ear, which, together with the surrounding parts, should be carefully cleansed. There is nothing more that the author can suggest doing, and he has been well satisfied with the results obtained in fractures of the base treated in this way. He would not advise tamponing the nose in this manner as a prophylactic measure. The secretion of mucus from Schneider's membrane is only increased by the irritation of such a foreign body, even though it be a soft and pliant one, and the holding back of the secretion by the tampon can be no advantage. Only the presence of considerable hemorrhage should induce the surgeon to tampon the nasal passages.

It is necessary to do more in those cases in which a fissure of the base communicates externally through a wound in the roof of the skull. No matter how small this wound may be, it should be protected from becoming infected throughout the whole process of healing, and every effort made to have it close as rapidly as possible. By these means the entire fissure is protected, which would otherwise be exposed to infection throughout the whole period of suppuration, granulation, and cicatrization. In caring for a wound and fracture at the vault, splinters of bone that reach to the base have been removed.

Should the flow of cerebrospinal fluid from the ear become turbid or purulent, there is danger of a basilar meningitis, especially dangerous as there is little that can be done to prevent its progress. Wiping out the ear and tamponing it with iodoform gauze is a much better plan than the common practice of irrigating with astringents, and this should be repeated several times in the course of the day. If suppuration and inflammation are limited to the middle ear and the mastoid process, the surgeon may expect to obtain free evacuation of pus by means of the modern operation, which consists in chiselling open the latter, or by a more radical operation, namely, evacuation of pus from the middle ear or even the middle fossa of the skull.

Frequently necrotic pieces of bone have been removed from the ear or the mastoid process after opening the latter in the later stages following fractures of the base. Signs of inflammation at the surface of the mastoid process or distinct fluctuation at the same point or over the temporal bone above the concha warranted making an incision and led to the discovery of sequestra.

Severe cerebral manifestations and blood aspirated from the naso-pharynx into the air-passages in the case of a comatose patient may demand still further surgical interference in the shape of a tracheotomy. The author found it necessary to perform this operation immediately in 3 cases brought to the clinic in a cyanotic state threatened with asphyxia. In one of these cases the operation saved the patient's life, as he recovered from his fracture and brain lesion.

Finally, one word regarding the *treatment of cephalhydrocele* and defects of the skull following simple fractures of the skull occurring in children, which have already been mentioned. In many respects the manifestations, especially the nervous symptoms, produced by this complication are the same as those of porencephalon, and it seems to one that it would be worth while investigating whether there is not always a congenital defect of brain that lies at the foundation of these tumors that follow traumatism. To bring about their removal puncture followed by injection of iodine, incision with drainage, and dissection of the portion outside the skull, with or without drainage of the ventricles, have been recommended. In three operations during the past year, following removal of the cyst, the author closed the defect in the skull by a König-Müller bone-flap, once with good result, and in the other two cases with collapse and death.

INCISED, PUNCTURED, AND GUNSHOT-WOUNDS OF THE SKULL.

Incised Wounds.—Wounds of the skull present features depending on the instrument causing the injury. If the blade striking the skull be narrow and keen, the edges of the cleft bone are sharp; while if the wedge penetrating the skull be blunt and angular, the bone is not only divided, but is also forced apart, splintered, and comminuted. Whether a smooth, clean-cut wound of the bone be produced, or one combined with single or multiple fractures, depends therefore on the character of the instrument inflicting the injury. The immediate injuries sustained by the brain as the result of incised wounds are, like those of the bones, dependent on the edge of the weapon. A sharp blade may pass from the top of the skull through the bone and penetrate the brain without immediate loss of consciousness taking place; but the mere shock of a blow delivered with a blunt weapon may produce contusion of the brain or loss of consciousness as the result of concussion.

The keen "Schläger" of the students, and the excellent small arms of certain warlike races, as, for example, the Schaschkas of Tscherkessia, divide the bone clean and smooth with artistic skill. However, even these weapons may cause splintering of one or other edge of the wound, especially at the inner table, if the blow be not delivered forcibly enough.

According to the depth of the wound in the bone, *penetrating* and *non-penetrating wounds of the skull* may be distinguished. Injuries are further classified according to the direction in which a blow is delivered. Thus are distinguished: 1. Simple cuts and superficial scratches, limited to the outer table (the "Hedra" of the ancients). 2. Division of both tables by blows delivered in a direction perpendicular to the surface of the bone ("Ekkope"). 3. Oblique or horizontal blows, splitting both tables, but not completely cutting off a flap of bone ("Diakope"). 4. Complete solution of a segment of skull, in which the bone may remain attached to the soft parts or both be cut off at the same time ("Aposkeparnismus"). The first-named injuries are linear wounds, the latter flap-wounds and wounds with loss of substance.

Linear wounds are produced by blows delivered in a more or less perpendicular direction, and the edges gape in proportion to the thickness of the instrument. These wounds will tend to gape more where blows are delivered in a direction more or less at an angle to the surface. The edge of the wound corresponding to the superior edge of the blade is usually raised above the level of the opposite one; this is owing to its being actually lifted, and not because the lower one is depressed. When the direction of the blow is very oblique, approaching the horizontal plane, *flap-wounds* are produced, the free edge of which always has a circular outline owing to the spherical form of the skull, while the attached portion appears bent or broken in. The smaller the base of attachment, the nearer is the approach to a wound with loss of substance, in which a larger or smaller piece of the skull is knocked off, either in its entire thickness or only as far as the diploë. At the same time the soft parts covering the bone may be cut away, or they may remain attached to the rest of the skull with the loose fragment of bone remaining adherent to them.

Bone-wounds of the skull are combined with fractures, not only in the form of small splinterings of the inner table, but as a rule in the case of blunt, heavy, wedge-shaped weapons. There are also produced depression of the edges of the wound, breaking off of larger fragments, and fissures that are prolonged to quite a distance beyond the site of injury. This is especially the case in axe-wounds. In these cases one nearly always finds extensive comminution.

The majority of linear, and still more so flap-wounds, are combined with fissures, with very typical arrangement. From each angle of th wound a crack runs in the bone for some distance, following exactly th line of the meridian passing through the place of injury. If a blow b delivered in the direction of the coronal suture, fissures may reach as fa as the base; while in injury of the frontal bone delivered in a vertica direction, fissures have been frequently found prolonged to the roof o the orbit. In the case of blows delivered in an oblique direction producing wounds that approach flap-wounds in form, fissures ar formed, prolonging the line of a circle, of which the rounded free edg of the flap may be considered a segment. There can be no questio that wedging and flattening are combined in the production of thes fissures.

Course.—The course of sharply incised wounds seems to be mor favorable than that of fractures of the skull, as far as can be determine by the statistics of the War of the Rebellion, and the fact that in th pathological collections of hospital museums three or four times as man specimens of healed incised wounds are found than healed fracture It would seem a priori that the brain is more frequently involved in ca of fracture than in connection with incised wounds, and the significan of every injury of the skull depends on the complications of the bra and brain membranes. In case of incised wounds the surgeon may fir simply a very fine, hair-like division at the surface of a hemisphe while in fractures there may be produced contusions of more or le. extensive portions, infiltration with blood, and lacerations not necessaril limited to the site of fracture. The mere fact of a wound penetratin the skull, whether it be clean and smooth or contused and lacerated, in itself of serious import. Whether the brain be injured or not, infe tions materials may be carried to the delicate membranes covering th brain and serve as the starting point of a progressive purulent inflan mation, a meningitis. As in compound fractures, the greatest danger t life lies in meningitis; traumatic osteomyelitis comes second, bringin with it secondarily thrombosis of sinuses and pyæmia.

Hemorrhages following penetrating incised wounds are more easil recognized and more easy of access than the same injuries to vessels i connection with fractures. The longitudinal sinus is most frequentl involved, while very little has been reported regarding injuries of th meningeal arteries.

Prognosis.—Non-penetrating incised wounds offer a favorable prognosis. Naturally they are subject to tne same disturbances and dangers as similar wounds of the soft parts. The course of flap-wounds, particularly those complicated by splintering and comminution as the result of blows, may be a very long and tedious one. Portions of bone along the edge may become necrotic, and be thrown off by a slow process of exfoliation.

Flaps of bone produced by obliquely directed blows may become reattached, but there is always some loss of substance at the periphery owing to the breaking or rounding off of the edges, making it appear as if they had beocme contracted toward the base of attachment. This peripheral loss of substance is even greater if the border zone become entirely or partially necrotic. In case of penetration of the skull a cleft always remains, closed only by fibrous cicatricial tissue adherent to the dura.

Before asepsis was understood the disk of bone detached in the case of wounds with loss of substance was usually lost as the result of necrosis. Even in these times, however, instances of reimplantation were reported. The fragment of bone at times regained its original position and became attached to some part of the edge of the wound, or, having been displaced, it rested with its cerebral surface on the outer surface of the rest of the bone and became attached in this manner.

Diagnosis.—The diagnosis of incised wounds of the skull is easy, as wounds of the soft parts overlying them usually have a tendency to gape. On the other hand, it may be exceedingly difficult to determine whether in a given case a wound has penetrated, or whether extensive fissures and comminution are present at the same time, especially when the latter involve the inner table. Taking into consideration the length of a linear wound that gapes very little, one may be able to decide whether or not it has penetrated. If a wound in a given case extends over a large part of the vault, it must necessarily, on account of the spherical form of the skull, have penetrated at its middle portion. Any further diagnostic measure except these calculations, and noting the presence of pulsation in the blood filling the wound, are useless and may do harm. In the case of larger wounds that show considerable gaping, in which the fact of the wound-edges being far apart shows that the injury was inflicted by a broad, wedge-shaped weapon, it is safe to assume from the beginning that comminution of the edges has occurred.

Treatment.—The treatment of incised wounds is practically the same as that of compound fractures, to which reference has been made. In linear wounds with little gaping the method employed should be the same as in similar wounds of the scalp—thorough arrest of all hemorrhage and suturing with fine, carefully sterilized silk. The sutures should be placed close together, and close the wound except at one or two places. In most cases treated soon after injury the results were most gratifying. If, however, suppuration sets in, the sutures should of course, be partially or entirely removed, and the further treatment be that of wounds of the soft parts complicated by cellulitis and abscess formation.

Suturing of the wounds should also be attempted in those c
which after examination there remains some doubt as to the cor
of the inner table. If there were more opportunities to make post-n
examinations in cases that have recovered from penetrating wou
the skull, one would find frequently that reattachment of fragmer
taken place, especially when the bone is only partially detached.
suturing of wounds in doubtful cases, as indicated above, is amply
fied, the more so as under these circumstances the rapid union
soft parts covering the wound is the principal factor in preventing i
mation and necrosis of bones. Assuming that suppuration doe
place beneath the closed soft parts, it is easy to reopen the wou
prevent further danger. Hemorrhage from the longitudinal sinu
be controlled by a compress of iodoform gauze introduced throu
trephine wound, just as would be done if in trephining the mastoid p
the sinus be wounded. A favorable course, in penetrating w
involving the sinus, has been frequently reported; hemorrhage fro
meningeal artery requires more extensive interference. The wound
be enlarged by gouging or boring and the vessel ligated.

If a disk of bone is completely detached, and is only adherent
flap of soft parts by its periosteal surface, it is usually sufficiently
tached, and reimplantation should therefore be attempted. I
wounds of the frontal region are frequently inflicted in such a dir
that besides the soft parts a piece of the supraorbital ridge is at the
time cut off. Experience has shown that even these cases are c
of good union. In all cases, then, it is safe to count on the union of
ments of bone attached only to the soft parts, provided aseptic me
are carried out. By carefully observing the patient any damage f
ing a failure to obtain a good result may be guarded against; w
successful the period of recovery is very much shortened and the d
lying in suppuration of the bone is correspondingly diminished. S
the edges of the wound be much fractured, and larger fragments be l
from the inner table, and be more or less depressed, an incised w
must be considered a compound fracture and treated accord
Wounds should therefore be cleansed, trimmed, and prepared jus
they were fractures. And from the same point of view it shou
decided whether they are to be closed or left open.

If pieces of bone are chopped off together with the soft parts ext
from the surface, an attempt should be made to close the wound by a plastic
tion after reimplantation of the bone fragment. If it is available,
by the use of larger disks good results have been obtained by

Incised Wounds. — Pointed instruments, knives, daggers, l

foramen, injuring the optic nerve. Foreign bodies passing along the inner half of the floor of the orbit may be deflected toward the sphenoidal fissure, as a convex irregularity at this part of the floor of the orbital cavity obstructs the path in the direction of the foramen rotundum.

These fractures of the roof of the orbit are *perforated fractures* with fissures and splinters radiating from the point of penetration. When a foreign body passes through the sphenoidal fissure, it causes a fracture of the bones bounding the fissure. Penetration of the greater wing of the sphenoid has been observed.

A foreign body may penetrate either the upper or lower eyelid, or the eyelids may not be injured at all, as in its course it may pass between the eyeball and the tarsal conjunctiva, penetrating the reflected fold of the conjunctiva. The severity of an injury may be overlooked, especially if the penetrating body has broken off and remains embedded in the orbital cavity or even in the brain. In the case of a cane-thrust through the orbit into the cranial cavity the ferrule may be stripped off on its withdrawal and remain embedded in the brain. If a foreign body remain in the adipose tissue of the orbital cavity, and be of some size, it can usually be discovered after careful search. The position of the eyeball is usually somewhat prominent, or displaced in a direction away from the foreign body; this may therefore aid in the search for the latter. In the case of metallic objects, as ferrules of canes or umbrellas, an x-ray picture is indispensable, and determines not only the presence of a foreign body, but also its exact position and location in the orbital cavity or brain.

Treatment.—The treatment consists in aseptic closure of the wound, provided the presence of a foreign body has been excluded by the history, as, for instance, by inspection of the inflicting instrument. It may be assumed that in these wounds, as in a large class of gunshot-wounds, the profuse hemorrhage taking place at the beginning has been sufficient to wash out all infections materials that may have gained entrance. The eye should be closed and the whole region between the nose and orbital ridge padded out with soft gauze. Considerable pressure should be exerted by tightly drawn but well-padded bandages. Should a foreign body have been embedded for some time in a wound before it is removed, or the entrance of dirt, dust, etc., appears probable from inspection of the wound, and from its character or that of the inflicting instrument, it is better to forego the advantages derived from rapid healing and closure of a small wound, and open up as far as the site of fracture in the orbital roof by dividing the skin and orbital adipose tissue. The presence of hemorrhage and the small space occasioned by the necessity of sparing the eyeball make operative procedures difficult. The method of Wagner may be recommended, therefore, for removing foreign bodies and establishing a wide-open wound as far as the site of fracture. This consists in the temporary resection of a wedge-shaped piece of bone from the orbital ridge and the adjacent bones of the face, similar to the method of Krönlein for operating on twin-sac dermoids of the orbital cavity. All bleeding having been stopped, the cavity of the wound should be filled with iodoform gauze, and according to the amount of saturation this may be left in place or changed repeatedly until the wound ceases to show signs of inflammation and the temperature returns to normal. The flap of bone and soft parts that were turned aside should then be replaced. Very rarely the lamina cribrosa has been broken by punctures of the nasal passages.

Gunshot Wounds.—The modern projectiles of small firearms that have been introduced into all the larger armies are characterized by their small calibre, their hard shell (mantle), and their high initial velocity. While the soft-lead bullet of the Russian army used in the last Turkish war attained an initial velocity of 390 metres (1200 feet) per second, the steel-mantled, hard-lead bullet of the German army attains 640 metres (2000 feet) per second. This great increase in the initial velocity is the principal factor in explaining the peculiarities of the injuries produced by these projectiles. Formerly dependence was placed on observations made in actual warfare. At the present time the action of projectiles is studied by shooting at the human cadaver and at living animals. Among very extensive researches reference will only be made to the works of Kocher, P. v. Bruns, and that of the medical department of the Imperial Royal Prussian War Department, published by v. Coler and Schjerning. They explain the laws of gunshot-wounds of the skull and place them on a definite basis.

In gunshot fired at very short range the skullcap, together with the scalp covering it, is torn into many pieces which with the mangled brain are scattered to quite a distance. At a range of 50 metres (160feet) the scalp is preserved and continues to hold the skull together, though the latter is broken into many fragments. The scalp shows two defects, with lacerated edges, from which brain-tissue exudes: the wound of entrance and that of exit. At a range of 100 metres (325 feet) the destruction of the skull is somewhat less, though two zones of comminution can be found grouped about the wounds of entrance and exit. The lines of fracture are in part arranged radially, in part encircling the bullet-hole like a series of bursting and bending fractures. The fissures may become united with one another, forming a network spread over the entire skull. The diameter of the wound of exit in the skin does not exceed 20-30 mm. At increasing range the damage done by the projectile continues to grow less. The zones of comminution do not run into each other, but are more sharply circumscribed. At a range of from 800 to 1200 metres (2600 to 4000 feet) the fissures encircling the bullet-holes disappear, and only the radial fissures are present; these disappear at a range of 1600 metres (5200 feet) and upward, except that there is one fissure connecting the wound of entrance with the wound of exit. Even this is no longer present at a range of from 1800 to 2000 metres (5600 to 6500 feet); at this distance there are clean-cut bullet-holes. It was not until a range of 2700 metres (8700 feet) had been reached that the skull was not perforated and the bullet remained embedded in the brain. Naturally individual injuries do not always bear the same accurate relation to the given distance of range, in the first place, owing to special circumstances, as, for example, the varying thickness of the skull in different individuals. and furthermore on account of the fact that the angle at which a projectile strikes an object is also variable. The degree and form of injury are constant only up to a range of 800 metres (2600 feet). The injuries

Fig. 33.

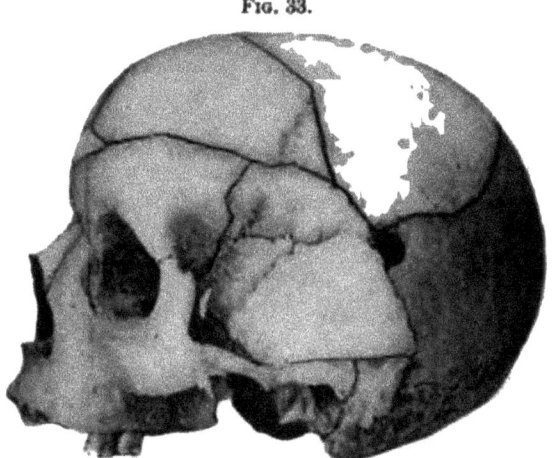

Gunshot-wounds of the skull.

Fig. 34.

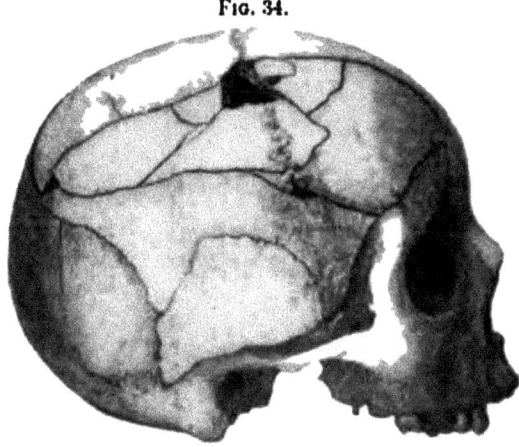

Gunshot-wounds of the skull.

of the dura mater are analogous in their character to those of the skull. If the latter be completely shattered, the dura is correspondingly torn to pieces. If the skull be broken into many fragments, but still held together by the soft parts, there are lacerations as long as 10 cm., corresponding to the wounds of entrance and exit, besides a number of shorter ones corresponding to the longer fissures. At increasing range these grow less and less, being limited finally to two defects at the points of entrance and exit. In the case of short range up to a distance of 100 metres (325 feet) the entire brain is severely injured in the form of diffuse hemorrhages and areas of contusions, the ventricles being filled with blood. This lesion is present even when a projectile traverses only the bone, when, for example, it ploughs along the base. A projectile passing from the mouth through the anterior fossa of the skull and out at the forehead produces less extensive local damage than one traversing the skull from the forehead to the occiput. With increasing range the local injuries of the brain become less severe, until finally the sinus produced by the bullet has a smaller diameter at its middle portion than at either the wound of entrance or exit. A further factor not present in ordinary fractures is responsible for the explosive or expansile effect produced by

Fig. 35.

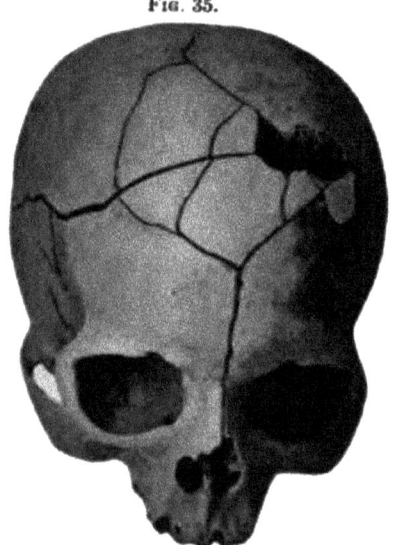

Gunshot-wounds of the skull.

short-range shots. This is the hydrodynamic action on the part of the semifluid brain. It is known from the experiments of v. Coler and Schjerning that this explosive action at short range is in proportion to the active force with which a projectile arrives at its destination.

The expansion produced in the skull may be illustrated by a projectile fired into a vessel of lead or tin filled with water or plaster. Water or a semifluid substance like wet plaster, soft brain, or sand mixed with water, transmits pressure received equally and without loss in all directions. A certain amount of the energy possessed by the penetrating projectile is transmitted to the water filling the metallic box. In this way it becomes possessed of energy which is exerted against the wall of the vessel, stretching and bursting the same. It is not simply the action of hydraulic

pressure, but the hydrodynamic action of the active force of the projecti
transmitted to the contained fluid. If the leaden vessel closed on all sid
be empty, it is simply perforated, just as if it had been filled with san
In both cases the walls of the vessel remain uninjured except for tl
perforations at the points of entrance and exit. The result is, howeve
entirely different if the metallic vessel be filled with water, plaster,
brain. In this case it is burst asunder and its walls bent from with
outward. That this is caused not by simple hydraulic pressure, b
by hydrodynamic force, is proved by v. Coler and Schjerning from t
fact that the bursting of the walls takes place in the vessel filled wi
water whether it be open or closed. Hydraulic pressure would cau
bursting only in case of a completely closed vessel. By determining t
degree of pressure the experimenters were able to conclude that t
velocity with which the water was thrown from the bursting vessel w
higher than it could have been had it been caused by hydraulic pressui

Fig. 36.

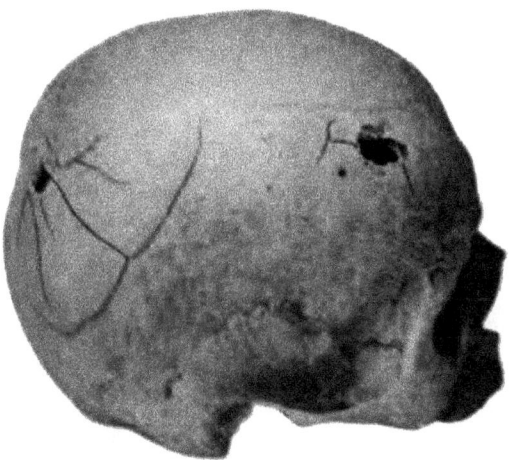

Gunshot wounds of the skull.

In the case of hydraulic pressure the bursting of the vessel would ha
to take place instantly at the moment of entrance of the projectile,
that when the latter reached the opposite wall the same would have be
already opened. In every case, however, in which the bent-out portic
of the lateral wall were put back in their original position, the hole
will was filled. It has been definitely settled from the above that
short-range shots with modern small-calibre projectiles the skull is bu
by hydrodynamic pressure. The contained brain has the necessa
physical qualities to enable it to take up the active force of the projecti
containing as it does the best degree of compressibility with the great
mobility of its molecules.

The gunshot injuries produced by the modern infantry projectiles
living human beings that have been reported in literature, as well

Fig. 37.

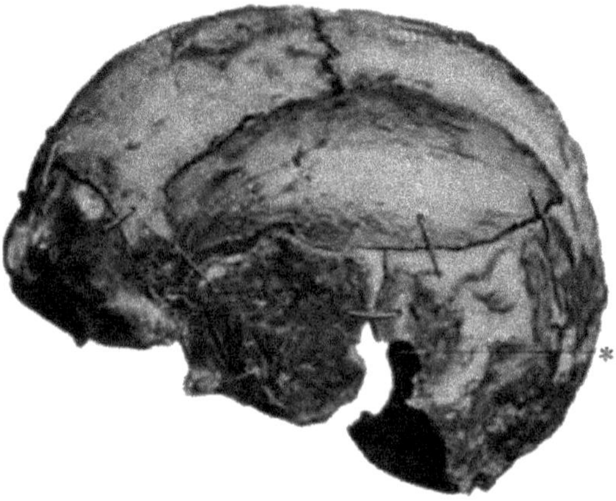

Fig. 38. Fig. 39.

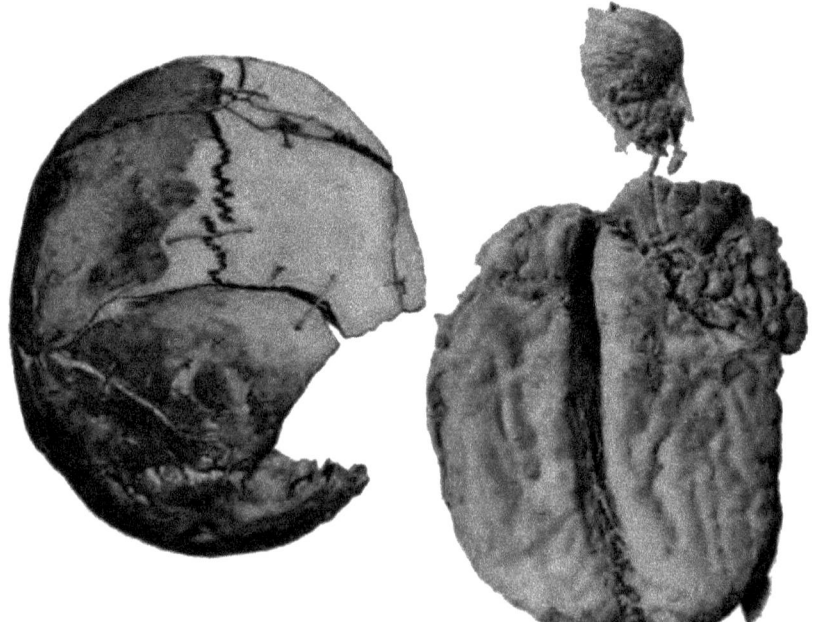

Exenteratio cranii. Gunshot-wound of skull (modern rifle, Swiss ordnance weapon, model 1890). Distance, 7 metres. Brain found lying on its base to the left of corpse at a distance of 20 cm. Its form was preserved. (Krönlein.)

Fig. 37.—View of skull from left side, * entrance wound.

Fig. 38.—View of skull from above.

Fig. 39.—Cerebral hemispheres, near it on left cerebellum.

those described by Deutsch in the army reports of the Royal Prussian Sanitary Division, principally cases of suicide, were produced at extreme short range and caused instant death. The cerebral lesions were as extensive as in experiments. In some cases the brain has been actually found completely removed from the shattered skull (exenteratio cranii, Figs. 37 to 39). It seems hardly possible that cerebral lesions produced by short-range shots can be compatible with life. Two such cases were, however, reported by Kröulein in which the shot had been fired at a very short range with full charge, but striking at a tangent, and had traversed only a small segment of the cerebral hemisphere. (Fig. 40.)

FIG. 40.

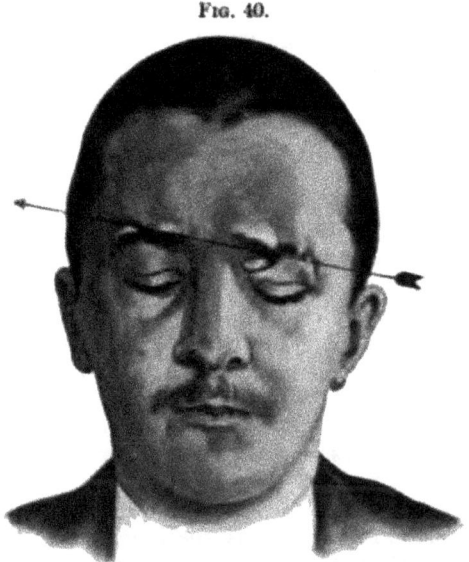

(Gunshot-wound of forehead. Total blindness of both eyes. Ordnance weapon, model 1871. Arrow indicates direction of bullet (tangential direction just above left orbital roof, destroying the left eye, then piercing inner and upper wall of left orbit in region of crista galli, wounding anterior pole of left frontal lobe).

The bursting of the skull and the destruction of the brain were observed even in the Franco-Prussian War during close combats, especially at the battle of Le Bourget. At that time the French were accused of having used explosive bullets. The relatively low initial velocity of the Chassepot projectile (420 metres – 1300 feet—per second), as compared with that of the modern small-calibre, completely mantled projectiles, was compensated for by the change in shape produced in the soft-lead bullet. For that reason these were almost as effective as the modern infantry projectile, in spite of only about half the initial velocity. The important part played by this change in shape was shown in the early experiences of the English in Afghanistan. The English "full-jacketed bullet" produced such smooth, clean-cut wounds of the soft parts and bones that the enemy, though wounded, were not stopped in their wild, onward rush, and were exceedingly dangerous to their opponents before falling to the ground. If, however, the nickel jacket covering the lead core was filed away for some distance from the point (Dum-dum projectiles—soft-nosed bullets), its effect was entirely different. At a range at which the full-mantled bullet would produce only smooth, narrow wounds they produced lacerations and contusions of the tissues. V. Bruns found in gunshot experiments with Dum-dum bullets that at short range they produced injuries far more terrible than those caused by the full-mantled bullet. Skull and brains were changed into a heap of splinters mixed with particles of soft tissues. The action of the deformed projectile is combined with that produced by the high initial velocity ("active force"). The injuries produced by such gunshots do not require the services of a surgeon. Surgical attention is only required in those wounded at greater range. The author observed injuries of this kind in 28 skulls collected during the Russo-Turkish War, which have been described with illustrations. Their character is determined not only by the elasticity of the skull, but also by the wedge action of the projectile, which was referred to in explaining the mechanism of certain incised wounds of the skull. Injuries like those produced by the German infantry rifle in experiments at 100 metres or more the author has seen only in those left dead on the field or in soldiers brought in a dying condition to the dressing stations. Numerous fissures radiate in all directions from the irregular, angular, comminuted wound of entrance, uniting again at the wound of exit, which is similar in appearance. In their course they communicate with each other by other fissures dividing the intervening surface of bone into a number of fragments, a sort of mosaic that is very difficult to fit together again after the skull has been macerated.

The majority of the soldiers wounded in the skull showed grooved and gutter-shaped gunshot-wounds, the latter being principally penetrating furrows or elongated losses of substance. These injuries, which were produced by bullets striking more or less at a tangent, showed certain peculiarities. On studying an extensive collection of them, as the author had the opportunity of doing in 20 specimens of this kind, one can always notice that at one point of the gouged-out loss of substance the edge of the defect is more sharply cut or smoothly broken than in the rest of the furrow. This point is always at the end of the groove pointing toward the direction from which the bullet came, and marks therefore the site of impact. Further, there are found about this point one or two concentric circles starting from and coming back to the same point. The mechanism in the occurrence of these circular fissures is the same as in the similar circular fissures occurring in connection with bending fractures produced by blows with blunt instruments, such as hammers and bolts. A bullet entering the skull at an angle at first presses in the skull and then proceeds to produce fracture. The portion of the skull depressed by the forcible impulse of the projectile undergoes the same changes as are produced in connection with less degrees of violence.

It is bent in, broken at the periphery of the depressed area, and returns to its normal position. At the point where the bullet having broken out a piece of the skull leaves the same, the changes produced are as constant as those described at the point of impact. At this place there is always an irregular fracture, with comminution, as well as a few or numerous fissures. Some of the detached splinters are forced by the bullet under the edge of the bone or into the brain, other splinters may remain embedded in the soft parts, and still others be torn away with the projectile.

Fig. 41.

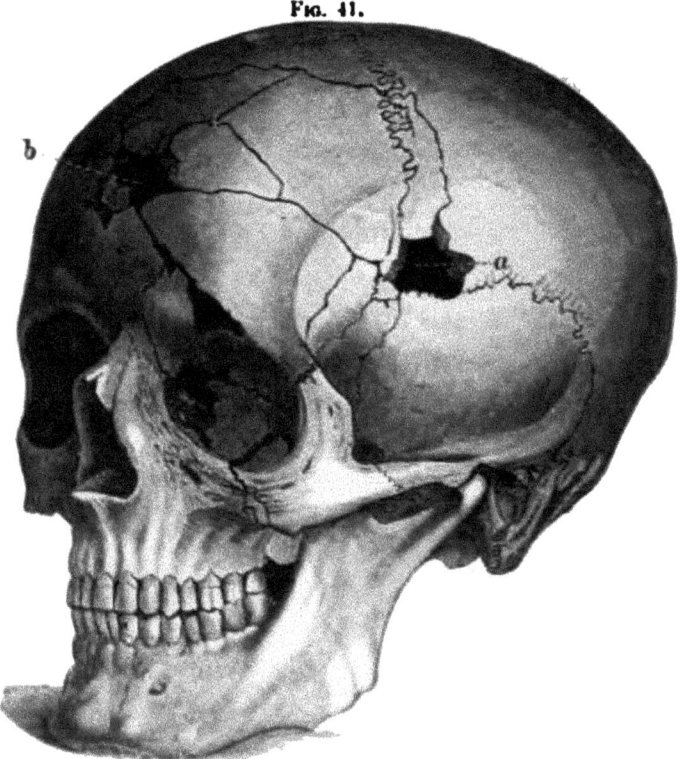

Gunshot wound of skull.

The comminution of the inner table is more extensive at the site of impact than at the wound of exit, where, however, the outer table is more seriously damaged. The outline resulting from comminution of the bone may vary very much. At times the wound of exit is broader than any other part of the loss of substance, at others narrow and elongated.

The illustration Fig. 42 shows the above-described conditions. A bullet struck the skull of a commanding officer in front, in the direction indicated by *a*. Two fissures, *b* and *c*, extend from the broader end and are joined by a third transverse fissure. At the latter end of the defect

the outer table is not so sharply cut as at *a*, but irregularly
Two large fragments of bone had been forced under the ε
fracture. This case possesses additional interest owing to tl
at the same time both orbital plates were fractured. T
b and *c* may therefore be considered beginning bursting fι
well as the fissures, and comminution of the orbital plates. T᾽
impact of the bullet altered the shape of the skull as a whole,
by its bursting along the line of the affected meridian. T
furrow surrounding the anterior end of the loss of substance i
fracture, in the same sense that the fissure connecting *b* and
also follows a circular course. In other cases numerous raι
extended in all directions from the site of a projectile that ϊ

FIG. 42.

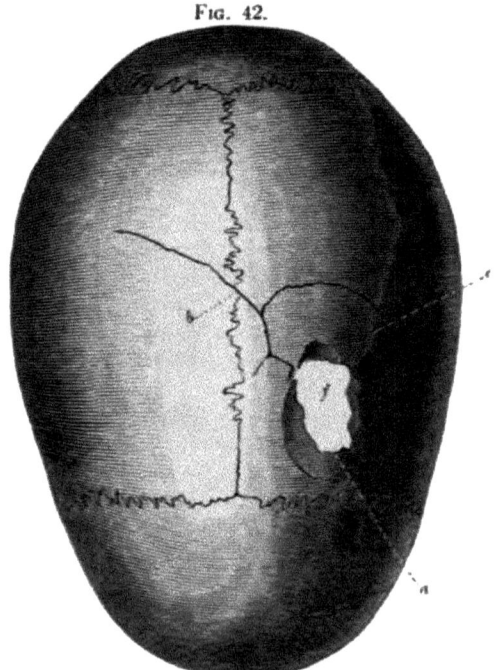

Gunshot-wound of skull. *a.* Point of impact. *b, c.* Two fissures leading tl

embedded in the skull. These can unquestionably be refe
wedge action of the penetrating foreign body. The authι
specimens in which the projectile remained embedded and st
bone. This condition is shown in the illustrations (Fig. 43),
Stromeyer's *Maximen der Kreigsheilkunst.* It is easily com
that a soft-lead bullet may be cut, split, or completely divided
against a sharp edge of bone. For this reason it frequent
that portions of a bullet are found in the cavity of the woun
rest has been carried deep into the brain. Some of the lea

stripped off at the edge of a wound, remaining as a fine deposit with metallic lustre when examined by the eye or with the assistance of a lens, and giving the impression of having been cast in the bone. It is not only the irregularity of the edge of the fracture, the notches, and indentations that cause abrasion of the metal, but the soft consistency of the bullet as well.

Fig. 43.

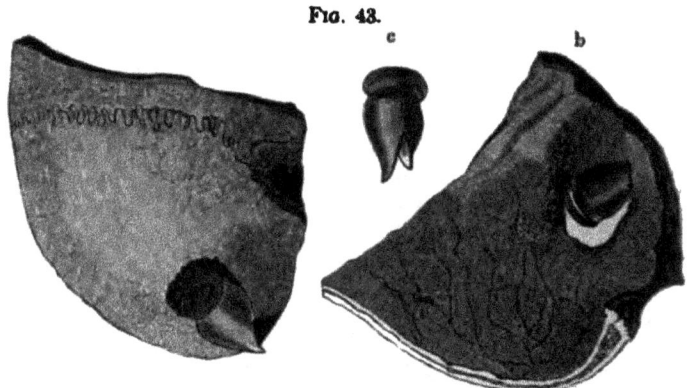

Gunshot-wound of skull. Projectiles embedded and straddling bone.

Ordinary pistol-shots and revolver-shots, even at short range, produce none or at most only short radial fissures, and one or two concentric ones about the hole resulting from the cylindrical bullet. They rarely traverse the entire skull so as to leave a wound of entrance and of exit,

Fig. 44.

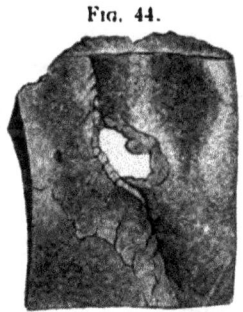

Showing wound of entrance produced by a small pistol bullet from without

Fig. 45.

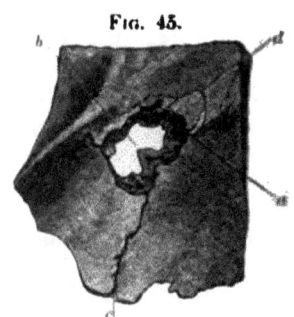

Showing wound of entrance produced by a small pistol bullet from within. a. Defect in the outer table. b. Defect in the inner table. c. Fissure. d. Detached piece of skull.

usually remaining embedded in the brain. Where there are two openings, their form is characteristic, and it is always easy to tell at once which is the wound of entrance and of exit.

The wound of entrance produced by a small pistol bullet in the case of a young suicide is shown from without in Fig. 44, and from within in Fig. 45; *a* is the boundary of the defect in the outer table, *b* in the inner table. On the internal surface will be found in addition a fissure, *c*, and a piece broken off at *d*. The difference in size of these defects is only determined by the usual direction of the shot from without inward. This may be demonstrated by firing at the skull of a cadaver. If a skull-cap, as it is usually removed from the head in autopsies, be freely suspended and shots fired at the convex surface, the inner table always sustains a more extensive opening than the outer; if, however, a shot be fired against the concave surface, the reverse results, and the hole in the outer table is the larger one. It can be easily demonstrated that the greater size of the hole of exit is not produced by the diminished velocity of the projectile. If two boards be set up with a space between them, and a bullet fired through both, the hole of exit in each board will be greater than the hole of entrance. In the case of the skull the wound in the outer table is made by the foreign body itself, while that of the inner table is caused not only by the bullet, but also by the fragments of bone broken from the layers of bone already traversed: the external table and the diploë. The internal opening is not only larger, but is also usually irregular in outline, with a notched and broken edge owing to the fact that it is produced, not by a spherical projectile alone, but by splinters and fragments carried along with it. Should a bullet penetrate the entire skull from one side to the other, the outer table will be more extensively comminuted than the inner for the reasons just explained. The ordinary 5 to 9 mm. revolver bullets have only a very small momentum. Where this is greater, as, for example, in the army revolver, and still more so in the Mauser magazine pistol, pistol-shot wounds are similar to those produced by the modern infantry rifle. The steel-mantled bullet with hard head-core of the magazine pistol has a higher velocity than the Chassepot rifle, that of the former being 425 metres (1300 feet). It produces less shattering than the latter, however, not because of its smaller dimensions, but owing to the fact that on account of its mantle it is not deformed. In the case of short-range shot-wounds of the skull destruction of bones and soft parts is not so extensive as that produced by the projectile of the model 88, because of its lower initial velocity. The injuries produced by the pistol at short range correspond to those produced by long-range rifle-shots. The effect produced by the pistol at 10 to 100 metres (32 to 320 feet) is about like that of the rifle at 1000 to 1600 metres (3200 to 5200 feet), according to v. Bruns. Pistol-shots of the skull exert a decided explosive action, though at a range of from 10 to 100 metres (32 to 320 feet) the force appears much diminished.

Treatment.—The treatment of gunshot-wounds of the skull cannot be considered apart from the accompanying cerebral injuries. Any measure directed toward the bones can only be considered as a solution of part of the problem. The points that might be brought up here will nearly all be discussed in the chapter devoted to Injuries of the Brain.

Though the danger of wounds of the brain produced by the modern infantry rifle is very serious, there are still a number of those struck in the head that remain alive and are brought to the dressing stations. In

It is bent in, broken at the periphery of the depressed area, and returns to its normal position. At the point where the bullet having broken out a piece of the skull leaves the same, the changes produced are as constant as those described at the point of impact. At this place there is always an irregular fracture, with comminution, as well as a few or numerous fissures. Some of the detached splinters are forced by the bullet under the edge of the bone or into the brain, other splinters may remain embedded in the soft parts, and still others be torn away with the projectile.

Fig. 41.

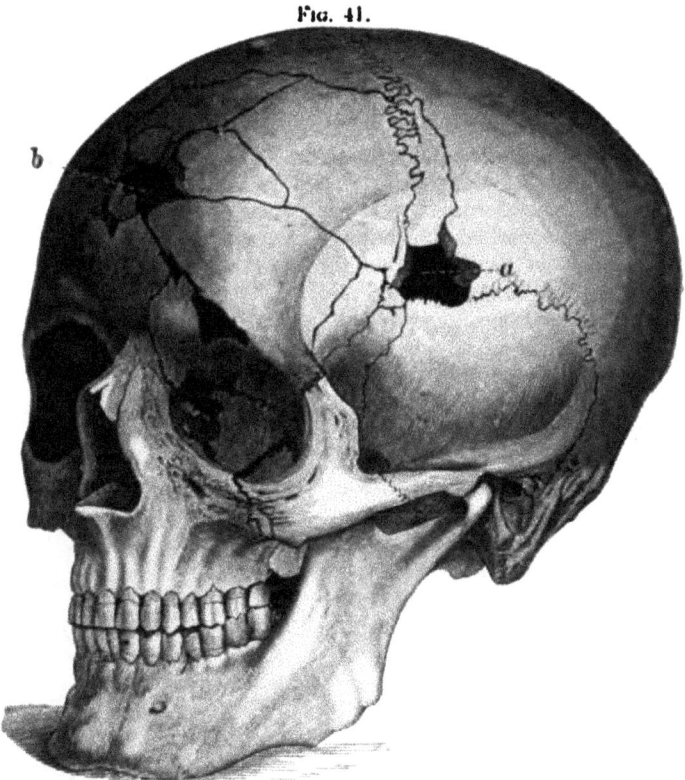

Gunshot-wound of skull.

The comminution of the inner table is more extensive at the site of impact than at the wound of exit, where, however, the outer table is more seriously damaged. The outline resulting from comminution of the bone may vary very much. At times the wound of exit is broader than any other part of the loss of substance, at others narrow and elongated.

The illustration Fig. 42 shows the above-described conditions. A bullet struck the skull of a commanding officer in front, in the direction indicated by a. Two fissures, b and c, extend from the broader end and are joined by a third transverse fissure. At the latter end of the defect

station, is infection, and care should be taken to prevent any further sources of infection from coming in contact with the wound. For this reason Langenbuch recommended tight closure of the wound by primary suturing. The author cannot endorse this suggestion, as blood and secretions flow from gunshot-wounds for some time, and are the best method of removing infections germs. By suturing, this flow is stopped. Only such form of occlusion as will permit free drainage of the wound secretions during the first stages is applicable—that is, packing with sterile absorbent dressing materials, regardless whether they are impregnated with antiseptics or not. If it were possible to protect the wound with a tampon of iodoform gauze inserted a little way, while the surrounding parts are being shaved, it would certainly be recommendable. There is not time to do more even at the most favorably located dressing stations. It is only possible to pack, apply compresses, and bandage with sterile hygroscopic dressing materials. If the dressing be removed at the first hospital station to which the wounded man has been removed, and the wound and general condition of the patient are good, it is wise to continue the same method. If, however, the wound shows signs of inflammation, more is necessary, and the same radical treatment should be applied as was suggested for infected localized fractures of the vault of the skull, namely, thorough and extensive opening up in all directions and antiseptic packing with or without drainage.

In the treatment of recent gunshot-wounds of the skull in time of peace the circumstances are different. Disregarding once more the brain, particularly rapidly increasing intracranial hemorrhage, the treatment of gunshot-wounds of the skull is analogous to that of gunshot-wounds of extremities and joints. In small cutaneous wounds the surgeon never thinks of making an incision, even if he believes in the effectiveness of antiseptic irrigations, but closes the wound under aseptic precautions, with good results; in the case of larger wounds, however, he makes such changes in the same as will promote proper

Fig. 50.

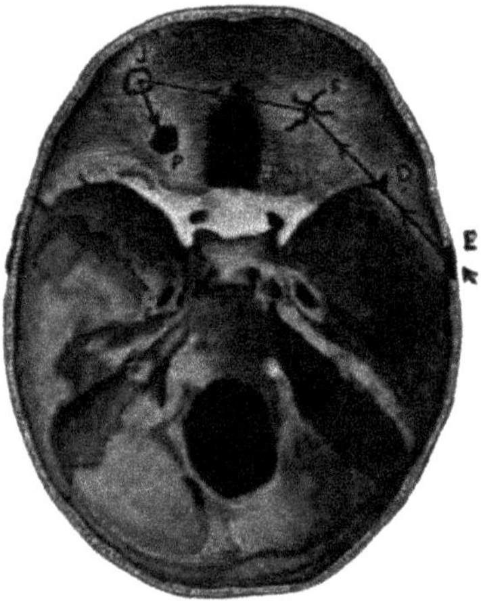

Bullet wound, temporal region (revolver, 7 mm.). Course of bullet: R. Entrance wound. D. Deflect in sphenoid. F. Fissure in orbit. I. Impression of bullet in bone. P. Misshapen bullet.

union. The trimming of recent wounds is not done for the mere purpose of disinfection. Undermined edges and pockets are opened up and divided not for the purpose of being able to apply antiseptics, but in order to arrest thoroughly all hemorrhages and to remove foreign bodies or detached fragments of bone, and above all else to provide free drainage for all wound secretions and their absorption by dressings. T accomplish this it may be necessary to enlarge the wound of the skul' when it is filled with pieces of brain and blood-clots, by means of chis and saw. The author has used this method, as Burkhardt suggestec with good results, and has even employed temporary resection of th skull to open up the cranial cavity.

In one case at the author's clinic v. Bramann enucleated an ha been traversed by a bullet, removed the comminuted orbital th entire outer wall of the orbit, and bringing down a large flap of ski from the frontal and temporal regions, covered the brain that was expose at the bottom of the wound, obtaining primary union of the entire flaj After eight years the author had the opportunity of satisfying himself the good health of the patient and the firm union of the flap. In th case a large portion of the temporal, frontal, and basal surface of th anterior lobe of the brain was covered by a plastic operation, the forms tion and displacement of a skin-flap, and thus protected against infectio after the manner suggested in the treatment of compound fractures the vault of the skull. Small cutaneous wounds such as are produc by revolver-shots and frequently met with in time of peace, the autho has for years treated according to one method regardless whether th bullet was embedded in the brain or not, and has every reason to fee satisfied with the results obtained. After thorough cleansing of th scalp, during which the wound is protected by being loosely packed witl iodoform gauze, he applies an aseptic occlusive dressing. When this i removed after from eight to fourteen days the wound has usually healed Up to 1895 he had obtained this result in 19 of 24 patients. Legge concluded from observation of 43 cases in the hospitals of Munich, an H. Graff at Eppendorf in 9 cases treated with and in 9 cases treated with out trephining, that "simple expectant treatment with aseptic dressing gave better results than primary trephining." There is one objection t this method. If the projectile has not penetrated the skull and remain embedded in or outside the skull, it is more simple to make an incision which is always a superficial one in the case of the head, and to extrac the bullet. By means of the x-ray the superficial or deep location of foreign body can easily be determined.

In the last two cases at the author's clinic the projectile was found i the one case immediately in front of the squamous portion of the tempora bone and in the other case in the frontal region. In both cases it wa excised; the wound, treated according to former methods, was not suture nor closed, but simply packed with iodoform gauze, and covered witl sterile absorbent dressings.

The author has found no occasion to remove at a later stage bullet that had remained embedded in the brain. This is only necessary whet they cause further disturbance, such as secondary hemorrhages and cere bral abscess.

CHAPTER V.

RHACHITIS OF THE SKULL.

THE most prominent change produced by rhachitis of the skull at the beginning and height of the disease is an excessive absorption of bone and the development of imperfect, non-calcified bone in the bones of the vault. These changes are less extensive and less noticeable in the cartilage composing the base.

The changes in the bones characteristic of rhachitis occurring at or before the fourth or fifth month affect the skull, the teeth, and the ribs. The head is really not larger than that of a healthy child at the same age, but it appears to be large when compared with the rest of the skeleton. In addition there is the miserable general appearance of the child, the atrophy of skin and muscles, especially of the face, both of which help to bring the head into greater prominence. The anterior fontanelle is open in all cases and larger in all its dimensions than that of non-rhachitic children. While usually closed at the end of the first year, at the very latest at the end of the fifteenth month, in rhachitis it may remain open much longer—as late as the third year or even later. The most important symptom, however, is the soft consistency of the bone along the lines of sutures and the occurrence of circumscribed soft areas in the occipital regions, which offer about as much resistance to pressure with the fingers as a thin card and can be depressed with little effort, but return promptly to their former position. This soft consistency of the occiput was first brought to the attention of physicians by Elsasser, and the name "craniotabes" was applied to rhachitis of the skull. The greater the degree of softness, the more will the occipital bone be flattened. While the occiput remains soft and flat, the parietal and frontal bones appear thicker; the tuberosities, in particular, become more massive and prominent. Owing to this the vault of the skull loses its spherical form and becomes square and angular (*tête carrée*).

On examining bones taken from the cadaver and holding them up to the light, the soft areas in the occipital bone appear as thinned spots, with only a fine, sieve-like layer of bone, or with the periosteum in intimate contact with the dura. The portions of bone bordering on the lambdoidal, sagittal, and coronal sutures have a similar appearance. On the parietal and frontal bones, on the other hand, are found pink or purplish growths, appearing like a delicate, porous deposit. If the periosteum, which is somewhat reddened and thickened, be stripped from the

(127)

outer surface of bone, this deposit will remain adherent to its inner surface in the shape of small plates or needles. Microscopical examination of these shows osseous tissue, with little or no deposit of lime, very widely scattered. The rhachitic hypertrophy is never exactly symmetrical, but is always developed more on one side than on the other. The illustration (Fig. 51), taken from Heinecke's work, is a faithful representation of this condition. Beneath these dep developed compact layer is much atrophied, and a than it ought to be.

These changes can be explained by the peculiarities of the rhachitic process. In the posterior portions we find absorption of fully developed bone which may proceed to such a degree that the external and internal periosteum may be in contact wth each other. In the anterior portions of the skull, however, the prominent feature is a development of

Fig. 51.

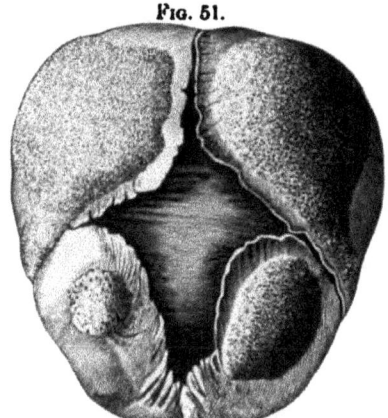

Rhachitic hypertrophy.

bone-tissue very poor in lime, especially in the central portions and in the neighborhood of the tuberosities. Although processes are sent out from the thin, soft, peripheral portions of the cranial bones, there is not sufficient bone developed to bring about closure along the sutures. For this reason the fontanelles remain unclosed and are more extensive than usual. The difference in character between the anterior and posterior portions of the skull can easily be explained by the continued pressure against the latter caused by the constant dorsal position of the child. The internal surface of the occipital bones shows much deeper digital impressions than does the frontal, as if the weight of the brain had pressed upon the bone in the back, while in front it had fallen away. The pressure produced while lying down may favor the process of absorption in the posterior position, while at the sides and front of the skull where there is no pressure the development of new bone-tissue goes on unchecked.

At the base of the skull, which is cartilaginous in character, irregular ossifications and deposits of bone are usually found only at its outer, inferior surface, and even here only in isolated areas and widely scattered. Noticeable features about the skeleton are the marked excavation of the middle fossa and the flattening produced in those portions of bone surrounding the posterior half of the foramen magnum.

The question whether rhachitis could originate during fœtal life was brought up and affirmed by Virchow, who found in children dying at the second week after birth a fully developed rosary and an irregular line of ossification at the anterior ends of the ribs. Kassowitz made investigations on the bodies of stillborn children, or those dying soon after birth, regarding this favorite site of rhachitis, and he came to the conclusion that congenital rhachitis was the usual, if not the exclusive, form of the disease, for he found it in 89.5 per cent. of his cases. As the result of

Fig. 52

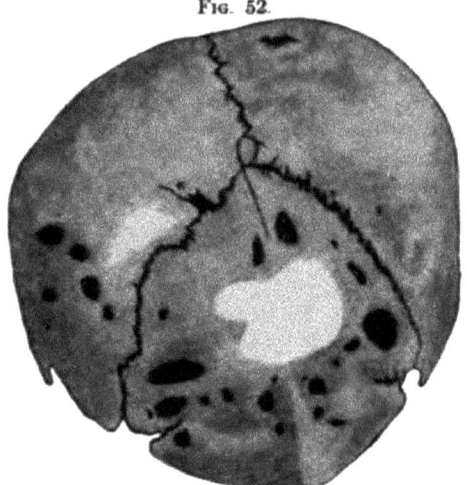

Craniotabes (rhachitis). (Bruns.)

later investigations, however, notably those of Boher and Tschistowitsch, it has been shown that moderate alterations at the junction of the ribs and costal cartilages cannot always be considered a sign of rhachitis, and further that these may frequently be confused with syphilitic osteochondritis occurring in the same place. Nor is the congenital soft consistency of the bone along the sutures a sign of rhachitis. This is always present in the newborn, but rapidly disappears. In addition there are two congenital affections, with disturbances in the development of the cranial bones that are very similar to rhachitis, and yet, according to the researches of Kaufman and Eberth, they are sharply distinguishable. Quite commonly chondrodystrophia or achondroplasia has been mistaken for rhachitis, and quite frequently osteogenesis imperfecta and fragilitas ossium congenita have been included under the same heading. As long as chondrodystrophia of the extremities was not differentiated

from rhachitis, the large fontanelles and the soft borders of the lambdoidal and sagittal sutures were also put down as rhachitic manifestations. At present, when certain distinguishing points in the relation
of the epiphyses of the long bones have been discovered and can at
any time be made visible by the x-ray, it should be easy to distinguish
even in the bones of the skull these two diseases of growing bone that
are so unlike in their outward manifestations. It remains in doubt
still, according to Ziegler's investigations, whether we have to distinguish
from early rhachitis an osteotabes infantum, which begins as a primary
disease of the medulla and is characterized by disappearance of bone
substance that had already been developed.

In imperfect osteogenesis of bone there is, as in rhachitis, the soft
skull that has become flattened owing to the dorsal posture of the
child. The parietal bones, however, are wide apart, especially in their
posterior portions, leaving a large triangular area between them which
is filled with a membranous fibrous tissue containing numerous small
plates of bone generally arranged radially. A similar membrane replaces
the upper half of the occipital bone, and membranous tissue divides the
mastoid process from the squamous portion of the temporal bone. In
other cases only the edges of the cranial bones, especially the frontal,
temporal, parietal, and occipital, show absence of ossification, while,
in the opposite extreme, cases may be observed in which the bones
are almost entirely membranous, only a fine network of bone trabeculæ
being left on examination. Even the bones of the base are as thin as
the feeling of a skull possessing the above-mentioned qualities with an x-ray examination, will determine the diagnosis;
the traces of multiple intrauterine fractures with and
callus will confirm the suspicion of osteogenesis
of the skull.

that is, originating during fœtal life—occurs
At the same time it is certain that the roof of the skull,
the junction of the costal cartilage, are involved as the
rhachitis occurring even before the end of the
The most frequent as well as most serious complication
occurring at this early period in parts of the body
spasm of the glottis (laryngismus stridulus). The
the more marked are the changes in the skull,
of the latter alone the diagnosis can easily be
symptoms, night-terrors, and various dis-
perspiration of the head sets in, which may be
under the child's head are saturated, while
portions of the body is hot and dry. At
relative to touch. Children who formerly
crying every fifteen minutes. Chang-
them immediately, but only for a
against the pillow and bury them in
in the arms of the nurse, it will
in a sitting posture, undoubtedly

general osteomalacia, but belongs rather under the head of fibr
ostitis deformans, to be described immediately below.

Though the bones are apparently hard and thick, the processes go
on in the interior in the way of bone formation and absorption, with
any changes on the surface or alteration in form, are more marked tl
in any part of the body. The thickening and deformity of bones occ
ring spontaneously and progressing gradually have been clearly explaii
in the works of Paget and v. Recklinghausen on ostitis deformans a
its relation to osteomalacia. Marked deformities of the skull occur
the course of both. Virchow demonstrated before the Berliner Naturl
scher Versammlung in 1886 a case of excessive hyperostosis of the sk
with hyperostosis and curvature of the femur, besides ivory-like b
processes at the angles of curvature, large fibrocartilaginous areas, a
cysts. V. Recklinghausen made independent investigations of g
importance bearing on this specimen, regarding cysts and fibrous aı
of the occipital bone and in the bone-marrow of most of the hollow boɪ
These findings, as well as the occurrence of real sarcoma in simili
changed bones, and finally the connection of the new growths in seco
ary diffuse carcinoma of the bones, led v. Recklinghausen to investiɣ
the manifestations common to both diseases. As a matter of fact, Pag
"osteomalacia chronica deformans" can hardly be distinguished fɪ
v. Recklinghausen's tumor-forming ostitis deformans. In both cases
bone-marrow had been changed into fibrous connective tissue, especi
at the angles of curvature, and the changes from marrow-fat tissue i
real fibrous tissue is shown in all the different stages, with this differe
that in v. Recklinghausen's cases the changes in the marrow were m
marked and had gone on to the formation of cysts and the developm
of sarcoma. In Paget's description the changes in the skull play
most important part. The bones consist almost entirely of a bright-ı
soft substance that is easily cut, and which is bounded externally a
internally by a thin layer of compact bone. At the same time they
markedly thickened, for which reason the forehead of the patient is bɪ
and very convex, the hollow of the temple is raised up, and the occi
projects considerably. In this way the head, which is usually bɪ
appears remarkably large, with thickened superciliary and orbital ridɟ
Taking into consideration the asymmetrical arrangement, accordinɟ
which one-half of the skull is affected more than the other, and
irregularities and protuberances of the surface, this deformity is eaɪ
recognizable. In no other case was the skull alone affected.

The curvature of the lower extremities causes the total length of
body to be much diminished. This is caused in part by the kyphɪ
of the vertebral column. After the bones of the lower extremities,
clavicle was most frequently affected, being markedly thickened a
broadened.

No successful treatment of deforming or tumor-forming ostitis has
yet been reported, though many methods have been suggested and tri

Senile Atrophy.—Senile atrophy of bone resembles in its finer p
cesses the absorption of bone of neurotic origin, as, for example, tl

form occurring in some varieties of insanity. Senile atrophy of tl
is usually eccentric. The trabeculæ of the diploë are absorbed un
have nearly disappeared, while the cortical plates become thinner
porosis or porotic atrophy). As the bone retains its original fo₁
changes going on in its inner structure will escape the notice of th₁
cian unless some act of violence, such as blows or kicks, produce f
with depression, which has been observed occasionally in apopleci
paralytics.

If this eccentric atrophy be limited to single areas of the skul
will result depressions similar to those produced by pressure of p
ating Pacchionian bodies. Hollows of the bone on the external

FIG. 53.

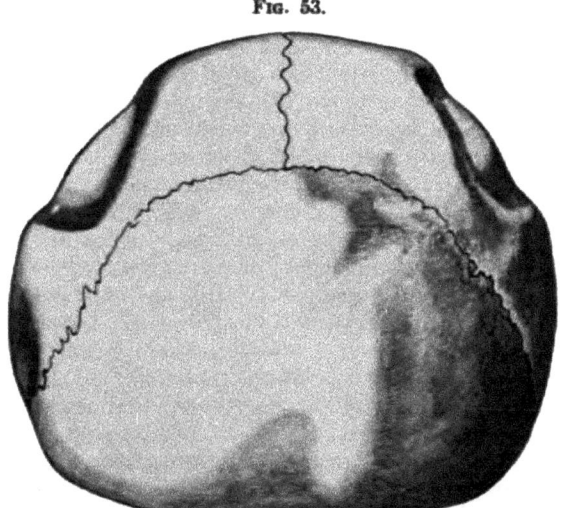

Senile atrophy of vault of skull. Defect in external table in middle portions of pariet₁
one-third natural size. (Ziegler.)

are produced only by very vascular tumors, such as racemose anei
never by sebaceous cysts. The hollows occupied by dermoi₁
are the result of impaired development of bone, in the san
that congenital lipomata are frequently found located in a h₁
the bone.

A peculiar form of atrophy is presented by symmetrical dep₁
.n both parietal bones in the region of their eminences which ₁
with occasionally in old people. Owing to the fact that at ti₁
portion along the edges slopes off toward the central portions, th
be mistaken for depressed fractures or even syphilitic affection₁
skull. Their real character can, however, be determined by the
metrical occurrence, the history, and other symptoms of the di₁
injury in regard to which the question would arise. (Fig. 53.)

TUMORS OF THE CRANIAL BONES.

Osteoma.—Only fibrous tissue exostoses occur on the vault of skull, as the development of cartilaginous exostoses takes place on those parts of the skeleton that are originally formed of cartilage where the latter exists for some time—that is, at the site of transit cartilage surfaces. Compact ivory-like exostoses are more frequ met with on the skull than spongy ones. The distinction between toses originating in the periosteum and enostoses developing from marrow of the diploë cannot be made in the case of the skull, fo enclosed osteomata of the frontal and nasal sinuses classed with latter originate either from the periosteum or the cartilaginous rudi of the ethmoid bone.

The favorite site of exostoses of the vault is on the frontal or par bones. They are located on the external or internal surface of the or on both. In the latter case dense sclerotic tissue, the parenchym the growth, is found in the diploë separating the external and int portion. Though generally single, exostoses may be multiple, like illustrated in Virchow's work on tumors, so that a large portion o skull may be studded with these wart-like bony tumors. These exos of the skull vary greatly in size.

Pedunculated growths are also found. They have a broad base the shape of truncated cones or are spread out like mushrooms slender stems. Smaller tumors usually have a smooth surface, whil larger kind are rough, warty, and prickly. The smooth forms, whic are generally found on the external surface, while the nodular or tite forms usually occur on the internal surface of the bones. Both are covered with a very thin layer of periosteum and dura. The ve like osteophytic deposits found on the inner surface of the skull in w who have died during pregnancy or the puerperal period are well kn These may be of every size and form. The surface may be smoot nodular and lobulated.

A large, if not the largest, specimen of exostosis is shown in Fig taken from an illustration in v. Volkmann's *Diseases of the Orga Locomotion.* The exostoses in this case were developed both extern as well as internally, to a considerable degree, appearing like a mas tubers and nodules. The neighboring cranial bones were thick and I on cross-section.

Traumatic origin has been frequently claimed in the case of t exostoses, but has seldom been proved.

Exostoses of the orbit are of special interest. Their favorite site i the labyrinth of the ethmoid bone and the neighboring sinuses of frontal and sphenoid bones. Though surrounded by bone they are enostoses, as they arise in a cavity situated within the bone, and n necessarily therefore be enclosed by the wall of this cavity, which may occupy to a considerable extent. In so far they resemble enosto but they do not originate in the diploë, but from the periosteum un lying the mucous membrane lining the cavities of the frontal sinus it is possible that they result from the remains of fœtal cartilage, as it is well known that the ethmoid is derived from this kind of tissue. Accordingly they ought properly to be called encapsulated osteomata. Knowledge of their development and clinical aspects is owing to the works of Arnold and Bornhaupt. The latter collected 49 cases of encapsulated exostoses of the bone sinuses, to which Tichof added observations on 29 cases. All osteomata of the frontal sinus are composed of a hard, ivory-hke shell enclosing a central spongy portion. The former

Fig. 54.

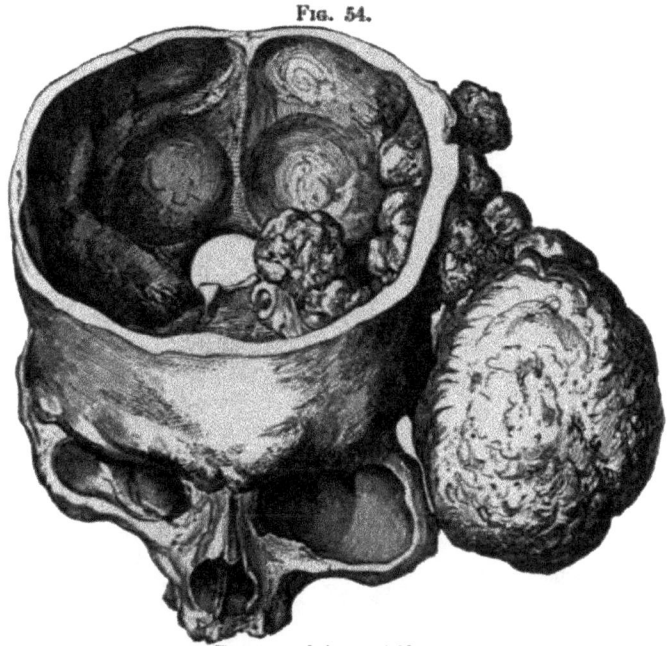

Exostoses of the cranial bones.

exceeded the latter in quantity to such a degree that the central nucleus might easily be overlooked. The form of these tumors is apparently dependent on the resistance met with in the course of their development. They distend the walls of the bony cavity in which they are placed, finally breaking through at different places. These perforations usually occur externally and anteriorly through the vertical plate of the frontal bone or inferiorly through the roof of the orbit. They may be unilateral or bilateral.

Symptoms.—Clinical manifestations of osteoma of the frontal sinus usually begin to be noticeable at the time of puberty. It begins as a diffuse swelling gradually becoming more prominent, situated at the inner angle of the orbit in the case of unilateral growths; in the middle of the forehead when they occur bilaterally. The swelling has the same appearance as that caused by effusion and empyema of the frontal sinuses. Such collections of fluid frequently complicate osteoma, especially when the efferent canal has been displaced or obstructed by the growth. As soon as the tumor encroaches on the orbit the displacement of the eyeball downward, forward, and a little outward is characteristic.

Fig. 55.

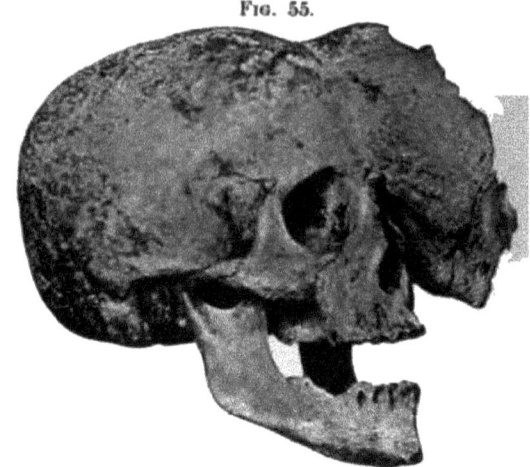

Osteoma of skull. (Mudd.)

Fig. 56.

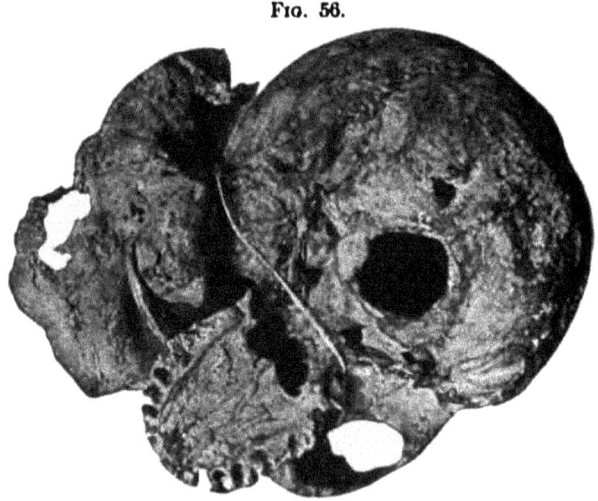

Same, seen from below.

The slow growth of these tumors explains the absence of symptoms due to cerebral pressure, even after they have invaded the cavity of the skull.

Free exostoses located on the walls of the orbital cavity are less frequent than the encapsulated variety. These hard, sharply circumscribed, bony tumors have the same anatomical structure as the enclosed forms. They are most frequently located at the supraorbital ridge and, in distinction from osteoma of the frontal sinus, more at the lateral portions. Another point of difference is their rough, irregular surface and the fact that they are more sharply set off from the neighboring bones.

Diagnosis.—The diagnosis of orbital—that is, frontal and sphenoidal —exostoses is based on their slow growth without pain, the typical swelling of the bones, the displacement of the eyeball, and the invasion of the cranial cavity and the nasal passages. In the beginning they may be mistaken for central sarcoma, later for empyema of the frontal sinus. The latter frequently follows as a complication. An important point in the differential diagnosis is the extremely slow growth of these tumors. Symptoms of effusion into the frontal sinus may help to distinguish between mural and encapsulated exostoses of the orbit, as these occur only in connection with the latter. Dpengel points out that the occurrence of a fistula opening externally, provided the existence of an exostosis has been determined, is a positive sign that the growth originated in the frontal sinus, as the skin never becomes ulcerated over the mural exostosis even when the latter attains considerable size. In some cases, according to Tillmans, inflammation of the frontal sinus has produced complete separation of the exostosis from its base of attachment, causing it to lie freely in the cavity of the sinus like a sequestrum or "dead osteoma." If a probe be passed into such a fistula, the hard, bare bone that is felt might lead to the conclusion that there was necrosis of the wall of the sinus. Osteoma of the sphenoidal sinus advancing forward will, owing to its closer proximity to the optic nerve, be more likely to produce impairment of vision. Otherwise the eyeball, though displaced by mural or encapsulated exostoses, retains its form and functions.

Exostoses of the vault of the skull are easily recognized, and are only liable to be mistaken for central sarcoma in the early stages of development. Their slow growth, their sharply defined boundaries, their conical and mushroom shape, cause them to be unmistakable. If there is an exostosis on the inner surface corresponding to the one on the outer, or, more properly speaking, when the external one traverses the entire thickness of the skull and extends into the cranial cavity, cerebral symptoms may be present, particularly in affections of those portions of the skull lying over the motor area. The early operations for epilepsy were directed toward the removal of these tumors. If the bone be smooth and even on the outer surface, the existence of an exostosis on the inner surface can be determined only by the presence of cerebral symptoms. In such cases the diagnosis is the same as that of cerebral tumors occurring in cases in which there are no changes in the skull.

Treatment.—The treatment of osteoma of the skull, including exostoses of the orbit and frontal sinus, requires radical removal, providing the size of the tumor permits it. The necessary incisions of the bones and soft parts are, generally speaking, the same in all cases, as they must be made with the object of exposing the tumor and to chisel or saw it away as close as possible to the surface of the bone from which it projects.

traverses the bone, it can only be removed by resecting a portion of roof of the skull, which operation will be discussed more fully in chapter treating of sarcoma of the skull.

Operations for osteoma of the orbit have not been regarded with favor on account of the high mortality rate, which Berlin estima 38 per cent. At the same time it is not justifiable to place all su operations in one class when making these calculations. If an opera is able to reach the base of a mural exostosis at the roof of the or and to remove it, as Knapp was able to do, the prognosis will be m favorable.

Many unsuccessful removals, such as those reported by Berlin, w done before the days of antisepsis. With the modern methods of p venting infection, no surgeon should hesitate to expose the infer surface of the frontal lobe of the brain. According to Durante, ev sarcoma of the base of the skull has been attacked in this way and go results obtained. In operations on tumors of the frontal sinus there a not only great technical difficulties to contend with, but also the difficu in applying antiseptics, owing to the fact that in opening the frontal sir the nasal passage is opened as well, and frequently the exostosis is fou bathed in pus. It is therefore easy to understand why of 15 cases operation on osteoma of the frontal sinus invading the cranial cav collected by Chipault as late as 1894 only 5 were successful; in t remaining 10 cases the patients died of a purulent meningitis or cereb abscess. There was also the additional fact that, prior to Bornhaup work, the anatomical relations of encapsulated osteoma were very imp fectly understood. Attempts were made to chisel away the portions of t tumor projecting into the orbital cavity, thus never getting beyond or the limits of the growth. Since then it has been learned that it is necessa to open up the bony capsule surrounding the tumor and attempt remove it at its base of attachment. By proceeding in this manner near all operations on encapsulated orbital osteomata have been successf (Nakel). The methods employed are the same as those used in empyen of the frontal sinus. An incision is made horizontally from the root the nose immediately above the supraorbital ridge toward the templ From the horizontal incision another is made vertically in the middle the forehead. If the tumor has not broken through the anterior wall the frontal sinus, the latter is removed by means of chisel, hammer, Luer's forceps. By pinching off the bone toward the orbital cavity th latter is opened up and the tumor pried out with an elevator. If th growth be of considerable size, it is usually necessary to remove th posterior wall of the frontal sinus or the roof of the orbit. Immediat closure of the wound with the flaps of soft parts should be done onl when there is no fistula in the skin and no inflammation of the sinus In the latter case packing with iodoform gauze is indicated. The autho would suggest that in all cases this be used in the median incision whicl communicates with the nasal cavity.

Leontiasis.—A number of specimens preserved in museums as e:
ples of excessive craniosclerosis are characterized by an enormous tl
ness of the cranial bones, accompanied by obliteration of the spac
the diploë. The specimen in the Dupuytren museum has been
quently described, and is similar, as are all of them, to the one sb
in Fig. 57, taken from Volkmann's *Diseases of the Organs of Loc
tion.* This thickening is usually uniform in character. Cases do oc
however, in which certain portions project more prominently, and t
have been described as tumor-like hyperostoses.

The cranial bones may attain a thickness of from 4 to 5 cm., v
the bones of the face are developed to such a degree that the weigl
the macerated skull will be five times that of the normal skull.
deposits of bone on both surfaces, but particularly on the inner,

Fig. 57.

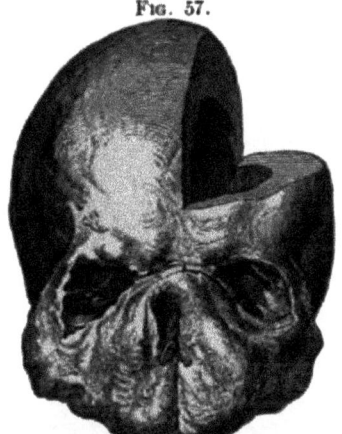

Leontiasis of the cranial bones.

cranial cavity is diminished in size and the orbital cavity filled up;
nares become tenosed and immovable, and the vessels and nerves lea
and entering the skull are pressed upon.

The progress of the disease is very slow and gradual. The au
observed in a boy in whom the deformity was noticeable at the t
year, that five years later there had only been an extension of the pre
to bones not previously affected, but no increase at the site of the orig
thickening. This corresponds to the history of development in a
of Forcade which has become more generally known than any of
It was that of a boy who had been well up to his twelfth year, at w
time his father, it seems, had opened the lachrymal sac at the inner a
of the right eye on account of distention due to a blennorrhœa. Sh
afterward there was noticed a swelling the size of an almond over
nasal process of the right superior maxillary bone, which increase
such an extent that in the course of fifteen years the nose was ent
stenosed. The inferior maxilla then became thickened, remaining

mal only at the articulations and the alveolar processes. The superior maxilla, the walls of the orbit with the exception of the roof, the hard palate, and the zygomatic processes were affected and became shapeless masses. Exophthalmos developed, causing myopia. There also resulted difficulty in speech, blindness, and psychical degeneration approaching total idiocy. The patient lived until he was forty-six years old.

Neither traumatism nor syphilis can be ascribed as a cause of this very typical disease. In several instances erysipelas of the scalp seems to have favored an increase in the thickening of the bones, the latter taking place regularly with each attack of erysipelas. These circumstances led Virchow to consider the disease as analogous to elephantiasis of the soft parts of the extremities, and caused him to designate it as leontiasis of the bones, it being believed that chronic inflammatory processes of the bones could in the same manner bring about an hypertrophy of osseous tissue.

FIG. 58.

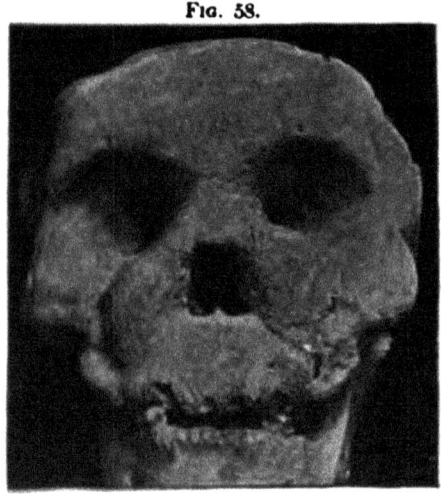

Leontiasis: skull of a Chinese woman (U. S. A. Museum, No. 10680). (Park.)

Leontiasis begins, as a rule, in one of the bones of the face, and often escapes notice for some time. The patient suffers no disturbance during the first years of its course. There is no pain, no loss of function; only the thickening of the bone becomes evident. Then exophthalmos develops. The displacement of the eyeball and the stretching and pressure on the optic nerve are followed after considerable time by amaurosis and phthisis bulbi. Later, disturbances in respiration and loss of the sense of smell are brought about by stenosis of the nasal passages. To these are added headache, at first in remittent attacks, later becoming continuous. Neuralgias, convulsions, and paralyses are caused in part by diminution in the size of the cranial cavity and also by pressure on the nerves passing through openings at the base of the skull. Finally, psychical disturbances predominate, leading to complete dementia. In all cases the course of the disease covers a period of many years, as in the case described by Forcade.

Symptoms.—The clinical picture in the stage of full development establishes the diagnosis without question. There might possibly be a likelihood of mistaking the disease for acromegaly. However, the latter always begins at the epiphyses of the bones of the lower and upper extremities, even if the bones of the face are subsequently involved. It is only necessary to note the site of origin of the disease to distinguish acromegaly from leontiasis, which is always limited to the bones of the cranium and face. A doubtful diagnosis might be occasioned by syphilitic hyperostoses of the skull and face. The latter, however, are never so uniform and extensive as general craniosclerosis. There are also the accompanying syphilitic manifestations in the face of syphilitic patients—keratitis and iritis, ozæna, ulcerations of the hard palate, and irregularities of gummatous ostitis of the roof of the skull. Differential diagnosis from Paget's ostitis deformans can always be made on account of the deformities of the extremities present in the latter disease.

Treatment.—No therapeutic measures have so far been successful in leontiasis. In all cases in which improvement followed the administration of potassium iodide and mercury the disease was not general craniosclerosis, but syphilitic partial thickening of the bone.

Echinococcus.—Of 52 cases of echinococcus of the bones described by Gangolphe, only 4 involved the cranial bones. Three were in the frontal and one was sphenoidal, filling the cavity of the sphenoid. In all cases the cysts were unilocular. The description of echinococcus of the frontal bone by the elder Langenbeck and Keats was for a long time the basis of a clinical picture of echinococcus of the bones in general. The sac, the size of a man's fist or even larger, was located between the two tables of the frontal bone, of which the inner was thickened and the outer considerably thinned. The four cases collected by Gangolphe occurred in individuals seven, seventeen, and eighteen years of age, with a very gradual development of the disease, originating probably in earliest childhood. There was no disturbance beyond the thickening of the forehead over and extending a little beyond the anterior wall of the frontal sinus. In Langenbeck's case the thinned external table crackled like parchment when pressed upon with the fingers. In one case there was a fistulous tract leading into the interior of the sinus. Observers have reported at length in regard to disturbances of vision in their patients.

Diagnosis.—The diagnosis can only be made with certainty if the examination of the fluid trickling from a sinus shows the characteristic booklets. In general, chronic purulent inflammation of the frontal sinus or osteoma would be more likely to be suspected than echinococcus. Myelogenous sarcoma would show a decidedly more rapid growth.

Treatment.—Operative treatment is the only one applicable. The skin is divided and procedures adopted similar to those employed in osteoma of the frontal sinus. After removal of the anterior wall of the sinus, instead of finding a solid tumor, the sac of the cyst is discovered. The wound cavity should be filled with iodoform gauze, and drainage of the

secretions collecting in the nasal passages provided for by openir
the communication between the latter and the frontal sinus.

Sarcoma.—Tumors composed of sarcomatous tissue occur prin
on the skull, and are, like all other sarcomata of bone, periostea,
peripheral, or myelogenous and central. During recent years V
wange has collected observations on anatomical structure, and Fro
on clinical features. The former reports 88 cases, and the latter 47
which were his own. Compared with those of the extremities, sar
of the head rarely occurs. Males were affected in about 60 per ce
the cases; females in 40 per cent. Every age seems equally dispos
the development of the disease. According to both authors, the tem
bone is most frequently affected; after this the frontal, parietal,
occipital. Of Weisswang's cases, 23 had undoubtedly originated i
periosteum, 40 in the bone-marrow. The result of microscopical e
ination in 18 of the former showed most frequently spindle-cell
round-cell sarcoma; 3 showed osteosarcoma and 3 chloroma.]
examinations of the myelogenous type the results were about the ?
except that giant-cell sarcoma was more frequently reported, as wen
round-cell and spindle-cell sarcoma, showing a scattering of giant
while alveolar sarcoma, osteosarcoma, and chloroma were second i
latter class.

Etiology.—In regard to the etiology, several instances have been
ported in which traumatism immediately preceded the development
a tumor. Such was reported in Grünberg's communication. No
nection, however, was found to exist between the two, nor are
conclusive examples to be found in Löwenthal's collection.

Course.—The course of sarcoma of the skull, when not interfered
is the same as that of sarcoma of the bones in other parts of the t
Periosteal as well as myelogenous sarcoma grows rapidly and soon l
to death, owing to destruction of the brain and the formation of nume
metastases. Peripheral sarcoma offers a less favorable prognosis
does central sarcoma. The richer in cells the tumor, the more dange
it is. Sarcoma of the skull of many years' standing is always a spin
cell sarcoma with an abudant fibrous connective-tissue stroma. O
average, most cases of sarcoma of the skull end fatally in from on
two years.

The early development of sarcoma of the cranial bones usually esc
notice. A swelling is discovered casually, or on account of difficult
combing the hair. As it grows rapidly, the patient is led to seek surj
aid. Even at this stage the surgeon is confronted by the question whe
he has to deal with a sarcoma of the bone or a perforating sarcom
the brain.

As long as sarcoma of the dura remains enclosed within the cavit
the skull its clinical features are those of cerebral tumors, with whic
will be discussed in a later chapter. From the moment, however,
tumor appears on the outer surface of the skull it should be distinguis
from similar sarcomata of the bones. In most cases, though not in
this is possible.

The fungus duræ matris, by which old term these tumors were designated, has until quite recently been often considered a primary carcinoma of the dura, probably because here alveolar sarcoma is so frequently found, as is also a class of tumors closely related to the latter, the endotheliomata originating in the lymph-spaces of the dura. The majority of the new growths, however, are spindle-cell sarcomata. Those arising from the dura are characterized by stratified lime concretions scattered throughout the growth, which originate in the cells themselves and are described in the beginning as laminated formations, of glassy appearance, without any deposit of lime having taken place at this stage. It is only later, when the centre of the formation takes on a dark-blue stain and the peripheral portions a red one, that lime is deposited to any extent.

Fig. 59.

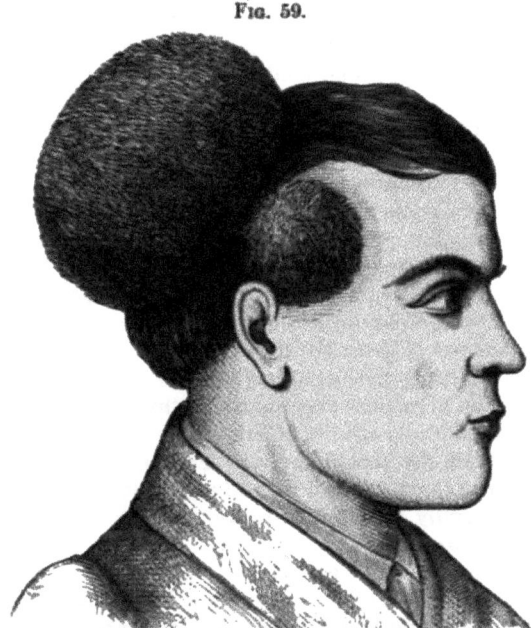

Sarcoma of skull.

Symptoms.—The symptoms of sarcoma of the skull, including perforating tumors of the dura, may be divided into local symptoms of a tumor of the vault of the skull, the extrusion of the growth, and the central disturbances.

On the skull a broad, immovable, adherent swelling is felt and seen, the appearance of which as it exists beneath the unchanged hairy scalp is depicted in Fig. 59, taken from the work of Heinecke, which has been frequently quoted. Even when a growth has attained the size of that shown in the illustration, the skin over it is freely movable, though extensively traversed by a network of veins. The rich vascular supply of a

peripheral sarcoma is frequently shown in distinct pulsation p
by dilated tortuous arteries. As the growth increases in size it
more firmly adherent to the overlying skin, and the latter bec
thin that the new growth, with its numerous bloodvessels, become
through it. The surface may become necrotic, there being found
ous ulcers with a smooth floor of a dirty yellowish-red color
surface may become gangrenous and, as the result of external
the slough be thrown off, followed by hemorrhage. In oth
spongy protuberances grow up through the defective skin. The
easily, and this has led to the use of the term "fungus." Finall
tion of these spongy growths may proliferate, slough off, and
deep, crater-like ulcer.

Sarcoma of the skull shows a tendency to increase in size a
early stage of development. This takes place in the form of se
nodules, located at first near the base, and later forming at some
from the original tumor. The tendency to local dissemination
diseased bone explains the frequency of recurrences. The tenc
develop secondary nodules can only be determined by micro
examination, and will therefore escape the notice of the operato
growths of sarcomatous nature take place from these rudimentary
In the case shown in the illustration a secondary nodule of qu
siderable size may be seen close to the original tumor. All
belonging to this class of sarcoma have a strong tendency to forn
tases in other parts of the body, both in bones and in the visce

In the case shown in the illustration only ten months elapsed,
ing to Heinecke's report, from the time the original tumor devel
the occiput to the time the secondary growth in the temporal
became noticeable. On close examination a third tumor, the si
apple, was found on the ninth rib, which, judging from its size, p
originated at about the same time as the second one. The
showed numerous tumors in the dura and several large ones in th

Metastases generally occur in the lungs, while the lymph-glan
rule are not involved.

Cerebral symptoms may be general, such as headache, vomitin
pulse, and the results of cerebral pressure. These may be accom
by localized cerebral symptoms. The latter are rarely present
the former. Thus, in the case of a woman from whom the author
a sarcoma by extensive resection of the vault of the skull, tl
symptom of a recurrent growth developing shortly after operati
aphasia. It is important, as hearing on the place of origin of a
to note whether cerebral symptoms appear before the developme
tumor becomes noticeable or whether they appear at a later sta

Diagnosis.—In the diagnosis of sarcoma of the skull it should b
in mind, first, that primary carcinoma of the bones and dura mat
not occur, for the reason that epithelial cells from which these
originate are absent. Researches of v. Volkmann "on certain ch
tumors that must be distinguished from sarcoma" have borne o
conclusion. Even Heller assumed that the growth illustrated in

was a carcinoma until repeated examinations of the specimen by Boström, according to Heinecke, showed it to be an alveolar sarcoma.

Only in the early stages and under conditions rarely present is it possible to determine whether a sarcoma of the skull is myelogenous, periosteal, or arises from the dura mater. If the surface be hard and bone-like, it can only be myelogenous sarcoma or, possibly, a local hyperostosis—that is, periostosis. The history of the case and, when there is doubt, further observation aid in making a differential diagnosis; for instance, in central sarcoma the surface soon becomes altered. There are later softer areas which bulge outward more prominently. The new growth soon breaks through the outer bony wall and proliferates. Quite frequently the summit of the tumor is soft, while the peripheral portions remain hard. In this way the appearance is very similar to that of

Fig. 60.

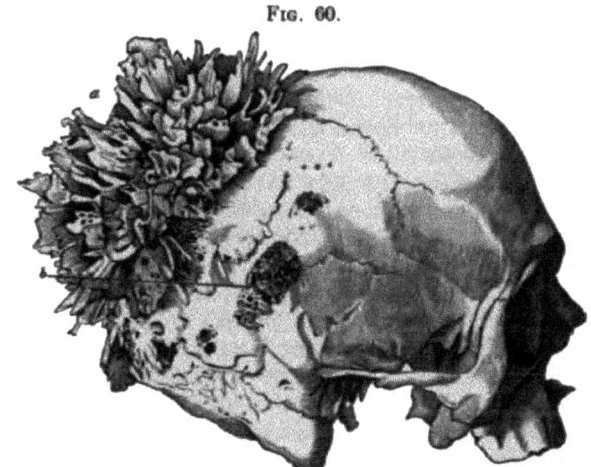

Skeleton of an osteosarcoma of vault of skull. *a.* Skeleton of main tumor mass. *b.* Caries of bone, with bone spicules at site of secondary tumor.

perforating sarcoma of the dura. The latter, however, never lifts up the bony wall of the skull, but destroys it by a process of ulceration, a solution of bone progressing from within outward. It is therefore surrounded after perforation by a bony ring. The latter, however, is on a level with that of the general surface of the skull, and does not, as in the case of myelogenous sarcoma, extend from the base of the tumor toward its summit. Even in specimens from the cadaver in which the growth has attained an enormous size this peculiarity is distinctly noticeable. Within the limits of the growth originating in the diploë there is noticed a divergence of the outer and inner tables, as if they had been forced apart, while within the limits of a sarcoma originating from the dura there is a jagged, notched edge of bone in each table, but the latter is not any further apart than usual. As the soft, spongy tissue of dural sarcoma can be compressed, the sharp edge of bone at the site of perforation can be easily

felt. If every periosteal sarcoma were composed only of soft tis
would be easy to distinguish it from myelogenous sarcoma as lon
latter still possessed a bony shell at the basal portion, if not at the s
However, osteosarcoma of periosteal origin, a growth that occi
quently, has a bony feeling also, both at the periphery and at the
of the tumor. The latter possesses no bony shell, but numerous
and spicules of bone extend into the interior of the tumor from th
its attachment to the sclerotic and thickened bone. (Fig. 60.) A
these growths have a firm skeleton composed of thick trabecu
plates. This condition has been observed in very small specimer
palpation these tumors give the impression that they have a bony c
and this leads to mistaking an osteosarcoma for a myelogenous sa
As the latter breaks through the capsule in several places at th
time, the examining finger meets with resistance only here and thei
the case of osteosarcoma of periosteal origin. These two forms, th
cannot always be distinguished from each other during the first s
development. The most certain indication of the origin of a new
in the diploë is the presence of the bony wall rising above the level
surface of the skull and extending toward the summit of the
When the tumor has attained an enormous size, the presence o
bony areas on and in the tumor points to osteosarcoma. As this
is always of periosteal origin, such a tumor would be a periost
coma, for a myelogenous sarcoma that had attained any noticeal
would have lost its bony capsule.

Sarcoma of the *dura mater* are recognized in exceptional cases
the above-mentioned peculiarities of the gap in the skull, its si
within the plane of the surface of the bone, and its sharp outlir
a rule it is diagnosticated earlier and by other symptoms. If pre
existing symptoms, especially those of intracranial pressure, dis
as soon as or soon after a tumor appears at the surface of the sk
surgeon is safe in assuming that the growth in a given case ori
from the dura. Such a tumor begins to develop within the cranial
and brings about symptoms due to encroachment on the intra
cavity. As soon as the tumor makes its exit from the interior of th
the diminution of space and the combination of symptoms resultin
from cease. In the second place, perforating dural sarcoma usual
sates as a result of the pulsation of the brain being transmitted to
the third place, such a tumor may be forced by pressure into the
cavity, causing temporary headache, slowing of the pulse, and
consciousness. If these three symptoms be present the surgeon ca
certainty diagnosticate sarcoma of dural origin that has perforat
skull and continued to proliferate outside the cranial cavity. Conv
he cannot, however, exclude the dural origin of a growth in cases in
these characteristic symptoms are absent. The isthmus of a tumc
be so closely adherent to the edge of the defect in the skull that r
sation of the brain can be transmitted to it or that pressure canno
the growth into the cranial cavity. Under the same circumstan
cerebral symptoms do not diminish; on the contrary, they are inc

if the tumor grows toward the brain as well as outward through the bone. The presence of cerebral symptoms accompanying a tumor on the surface of the skull has no bearing on the differential diagnosis under discussion, for periosteal as well as myelogenous new growths may proliferate inwardly as well as outwardly. Only a short time ago the author removed a deep periosteal tumor traversing the bone. Cerebral symptoms were present, and the question arose whether the new growth had developed on both sides simultaneously, as Arnold has shown to be the case in myelogenous sarcoma, or whether it had traversed the bone from the outside. The diagnostic importance of cerebral symptoms depends upon the fact that they occur before the tumor becomes noticeable, and disappear after it has made its appearance on the surface. As soon as the tumor reaches the surface of the skull it spreads out to an extraordinary degree, the defect in the skull becomes completely covered, and there is no longer anything to distinguish it from periosteal and myelogenous sarcomata, which similarly proliferate and attain an enormous size.

Fig. 61.   Fig. 62.

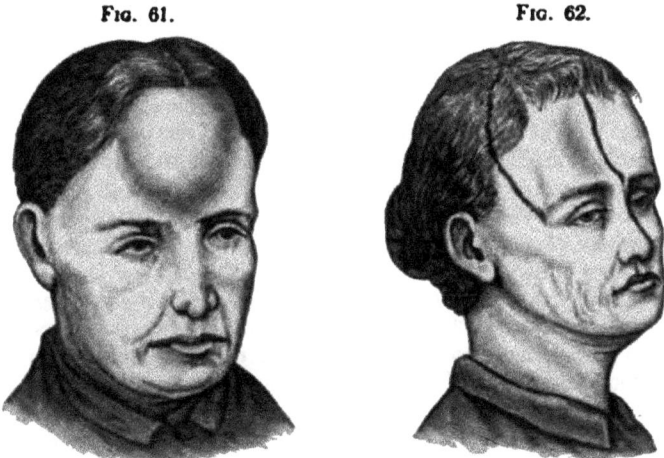

Sarcoma ossis frontalis before and after excision.

The *base of the skull* is not so frequently the site of sarcoma of the bones and dura as is the vault of the skull. However, the respective forms of new growth develop there either after the manner of other intracranial tumors, and belong therefore to the class of basal cerebral tumors, or else they grow into the orbital cavity or nasal passages, and belong clinically, for this reason, to the tumors of these regions.

In addition to primary sarcoma, which is the more important because of its frequency and clinical significance, there are secondary metastatic sarcomata of the skull, secondary to sarcoma of other bones, and in some cases to tumors of the kidneys and thyroid. Only in those cases in which there is a primary sarcoma of the ribs, pelvis, or long bones, and in which at the same time there are other metastases, such as those of the lungs, is it safe to conclude that any tumor of the skull is a second sarcoma. Secondary carcinoma occurs also in this location follow carcinoma of the breast or lungs. In all such cases it is characteri by being more sharply circumscribed than a primary carcinoma.

Treatment.—The treatment of sarcoma of the cranial bones and proliferating dural sarcoma consists in dissection and removal of entire new growth whenever circumstances permit. · If a tumor be large size, or if secondary nodules are scattered over the surface of skull, not to mention metastases in other parts of the body, exten: operative interference is positively contraindicated. An operation also contraindicated in a case in which a sarcoma has existed for so time and the patient presents a cachectic appearance, for under s circumstances it is always a sign of advanced degeneration, and in probability of extension of the disease. In all other cases operative in ference should be attempted. At the present time, when the succes removal of brain-tumors is frequently reported, surgeons do not besit to remove the dura mater or even some of the adjoining layers of brain itself.

The author has done extensive resections in 4 cases of cranial in 1 of these the patient died. The tumor had proliferated siderable depth into the occipital lobe of the cerebrum and bleeding which resulted caused collapse. The 3 other recovered. Two died at the end of one and a half and two tively, as a result of recurrence of the growth. Regarding the third he was not able to obtain any information. Grünberg investi the histories of all operations published during the last two dec Twenty-two operations were performed on 17 patients. In 3 cases or more attempts at interference were made necessary by recurrence the growth. Of these 22 operations, 5 were not completed, partly cause of hemorrhage, partly on account of collapse, and, partly, ow to the too great extent of the growth. The operation was complet 17 cases. Three of the patients died as a result of the operation, de being caused by the entrance of air into sinuses, thrombosis of sinus, cerebral abscess. In 7 cases recurrence took place soon after the op tion. In 2 no information was obtainable. Of 17 cases, 5 were app ently permanently cured, which is a good result considering the certai fatal termination otherwise.

The skin incision should extend over the summit of the tumor around any thinned or ulcerating areas. If the tumor has not brol through the periosteum, the soft parts should be dissected away on eitl side until the base of the growth and its attachment to the bone or 1 defect in the skull have been exposed. Even this step in the operati may cause considerable hemorrhage. It is therefore advisable, as I been already suggested, to cut off the blood-supply to the scalp means of a stout rubber band wound tightly about the head in the pla of the frontal and occipital bones. The periosteum should be incis about the base of the tumor at a distance of not less than 1 cm. exceptional cases only is it possible to lift off the tumor with the perioste by detaching the latter by means of periosteal elevators, beginning at the site of the incision. Even in those cases in which the new growth has originated in the periosteum it has invaded the superficial or deep layers of bone, under which circumstances the latter is characterized by its dense, sclerotic structure. It is necessary therefore to use the chisel in most cases. Portion after portion is broken off with a gouge until all diseased tissue has been removed and sound bone fills the bottom of the wound. The latter may be hard and dense like ivory. If the growth has traversed the bone, or be located on both surfaces of the bone, or if it has originated in the marrow or from the dura, the bone must be resected after incision of the periosteum. This is best accomplished by means of an electromotor circular saw. Of course, the chisel may be substituted for the saw, or a hole may be bored to the dura with a Doyen's drill and from this point the bone cut through with a Dahlgren forceps. This bone incision should be carried completely around the base of the growth, where it is attached to the bone or where it emerges from the skull, and the circumscribed portions of bone loosened and removed. In most cases that portion of the new growth directed toward the cranial cavity can now be removed without difficulty. In some cases, however, it is necessary to break up the bony ring resulting from the bone incision in order to obtain sufficient room to inspect properly the interior of the skull and the surface of the dura mater. Should the limits of the tumor extend beyond the dura, which was the condition in the third case in which the author operated, the dura must also be cut through about the circumference of the tumor, and the growth enucleated by means of a blunt dissector or the finger of the operator. This step will be all the more serious and difficult if the growth extends deep into the brain or if it is intimately or diffusely attached to the convolutions of the latter.

The final step in the operation is the arrest of all hemorrhage. This should be very carefully carried out. Not until all intracranial vessels have been tied or transfixed should the rubber tube about the head be loosened. Attention should then be paid to all spurting vessels of the scalp. As in all cases there is a considerable loss of blood, and as such extensive interference is liable to produce a condition of shock even without hemorrhage, it is not advisable to attempt any further operation with the intention of closing the defect in the skull. It is better to postpone even the closure of the soft parts in order to prevent any risk to the patient through secondary hemorrhage, and simply pack the cavity of the wound down to and into the brain with iodoform gauze. If the further course is favorable and the patient recovers promptly, the gauze packing may be removed on the fourth day. If the wound appears clean and healthy, the dissected scalp may be laid over the defect in the bone and united by secondary sutures. If much skin has been removed from the surface of the tumor, a plastic operation should be performed for the purpose of covering and closing the wound. One or two flaps with a broad base are prepared from tissues in the immediate vicinity of the wound and placed over the defect in the skull that is to be covered. The wounds should be protected by layers of sterile gauze after the first as

well as after the second operation. The author never ventures to atte
bony closure of the defect in the skull until some time has elapsed
year or so—when the danger of recurrence has passed   In the m
time the head of the patient can be protected by a cap fitted witl
aluminum plate.

SYPHILIS OF THE CRANIAL BONES.

Manifestations of *hereditary syphilis* are met with in the skull of yo
children in those cases only in which there is a recurrence following
subsidence of a primary attack.   In such cases it is usual to find g
mata in addition to those disturbances belonging to the "condyle
tons" period. (Fig. 65.) The same symptoms of the disease are fo
in young children as those occurring in the adult in syphilis *tar*
Darier and Feuland observed extensive gumma formation in the co
of recurrence in an eleven months old child in whom typical beredi
syphilis had first shown itself during the fourth month. When vise
syphilis of the fœtus manifests itself in the nursing infant, the sku
as a rule not involved, in spite of the frequency of osteochondrit
the long hollow bones.

The skull is most frequently affected in *acquired syphilis d*
later stages, very rarely at the time of the first manifestations.
tion to macular and papular lesions of the skin and mucous
there may be felt and seen deep swellings located on the skull,
true gummatous periostoses. These disappear, however, as a
ing no trace. They cannot be considered the result of a simple
titis, as all syphilitic lesions of the skull are divided into g
inflammation of the periosteum and gummatous inflammation
marrow of the diploë. Both forms of disease may run their course
out producing suppuration. Both may, however, be followed by
ration as the result of other processes and fresh disturbances, so
their course the surgeon must distinguish those that suppurate
that do not.

The most infrequent and mildest form of periostitis occurs,
syphilitic affections of the head, on the anterior portions of the
especially the frontal and parietal bones. Convex tumors form of
elastic consistency, the skin overlying them being unaltered and fi
movable.   They vary in size from that of a five-cent piece to that
dollar. There may be only one or a large number of such swelli
When these develop rapidly and suddenly, as is the case in the early st
of syphilis, they may be quite painful, causing the patient to believe
he had bruised his head against the bedpost. When they occur du
the later stages of the disease, their development is quite slow and
be unnoticed. They subside promptly under mercurial treatment,
appearing within a few weeks. Left to themselves, they continue
months and may leave permanent thickening of the periosteum.
may be in the form of low, flattened swellings, or nodular deposit
bone on the outer surface of the skull. There is as a rule a good

of sensitiveness at first, but in the course of time it disappears. When a number of periostoses exist close together, the picture will be that of a hyperostoses of the entire portion of the skull in which they are situated. The opinion has been held that this circumscribed periostitis should be considered a simple inflammation and distinct from a gummatous process, because it occurs during the early stages of syphilis and in connection with surface manifestations of the disease. It has been further held that, acting like a simple traumatic periostitis, the process subsides or gives rise to the development of circumscribed areas of new bone or a periostitis ossificans. This distinction cannot, however, be maintained, for if periosteum be stripped from the bone, as has been occasionally done following unnecessary incisions, small processes will remain adherent to it, corresponding to the tufts of vessels dipping into the Haversian canals, which show on microscopical examination the character of gummatous infiltration—free nuclei, leucocytes rich in chromatin, and possibly giant cells. The rapid and complete disappearance of such swellings shows that the development of the syphilitic tissue has gone on only to a slight degree before fatty degeneration and reabsorption take place. Its presence is sufficient, however, in a certain sense to stimulate a reactionary productive inflammation of bone similar to that produced by the irritation of other growths, such as fibroma or carcinoma, and which results in permanent periostosis or partial hyperostosis.

The further development of such periostoses results in extensive deposit of gummatous materials in the deepest layers of periosteum. These circumscribed swellings rising above the level of the skull, known as syphilitic nodes, and at times erroneously called exostoses, consist of a deeper, firmer, and denser portion, and an upper, usually smaller, soft, almost fluctuating portion. On macroscopical examination they show the character of true gumma—soft, jelly-like, pale-red tissue, with small, yellow, opaque inclusions. Even new growths of this extent may be entirely absorbed. They may, however, invade the bone further, become necrotic, and lead to suppuration. In the former case the soft summit of the cone-shaped swelling becomes depressed; the tumor becomes flattened and disappears in the course of time. Should suppuration take place, the skin overlying the swelling becomes thinned and reddened, and the accumulated pus and broken-down gummatous material breaks through, unless evacuation be previously accomplished by surgical interference. The edges of the wound have a tendency to gape on account of tense infiltration of the peripheral portions. Infiltration appears as a yellowish-gray deposit in the deeper portions of the ulcer, which is gradually thrown off in the course of ulceration either in the form of fragments or long necrotic shreds. The edges of the ulcer are undermined and its floor is composed of exposed bone. Necrosis of the bone may be produced by this gummatous periostitis in the same way that it is produced by the invasion of an ulcerating gumma of the skin.

The bones themselves become affected either secondarily by extension from the periosteum, or primarily by the development of gummatous tissue in the marrow-spaces of the diploë. The gummatous tissue fol-

lowing the periosteal vessels into the Haversian canals causes the
to become enlarged. This gives an appearance of a large group o
vessels in the compact layer of the surface of the bone. In the
of time these openings increase in size, the portions between the
absorbed, and there results a depressed area of a worm-eaten appea
filled with a mass of gummatous material. This necrotic proces
extend over quite an area and to a considerable depth, involving
portions of the skull. If this process involves both surfaces of the
as is not uncommon, the changes produced may be of such a deg
illustrated in the specimen taken by Heinecke from the collect
Erlangen. (Figs. 63 and 64.)

Fig. 63.   Fig. 64.

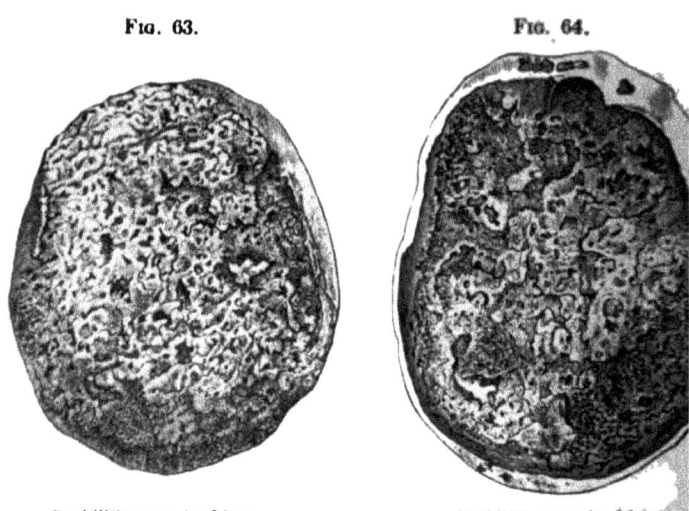

Syphilitic necrosis of bone.   Syphilitic necrosis of bone.

Whenever gummatous deposits are produced in bones they
the development of a permanent new growth of bone along their
daries. The trabeculæ, bars, nodules, and elevations, grooves and
lows seen on both surfaces of the specimen in the illustration ar
results of such bone production, not the immediate effect of
syphilitic poison, but a process of demarcation surrounding the sp
deposits.

The same gummatous growth which follows the vessels of the dis
periosteum into the bone may develop in the marrow of the diploë,
the periosteum remains unchanged. The bony partitions and trahe
of the spongy layer of bone disappear and the alveolæ filled with
matous material are opened up and communicate with each other
process being like that of any other bone inflammation that resul
osteoporosis. While in the interior portions of the bone the structu
weakened at one or more places, there is an active production of
bone beneath the periosteum and in those portions not affected by

matous infiltration. The bone surrounding and overlying the diseased area becomes thickened and dense. These two processes, that of bone absorption and bone production, constitute gummatous ostitis of the skull. There results a peculiar picture. The places on the macerated skull out of which the gummatous material has fallen look like the burrowings of the ship-worm, while between them are comb-like or reef-like elevations, the osteophytic processes.

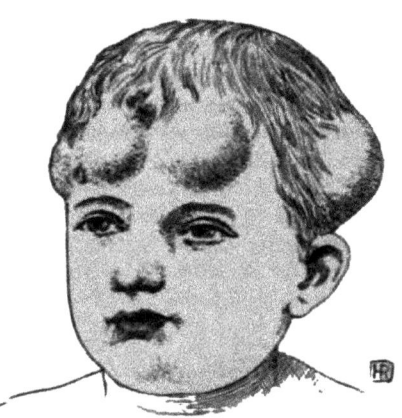

Fig. 65.

Hereditary syphilis; gummata of the cranial bones. Child, aged eighteen months. (Koplik.)

Even such extensive destruction can take place without suppuration and without involving the skin. The gummatous deposits undergo cheesy and fatty degeneration and are absorbed. The resulting defects of bone are to a large extent, but never completely, filled as the result of the reactionary periostitis and ostitis. The skin overlying the bone, usually deprived of hair at the beginning of the process, together with the remaining layers of the scalp, sinks to the bottom of the grooves and hollows on the surface of the skull, and the irregularities left as a result of the disease are only perceptible by digital examination.

Frequently, however, the course of the disease is quite different when gummatous and productive ostitis are followed or accompanied by suppuration. Whether this be caused by an excessive proliferation of leukocytes in a gumma or, as is more probable, by some infectious materials carried in the circulation, is of little importance. As a result of suppuration the destruction of tissue is far more extensive, and there is more danger of an abscess, which may not only spread beneath the skin, but also extend to a great depth and invade the brain-membranes. The areas of gummatous infiltration become liquefied and discharge as broken-down masses together with the fluid pus. At some points pus may burrow through the entire thickness of the necrotic bones. If this takes place at the periphery of a portion of the skull, the latter will be cut off from its source of nutrition and destroyed *in toto*. In this way most syphilitic necroses originate. They are characterized by two peculiarities. At times the surface appears worm-eaten, full of little depressions, and traversed by numerous tunnel-like holes reaching as far as the dura. The pulsations of the brain may be frequently transmitted to the stagnant pus filling the latter. At other times the sequestra are conspicuously heavy, dense, and firm, like ivory. This sclerosis corresponds to the places in which the bone-forming inflammation surrounding the gummatous islands and processes has attained a considerable degree of

development. Thus the results of two co-existing processes, character-
izing syphilitic inflammation of bone, are combined in the sequestra they
form. It usually requires years before these are thrown off by a process
of suppuration or granulation. At times they may be observed for a long
time lying within an ulcerated defect of the skin. The dura is dissected
from the inner surface of the sequestrum by the accumulating pus, which
does not, however, collect in any large quantities, as the numerous openings in the sequestrum afford an easy means of exit. The dura itself
becomes thickened and contracted, so that it is detached from the skull
not only immediately beneath the sequestrum, but also for quite a distance beyond. At times one may, after removal of a sequestrum, look
into the cavity of the cranium, or introduce a finger between the dura
and bone. After the sequestrum has been thrown off there remains a
large defect of bone, the edges of which are elevated like a wall and
divided by clefts into hills and valleys placed side by side, while for a
considerable distance the irregular
wave-like surface of the bone shows
where the gummatous ostitis has run
its course. The accompanying illustration (Fig. 66), taken from Heinecke's work on the diseases of the
head, in the *Deutsche Chirurgie,* shows
this condition very clearly.

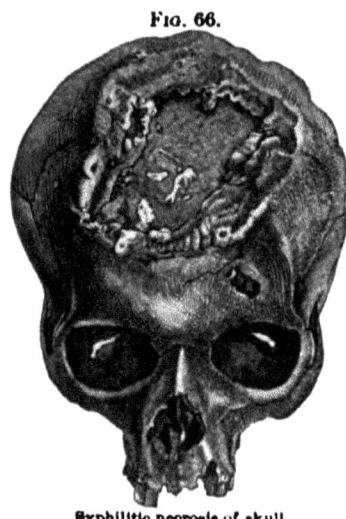

Fig. 66.

Syphilitic necrosis of skull.

At the bottom of the defect is the
hard, thickened dura mater, covered
here and there with a thin sheet of
newly formed bone.

One occasionally observes in the
skull, as elsewhere in the body, that
the pathological process in "syphilis
tardive," especially if it goes on to
ulceration, is not limited to one tissue or organ of the affected portion
of the body, but is regional—*i. e.,*
attacking and invading all structures
in a given region. It very frequently happens that when there is a serpiginous ulcer of the skin of the chin the bone of the lower maxilla
beneath it becomes thickened as the result of a gummatous ostitis.
Gummata also are found in the genioglossus and mylohyoid muscles,
as well as deep ulcers in the anterior portions of the tongue. In the same
way, kidney-shaped and horseshoe-shaped ulcers of the scalp are followed
by gummatous periostitis and ostitis of the skull, pachymeningitis, with
the formation of gummata which may invade the brain, or very extensive
inflammation of the arteries, with distinct, superficial degeneration of
the brain itself. In the course of years these ulcerative processes cause
the death of the patient, either through the increasing cachexia or
through the above-mentioned invasion of the brain. The exhaustion and
emaciation proceed rapidly when amyloid disease of the kidneys and

amyloid degeneration of the mesenteric vessels are an early complication.

Non-purulent syphilitic ostitis of the larger bones of the extremities frequently brings about extensive development of new bone—syphilitic hyperostoses. In these cases the process of proliferation is so predominant that the gummatous deposits seem insignificant in comparison. This does not, however, occur when the disease affects the cranial bones. At the same time syphilitic hyperostoses of the cranial bones are frequently spoken of. Isolated nodes have erroneously been described as exostoses, but in these, as well as in the diffuse thickening surrounding areas of bone affected by gumma, softening and necrosis always pre-

.FIG. 67.

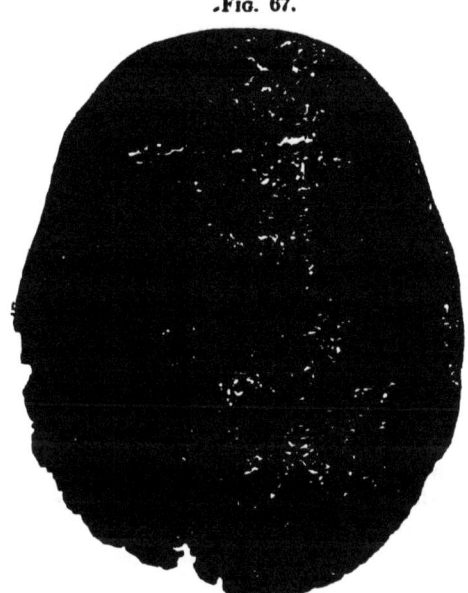

Syphilitic caries of cranium. (Bruns.)

dominate. Destruction is always more extensive than production. Between nodules, swellings, ridges, and spines, which project from the outer as well as inner surface, there are found hollows and grooves of considerable breadth. A uniform swelling is in most cases the result of an early periostitis, and will in such cases be tense and elastic rather than hard and bony. In his work on tumors Virchow emphasizes the fact that syphilis does not cause any special form of hyperostoses of the cranial bones and that the partial hyperostoses of the cranial bones and the bones of the face, regarding which he cites a number of instructive descriptions which cannot be referred to the above disease. According to the opinions of the author, traumatism plays an important part in their occurrence.

Treatment.—Ever since Fallopias first referred the above chai the skull to previous attacks of "grande virole," specific antisy methods have been suggested and used in their treatment. The of mercury is most noticeable in the case of early periosteal deposi even in the most severe forms the three drugs, iodine, mercur potassium, have produced excellent results.

In addition to the above, local surgical treatment may be exte employed. Acute recent swellings of the periosteum occurring the early stages of syphilis should not be interfered with, as they ably disappear under general treatment. Local surgical measures case of gumma occurring during the later stages of syphilis may l ployed with advantage. When there is a solitary node situated frontal or parietal region which shows no tendency to distribute specific general treatment has been kept up for a week or ten. advisable to open it as soon as fluctuation becomes distinct, and away all tissue as far as and even including the bone. The wound be kept open and packed with iodoform gauze for a few days. Fol this the author uses a dressing of blue ointment spread on stripes and inserted into the cavity of the wound in such a way that every of the latter comes in contact with the drug. As a rule, healthy lations begin to grow very quickly, and in rare cases only will th of the ulcer take on a bacon-like appearance and the walls become mined. Under the latter circumstances the surgeon will have to the measures indicated in the case of purulent gummatous os extensive portions of the skull. The author has frequently obse syphilitic node become softened, and at the same time increase i especially under potassium iodide treatment. If such a node be o and all diseased tissues, soft and hard, scraped out, the wound res from the operation will usually heal rapidly, general treatment continued meanwhile.

Diffuse gummatous, even purulent, ostitis of the cranial bones s be given only general treatment. In these cases there are no so areas or collections of fluctuating, broken-down material. Very can be done locally except to cover with mercurial plaster the p of the skull that appears to be diseased. Unna's gray mull plaste the most serviceable for this purpose. The hair must be closely s before these are applied. The plasters should be changed every t three days, and the material that remains adherent to the skin s be washed off with ether in order that the scalp may be shaved time. The small "clipping machine" has the advantage of not inj the skin and produces less irritation. If the scalp is not reddene application of the plaster is repeated; if it is reddened, it will be a sary to treat the eczema caused by the former application.

Purulent gummatous inflammation must be treated surgically thr out, as suppuration will continue and increase as the result of mc less necrosis constantly going on in the areas of gummy deposits pying portions of the skull. According to Wallet, in addition t dangers of the destructive period, those of phthisis and amyloid di of the kidneys and the local affections must not be forgotten. Of 45 patients belonging to this class, excluding 5 who died of some intercurrent disease (variola, peritonitis, pleuropneumonia), 19 died from the immediate effects of the disease, as follows: 1 of erysipelas, 4 from exhaustive suppuration, 14 from brain complications, viz., cerebral pressure, encephalitis, and cerebral abscess. The author does not believe that it is justifiable to postpone the application of surgical measures until cerebral symptoms necessitate trephining and searching for gummatous deposits and collections of pus in the brain. Intractable suppuration and obvious necrosis at the bottom of fistulous openings indicate operative interference. Syphilitic ulcers of bone should be treated precisely as kidney and horseshoe-shaped ulcers of the skin. There are two reasons why this has not been done more frequently. In the first place, owing to death taking place as the result of removing sequestra—which is not so easy as it would seem—for frequently processes of bone extend beyond the line of demarcation nearly to the centre of the necrotic area and hold the latter like clamps. In the second place, there may be firm adhesions between the fragment and the dura mater. In removing the former the latter may be torn through and the pus contained in the cavity of the ulcer is brought in contact with the pia mater of the brain. Further, the fact has been frequently brought forward that an apparently necrotic portion of the skull may become entirely surrounded and traversed by healthy exuberant granulations as the result of general treatment, complete recovery taking place rapidly without further interference. That which had appeared lost and destroyed still retained vitality and power of growth. It is perfectly proper, therefore, to treat patients with ulcers of the skin and bones with inunctions and potassium iodide for a time; but it is not advisable to wait too long before dividing fistulous tracts and undermined edges in order to expose suppurating surfaces of bone and to scrape the latter thoroughly. As the bone is frequently hard and dense, like ivory, a broad-edged periosteal elevator held at an angle may be of more service than the sharp spoon. It is never necessary to scrape away more than the superficial layer of honeycombed necrotic bone. Hofmeister correctly expresses the opinion that production of new bone around a sequestrum is not only the cause of delayed separation, but also a factor in keeping up continued suppuration owing to the fact that the bony partition causes a retention of secretions. This explains why the removal of the superficial diseased layer of bone exerts such a favorable influence on the progress of recovery. In this case also the wound is closed with iodoform gauze for a few days before dressing with mercurial ointment.

The removal of an extensive sequestrum should not be postponed too long. The existing difficulties and the impending dangers may be overcome by care and patience in operating, though at the same time it is necessary to consider the tendency of destructive inflammation surrounding a sequestrum to spread. It is easier to decide upon removing even very large pieces of bone, as, for example, half of a frontal bone, together with portions of the adjoining parietal, after noting the experiences of

Willemer, Goa, and Hofmeister in regard to regeneration of bone f(
ing such operations. They report remarkable results, considerin
extensive defects produced in the skull. In the case of a seventeei
old girl a defect covering an area of 150 square centimetres was pro
in the frontal bone by the removal of a sequestrum. After ten yc
had very nearly disappeared, being less than 4 square centimet:
area. It seems probable, according to Hofmeister's microscopical (
ination, that the dura mater plays the most important part in thi:
duction of bone, the process being similar to that taking place i
rather rare instances of traumatic defect of the skull being filled up
new bone.

TUBERCULOSIS OF THE CRANIAL BONES.

Tuberculosis of the roof of the skull is not so rare as was for
supposed. Since v. Volkmann gave a typical picture of the disea
has received more attention from surgeons. Tuberculosis of th
cranial bones and tuberculosis of the mastoid process are distingui
As the latter is in many respects similar to the suppurative pro
taking place in the cells and antrum of the mastoid process and resei
the latter in the manner of extension into the cavity of the sku
description belongs more properly to that of diseases of the ear.
surgeon therefore is only concerned with tuberculosis of the vault (
skull. It occurs either as a circumscribed disease of the bone or
diffuse development of tuberculous tissue extending for some dis
in the diploë as well as between the periosteum and bone, and under
early cheesy degeneration.

Circumscribed tuberculosis usually occurs only at one place o
skull, but the author has seen as many as seven foci, and Israel re
seeing five at one time on the skull of a child. Ménard found twenty
tuberculous foci on the skull of a child. As a rule in such case
only is the skull the seat of the disease, but other parts of the bo
well—bones, skin, and lymph-nodes—are involved. In 3 of Israe
cases there was a very extensive general tuberculosis; in the fourth
in addition to tuberculous foci of the vault of the skull, there was t
culosis of the petrous portion of the temporal bone. Tuberculous le
of other bones may be looked for in the orbital ridges and in the l
as well as in the temporal process of the malar bone. In this situ
there may frequently be found one or more fistulæ from which the
discharged a thin, purulent fluid, and at the bottom of which dead
may be detected with a probe.

Tuberculosis of the cranial bones, especially the circumscribed
begins very probably in the marrow cavities of the diploë, where
liferation first sets in about the vessels with the formation of giant
This is followed by caseation and suppuration, as well as by necros
the lamellæ of bone that have become infiltrated with tuberculous
The latter is characterized by extending through the entire thickne
the skull, so that externally the periosteum and internally the dura

separated from the bone by a collection of pus. As a result of this process there is a perforation of the skull at the site of this necrosis. This
circumstance led Virchow to call the disease perforating tuberculosis of
the bones of the skull. Clinically the latter presents the picture of "cold
abscess," situated as a rule in the frontal and parietal regions. The
abscess may frequently attain considerable size, is always soft, without
much tension, and covered by purplish colored skin. In a relatively
infrequent number of cases the process does not go on to abscess formation. There is simply a growth of fungoid tuberculous granulation tissue
beneath the thickened periosteum and in a shallow groove in the surface
of the skull. Under such circumstances a sensitive, circumscribed, semi-
fluctuating swelling appears, very much like syphilitic gumma, except
that it is usually larger and the skin covering it generally becomes reddened earlier. Though there might be liability of mistaking such an
affection for a syphilitic lesion on account of the perforating necrosis
occurring during the later stages of development, in a given case the
differential diagnosis is difficult only in those cases in which syphilitic
nodes are characterized by extensive and distinct fluctuation at their
summit, a condition rarely met with in periosteal gumma. Moreover,
as tuberculosis usually occurs in children and syphilis in adults, it is only
under unusual circumstances that it is impossible to arrive at a correct
conclusion. On opening such an abscess, a thin purulent fluid escapes
which is filled with a number of tissue fragments, or there is found a
mass of spongy granulations filled with cheesy foci. After the abscess
cavity has been scraped or wiped out, it is easy to recognize the diseased
bone as a sequestrum of the size of a pea or a bean, of an opaque white
or dull-gray color, surrounded by an irregular line of demarcation. The
pus filling the abscess may pulsate distinctly—a sign that the skull has
been perforated. These tuberculous sequestra, as distinguished from
syphilitic sequestra, are easily removed by a blunt dissector, periosteal
elevator, or simply with a spoon. Following their removal, the dura is
exposed covered only with a layer of pus, cheesy material, and broken-
down granulations. Occasionally a sequestrum is absent or it does not
involve the entire thickness of the skull. In still other cases there is a
small opening in the skull filled with tuberculous pus and traversing the
entire thickness of the bone. Finally, in a fourth class, no sequestrum
is developed and perforation does not take place. Only a limited and
superficial area of the outer table of bone appears involved in a cheesy
growth, which to a very slight extent invades a few spaces of the diploë.
When a subperiosteal abscess is of considerable size, the tuberculous
process also extends for considerable distance on the inner surface of the
skull in the neighborhood of the necrotic area of the bone. These cases
represent the transition to infiltrating tuberculosis of extensive portions
of the skull. The spaces of the diploë covering quite a large area are
filled with cheesy material and the dura underlying the diseased portions
of bone is separated from the latter by purplish-soft or friable granulations. The external soft parts are as a rule broken down and the site
of numerous fistulous tracts which lead to the diseased bone and are

and form abscesses.

Prognosis.—The prognosis of circumscribed tuberculous ostit cranial bones is always better than that of the diffuse form; bu the former it will depend largely on what other parts of the body organs are involved in the tuberculous process.

Clemens reported 16 cases operated on by König and obse some years afterward. Of 12 patients who were suffering fro1 culosis of other parts of the body at the time of operation, 9 d a few years; 1 died of a purulent meningitis, and 2 were livin end of ten years. Of 4 cases in which the disease was limited to th bones, 1 died of a general miliary tuberculosis complicating the of the skull, 1 died of some other intercurrent disease, and 2 li

Treatment.—The danger of long-continued ulceration, progres semination of the tuberculous process in and beneath the bones, as the constant danger of meningeal complication or cerebral justify radical surgical interference. As a rule an attempt is 1 prevent the development of general tuberculosis by destroying the focus. According to this rule, every abscess or tuberculous gr: of the head should be extensively incised and the abscess cavity c cleaned out with a sharp spoon. A sequestrum extending p wholly through the bone should be removed with the aid of a chis necessary, in order that old and recent tuberculous growths carefully scraped away about the dura as well as beneath the peri In order to accomplish this purpose, it may be necessary to p' pieces of bone from the edge of the site of perforation in order to (the extent of the tuberculous process on the inner surface anc beyond it. The whole cavity should be filled with iodoform ga this left in place for several days. As soon as healthy gran develop, the skin may be laid over the defect in the skull and place by an ordinary dressing or by secondary sutures. The should be kept partially open in order to secure drainage and to the accumulation of wound secretions over the dura and bene periosteum.

In the case of the boy mentioned above the author found that of the seven places the wound healed rapidly and smoothly, alth every one of them the dura had been reached in the process of s and removal of sequestra. Furthermore, there was complete bony of each of the seven defects of the skull. The boy came to th five or six years later for the removal of tuberculous glands of th At the sites of the previous openings in the skull white movabl scars limited to the skin were found. The defects had been con filled in with new bone, leaving no trace of the original operations complete filling of gaps must be considered a peculiarity of circum tuberculosis of the skull. It was also observed by Israel. A case established a basis for this conclusion. It was that of a fi old boy with a soft, elastic tumor of the parietal bone. Consid a tuberculous granuloma, the author made an incision. It cont1 few granulations, in the middle of which was found a disk-shaped piece of bone, 1.5 cm. in diameter, with a ragged, irregular border, and cheesy infiltration of the diploë. Its outer surface could easily be recognized as the outer table; its inferior surface as the inner table. Having removed the sequestrum search was made for the gap in the skull out of which it had been forced by the growth of granulations. None such could be found. The skull was completely closed and intact. The bone beneath the periosteum that had been raised by granulations was smooth and sound. It must be assumed, therefore, that after the extrusion of the sequestrum without suppuration the perforation of the skull was completely filled with new bone at a time when the sequestrum had not been thrown off.

Recovery after surgical interference is not always rapid. Even under such conditions recurrence, tedious, carious ulceration, and continuous development of fresh fistulous tracts have been frequently observed. Such recurrences demand further interference and repeated scraping, which should not be postponed too long, as they certainly do more to save the general strength of the patient than long delay.

The attempt to remove extensive portions of the skull diffusely infiltrated with tuberculous tissue is unsatisfactory on account of the wide distribution of the disease; and the run-down, anæmic patients are unable to bear the loss of blood that is unavoidable in such procedures. In more than one instance it has been found necessary to leave an attempted operation unfinished.

ACUTE OSTEOMYELITIS OF THE CRANIAL BONES.

Acute osteomyelitis, called spontaneous, occurring in the long hollow bones of children and young people was well known for some time before it had been observed and described in flat bones. Attention was directed to the latter by the observations of disease of the ilium and scapulæ which had erroneously been described as periostitis of these bones. This so-called periostitis was found most extensively developed at places where the periosteum was least abundant, as, for example, when tendons were directly inserted in thick layers of spongy substance.

Although Chassaignac reported the history of a case that was undoubtedly one of acute spontaneous osteomyelitis, and Jaymes collected observations on 15 similar cases, Lannelongue was the first to offer positive evidence of the occurrence of the disease in the flat bones of the skull. He cultivated *Staphylococcus pyogenes aureus*, the specific cause of the disease, from pus obtained from a subperiosteal abscess in the temporal region. In a case recently published Fischer found at autopsy pus in the marrow-spaces and the dura separated from the bone by a collection of pus. The description reminds one of the picture that Pott described as a result of contusion of the head. According to the opinion held at that time regarding the etiology of inflammation, acts of violence were in themselves considered responsible for all subsequent changes. At the

present day it is known that an infiltration of blood filling the
spaces of the spongy layers of bone is not the cause of necrosis
puration, but that the latter is brought about by small excoriati
abrasions of the skin which offer a means of entrance to pyogeni
isms.

It is characteristic of all cases of myelitis, including those of th
that they apparently originate spontaneously. However, in son
the point of entrance of the specific cause of the disease may be
ered, as, for example, a recent furuncle, circumscribed celluliti
nail-bed, a small, unnoticeable wound of the scalp, or an abn
the skin overlying a subcutaneous hæmatoma. The latter is fre
referred to in descriptions of the disease. Thus, a child may fal
striking the head and sustaining a circumscribed extravasation
and, at the same time, lacerations and abrasions of the skin o
it. These excoriations become skinned over and the hæmatoma b
contracted, but two or three days after the accident there is a cl
lowed by a rise of temperature exceeding 40° C. (104° F.).
symptoms of the disease are those of an infectious disease, a
attending physician, having satisfactorily excluded pneumonia,
attention being directed to the head by pain, located at the sit
contusion or on top of the head or the back of the neck, susp
acute tuberculous meningitis. As in other forms of acute osteo
the child falls into a typhoid state; the general senses are impaire
are alternating dizziness, stupor, and mild delirium; the skin
jaundiced, the tongue brown and coated; the abdomen distend
pulse frequent, easily obliterated, and irregular. The disturbances
more severe in character, and in the course of two or three da
appear swelling and redness of the soft parts, located, accordin
histories of nearly all cases, at the site of the previous injury. Th
toms of the disease during its further course are determined by t
mation of an abscess, intracranial complications, and necrosis
cranial bones.

In the case of the sternum and ilium, when infection of the
in the spongy portion of these bones takes place, the periosteum
quently raised only on one side of the bone. In the bones of th
this usually takes place both on the inner as well as the outer s
The skin overlying the outer abscess becomes reddened. This is
earliest on the forehead and over the mastoid process. The sof
become œdematous, the eyelids swollen, the scalp adherent and i
able; it feels doughy and sooner or later fluctuation becomes
at one or more places. The extrusion of pus beneath the te
muscle and into the orbital adipose tissue was mentioned by Chass
Surgical measures should anticipate spontaneous rupture of an a
On incision there is usually discharged a pale brownish-red pus o
consistency and containing an abundance of fat. At the bottom
wound or site of rupture bare bone is found, a fact which can be d
strated by means of a probe or examining finger. In this way n
originates. This has been considered such a prominent feature b

authors that the disease, as a whole, has been characterized as an acute necrosis of the cranial bones.

These regular or cardinal symptoms may be followed by a number of cerebral disturbances. They are caused principally by collections of pus between the bones and the internal periosteum or dura. Inflammation may extend through the dura mater, set up an acute purulent meningitis, and cause rapid death. General convulsions, like those accompanying meningitis produced by other causes, will betray the serious turn of the disease. Besides meningitis there is the danger of thrombosis of the longitudinal and cavernous sinus extending to the jugular vein, as well as the development of pyæmic symptoms.

By opening an abscess the immediate danger is passed. The temperature and threatening cerebral manifestations having subsided, the chronic stage sets in, during which the course is determined by the fate of the sequestrum. Even here it may happen that cerebral complications or a cerebral abscess produce the most prominent symptoms.

Extensive necrosis frequently takes place with extraordinary rapidity —a sign that it was originally caused by an affection of the marrow of the diploë, and not by a simple exposure of periosteum. The separation of the sequestrum and the development of products of repair go on very slowly, for in osteomyelitis, as in traumatic necrosis, there is a want of nutrition. Only moderate thickening or numerous osteophytes appear in the vicinity of the sequestrum, but there is no tendency to form an involucrum. While during the acute stages there is a strong tendency on the part of the suppurative process to extend and spread to the intracranial organs, this is absent during the later stages. Cases have been reported in which there was a gradual separation of a sequestrum, requiring fifteen years, without cerebral abscess or sinus thrombosis developing during this long period. The granulations surrounding the necrosed portion of bone may have acted as a protective barrier.

Tuberculosis of the cranial bones, like osteomyelitis, may originate in the marrow of the diploë, but the process is always a chronic one, never acute. Gummatous disease of the bone-marrow is also chronic in its course. As staphylococcus osteomyelitis always results in extensive necrosis, it might in its later stages be mistaken for the late forms of syphilis, but never for the sharply circumscribed necrosis of the cranial bones produced in tuberculosis. The acute onset and the relatively rapid development of necrosis are important points in differential diagnosis. Of similar import are the affections of other parts of the body in tuberculosis and syphilis.

Prognosis.—The prognosis of acute osteomyelitis of the cranial bones is necessarily serious. The high temperature and severe general symptoms usually present during the first few days of the disease may in themselves cause death in a manner similar to that resulting from rapidly developing septicæmia. The intracranial complications are equally serious. These are meningitis, sinus thrombosis with pyæmic abscesses, as well as cerebral abscess, the latter, however, having been observed in only one or two instances.

Treatment.—Therapeutic measures are clearly indicated from th
set, and should be radically carried out. Even when the diagnosi
between osteomyelitis or circumscribed cellulitis, an incision is a
indicated. This frequently limits the purulent process and preve
spreading to the contents of the cranial cavity; at the same time i
terminate the acute stage with its attending dangers. After makin
or two extensive incisions and exposing the bone, the latter shoul
be opened throughout its entire thickness in order to expose the
for the periosteum of both the internal and external surfaces are
rated from the bone by a collection of pus. This must be evacuate
provision made for continuous thorough drainage. After this has
accomplished the surgeon may expect separation of the sequestrum
hope for a limitation of the necrotic process on both the externa
internal surfaces. This cannot be expected if a considerable amo
pus has been present for any length of time.

Removal of a sequestrum should not be delayed once a line of de
cation has been established separating healthy and diseased ti
Even if at this time there exist bridges of communication betw
sequestrum and the surrounding bone, it should be removed. Thi
usually be accomplished by a few strokes with a chisel. At first the
should be applied well within the limits of a sequestrum at those
where the boundary between dead bone and sound bone is indi
After the removal of the larger portion of the sequestrum the ed
the remaining bone can be trimmed off with Luer's gouge forcep
a sequestrum has become separated and is distinctly movable, it m
extracted without difficulty. An elevator is introduced along the li
demarcation and the edge of the loosened fragment of bone is
sufficiently for it to be seized with sequestrum forceps. A vigorou
on the forceps will bring away the piece of dead bone. A seques
is more extensive along the inner table than along the outer. Suffi
of the latter should be chiselled away to facilitate extraction of the
ment.

A classical description of acute periostitis was given by Graves in
This corresponds in every feature with the picture of primary osteo
litis, and for that reason alone the surgeon is justified in expressing
doubt as to the independent occurrence of acute purulent periostitis
has good reason to consider the latter as only part of the osteomy
Even purulent inflammation of the periosteum following cellulitis o
scalp, or a compound fracture of the skull, is only indirectly the rest
the infection. The latter always attacks first the loose connective ti
or even the pia mater, the periosteum becoming involved later.
symptoms of the periostitis are obscured, however, by the picture
diffuse spreading inflammation.

CHAPTER VI.

INJURIES AND DISEASES OF THE BRAIN, ITS MEMBRANES AND VESSELS.

By Prof. Dr. E. von BERGMANN and Prof. Dr. R. U. KRÖNLEIN,

IN CONJUNCTION WITH

Dr. SCHLATTER and Oberarzt Dr. P. WIESMANN.

CONGENITAL SURGICAL DISEASES.—CEPHALOCELE.

By Prof Dr. von BERGMANN.

CEPHALOCELES are congenital tumors found on the external surface of the skull. They are covered with skin and communicate with the cranial cavity through a defect in the bony wall of the skull. Cephalocele occurs about once in 3500 to 4000 newborn children, and is always found in certain definite situations on the skull, in the median line, either in the occipital region or in the region of the glabella and root of the nose. The latter is the most frequent site. Rare forms of cephalocele occurring at the base of the skull need only mention. They emerge through a cleft between the body of the sphenoid and the ethmoid bones and project into the nasal cavity. They may be mistaken for nasopharyngeal polyps occurring in the same region, and in one case this error has led to the performance of a fatal operation. Basal cephaloceles have only an embryological significance and are of little clinical interest. *Occipital cephalocele* is either *superior* or *inferior* according to whether it emerges above or below the external occipital protuberance. In superior cephalocele the hernial opening may communicate with the posterior fontanelle; in inferior cephalocele with the foramen magnum. Frontal cephalocele may be *nasofrontal*, where it emerges above the nasal bones, in the region of the glabella; or *nasoorbital*, where it makes its appearance at the inner angle of the eye; or *nasoethmoidal*, where it is situated below one of the nasal bones. The clinical picture of a large nasofrontal cephalocele is shown in Fig. 68 taken from v. Bruns' *Atlas*. The accompanying illustration (Fig. 69) of an inferior occipital cephalocele is also taken from the same work. The latter tumor was divided into halves by a fissure.

All three forms of frontal encephalocele communicate with the cranial cavity through the horizontal plate of the ethmoid. The examination of small hernias shows that the funnel-shaped opening in which they are situated is formed by a part of this plate; for externally they are

(165)

bounded by the frontal bone, internally by the remains of the plate the ethmoid; and if there exist two hernias at the same time—a p occurrence—they are divided by a plate of bone belonging to the cri of the horizontal plate of the ethmoid.

Fig. 68.

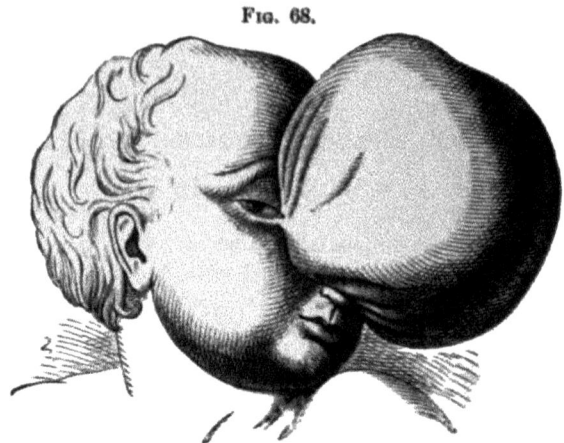

Nasofrontal cephalocele.

Anatomy and Etiology.—The anatomical and etiological features c be clearly understood only by studying their analogy to similar cys forms of spina bifida. One may consider them as a class of defe

Fig. 69.

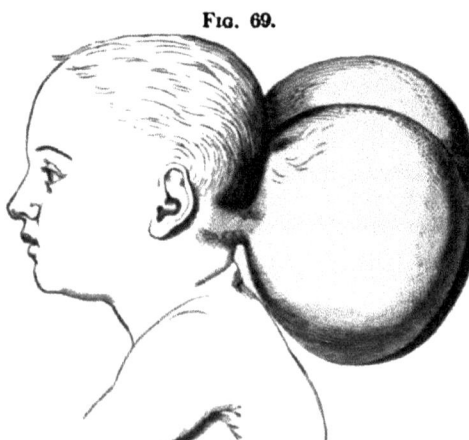

Inferior occipital cephalocele.

of the skull originating in the same way as do myelomeningocele, mye cystocele, and meningocele of the back from defects of the verteb column.

The most frequent and at the same time most typical form of encephalocele is *hydrencephalocele*, which is identical with *myelocystocele*. These tumors are covered with skin which remains unaltered where the swelling is of moderate size, but where this swelling is considerable the skin presents on the summit of the elevation the signs of atrophy due to stretching. The arachnoid membrane is found just beneath the subcutaneous connective tissue, as pericranium, skull, and dura mater are wanting. Dura mater and pericranium merge into one another at the base of the tumor. The arachnoid membrane covering the growth is always thickened and frequently otherwise altered, being particularly the seat of cystic degeneration, as is soon to be mentioned. Passing still further inward there is found a layer of nerve-tissue derived from the brain, enclosing a cavity of greater or less extent filled with cerebrospinal fluid. This cavity invariably communicates with one of the ventricles of the brain. In frontal cephaloceles it communicates with the anterior horn, in occipital cephaloceles with the posterior horn of the lateral ventricles. Connection with the fourth ventricle has been found in a few very large specimens. Encephalocystoceles are therefore to be considered as protrusions of a lateral ventricle. The typical form of growth described above is subject to three changes. In the first place, during fœtal life, that portion of hernia lying without the skull may become reduced and only a portion of the brain-tissue surrounding the cavity filled with fluid remains beneath the three coverings: skin, fascia, and arachnoid. The entire contents of a tumor would under such circumstances include only one or two cerebral convolutions. Such tumors containing only brain-tissue and occurring exclusively in the region of the glabella as small hemispherical naso-frontal hernias have been called *kenencephaloceles* by Heinecke, since they are not cystic in character. They must be considered as encephalocystoceles undergoing retrograde change. In the second place large cysts develop in the arachnoid, as has been mentioned, occasionally solitary, more frequently multiple, just as beneath the arachnoid in myelocystocele there is frequently found a collection of fluid. The latter are called *myelocystomeningocele*, the former *encephalocystomeningocele*. In the third place, the layer of brain-tissue surrounding the continuation of the ventricle into the tumor is occasionally absent, and there remains beneath the arachnoid a layer of epithelium identical in character with that of the ependyma lining the ventricles. The thickness of the layer of brain-tissue varies. At times it is 1 cm. or more thick, at others its presence can only be confirmed by microscopical examination. If even these remains disappear, the layer of ependyma alone forms the wall of the continuation of the ventricle, as first demonstrated by Muscatello, being attached directly to the inner surface of the vascular tissue composing the arachnoid. It consists of a layer of ciliated cylindrical epithelium without nerve-fibres or nerve-cells. These forms are obviously encephalocystoceles also. They have, however, not always been considered as such, having, as a rule, been classed as a variety of cephalocele—*i. e., meningocele.* They were

supposed to be due to the separation of the pia mater followin
lation of serous exudate. Taking into consideration the fa
means of communication between the ventricle and the free
cystocele of Muscatello is usually very narrow (in a specimen
by the author it is hardly possible to pass a probe through th
or may be entirely obliterated, it is quite conceivable that
have been described as pure meningocele without considerin
sary to make a microscopical examination of the lining o
Since the latter has been more generally done fewer cases
reported in which the cyst-wall was composed of only skin, f
arachnoid membrane. If such forms do occur, they are un
cases of pure meningocele; but in all probability they have
from the above-mentioned class of encephalocystomeningoc

FIG. 70.　　　　　　　　　　　　　　FIG. 71

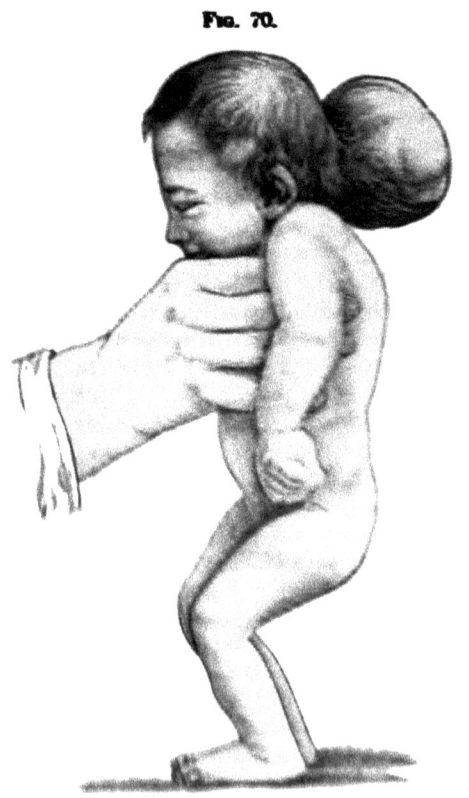

Encephalocystome

Encephalocele.

protruding proc
ventricle surrou
brain-tissue ha
ceded, there rem
the cystic fr
about it, or
large cyst in
arachnoid tiss
rounded by th
ened pia mater a
senting the men
described by o

thors. Accordingly all cephalocele should be considered as
from encephalocele communicating with a ventricle, and le
loceles as well as meningocele as two examples of retrograde

PLATE I.

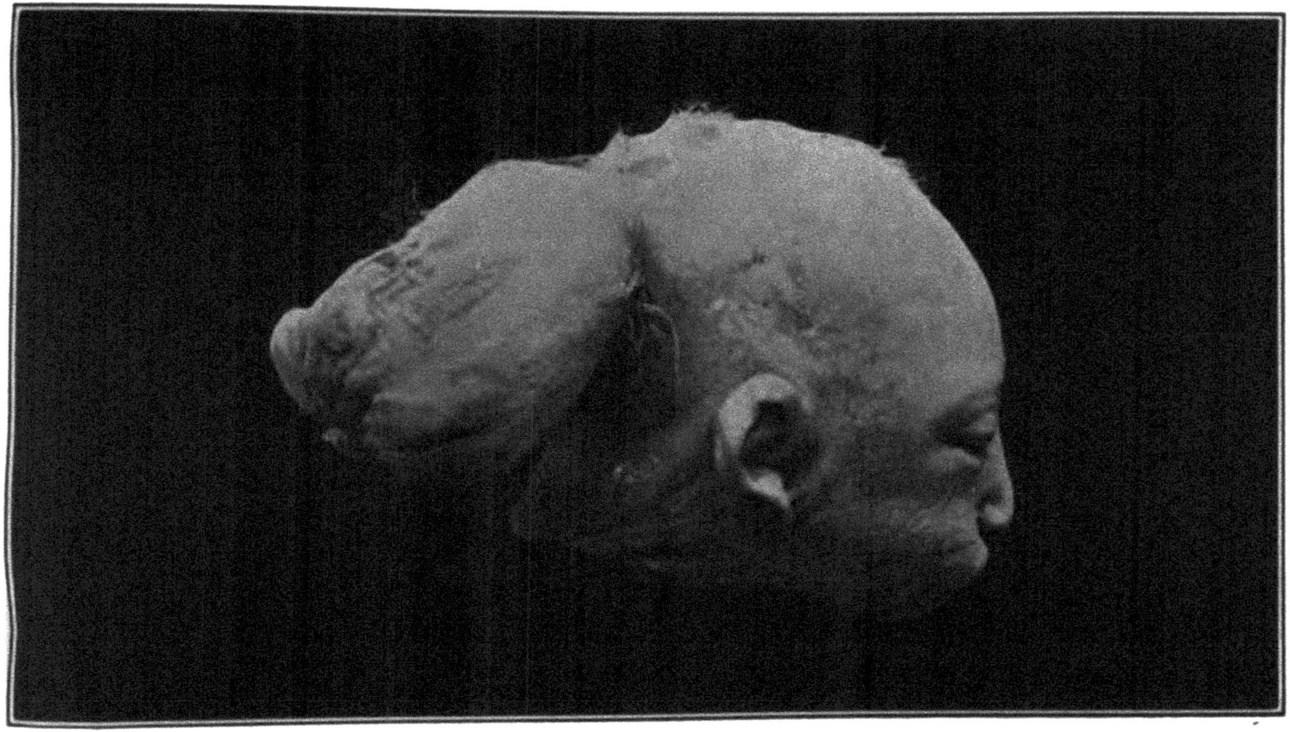

Large Encephalocele.

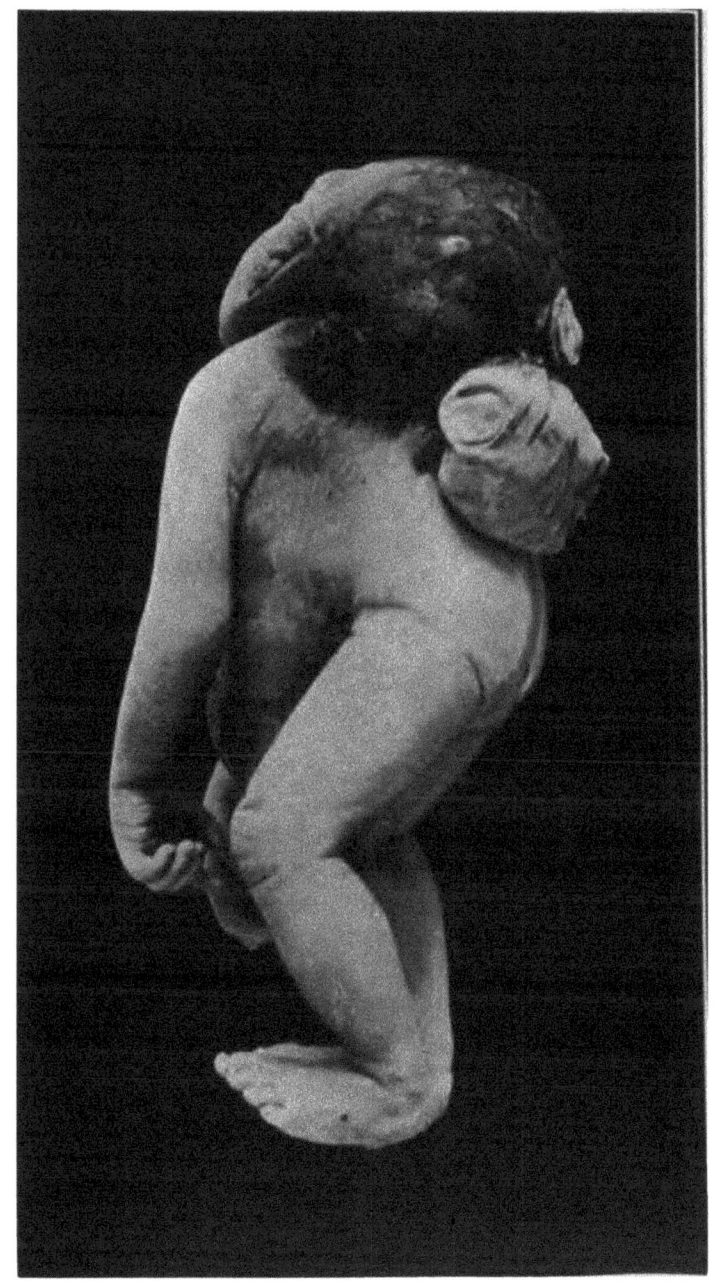

with encephalocele, regarding whose ultimate fate information was obtained by Miller, all died before the end of the first year, usually by bursting of the tumor. Up to the year 1889 it was believed that only pure meningoceles not communicating with the ventricles should be operated upon, but it is possible that even at that time many communicating encephaloceles, in the sense of Muscatello's description, were removed without disastrous results. It was not until after it had been demonstrated that brain-tissues governing important functions and even large portions of the brain could be removed without danger that it was considered possible to remove deliberately portions of brain prolapsed and lying within an encephalocystocele. Schmidt was probably the first to attempt this. Since then many such cases have been operated upon and with excellent results. In 1893 Diakonow collected histories of 27 operations with 17 recoveries, and in 1896 Lyamschow collected 62 with 33 recoveries. Of 10 cases of the author's, operated on in earliest infancy, only 2 died. In both cases there were very large occipital tumors, of which one extended over a cleft in the skull reaching from the occipital protuberance through the foramen magnum to the fourth cervical vertebra.

After thorough preparation of the field of operation, two crescent-shaped flaps of skin should be made from the base of the tumor. These must be sufficiently large to cover the defect left after removal of the pedicle. The flaps being held by sharp retractors, the pedicle is followed to the defect in the skull, which is usually roughly circular in outline. The tumor is held tense and cut off 2 to 3 cm. above the bone. At the same time a considerable quantity of fluid may pour out. This should be prevented as much as possible by pressure with the finger or a plug of fluff-gauze, as well as elevating the head of the patient. The edges of the divided sac should be rapidly turned into the cleft in the bone and sewed together, the needle being passed through only the base of the inverted sac. According to the size of the hole in the bone, more or less of the connective-tissue covering of the underlying portion of the sac should be preserved, in order to be able to turn in sufficient of the sac securely the defect. Over the first row of sutures, which should be formed there is placed a second row. If deemed advisable, one may dissect off two flaps from the connective tissue covering the encephalocele and suture them over the defect. These may be secured with sutures passed to the adjacent periosteum. In carrying out this suturing it is obvious that the portion of the covering to be used should be thick and strong. The two skin-flaps are then replaced. In cases in which an encephalocele is of considerable size, containing much fluid, and probably a large channel of communication, it is advisable after dissecting away the two skin-flaps to clamp the pedicle to prepare the flaps of tissue to be used for the inversion of the defect and pass the sutures, so that as soon as the tumor is removed it may be possible rapidly to turn in the edges or the opening of the sac closed. In cases in which the pedicle is narrow, and the cleft in the bone narrow, the former may

Congenital hydrocephalus, child one year old. Circumference of head about the two-fifths natural size.

in measurements of the head in normal cases. The maximum circumference of the skull in newborn children should not exceed 37, the length of the occipitofrontal diameter 12.5 cm. and that of the biparietal 10.2 cm. Larger measurements than these, and the fact they increase rapidly during the first few weeks, would lead one suspect hydrocephalic expansion of the skull. This expansion place not only along the separated sutures and fontanelles, but also the bones themselves. (Fig. 72.) The base of the skull alone does participate in the process of dilatation, which fact explains the peculiar shape of the hydrocephalic skull. The accompanying illustration (Fig. 73), taken from v. Bruns' *Atlas,* clearly depicts the condition described

different. In such cases the further progress of the patient depends
how severely and extensively the brain was injured during the pri
period of expansion of the head. When only moderately affecte
psychical functions may develop, and though they never reach a n
degree, and though such children are always defective mentally,
can be brought up. There are cases in which normal mental p
were developed and the power of memory left nothing to be de
This must be regarded as recovery even if the shape and size c
head remain abnormal. A subsequent diminution in size has

FIG. 74.

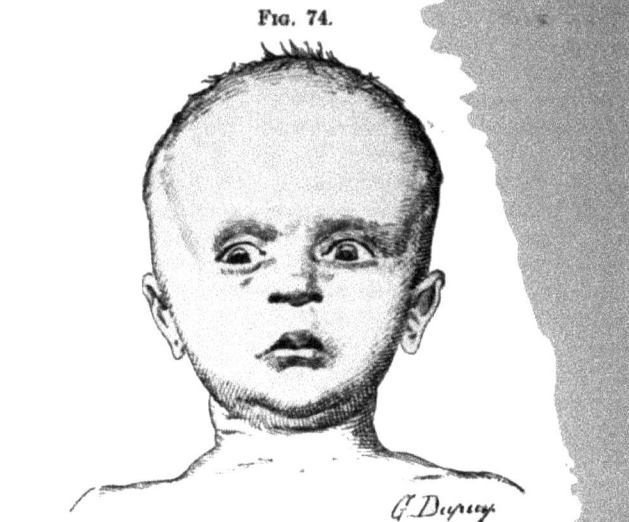

Congenital internal hydrocephalus. Infant, nine months of age. (Koplik.)

been observed. On the other hand, the head has continued to inc
in size after the progressive accumulation of fluid had ceased to
place, and the child continued to develop physically and men
As a rule children born with hydrocephalus are weak-minded
remain so. Wyss followed the histories of 41 such cases admitte
the canton hospital of Zurich: 31 died early; 10 of those surviving
between the age of three and twenty-one years; 7 had learned to
only between the ages of six and ten years; and 5 were able to g
school. A large number of those born with hydrocephalus die du
parturition. According to Hohl, 63 out of 77 cases require artif
means of delivery.

Diagnosis.—The diagnosis of hydrocephalus is generally easy
can usually be made at the first glance. There are only two condit
from which it may have to be differentiated. The first of thes

rhachitis. During the early stages of rickets the skull is generally not enlarged. The two diseases have in common therefore the soft consistency and flexibility of the edges of bone along the sutures, and not the unusual size of the head. Many cases of acquired hydrocephalus, on the other hand, easily lead to confusion with rhachitis. In the first place, owing to the fact that the two diseases may coexist, that is to say, in cases of hydrocephalus in older children rhachitic disturbances may show themselves on the thorax, vertebral column, and on the extremities. Further, suspicion might be aroused by the unusual size of the head in some cases of rickets, that the increase in size was due to dropsy of the ventricles, especially when the large, open, anterior fontanelle is markedly prominent and tense.

The differential diagnosis between congenital and acquired hydrocephalus is also important in determining the further course and treatment of the disease. A mistake is very liable to be made, for every secondary effusion into the ventricles, resulting either from meningitis, spina bifida, cephalocele, tumor, porencephalus, or other disturbances in development, may produce an expansion of the skull as long as the fontanelles and sutures remain open, thus simulating the condition produced by congenital effusion into the ventricles. The difference between the two is, first, that the congenital affection is discovered at or soon after birth. At the same time it must be remembered that only cases with moderate hydrocephalus can be born alive or with power of life, but that even in them the size of the head is abnormally large and shows a rapid increase in size during the first week. In the second place, a cause for acquired hydrocephalus can always be found. It may happen that in cases in which repeated exacerbations of growth take place the mother or nurse may date the beginning of the disease from the time of the last exacerbation, and thus lead the physician into error. This, however, is rarely the case, for it is usually easy to determine the fact of meningitis having preceded the beginning of an acquired hydrocephalus.

Treatment.—The treatment of hydrocephalus at the present time leaves a great deal to be desired. The problem is to restore the equilibrium between secretion and absorption of the cerebrospinal fluid in the dilated ventricles of the brain. That this can take place is demonstrated by those cases in which without medical treatment or surgical interference the dropsy of the ventricles and the increase in size of the head cease. Since the dangers of puncture have been removed through aseptic methods, this minor operation has been frequently carried out. Several favorable reports have been received where the operation was done as many as thirty times in a single case at intervals of five to ten days. Rehn showed before the "Congress für innere Medicin" two instructive cases in which cure had been effected by this measure. Puncture is made either in the skull or in the spine. In congenital hydrocephalus the skull is always selected, the site chosen being the coronary suture, to the right or to the left of the fontanelle, about midway between the base and the top of the skull. The head

having been prepared in the usual way, a Pravaz needle is th
until the spurting of a stream of fluid shows that the lateral v
has been entered. About 30 to 60 c.c. of fluid are allowed to fl
and the needle withdrawn; a small compress of gauze is pressed
the wound until blood ceases to ooze. A second smaller comp
gauze is then applied and held in place by strips of adhesive pla
The lateral ventricle may be reached by other methods. These
will be discussed in considering operations for cerebral pressure
tempts at evacuating hydrocephalic fluid by puncture of the spina
may also be recommended. Opposed to the latter, however, a
experiences of O'Carroll, who found in two children that the fo
of Majendie was closed. Where no communication exists betwe
ventricles and the subarachnoid space of the spinal cord, lumbar
ture is of no service. The fact that after puncture of the spinal
and dura, as the author has done in cases of congenital hydrocep
not a drop of fluid is obtained, is explained in this way.

It has frequently been held that the effect of puncture mi
assisted by compression of the skull. This has, however, not been
out by experience. Neither is puncture combined with the inject
iodine solutions certain or without danger. Keen has attempt
cure of congenital hydrocephalus by long-continued drainage
punctured above the external auditory canal, and before withdr
the hollow needle introduced a dozen strands of sterilized bors
through the needle. After four days the needle was introduce
similar manner into the lateral ventricle of the opposite side
rubber tube introduced. Evacuation was too rapid, and the child
into convulsions and died. Broca has collected all cases of dr
of ventricles in hydrocephalus that have been reported to the p
time, in order to demonstrate that in not a single instance did the
survive the interference; moreover, that all died in a very short ti

CONCUSSION OF THE BRAIN (COMMOTIO CEREBRI).

Hurd (1877) classed among the effects of contusion of the head a
of disturbances which was neither dependent on a fracture of the
... a tear of the bloodvessels, but was so transitory and of such
intensity that an actual wounding of the brain could not be its u
lying cause. It is not remarkable that in times when a distinctior
... between diseases of function and of matter less was asked s
the ... alterations which the brain suffered, if the brain
... went dynamic atony and paralysis" or "suffered a mole
displacement."

Later, when autopsies were more often made on those dying of
... a riddle was presented which has only recently been so
... over and dangerous brain symptoms had been observed di
... autopsy was unable to show the slightest trace of visible alter
... of the deceased, even after the most painstaking examina

On other occasions patients were seen in whom all brain symptoms were absent, in whom neither the psychical nor the general sensorium, neither the motor nor the sensory functions, had suffered, and yet an entire frontal lobe or some other part of a hemisphere was crushed to a pulp. The extent of contusion of the brain would, perhaps, not have been realized had not the patient succumbed to other injuries—a rupture of the intestine or a pneumothorax, for example. On the one hand, notwithstanding the severest brain symptoms during life, not the slightest discoverable anatomical alteration in the brain; on the other hand, notwithstanding an absence of all brain symptoms, extensive and striking destruction of brain substance. The lack of anatomical findings and a theory advanced in the last century of the occurrence of fractures of the skull at a point remote from the acting force created the doctrine of the traumatic concussion of the brain, not yet forgotten and deemed satisfactory only a few decades ago. The vibratory waves spreading over the bones ought to come together at the opposite point of the sphere, and their effect be so augmented by interference that the continuity of the bone would be broken at this point. It can be easily understood that this doctrine of vibrations led surgeons to accept the same theory for the brain itself. The vibrations of the skull, it was thought, shook the brain until it was shrunken and sunk in its capsule. This was a particular effect which Littre asserted he had seen in a certain autopsy, and for which he constructed a corresponding and special clinical picture —a permanent, fatal, or transitory paralysis of the most important brain functions, of consciousness, of circulation, and of respiration. Littre shrinking of the brain has long been known as a post-mortem phenomenon dependent on the distribution and flow of the cerebrospinal fluid after death. And physics has given us more accurate information concerning the destructive vibrations of the brain. That the head, after every blow that strikes it, passes through a series of vibrations before it comes to rest is self-evident. But it is not these after-vibratory movements which do harm to the brain and its contents, but the first blow is and remains the sole cause of the traumatism which the brain suffers. The vibrations following this first impact cannot go far with the same force, acting on bones, nerves, blood, and lymph, for, communicated from layer to layer, they are quickly lost, transferred as they are to such heterogeneous materials as those just mentioned. So that all the theories formerly connected with brain concussion are no longer advanced. The brain is neither shrunken nor broken up by immediate or progressive vibrations.

The main fact of a profound depression of all recognizable brain functions, especially the consciousness, after a severe brain injury, nevertheless holds good, as well as the immediate passage of this cessation into death or health—a rapid extinction or a rapid and complete recovery. This is the clinical conception that we at present connect with the old designation of brain concussion. The diagnosis of concussion of the brain is based to-day on a thoroughly distinct clinical picture, in its development, as well as its subsequent course, in its invasion and its de-

180

alina, at the beginning as well as at the end. The patient is a unconscious—he hears, sees, feels nothing. His expression is the is deep sleep. But not only are the higher psychical functions p depressed, but also the automatic apparatus hidden in the oblongata is attacked. The unconscious patient breathes at times at times irregularly. Deep respiratory efforts alternate with ficial or at times respiration ceases entirely, to begin again after with deep spasmodic inspirations. The pulse becomes less freq beats sinking to 40 or even less in the minute. If the patient worse and the end approaches, then the pulse, which has g become smaller, begins to beat more rapidly. The rapidity in and it gradually grows weaker and weaker until it stops altogethl on the contrary, the patient becomes better, the pulse first recov returns to its normal frequency, while the general sensorium co deranged and disturbed. When the separate manifestations of a appear in such definite order, it is justifiable to suppose, as an imi cause, the self-same disposition of the affected organs. The abi consciousness while life continues is known as an inhibitory pro the cerebral cortex, for it is this cortex that brings into connection which are in a position to excite conscious manifestations on acc its many-sided relations to the motor and sensory provinces of th periphery, to the ganglia of the brain and to the cerebellum. account it is recognized as the organ of consciousness. A cessa consciousness must consequently be considered as a disease of th brain cortex, and indeed as a depression or paralysis of it. The n need of the cerebral cortex is just as active as its sensitiveness i Slight impressions can abolish the entire function, impressions need not touch other parts of the brain, but rather leave them qui undamaged. The heart is the last to die, the cerebral cortex t exhausted, for the heart continues to beat even after a poison, for ple, the deficiency of oxygen in the blood in lung diseases, has ben for a long time the general sensorium. It is self-evident that th sensitive part of the brain first suffers. After a fall on the he injured person is confused, unimpressionable, pale, weak, dull, anc great violence, somnolent; he lies in stupor and coma; consciousn been interrupted and has vanished. During the comatose state th matic apparatus in the medulla continues to act. It is not para on the contrary, in contrast to the cerebral cortex, it is stimulated. slowing of the pulse, as is known from the well-recognized expe of the Weber brothers, is an irritation phenomenon. While one of the brain—the cerebral cortex—is paralyzed, another portio which conceals the vagus centre, is in a condition of stimulation by side irritation and paralysis, and both manifestations of ane a same cause. The main fact of this coincidence of symptoms of irr and paralysis has been determined and is explained by a series of ments which have been made on the convulsive, vasomotor, and centre by sudden disturbances of nutrition. Such experiments hav carried out under the author's direction by Bastgen. The anæmia brain was caused by widely disseminated capillary emboli, brought about by the injection of fat into the peripheral end of one carotid, and then the frequency of the pulse and the blood-pressure measured by a registering apparatus. A few seconds after the beginning of the injection a slowing of the heart-beats began, so that in the course of two minutes the frequency of the pulse was only 53 per cent. or even 25 per cent. of the normal pulse-rate. At the same time there was a rise in arterial blood-pressure, which reached its highest point in the course of two minutes. After that time both frequency and blood-pressure changed. Then came an instant in which the circulation of the animal seemed to have regained the normal. Instead, however, of persisting at this point, the blood-pressure dropped until it reached the zero line, while the pulse increased in rapidity until it came to a stop in death. Bastgen's experiments show plainly that brain anæmia caused by fat-emboli brings about two conditions in the heart and bloodvessels, viz., first, a period with increased blood-pressure and slowing of the pulse, and, second, with a diminution of the blood-pressure and an acceleration of the pulse. This is the way in which one and the same cause can bring about first an irritation and then a paralysis.

Some patients lie only faint, weak, benumbed, without slowing of the pulse. The blow which struck them has affected only the cerebral cortex; its action was too slight to affect the vagus centre, which did not feel it, and consequently permits the heart to go on quietly working. In other cases the patient is completely stupefied and his pulse-rate markedly lowered, in which case greater violence has taken place sufficient to paralyze the cerebral cortex and to stimulate the vagus centre. If even greater violence has been inflicted, the patient lies in the deepest coma and is completely unconscious, and, in contrast to the other cases, the pulse is accelerated. Here both regions of the brain, the cortex and the vagus centre, are paralysed, the latter after a transitory and therefore unnoticed stage of irritation. The hurried pulse becomes smaller and less easily felt, faltering, and irregular, until it finally ceases to beat. These are the most severe cases of brain concussion in which the patients act as if deeply narcotized, and their pulse shows an acceleration instead of a retardation. The danger is great because this combination of deep unconsciousness with acceleration of the pulse is characteristic of the terminal stage of paralysis. In the clinical analysis of these cases, it is permissible to consider the processes going on in the brain as disturbances of nutrition of the entire organ, and not of any particular part. It may even be assumed that the brain is not only affected in its entirety, but equally so in all its portions, the same degree of disturbance acting according to the irritability of the different portions of the nervous system, in one instance as a stimulant, in another as a depressant.

Every blow striking the hollow skull changes its form momentarily, even if it does not succeed in breaking it. By virtue of its elasticity it immediately resumes its former shape, as has been seen in the section on Mechanism of Fracture of the Skull. Owing to the fact that nervous tissues and the bony skull possess different degrees of elasticity, the same

the skull, whether the latter be fractured or not. Shock
is therefore considered the cause of that group of symp...
as concussion of the brain.

According to the above, the idea of concussion w...
coincide etiologically with that of contusion of the b...
of fact, in his recent exhaustive work on cerebral c...
has proposed that the old term be dropped entirely and ...
be substituted therefor. The author has no objections to ...
bral concussion as a form of contusion or crushing, and t...
the respective section on head injuries, if clinical exp...
teach otherwise. Owing to the fact that a patient may sim...
pletely recover from such severe cerebral disturbances, and ...
fact that such a patient continues to remain in perfect heal...
easy to assume a solution of continuity of the brain as a ca...
symptoms observed. As the patient recovers consciousness with...
minutes, one can only think of a momentary effect that disapp...
leaving traces. When pain is experienced in a bruised finger, the ...
does not expect to find anatomical lesions of the nerve stim...
site of the injury. In addition there is the fact that affect...
central nervous organs have been produced experimentally witho...
sioning any discoverable solution of continuity of their subst...
fore surgeons have been led to accept a physiological basis for the ...
This was furnished by Koch and Filchne, and even at the pr...
time the author considers their researches of the greatest import...
Both experimenters conceived the idea of producing the same effe...
a series of light blows as by one severe blow. By this method of i...
tigation all disturbing and confusing complications were excluded,
cases of pure concussion (commotion) were actually produced in w...
there was a momentary and immediate effect on the nervous tis...
For one stunning blow there was substituted a series of light blows,
the complete picture of concussion was produced in animals without
anatomical lesions of the brain. The temperature of the animal fell
degrees, respiration was shallow and slow, and the pulse-rate was als...
from 58 to 36 beats a minute. The animals were powerless, and c...
be placed in any position without resistance, as if absolutely and c...
pletely unconscious. On autopsy no rupture of any vessels was fo...
The parenchyma of the brain, the medulla, and the spinal cord w...
absolutely free from contusions or other mechanical lesions. In
animals which had received blows there was a complete and fully de...
oped picture of cerebral concussion, and yet there was total absenc...
any discoverable cerebral lesion. Witkowski also was able to proc...
pure concussion in a frog by a single blow. Any frog could be brou...
into a state of unconsciousness and paralysis if the head were str...
against a hard substance. Witkowski removed the central nerv...
organs from animals that had been stunned in this way, and harde...

them, but could not discover anything abnormal even on microscopical examination. Neither could Polis discover any microscopical or macroscopical lesions in the brains of animals he had subjected to the experiment of repeated blows.

Koch and Filchne's researches have made clear the pathogenesis of cerebral concussion. No one centre included in the brain is affected by itself, but all are altered in the same way and at the time of the act of violence. As the result of a displacement of the brain, through blows or knocks, the nervous tissues as such are directly affected and injured. This injury is manifested in the experiment of repeated blows on an animal by all centres being at first stimulated and then by exhaustion and paralysis, and the longer the blows are kept up, the greater the degree. Regularly, whenever during the period of excitation the blows with the hammer were interrupted, the activity of the respective centre sank still further, to be elevated again more or less rapidly. The stimulation during the time the blows were delivered and the depression immediately after they were interrupted could be repeated several times. That is, if the blows were delivered again after the first interruption, the action of the centre would be increased, or, in other words, stimulation would be produced, and after the second pause inhibition and exhaustion would again set in, but every time the experiment was repeated stimulation would become less and depression greater.

It having been definitely established by the researches of the above-mentioned investigators that death may result from cerebral disturbances caused by traumatism even when no anatomical changes in the brain are produced, it appears convincing that these disturbances may produce similar effects even if other and more noticeable injuries have been inflicted at the same time. Accordingly cerebral concussion may be considered the sole cause of death or a contributory cause of a fatal termination. One would be inclined to ascribe cerebral concussion as the cause of death in those cases in which intracranial changes are so insignificant as not to account for death immediately or soon after injury. One would feel otherwise, however, in the presence of extensive brain injuries in which, for example, half or even a whole lobe has been crushed. But even in these cases it is necessary to remember that extensive cerebral injuries, large areas of contusion, frequently occur without causing any symptoms, and are at times found unexpectedly on autopsy in cases in which the patient happened to die of some other disease, such as erysipelas or pyæmia.

Cerebral concussion must be considered as a contributory cause of death even if other injuries, hemorrhages of the brain, or areas of contusion are often found, for very noticeable anatomical lesions are not necessarily the cause of death or even of the predominant clinical picture. For this reason when destruction of an entire lobe of the brain is found on post-mortem examination, and this is given as the cause of death in the autopsy record, it should be remembered that it may have played no part in producing a fatal result, the latter being more probably due to an accompanying cerebral concussion.

The idea of pure cerebral concussion is retained for the reason that it passes over quickly, leaving no trace, because in experiments on animals all its peculiarities are reproduced, and finally because in numerous instances no anatomical lesions have been found in the brain of individuals that have died as the result of cranial injuries. The last condition might be explained by fatal disturbances of circulation such as the action of cerebral compression on the vasomotor centre, either a vasomotor spasm, (Schultén) or a vasomotor paralysis (Fischer). However, as the existence of nerves in the cerebral vessels is doubtful, it cannot be held that they can exert such powerful influence from any one point of the brain.

In the author's opinion the rapid *restitutio ad integrum* would lead one to believe that instead of a permanent disturbance, a transitory material disarrangement within the central nerve-tissue was responsible for concussion of the brain. The constant clinical manifestations lead one to hold the same opinion. Although it is true that the description and histories of cases of cerebral concussion are variable and contradictory, it is equally true that the whole mass of observations presents a constant clinical picture—the regular combination of slow pulse and loss of consciousness. In this sense cerebral concussion is something apart—a combination of symptoms governed by the same conditions and with a character of its own. If this cannot be granted, cerebral concussion resolves itself into contusion of the brain, or, as Kocher has recently suggested, into acute cerebral pressure.

One thing, the author readily concedes that, assuming a common cause (the change in form of the elastic skull as the result of external violence), concussion must very frequently be combined with contusion. Under such circumstances there is not a constant clinical picture; on the contrary, the symptoms vary according to the site of the contusion, whether it be extensive or limited, single or multiple.

According to prevailing ideas, differences exist between cerebral concussion and cerebral pressure on the one hand, and cerebral contusions on the other. In the one case there are always the same symptoms coming and going in regular order; in the other, on the contrary, there may be convulsions, paralyses, disturbances of speech, of facial muscles, hearing, respiration, or circulation. As a rule in any given case a combination of general symptoms and those due to localized cerebral injuries are found. The clinical analysis of such cases must aim at differentiating the symptoms due to the one or the other disturbance produced by the same act of violence. The surgeon must determine which are produced by the immediate effect on the central nervous organ (concussion), which are due to disturbance of circulation (compression), and which are the result of destruction of brain-tissue (contusion).

Marshall, Hauser, Friedmann, and others believe that immediately following an injury, called by the author concussion, no changes can be discovered in the nervous tissues, but that later degeneration of these or of the vessels supplying them follows. Thus they establish a remote effect of what was originally considered pure concussion. Durante,

upon the skull in a certain direction, in order to determine in v. manner this was transmitted to the brain. The author is unable describe here in detail these investigations, which were carried out Kocher and Ferrari. The greatest degree of displacement and the i violent compression of the brain take place in the direction of diminished diameter of the ovoid of the skull corresponding to direction of the blow. However, the effects of transmitted violence displacement are felt not only in this one direction in which ther the greatest degree of motion, but also in a direction perpendicula this one, and to a certain extent in all directions, owing to the consistency of the brain and the contained cerebrospinal fluid.

Tillman considers the above experiment an explanation of the and most important symptom of concussion, namely, unconsciousn He believes that the brain, enclosed in its air-tight capsule of bone, is in motion by the force of a blow directed against the skull. As white substance possesses a higher specific gravity than the gray continues to be in motion a longer time than the latter. The re is that if any severe violence is inflicted upon the skull, there is a tortion along the boundary between gray and white matter which cat the loss of consciousness.

The momentary paralyzing action of a severe blow on the he especially if it be delivered on the vault, Kocher seeks to explain the experiment carried on by himself in connection with Curti Munslund, and Saltikoff.

Thus, according to Kocher's description, the cerebral injury p duced by violent blows, as illustrated in these experiments, is an ac anæmia, besides microscopical and macroscopical areas of contusi with and without laceration of bloodvessels caused by the sudden placement of cerebrospinal fluid and blood. In no case, howe would all the centres be uniformly involved. As far as circulat disturbances are concerned, there would be a constant clinical pictu with cessation of respiration and circulation and loss of consciousn When, however, small or extensive areas of contusion are pres there are the variable symptoms of cerebral contusion, into which th would be a gradual transition, and the limits of which can only determined arbitrarily.

Symptoms.—The clinical manifestations of cerebral concussion primarily disturbances of consciousness, loss of intellectual pow going on to a state of stupor or coma; loss of muscular power, imp. ment of sensation and reflexes, vomiting, exhaustion, slowing of pul inhibited respiration. Cases may be divided into mild and severe.

After a fall or blow the patient loses his senses; there are dizzine flashes before the eyes, and buzzing in the ears; consciousness is l entirely; there is complete exhaustion, the knees give way, and the ar hang down relaxed. The face is pale, the eyes are fixed and expressio less, the eyelids closed. Respiration is so shallow as to lead one believe that the patient has ceased breathing entirely. The pulse hardly perceptible, small, thready, and slow. This condition is short duration. The pulse improves; this is followed by several deep respirations; the patient may vomit, open his eyes, stretch out his arms, and get up. On attempting to walk or stand he is unsteady, grasps his head, complains of pain in it and at the site of the injury, of buzzing in his ears, soreness of the entire body, and great lassitude. Such are mild cases. These symptoms having subsided, there are no further effects of concussion. Strength is regained and the patient resumes his former occupation.

Frequently there is more or less loss of memory. This has been described particularly by Bouillard and Gussenbauer. Most cases recover from the loss of consciousness with their minds clear, except that they remember nothing of the violence that produced their injury. There are, however, numerous cases in which a half-stupid patient answers questions regarding which he has no recollection whatever after he has recovered. Still further, the loss of memory may extend to events some time previous to the injury. The author's assistant, Nasse, was thrown against the iron beam of the ceiling by an explosion at the moment he was entering the ward in making his morning visit and sustained a compound fracture of the skull. Although he recovered consciousness completely fifteen minutes later, he could not remember the work he had been doing in his room an hour before, neither did he remember that he had left his bed, had taken breakfast, and put on his clothes. In other cases a defect of memory extends back several days, although in other respects the patient may be psychically normal. This retrospective amnesia may be temporary or continue for some time. In the former case, recovery takes place in the course of a few days or weeks, memory of those events nearer the time of injury being the last to be regained. In the second case the defect in memory may remain to its original extent, or memory returns in part, but memory of those events happening immediately before the injury remains permanently lost.

In the same category may be placed other circumscribed functional disturbances which usually disappear, but may persist to a greater or less extent. Such are defects or weakness in the motions of the eyeball, as a result of which the eye in attempting to fix its gaze goes beyond the point aimed at; also disturbances of speech, stammering, and difficulty of articulation, inability to recollect certain words, confusion of ideas; further disturbance in co-ordination of certain movements, loss of equilibrium and purposeless movements in order to obtain support and maintain gravity. Finally, there must be mentioned interesting disturbances of metabolism and of the functions of the kidneys which have been observed to follow cerebral concussion—diabetes mellitus and insipidus, as well as albuminuria. All such disturbances are unquestionably not the result of pure concussion, but are brought about by the anatomical lesions of circumscribed portions of the brain and are, therefore, symptoms of cerebral contusion. As, however, cerebral concussion rarely occurs without being accompanied by such anatomical changes, small apoplectic foci, or lesions of nerve-cells and

nerve-fibres, such disturbances usually occur
corresponding functional centres are affected.
of such disturbances will, however, be taken up in the chapt
Wounds and Contusions of the Brain.

In severe cases of cerebral concussion the patient collapses
moment of injury and remains absolutely motionless as if in deep
He cannot be aroused, reacts to no external stimuli, nor attempt
defensive motion if the eyelids are raised and the conjunctiva tou
neither does he respond to painful cutaneous irritation. In all
however, the pupil, which may be contracted or dilated, contracts
exposed to intense light; and if water be poured into the moutl
movements of swallowing are carried out. The face is pale and su
The surface of the body, especially that of the extremities, is
Respiration is regular, but shallow and hardly perceptible, interr
at intervals by deep sighing inspirations. The pulse is small, som
irregular, and usually, though not always, slow. Feces and urine
be retained or are passed involuntarily. There is repeated vom
especially immediately following injury. This condition may cor
for hours, sometimes for days. Finally, respiration becomes d
heart and pulse beat stronger and fuller, the body regains its n
warmth, and at the same time consciousness and the power of m
return. The senses are unimpaired and questions are answere
plicitly and clearly. As a rule the above stage of *depression* is foll
by a stage of *exaltation*. The pulse increases in frequency, bec
hard, the surface temperature is increased, the face is red, the ι
are contracted, the eyes bright. The patient complains of head
restlessness, and pains in the limbs. The duration and intensi
this stage may be as variable as those of the preceding stage. Frequ
severe symptoms of congestion are developed, threatening a tran
to meningitis. If the symptoms continue for several days, the diag
of pure cerebral concussion is excluded. The longer the state of
continues, the more reason will there be for assuming that other i
cranial injuries have been produced. In such cases only can the
nosis of pure cerebral concussion be made with certainty in whicl
patient recovers rapidly after injury and regains complete conscious
Even then it is safer to be prepared for subsequent disturbances, fe
a very short time severe pressure-symptoms may set in as the
of extensive extravasations. In severe cases of cerebral concus
in which the clinical picture presented has continued for one or
days, the predominating symptoms may not, as has been mentic
be referred to concussion alone, no matter how typically they
be presented. Only in cases in which the dangerous symptoms
side rapidly can the occurrence of extravasation and consequent ii
cranial pressure be excluded; while conversely in those cases in w
the manifestations increase in severity from hour to hour, the ρ
becoming slower, coma more deep, and respiration intermittent, fui
disturbances are present, due to continuously increasing intracr
extravasation.

In the author's opinion there is only one criterion regarding pure cerebral concussion—*the transient character of its manifestations.*

Treatment.—The treatment of cerebral concussion is carried out at the present time according to definite lines, although formerly a matter of much dispute. No measures that would in any way depress the heart's action should be attempted; the surgeon must be satisfied with attempting to restore the bodily warmth. Hot-water bottles should be placed near the extremities, hot cloths over the abdomen and genitals, and the patient placed in a warm bed and heavily covered with blankets.

The head should be lowered, shaved, and carefully examined. The most important indication is stimulation of the heart. For this purpose cutaneous counterirritation should be employed; mustard plasters should be placed over the cardiac region; in the absence of the latter, a sponge wrung out in hot water may be placed over the heart. Hypodermic injections of ether and 10 per cent. camphor oil are recommended. The latter may be repeated ten or more times at frequent intervals. As the patients can often swallow fluids poured into the mouth, musk may be administered in large doses, especially when the pulse is alarmingly small and irregular. The most powerful stimulant is the faradic brush, as it instantly produces increase in blood-pressure. It may be passed over the soles of the feet or the palms of the hands. For the same purpose a few short inhalations of ether may be employed. The improvement in pulse indicates the efficacy of the means employed.

Excellent also is Kocher's suggestion that artificial respiration be applied for a time in case respiration fails entirely, becomes intermittent or very superficial. It should be kept up until respiration becomes deeper and the pulse stronger.

Should symptoms of congestion set in after the patient has recovered from the state of depression, the head should be covered with an ice-cap, unless other injuries necessitate the application of antiseptic dressings. If a dressing has been applied, the ice-bag should not be used, as it keeps the dressings saturated. Under such circumstances drastic purgative remedies should be employed. Dry cups applied to the back and front of the chest are also of assistance.

During the stage of congestion the patient is quieted very quickly by a subcutaneous injection of morphine, which is indicated at the same time on account of hyperæmia of the brain.

COMPRESSION OF THE BRAIN AND THE OPERATIONS FOR COMPRESSION.

Compression of the Brain.—The combination of symptoms called "compression of the brain" is a condition of great clinical and partienlarly therapeutic importance. It enables the surgeon to make a diagnosis of rupture of the meningeal artery or of a brain tumor, and is of

orrhage has lost consciousness. If the circulation of the brain becomes gradually slower, each centre is affected in order according to a scale described by Huguenin. The order of succession of the centres affected is as follows: the cortex, the corona radiata, the gray matter of the spinal cord, the region of the pons, and finally the medulla oblongata. Assuming that such an order exists, and, further, that the manifestations of such injuries follow a regular order, it is easy to understand that at a time when certain centres are paralyzed, others only begin to be affected. Therefore unconsciousness is seen in combination with general convulsions. It can be understood also that slight but sudden variations in circulation which exert no influence on other centres of the brain produce severe disturbances of the cortex, for that portion of the brain governing consciousness requires the greatest amount of nutrition and therefore is most sensitive to disturbances of nutrition.

Consciousness is lost more rapidly than any other function, and, *vice versa*, returns only after circulation has been fully restored. In clinical cases of cerebral concussion the symptoms present a varied picture, and this is true of cerebral compression. Many more cases are admitted to hospitals suffering from a variety of injuries to the skull and its contents than presenting a single form. The contraction of intracranial space caused by traumatism through intracranial extravasation and bone depression is seldom of so pure and uncomplicated a type as to present a clear clinical picture of cerebral pressure. Depression of bone is in most cases combined with contusion of brain-tissue, and in addition there is always cerebral concussion. In the same way intracranial extravasations of blood are complicated by cerebral contusions and fractures of the bones. For this reason it would have been impossible, in spite of careful observations, to determine the significance and part played by one cause in the presence of a combination of many causes, had not experiments been carried out in order to obtain a correct value for each one of the component manifestations. In this way it has been possible to demonstrate that pressure-symptoms develop in regular order, and that, generally considered, the same symptoms always correspond to certain degrees of pressure.

Restlessness, moaning, and headache, in the beginning, are followed by nausea, vomiting, unconsciousness, drowsiness, stupor, and coma. As soon as a condition of stupor sets in the heart action becomes slower. The slowing of the pulse is the most constant and distinct symptom of cerebral pressure. With increased pressure this becomes more distinct, but only within certain limits; if pressure exceeds a certain degree, the pulse, which may have become very slow, suddenly increases in frequency. The transition from a slow pulse to a rapid pulse is always preceded by changes in its rhythm. Instead of remaining regular and strong, the pulse became weak, small, and intermittent.

The initial slowing and final increase in frequency of the pulse show an involvement of the vagus corresponding to a stimulation during the first stage and depression during the second. Leyden demonstrated by experiment that the vagus was responsible for the changes in frequency

ining the eyes of the patient. The ophthalmoscopic examination shows, as was discovered by Graefe, swelling at the site of entrance of the optic nerve into the fundus of the eye—the choked disk mentioned above. The arteries leading into the eye from the internal carotid follow along the optic nerve, as do also the most important veins leading from the eye into the cranial cavity. The optic nerve is, moreover, surrounded at its entrance into the sclerotic by two sheaths: first, by the pia mater, which encloses between it and the nerve a narrow cleft communicating with the subarachnoid space and filled with cerebrospinal fluid; second, by dura. Between this and the external dense layer of the pia mater is a continuation of the subdural space. Whatever processes go on, either in the arteries and veins of the cranial cavity, or in the cerebrospinal fluid, may be seen or determined in the fundus of the eye.

Besides these symptoms of a general affection of the brain, injured individuals usually present signs of a localized injury referable to certain areas of the brain. These consist of a complete or incomplete loss of motion in one-half of the body. In the next chapter an injury which produces the typical picture of uncomplicated cerebral pressure will be discussed, namely, rupture of the middle meningeal artery, and in considering this these paralyses will be taken up more fully and their proper significance pointed out.

The immediate causes of cerebral pressure-symptoms are the same (initial stimulation and terminal paralyses of the cerebral cortex and the automatic centres) as those causing cerebral concussion. They are not produced, however, by a direct mechanical injury to the nerve-tissues, as in cerebral concussion, but are brought about by a slowing of the circulation in the cranial cavity which is the result of a diminution of space within the cranial cavity. Observation and experiment have both demonstrated this clearly.

We proceed from two premises: First, that after closure of the fontanelles the skull is a rigid, firm capsule, incapable of being stretched or compressed, so that the space containing the brain, its membranes and fluids, is unalterable. Second, that the nerve-tissues composing the brain are incapable of being compressed by those degrees of tension possible within the cavity of the skull. If one of the component parts of the skull contents, the nerve-tissues, cannot be compressed, a foreign body or a rapidly growing pathological mass will not find room within the skull unless the two other component parts of the cranial cavity, the blood and the cerebrospinal fluid saturating the brain and filling the subarachnoid spaces, are forced out of the skull. Blood may find its way out through the sinus of the dura and the veins of the neck. The cerebrospinal fluid may leave the cavity of the skull by finding accommodation in the distensible spinal canal. Experiments have been carried out for the purpose of proving these premises and possibilities and to place them on a satisfactory basis.

The constancy of the space within the skull has never been disputed. This cannot be said in regard to the incompressibility of the brain. Adamkiewicz declared that contraction of the intracranial space took

Consequently the pressure within the tube increases until it overcomes the compression and the current again flows from the tube. When this is repeated the distal end of the tube undergoes visible vibration. The result of this interruption of the current is that in the same space of time less fluid passes through the tube during the time that the experiment is carried out than under ordinary circumstances.

The velocity of the current in the elastic tube is diminished just as the blood-current is retarded within the inelastic cavity of the skull whenever the cerebrospinal fluid is subjected to increased pressure and the veins are obstructed at their exit from the cranial cavity. Cramer and the author were the first to discover the pulse in the sinus of the dura mater at a point where the internal jugular emerges from the skull, and the first to demonstrate it with the kymograph. At the same time Cramer demonstrated that the venous pulse observed at a point where the internal jugular vein leaves the sinus is not produced by the transmission of the arterial pulse through the capillaries, and that it is not caused by the contraction of the right auricle, but that it is the result of an intermittent increase of tension of the cerebrospinal fluid corresponding with systole and diastole of the heart. The same thing was demonstrated by Koch and the author, and later still more conclusively by Knoll by observations on the occipito-atlantal ligament. Mincke observed the same phenomenon in the cerebrospinal fluid following lumbar puncture. The author determined it in the case of a myelocystocele in which the fluid contained in the tumor was allowed to flow into a U-shaped tube. When the heart contracts in systole, the endocranial veins are made to contract by the increased tension of the cerebrospinal fluid surrounding them; during diastole they become dilated. This rhythmic action produces the venous pulse in the brain. Hill demonstrated this pulsation at the torcular; Ziegler, in the sinus of the dura mater.

The physiological increase in pressure of the cerebrospinal fluid does not disturb endiämorrhysis, compensation being provided for to meet this. Tension may increase markedly before cerebral circulation is interfered with, as in the case of intracranial pressure. The experiments of Cramer teach that even considerable increase of arterial pressure does not retard the intracranial circulation. Every increase of arterial pressure is followed by a corresponding increase of venous pressure with increase of intracranial circulation. Ziegler, Hill, and his coworkers demonstrated by means of measurements the relation of pressure in the right auricle, in the torcular, in the carotid or femoral arteries, and of the cerebrospinal fluid. They found that within physiological limits, or even under pathological conditions, the circulation of the brain behaved very much like that of the rest of the body. Every change in position of the animal influences the degree of tension and fulness of the intracranial vessels; every phase of respiration and every muscular effort is followed by corresponding changes in the intracranial circulation, and all this may happen without noticeable cerebral disturbance. That there is space in the skull for such a marked engorgement of the vessels

as occurs under the above-mentioned circumstances is made po
two arrangements: First, the escape of the cerebrospinal fluid
subdural space of the spinal cord. Second, by an almost instal
absorption of the cerebrospinal fluid. By these means an ii
amount of blood is accommodated within the skull under phys
conditions.

The *escape of cerebrospinal fluid* from the cavities and passage
the skull into the extensible spinal canal is an unquestionable
much so as the fact of this elasticity. Every one who has expe
occipito-atlantal ligament of a dog has observed the pulsation
membrane, by which is meant that following any increase of
of the cerebrospinal fluid the latter escapes into the distensible s
space. The escape of cerebrospinal fluid is only prevented wh
quantities of the fluid have already been forced from the crania
into that of the spinal column, and the elasticity of the ligai
apparatus of the vertebral column has been taxed to a high
While it was formerly believed that this escape of fluid into the s
space provided the principal means of accommodating an ii
amount of blood within the cranial cavity, Ziegler and Hill have
shown that cerebrospinal fluid is absorbed by the blood-capillarie
each systole of the heart, and that this action is quite considerabl
ever the tension of the cerebrospinal fluid is increased. Even A
was surprised to observe that more than 500 c.c. of water that h
injected into the subarachnoid space of a dog disappeared in k
two hours. It has been shown by the investigations of Naunyn
coworkers that cerebrospinal fluid is absorbed with extraordinary
almost immediately after its secretion. This may be explained
fact that absorption is performed not by the lymphatics alone, b
cipally by the bloodvessels. Hill and Ziegler both injected a sol
potassium ferrocyanide into the subarachnoid space of the s
animals experimented on in order to observe whether this sul
which is easily recognizable, would appear first in the lymph-ve
the neck or in the facial vein which carries away most of the
blood of the brain in animals. The solution appeared in the l
from six to ten seconds after injection, but only traces could be re
in the lymph-channels half an hour after injection. Absorptio
take place therefore through the living capillary walls, as Zieg
rectly concluded. This corresponds also with the results obtai
Haidenhain in his experiments on absorption in general. Abs
takes place everywhere, both in the cranial cavity and in the spina
In the former, owing to intracranial pressure, venous return thro
veins of the face and neck may be retarded. In the latter this
take place. The bloodvessels in the dural space of the spinal co
municate very freely with the extradural venous plexus of the
canal, and can therefore always carry away rapidly the blood co
in them.

Every physiological increase of blood-pressure in the cerebral
is directly transmitted to the cerebrospinal fluid surrounding the

permeating the entire brain. The escape of the fluid into the spinal canal, as well as its rapid absorption, affords additional space for an increased amount of blood within the cranial cavity.

Under pathological conditions the circumstances are different. Cerebral pressure must be considered a pathological process in this sense. It can only be brought about through a disturbance of the constant equilibrium between transudation and absorption of cerebrospinal fluid. As long as both factors acting in the presence of physiological increase of blood-pressure remain undisturbed, and the distention of the spinal canal and the absorption of the capillaries continue to act together, cerebral pressure of a pathological degree cannot be produced. As soon, however, as they fail intracranial circulation is disturbed in the sense of an adiämorrhysis—that is, there is a slowing of the blood-current.

The distention of the dural space of the spinal cord ceases to take place if cerebrospinal fluid be suddenly forced from the contracted intracranial cavity into the spinal canal, either by rapid extravasations of blood or experimentally by the injection of wax, for under such circumstances the dura will suddenly be stretched to the limits of its elasticity. From the very moment when this takes place the resistance on the part of the dural membrane reacts on the cerebrospinal fluid, producing pressure and causing a rapidly increasing tension. If under these circumstances the factor that produces a contraction of the intracranial space increases even to a small degree, the effect of this minimal increase is considerable and suddenly brings about an exceedingly dangerous state of affairs. The tension of cerebrospinal fluid is of a sufficiently high degree to produce compression of the veins emerging from the skull and brings about a slowing of the cerebral circulation. This is also true if absorption of the capillaries is interfered with. In a number of inflammatory diseases of the brain-membranes (meningitis tuberculosa and serosa) this is certainly the case, for the changes in the walls of the capillaries are an integral part of the inflammatory process. For that reason every inflammation of the plexus and tela is combined with exudation into the ventricles. The increased quantity of fluid causes an increased tension of the latter, as shown by the velocity with which the stream of cerebrospinal fluid will flow out if the ventricles be punctured in such cases. Every rapid increase in quantity of cerebrospinal fluid is necessarily followed by an obstruction and contraction of the efferent veins, thus bringing about intracranial pressure.

In addition to these two factors in the production of increased tension of cerebrospinal fluid, there is a third—the displacement of the brain, if an extensive extravasation of blood or a rapidly growing tumor, either within or outside the brain, makes demands on the intracranial space. Hill's experiments have taught the significance of these displacements in regard to intracranial pressure, and the same thing had already been noted by Bönninghaus. Hill believes that the cutting off of communication between the fluid in the ventricles and that of the subarachnoid space of the spinal cord regularly follow the occurrence of extensive extravasation at the convexity of one or both hemispheres. Whenever

he injected fluid at a pressure of about 100 mm. he was convincↄ
the cerebrum was forced against the tentorium, and that the cere
and the medulla were displaced downward to such an extent tha
were pressed against the edge of the foramen magnum. Support
Althanns' views regarding the free communication between cerebro
fluid in the different cavities both in the brain and in the spinal corↄ
injected warm salt solution through an opening in one parietal bↄ
the bottom of which the dura was opened. He used very slight pↄ
in injecting the fluid and employed other precautions in order to
accidental lacerations and the production of artificial channels of co
nication. He observed that under normal conditions the salt sↄ
injected into the cranial cavity could flow out of a hole drilled throuↄ
lamina of a vertebra at the bottom of which the dura had been oↄ
In such cases, however, as has been described, where foreign subsↄ
placed between bone and dura mater had pressed the cerebelluↄ
medulla against the edges of the foramen magnum, the experiment ↄ
as communication had been cut off. Assuming that absorption of ceↄ
spinal fluid takes place primarily through the blood-capillaries,
fact was conclusively proved by Ziegler's investigations, if communiↄ
between the fluid in the cranial cavity and that in the spinal canal ↄ
off, the absorption of cerebrospinal fluid will have to be performↄ
the capillaries of the cranial cavity alone. This however, is morↄ
they can accomplish, for, as a result of the tension of the cerebroↄ
fluid, the veins carrying blood away from the head are compressↄ
that the absorbed fluid cannot be removed. From this it is easy
how the rapid absorption of cerebrospinal fluid depends on a free
munication of all cavities, clefts, and channels containing the fluid
why in the event of an interruption of this communication the nↄ
relation between secretion and absorption of cerebrospinal fluid i
turbed, resulting in the production of the clinical condition knoↄ
cerebral pressure.

In the latter instance the increased tension of cerebrospinal fluiↄ
through the retarded circulation in the capillaries, even if fron
beginning the veins are compressed and obstructed where they en
from the cranial cavity and at the very place where the internal vↄ
pressure is lowest. The pressure of a foreign body encroaching o
cranial cavity is transmitted not only through the cerebrospinal fluiↄ
through the semifluid brain as well. It has already been menti
that the brain substance, like water, possesses the least degree of
pressibility combined with the greatest degree of mobility of its ↄ
cules, and that it makes no difference as far as the expansile actiↄ
gunshots is concerned whether the projectile be fired through a ↄ
tacle filled with water or with brain.

Schnitzler and Reiner objected to the views the author has exprↄ
regarding the action of cerebrospinal fluid in cerebral compresↄ
They were able to produce regular and distinct symptoms of intracↄ
pressure by means of local intracranial pressure exerted artificↄ
after all cerebrospinal fluid had been allowed to drain away. Deↄ

repeated the experiments and modified them with some improvement. He also opened the subdural space and drained away the fluid before injecting paraffin, and observed that in spite of the absence of cerebrospinal fluid there was produced the characteristic picture of cerebral compression, including the mildest as well as the most severe symptoms. Pressure exerted upon the surface of the brain is not transmitted by cerebrospinal fluid alone, but by the semifluid brain as well, even if the latter does not transmit force as perfectly and completely as does a fluid like water. It transmits force, however, unlike a solid, particularly as regards the direction in which force is exerted. Like water, it does this in all directions, not however undiminished but evidently lessened. For this reason Deucher found that in order to obtain the same results after flow of cerebrospinal fluid as would be obtained before, it was necessary to inject greater quantities of paraffin. In the case of the unopened skull the effect was noticeable after a few seconds, but when the fluid had been allowed to drain away several minutes were required. The more cerebrospinal fluid an animal possesses, and in this respect man seems to surpass other animals, the more readily will it transmit pressure exerted on a circumscribed portion of the brain-surface to the veins where they emerge from the skull. The less fluid, the more irregularly will pressure be transmitted, and in a proportionate degree its force will be diminished in the course of its transmission.

That portion of the brain lying immediately beneath the object producing pressure (blood-clot, paraffin mass) suffers most and is affected by direct compression of the capillaries. This explains the paralysis of the opposite side after laceration of the middle meningeal artery, which will be discussed in the next chapter. Injections of fluid into the subarachnoid space can only produce general cerebral compression, never local pressure. On the other hand, where there is an intrusion of a solid body between brain and the bone (including blood-clots in the category) a general as well as a localized cerebral compression is produced, the significance of the latter depending on the portion of the brain directly affected.

The same question is presented when the fundus of the eye is examined and an attempt is made to explain the significance of the visible changes present during cerebral compression. Gräfe had explained his choked disk by pressure on the cavernous sinus into which the central vein of the retina, as well as the superior ophthalmic vein, empty, the latter being formed by the posterior and short ciliary veins. A constant branch of the superior ophthalmic vein emptying into the anterior facial vein, to which attention has been called by Sesemann, might in the event of the channel to the intracranial sinus being obstructed serve to provide an unobstructed extracranial channel to carry blood from the ophthalmic vein and central vein of the retina. For this reason Schmidt-Rimpler and Manz were inclined to refer the stasis of the veins of the fundus and the swelling of the papilla to the increased tension of the cerebrospinal fluid in the arachnoid sheath surrounding the optic nerve. More

'The course of intracranial pressure depends upon its
depends, in the first place, upon whether the encroachment
nial space is a permanent one, or whether the condition pro-
apression of the brain becomes altered, either demanding
t in consequence of an increase in volume or less space as a
minished size. A depressed fragment of bone, unless it be
y operative measures, produces a permanent and constant
ent on the cavity of the skull. An extravasation of blood
t first until the bleeding vessel is closed either as a result of
coagulation of blood. A rapidly forming abscess progresses
ly and therefore produces constantly increasing intracranial
The important feature in judging pressure-symptoms is to
whether they are increasing or diminishing. According to
ey progress or recede, it can be determined whether the causes
hem are progressing or recedi g. In the former instance the
es an increasing danger ; in rthe latter case there is simply
ce that will cease sooner or later.
rmination depends largely upon the size of the body producing
Extravasation of blood from larger arteries may rapidly
extensive as to interfere with the entire cerebral circulation,
very large number of cases moderate extravasations are pro-
easing at first, but disappearing finally without having caused
t disturbance.
tion of time during which pressure is exerted is also of impor-
m experiments it is known that even a high degree of pressure
rne provided it acts only momentarily, while long-continued
inders recovery and finally renders the latter impossible.
he most severe, symptoms of general compression may dis-
oon as the factors causing contraction of intracranial space
d. Patients may recover completely from a condition of
i slow pulse even if the latter has continued for weeks. A
f deep coma, however, with complete muscular paralysis and
sensitiveness to external impressions, with dilatation of pupils
ir deep respiration, will terminate fatally unless some remedy
immediately. The onset of paralysis of the circulatory and
centres is a sign of speedy dissolution.
istency of pressure is as dangerous as an excessively high
ressore. When circulation is retarded to such a degree as to
st entirely ceased, the fluid elements of the blood escape
i walls of the vessels and enter the adventitial spaces, increasing
y of cerebrospinal fluid. In this way the tension of the latter
ier raised and its inhibiting influence on the movement of the
nt also increased. (Edema of the brain occurring in this way
ie compression of the brain and at the same time by an
process paralyzes the functions of the nerve-tissues. At all
mpf has demonstrated maceration and degeneration of the
ers in the peripheral nerves as a result of stasis of the
sirculation.

in this nor in any other of the author's cases was it possible to save the life of the patient. The only known case in which the operation was followed by favorable results was one reported by Freyan, who performed lumbar puncture and drew off a quantity of fluid that had existed under considerable pressure and which contained albumin, few pus-cells, and many tubercle bacilli; the patient recovered. Many operators report astonishing, but only temporary, favorable results; Fürbringer reports the results obtained in 37 cases as *nil*. Nevertheless, the momentary recession of the dangerous symptoms tempts one to perform puncture repeatedly, and the author would advise that it be carried out in the ventricles rather than in the lumbar portion of the cord.

The occurrence of serous meningitis or acute idiopathic hydrocephalus has for a long time been considered doubtful, but the experience of physicians familiar with the diseases of children points to this as a primary disease not dependent upon any new growth or cerebral abscess or a purulent meningitis, and forces us to distinguish it from the exacerbations of chronic congenital or acquired hydrocephalus. If all these pathological processes can be excluded, and there are present symptoms like those of a tuberculous or purulent meningitis, such as disturbances of consciousness, violent headaches, drowsiness, motor disturbances and paralyses, twitching of the legs or hands, stiffness of the back of the neck, high temperature, and, above all, bilateral choked disk, lumbar puncture should be chosen both for diagnostic and therapeutic purposes as being the more conservative procedure. Bönningham has reported a number of cases in which this operation produced rapid and permanent improvement.

Chronic acquired hydrocephalus, as contrasted with congenital hydrocephalus, is not a distinct disease in itself, but is the result of different intracranial diseases, such as acute serous and possibly tuberculous meningitis, or it may develop as a chronic process from the beginning. Cases of the first class, with acute onset, occur at about the end of the first or beginning of the second year. Those of the second class have a varied etiology. In this category must also be placed cases of serous effusion into the ventricles in rhachitic, perhaps also in syphilitic, children, cases of chronic hydrocephalus following encephaloceles and spina bifida, the accumulation of cerebrospinal fluid in one ventricle after inflammatory closure of the channel of communication with the other cavities containing cerebrospinal fluid, the filling of large porocephalic clefts with fluid, the same condition in other cases of loss of substance produced by traumatism or atrophy, and the dilatation of the ventricles in connection with cerebral tumors.

If chronic acquired hydrocephalus develops before closure of the sutures and fontanelles, it produces the same increase in size of the skull that is characteristic of typical congenital hydrocephalus. If it occurs later, when the skull has become rigidly and firmly closed, it exists without increase in size of the skull; in fact, even cases of microcephalus have been recently reported in which the ventricles were dilated and filled with fluid.

In this connection there are probably only two circumstances to l sidered—the time when the increase in size of the skull was first and the development of an acquired hydrocephalus after a previou intracranial inflammation. The latter is frequently obscured tl being put down as a disturbance of dentition. The diagnosis of effusion into the ventricles is always uncertain. Thus, acquired chronic hydrocephalus in adults has almost always been taken for i tumor, if for no other reason than that it very frequently comp the latter, its development being due in a great measure to tl placement of the brain produced by a growing tumor. Lumbai ture for the purpose of diagnosis, introduced by Quincke, is recommended in all such cases when marked symptoms of pi develop.

The different methods of drawing off cerebrospinal fluid in conr with the above-mentioned diseases are: 1. Lumbar puncture. 2 tricular puncture. 3. Drainage of the ventricles. 4. Drainage spinal dural sac.

1. In Quincke's puncture of the lower portion of the dural sac br two lumbar vertebræ, advantage is taken of the anatomical relati that region, carefully studied by him and later by Brauer. As the spinous processes of the lumbar vertebræ are placed borizo The space between two vertebræ, therefore, is found most easily median line, and the instrument, held horizontally, should be exactly between two spinous processes. At times the inferior edg spinous process is bent down to such a degree as almost to tou superior edge of the process lying beneath. Under such circumst which is made evident by the needle or trocar striking the bone better to pass the instrument obliquely from below upward inste horizontally. The point at which puncture can be most readily perf lies, according to Jacoby, in the median line behind, at a point the latter would be intersected by a horizontal line passing th the highest point of the crest of each ilium. As it is of importan only to make a microscopical, bacteriological, and chemical exa tion of the fluid obtained, but also to determine the pressure which it exists, the hollow needle may be connected by means of a of rubber tubing with a U-shaped manometer.

2. Puncture of one of the lateral ventricles may be performed l author's method through the frontal region or, as carried out by through the parietal region of the skull. The surgeon should loc the tuberosity of the frontal bone, make a small longitudinal incis little above and to the inner side of it, going through the soft part to the bone, and bore a hole through the skull with a layer bore. He should then pass a long hollow needle in a dir from below backward and a little downward and inward, push through the brain-tissue until the fluid flows out. Keen chose a po not more 1½ mm. above a line joining the supraorbital ridge and ext

occipital protuberance, and taken from this line 32 mm. behind the external auditory meatus.

3. Drainage of the ventricle was also first suggested by Keen. Henle has reported on the value of this procedure from Mikulicz's clinic. The technic has already been described. Drainage of the ventricles seems a rational method, especially in the case of the non-ossified skull, owing to the soft consistency of which a diminution in size is possible after removal of the fluid in the ventricles. This method is, however, exceedingly dangerous, for as long as fluid is oozing and saturating the dressings there is liability to infection and subsequent purulent meningitis. It has been mentioned that all attempts at ventricular drainage in the case of the unossified skull have ended fatally. In only one case in which the bones of the skull had become completely ossified was Broca able to bring about recovery. This was the case of a boy four years old. The drainage-tube must be passed through the trocar after the latter has reached the cavity of the ventricle, and must of necessity, therefore, be a very small one.

4. Instead of drawing off the fluid at one step by means of lumbar puncture, Essex Winter attempted to establish continuous drainage in the lumbar region. The result was fatal.

INJURIES OF THE INTRACRANIAL VESSELS.

BY DR. P. WIESMANN.

The principal vessels in connection with this subject are:

1. The middle meningeal artery and its accompanying veins.
2. The sinuses of the dura mater, particularly the longitudinal and transverse sinus and the torcular Herophili.
3. The larger veins of the pia mater emptying into the sinuses.
4. That portion of the internal carotid artery lying within the cavity of the skull.

The vessels of the diploë and the emissary veins hardly deserve special attention. Injuries of the jugular vein at the site of the posterior lacerated foramen and consequent accumulations of blood between the skull and dura occur so rarely that it is sufficient to mention them.

The significance of these injuries lies, in the first place, in the loss of blood; and in the second place, in the accumulation of extravasated blood within the cranial cavity, with consequent encroachment on intra-cranial space.

Of the above-mentioned bloodvessels, the middle meningeal artery possesses the greatest surgical interest, for it is most frequently the source of intracranial hemorrhage caused by trauma—in nearly nine-tenths of all cases according to Prescott Hewett—and at the same time injuries of this vessel produce the most typical combination of symptoms. Further, this injury is usually fatal under expectant treatment, while in proper cases operative interference is followed by the most satisfactory

PLATE III.

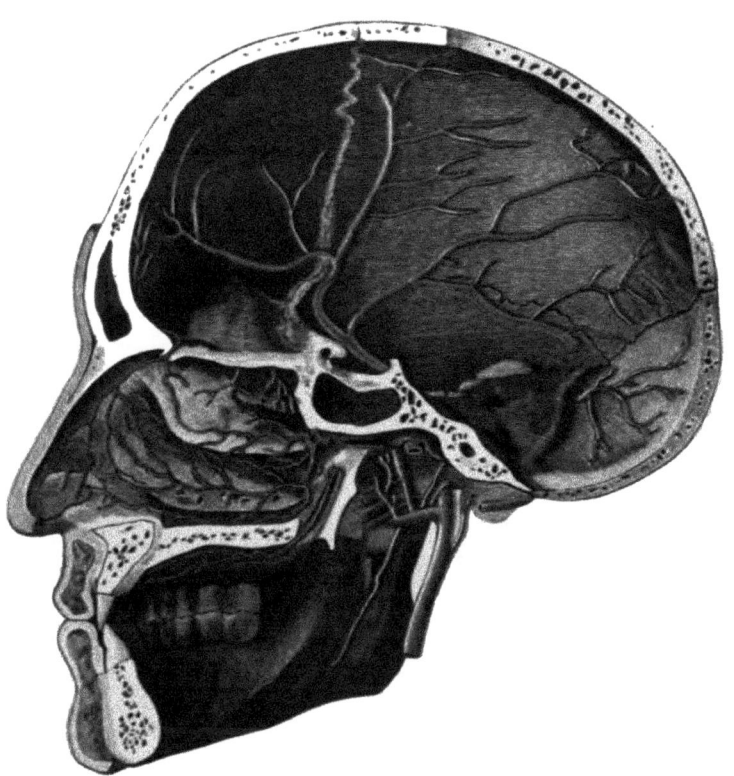

Arteries of the Skull and Nasal Cavities. (Spalteholz.)

the skull in the temporal region. Gunshot injuries of the artery were observed by Tylecote, Guthrie, B. Beck, Gross, and Otis. Ledderhose observed a case of injury from a shot-gun. Krönlein observed an injury resulting from a pistol-shot, in which case the bullet lacerated the posterior branch on one side in entering, and the anterior branch of the middle meningeal artery of the opposite side in leaving the skull. Moreover, in gunshot-wounds laceration of the vessel may result from fracture of the bone produced at the same time, the latter being the direct cause of the injury of the artery.

In the majority of cases, however, violence with blunt objects of various kinds produces more or less extensive bone injury, in the course of which and as the result of which the vessels are lacerated. In this connection two ways of occurrence must be considered. Either a comminuted fracture is produced, a splinter of bone transfixing the artery, or the latter is torn against the sharp edge of a fragment of bone. Thus, Coutagne observed in a case of stellate fracture of the parietal bone produced by a blow with a bottle, a longitudinal tear 1 cm. long in the anterior branch of the middle meningeal artery, caused by a sharp fragment of bone projecting inward. Even in cases of simple fissure, especially when the line of fracture runs across the course of the vessels, the latter may be cut into by the edge of bone if the latter be sharply depressed at the moment the fracture is produced. The most frequent mode of occurrence appears to be, however, that the vessels lying in the grooves in the bone are torn at the same time that the bone is broken, as the result of the deformity of the skull produced by violence with blunt objects. This is particularly liable to occur when the artery, instead of lying in a groove, is enclosed in a bony canal, which condition Krönlein found in three of his cases of injury of the meningeal artery.

Those cases are especially interesting in which injury of the meningeal artery is produced without any injury of bone—that is, without any fracture of the bone in the vicinity of the injured vessel. This occurrence has been positively confirmed by a series of reports upon autopsies and

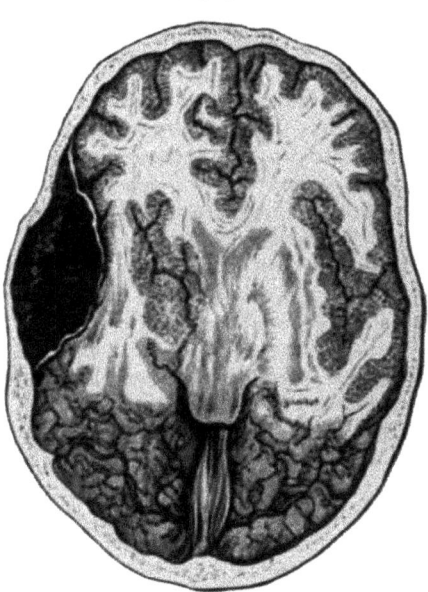

Fig. 75.

Compression following hemorrhage from the middle meningeal artery. (Helferich.)

operations. It is assumed that when the shape of the skull is c
at the moment of impact the vessel is stretched in the same direc
the molecules of the skull. While, however, the molecules of th
are not completely torn apart, and by virtue of their elasticity re
their former position, the artery, possessing less elasticity, suffer
tion of continuity. Not only the fact of the vessel being embed
the grooves in the bone, but also the fact that the artery is attac
the bone by numerous perforating branches makes this liable to h
According to v. Bergmann, especially bodies with a more or less :
cal form, if impelled against the skull and driving in the area of in
immediately rebound and allow the skull to assume its normal
without producing fracture; the artery, however, is torn.

Frequently, comparatively slight violence may produce such an i
as, for instance, blows with canes, fists, stones, etc. In such ca
discoverable injuries of the soft parts may be absent.

Less frequent, but of great diagnostic importance, are injun
vessels caused by *contrecoup*, cases in which laceration of the arte
produced, not on that side of the skull receiving violence, but at a
directly opposite or at a point some distance from the site of in
Thus in a case of Krönlein's the patient had fallen down the cellar-s
the direct result of violence being a contused wound over the
parietal bone, while on the left side there was produced a lacerati
the artery, no fracture of bones being present. These lesions as
plained by the change in form of the skull as a whole which results
considerable violence.

Finally, cases have been described in which both meningeal ar
were injured, the one probably directly as the result of the act of viol
the other probably through *contrecoup* or the extension of fissures t
opposite side. Such a case of double hemorrhage from injury of
middle meningeal arteries was observed by Krönlein. At the si
injury, produced probably by a blow with a cane, there was a co
nuted fracture with laceration of the middle meningeal artery; fror
comminuted area a fissure extended to the other side of the skull, inj
the artery on that side also.

Cases have been observed with lacerations of the trunk, and of s
branches; also cases in which the artery has been found torn thr
at the foramen spinosum.

Effects.—The natural consequence of injury of the meningeal a
is almost always hemorrhage; this is usually severe. In many case
circulatory disturbance dependent on shock may in the beginning
vent the escape of blood from the artery. As soon as, after a long
shorter time, this condition disappears and action of the heart bec
stronger, hemorrhage from the injured artery sets in. In a ce
number of cases there is absence of hemorrhage even after rea
takes place, or hemorrhage may be so slight as to produce no sy
toms, and it is only after some time has elapsed, frequently several c
that some cause, as coughing, mental excitement, or suppuration, bi
about secondary hemorrhage.

The effects produced, and consequently the entire clinical picture, are entirely different according to whether the blood can escape freely or accumulates within the cranial cavity. External hemorrhage takes place if at the site of the injury of the artery there is present a compound fracture of the skull through which the blood can find an outlet. In such cases even on inspection of the wound there can be seen bright-red blood pouring from the wound, or hemorrhage will suddenly set in during the toilet of the cranial wound—while removing fragments of bone, elevating a depressed area, chiselling off projecting edges of bone, etc. In the course of these manipulations the actual source of hemorrhage may occasionally be discovered and the spurting artery distinctly seen. Krönlein observed, in a case of laceration of the meningeal artery resulting from comminuted fracture, blood spurting from both the proximal and distal ends of the artery. Exceptionally in cases of complete division of the artery hemorrhage may be absent.

In the majority of cases there is intracranial hemorrhage, the blood usually collecting between bone and dura mater if the latter has escaped injury, causing a hæmatoma which is usually of considerable size. It is called supradural or, still better, extradural. The term hæmatoma of the dura mater is misleading and inappropriate.

The blood escapes from the artery under considerable pressure—80 to 100 mm. of mercury, according to v. Bergmann. The increasing volume of blood separates the tense dura mater from the inner surface of the skull. This may take place over a considerable area, and extend even beyond the lines of the sutures.

Hemorrhage continues until the artery is closed by a temporary thrombus, or until the extravasation of blood, encroaching on the intracranial space produces such a degree of intracranial pressure as to equal the blood-pressure within the artery and prevent further accumulation of blood. In this way it frequently happens that enormous quantities of blood accumulate. Extravasations amounting to 4 ounces have been frequently observed, while 5 to 6 ounces are not infrequent. Krönlein observed an extravasation weighing 9 ounces, and James Hill reports a case in which after trephining he removed from the same patient two clots of blood each weighing 6 to 7 ounces. As a rule the extravasated blood assumes the shape of a segment of a sphere, the convexity of which is directed toward the brain and which may frequently be several centimetres thick. Not infrequently the central point of the convex surface corresponds very nearly to the point of rupture of the bloodvessel, from which point the accumulating blood has dissected the dura from the bone uniformly and in all directions. (Fig. 75.)

Regarding the exact location of supradural hæmatoma, Krönlein has laid down important laws. He divides hæmatoma into *diffuse* and *circumscribed*, the former usually extending more or less over one entire half of the skull; the latter he divides according to the course of the three principal branches of the artery, into an *anterior* hæmatoma ("frontotemporale"), a *middle* hæmatoma ("temporoparietale"), and a *posterior* hæmatoma ("parieto-occipitale"). Of these, the middle

occurs most frequently, corresponding to the great vulnerabili
temporal region in the first place; and secondly, owing to the
of important arteries (the trunk and both principal branche
middle meningeal artery). The posterior hæmatoma followin
of the posterior principal branch is much less
frequent is the frontotemporal hæmatoma, caused by
anterior division of the anterior principal branch.

FIG. 76.

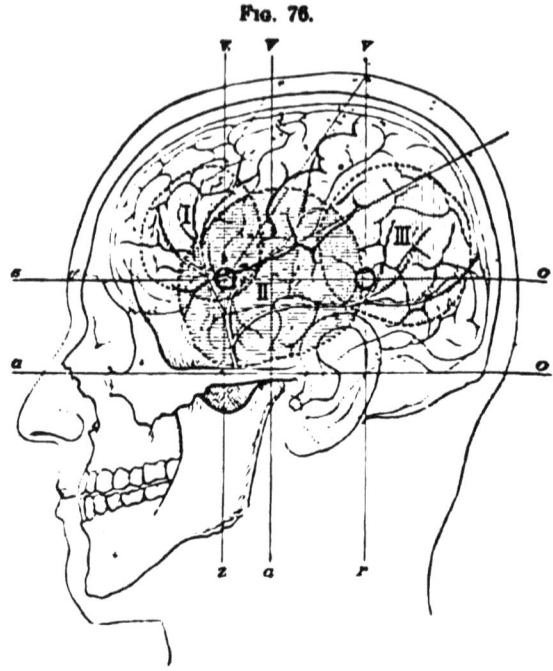

Scheme of hæmatomata of middle meningeal artery. I. Frontotemporal hæmatoma
poroparietal hæmatoma. III. Parieto-occipital hæmatoma. a. Auricular orbital (
line. s o. Supraorbital (horizontal) line. v z. Vertical zygomatic line. v s. Ventria
line. p r. Vertical retromastoid line. The two circles represent the places for trephin
ing to Krönlein. (After Krönlein.)

As a rule a necessary condition for the formation of supradura
toma is the uninjured state of the dura. If the dura be injure
may accumulate outside the dura. As a rule, however, the large
of blood flows beneath the dura mater. Here also there
formed an enormous blood-clot; more frequently, however, th
is spread in a thin layer in the subdural space. In a certain
of cases a part of the extravasated blood is situated above the
part below, and both portions communicate with each other th
slit-like opening in the dura. As a companion piece to this
bilocular hæmatoma, are cases in which the soft parts remainin

over an open fracture of the skull, blood collects on each side of the bone. Such cases occur particularly among children, in whom the firm attachment of dura to bone favors the expression of blood from the cranial cavity. Finally there are cases in which, besides laceration of the dura mater, there is injury of brain-tissue at the site of injury. Under such circumstances blood finds a path prepared by which to invade the substance of the brain itself, much as in cases of apoplexy.

Regarding the fate of the blood accumulating over the dura little is known. At all events it does not remain in a fluid state very long. On trephining or on autopsy it is usually found in the form of a compact hard blackish clot. In fatal cases death results so rapidly that marked changes in the extravasated blood cannot take place. In the cases that recover the blood-clot is usually completely absorbed, though the conditions for absorption of extradural hemorrhage are not by any means so favorable as they are for hemorrhage into and beneath the pia mater. It has been conclusively demonstrated by a case of Perrin that

Fig. 77.

Fig. 78.

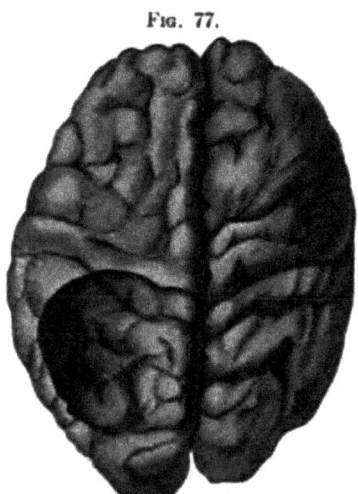

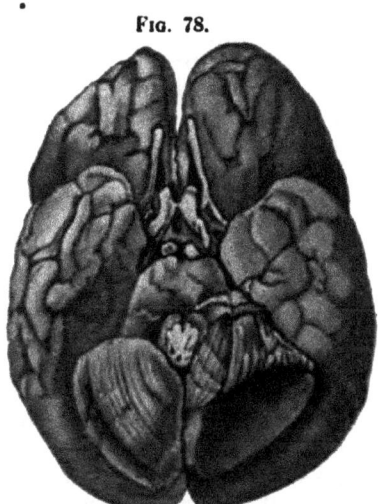

Depression in cerebral hemisphere following hemorrhage from middle meningeal artery.

Depression in cerebellum following hemorrhage.

even considerable extradural hemorrhage may be absorbed. The patient had been struck by a fragment of an exploded shell, with the production of typical symptoms of rupture of the middle meningeal artery. Three years later on autopsy a healed fissure was found intersecting the artery. Furthermore, blood-clots may undergo suppuration and decomposition, even in case of subcutaneous cranial injuries. Huguenin observed this, in the case of a patient dying eight days after injury.

The result of such large accumulations of blood in the cranial cavity is a typical change in form of the brain. Not only are blood, lymph, and cerebrospinal fluid displaced, but also the lateral walls of the ventricles are forced inward, the convolutions are flattened, frequently entire hemisphere is flattened out beneath the extravasation, or depre saucer-shaped. Figs. 77 and 78, taken from specimens in the Zu clinic, show such depressions, one being in one cerebral hemisphere other in the cerebellum. Those parts of the brain particularly aff are frequently noticeably dry as if squeezed out.

Rupture of the middle meningeal artery is frequently other cranial injuries. Very rarely an injury of a sin at the same time (cases of Guerlain, transverse sinus Wagner, longitudinal sinus). Accompanying injuries of the dura n are more frequent. From the point of view of diagnosis, and certain extent also of prognosis, the presence of contusions of the b tissue is important. The contusion of the brain may be in the : region as the injury of the vessel, and may also have been produce the same cause and mechanism: circumscribed,comminuted, or depre fracture. On the other hand, if produced by contrecoup, it may be : entirely different part of the brain, frequently at a point directly opp to that at which the artery was injured. Prescott Hewett assumes contusion of the brain always accompanies rupture of the middle me geal artery. But the absence of contusion of the brain has been repe in a large number of autopsies, and after investigation of a large nu of cases, so that it is a rule, rather than an exception, that the bra uninjured.

Symptoms.—The symptoms of rupture of the meningeal artery according to whether hemorrhage is *external* or *internal.* The fo were discussed in describing the pathological anatomy. Certain present symptoms which represent a transition into the second (where hemorrhage takes place internally, the latter being decidedl more frequent manner of occurrence. In these transitional cases he rhage either takes place beneath the external soft parts (pressu such an external hæmatoma producing symptoms of cerebral pres: or hemorrhage having been prevented by a temporary bandag followed later by a typical combination of symptoms. Cases o first kind were observed by Golding Bird, Holmes, Marchant, Krön cases of the second kind of Krönlein and Ledderhose.

The clinical picture is much more complicated in those cases in w extravasation of blood takes place between bone and dura. The s toms are all more or less referable to compression of the brain, a is only the manner of its development and the particular location blood-clot that determine a definite characteristic clinical picture.

The symptoms of intracranial hemorrhage from the middle menir artery are due in part to gradually increasing intracranial pres: and in part to localized pressure. The former, which may be c *general*, or, according to Kocher, *indirect*, symptoms, consist of dist ances of consciousness, changes in pulse and respiration. The la called *local* or *direct* symptoms, consist of disturbances of powe motion, possibly also of sensation, further disturbances of speech, char in the pupils as well as in the fundus of the eye.

PLATE IV.

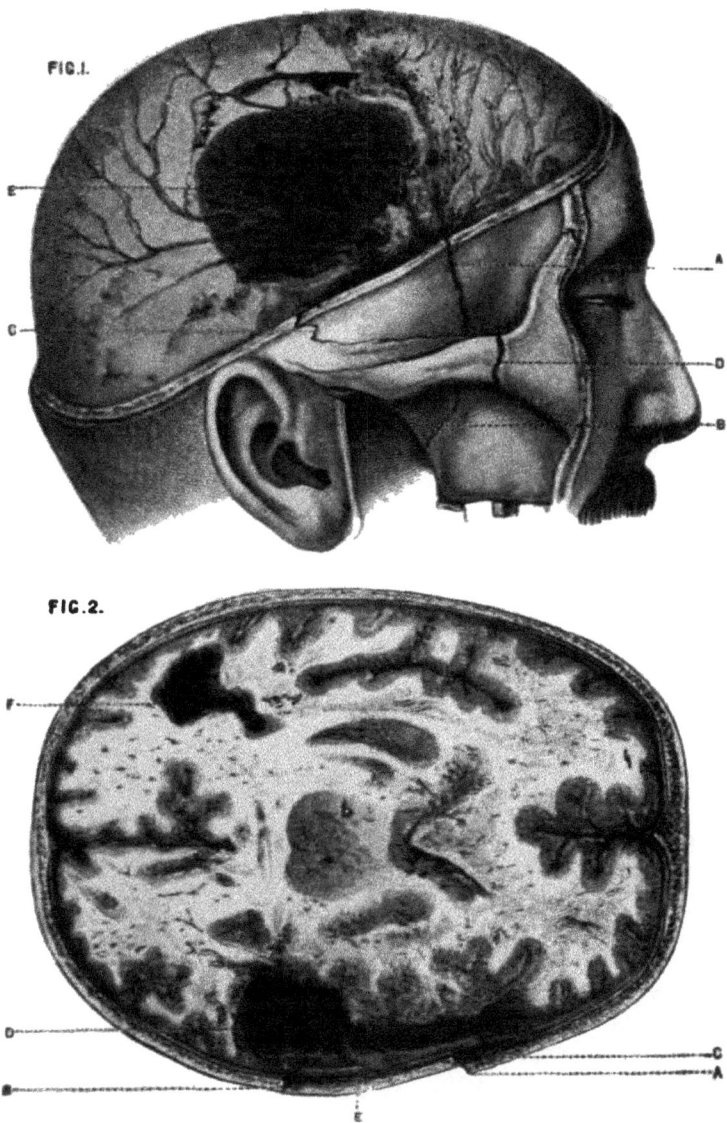

FIG.1.

FIG.2.

Fig. 1. Compound Fracture of Cranium, with Depression; Fracture of Bones of Face; Extradural Clot from Rupture of Middle Meningeal Artery.

Fig. 2. Horizontal Section of same, showing Depressed Fracture of Bone; C, Extradural Clot; D, Laceration of Brain-substance, with extensive Intracerebral Clot; F, same condition produced by *Contrecoup*. Punctate Hemorrhages and Minute Lacerations at Numerous Points, characteristic of *Contusion* of the Brain. (Anger.)

PLATE IV.

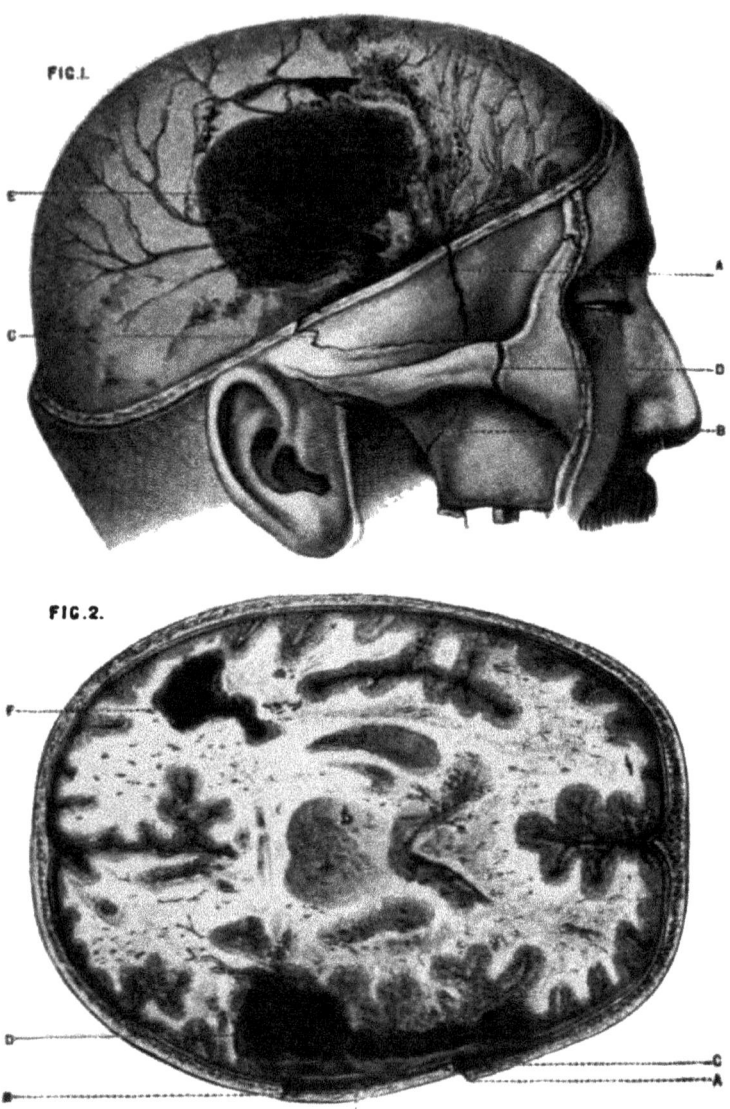

Fig. 1. Compound Fracture of Cranium, with Depression; Fracture of Bones of Face; Extradural Clot from Rupture of Middle Meningeal Artery.

Fig. 2. Horizontal Section of same, showing Depressed Fracture of Bone; C, Extradural Clot; D, Laceration of Brain-substance, with extensive Intracerebral Clot; F, same condition produced by *Contrecoup*. Punctate Hemorrhages and Minute Lacerations at Numerous Points, characteristic of *Contusion* of the Brain. (Anger.)

The most important symptoms are the *mental disturbances*, especially the so-called *free interval* which is characteristic of all extensive intracranial extravasations of blood. Besides the free interval other progressively increasing symptoms of compression of the brain are developed. After loss of consciousness immediately following injury, which continues for a greater or less length of time, combined with superficial respiration and a weak, rapid pulse, the result of concussion, the patient regains consciousness. Gradually, however, consciousness becomes lost a second time, the patient becomes drowsy and stupid, falls into a state of deep coma until, after a longer or shorter time, death takes place. J. L. Petit drew attention to these "primary and consecutive" cerebral manifestations and pointed out their relation to intracranial hemorrhage. At the same time that consciousness is disturbed the other symptoms increase in intensity, the pulse becomes slower, respiration becomes laboring and stertorous, and paresis sets in, finally terminating in complete paralysis. Not infrequently initial cerebral concussion remains absent, the patient retaining consciousness. He may pay no attention to the injury, continue his occupation, may walk for considerable distance, and it is only after some time that severe manifestations set in. Finally the typical free interval may be absent, or be obscured, as cerebral concussion passing directly into compression of the brain.

Kocher explains the free interval in the following way: As the result of hemorrhage there is an increased intracranial pressure which at first produces compression of the veins, these offering less resistance. The obstructed venous return increases blood-pressure in the arteries and circulation continues unimpaired. This "stage of complete compensation" corresponds to the free interval. The brain being supplied with sufficient blood, apparently carries out its functions in a normal manner, and the only sign of a pathological condition at this time may be headache due to increased tension of the dura.

The *duration of the free* interval is very variable, to which attention is particularly drawn, as attempts have been made to make use of this fact in differential diagnosis. This point will be discussed further in taking up intradural hemorrhage. In the majority of cases observed the free interval lasts a few hours, possibly as long as one day. Cases in which the free interval lasted three, four, or five days are extremely rare, and must be explained by special circumstances.

An important sign of gradually increasing intracranial pressure is changes in the frequency and force of the *pulse*. Decided slowing, hardness, and tension of the same—the so-called pressure-pulse—is common to other causes producing contraction of the space within the cranial cavity. If, however, the pulse is normal immediately after injury or during the free interval, and becomes slower after the lapse of some time, one would be pretty safe in assuming the existence of hemorrhage. During a later stage, just before death, the pulse becomes very rapid. At first, as the result of general pressure, the vagus centre in the medulla is stimulated; as the result of long-continued and increasing pressure the centre is finally paralyzed. The pulse-rate may fall ░░░░░░░░░ during the terminal stage it may reach a frequency of ░░░ ░░░░░.

The *change in character of the respiration* is a symptom ░░░░░░░ its significance and causes to the changes in the pulse. ░░░░ ░░░ stertorous breathing referable to circulatory disturbances in ░░ ░░░ brought about by general compression of the brain is a prominent symptom of intracranial pressure.

While, as has been mentioned, disturbances of consciousness, ░░░░░ in pulse and respiration, indicate the existence of general compression of the brain, and by their typical course enable the surgeon to conclude the presence of intracranial hemorrhage, there are a number of symptoms dependent upon marked compression and anæmia of certain areas of the cortex, which enable him to determine the location of hemorrhage in a given case.

Very frequently there are motor disturbances consisting of contralateral hemiplegias; they are especially pathognomonic of subdural hemorrhage resulting from injury to the middle meningeal artery, and are caused by pressure on the motor centres. In temporoparietal hæmatoma, the most frequent form, the central convolutions are the ones subjected to the greatest degree of pressure. These areas are the ones most frequently rendered anæmic, and that to a very high degree. At the onset localised anæmia of the gray substance gives rise to convulsions; these are soon followed by paresis of the opposite side of the body, while extreme degrees of anæmia lead to more or less complete hemiplegia. The arm-centre occupying the middle of the motor area, the arm of the opposite side is the part of the body affected first and the part that suffers most serious damage; while the leg of the opposite side, whose centre lies in the superior portion of the central convolution, suffers less disturbance and is never affected alone. In ░░░░ ░░░░ latter circumstance Jacobson has investigated 78 cases. As ░░░░ ░░ the region of the motor centres for the leg, the branches of the meningeal arteries have become quite small; they cannot cause very extensive hemorrhage in this situation, and so cannot produce serious ░░░░ of function of these centres. Isolated and marked facial ░░░░ ░░░░ to hemorrhage in front and below. In isolated paralysis ░░░░ arm there is usually hemorrhage producing pressure on ░░░░░░ of the central convolutions.

░░░░ cases have been observed in which apparently paralysis ░░ the opposite side of the body, but on the same side ░░░░ so-called cases of *collateral hemiplegia*. Recently ░░░ published observations regarding this condition. He ░░░░ he considers typical of collateral (uncrossed) hemi-░░ such cases collected from literature. In these the hemorrhage caused by trauma or brain injury, spon-░░░░ areas of necrosis, cerebral abscesses, or new ░░░░ ░░ Kidderhose: "It appears from study of such ░░░░ hemiplegia of the same side (not crossed) does ░░░░ with all kinds of brain lesions. Accordingly in cases in which the general symptoms and the presence of hemiplegia would lead one to make a diagnosis of lesion of one hemisphere, one must be prepared to find that in a certain number of cases the lesion will be found on the same side as the paralysis, and not on the opposite side."

Without entering too deeply into a controversy regarding the unsettled question of collateral hemiplegia, the author wishes to draw attention to the objections made by Oppenheim. According to him, it is in most cases only a question of faulty observation and error in judging the state of motility. The majority of individuals in whom diagnosis of collateral hemiplegia was made were examined while in a state of deep coma. The muscles of the opposite side were found to be in a state of tonic contraction, spasm, twitching or convulsion, etc., while the muscles of the same side were lax, immobile, and without tone. The latter circumstance, depending upon the state of coma and the flaccid condition of the limbs, was mistaken for paralysis, while the condition of contraction or convulsion of the opposite side was taken for one of healthy activity.

According to Ortner, the side can be determined in a state of coma by the fact that the muscles of respiration on the paralyzed side are also paralyzed, or their function at least considerably impaired. And, according to Ortner, the opposite side of the thorax always moves less during the act of respiration, whether the intracranial lesion acts as an irritant or a depressant. At all events this symptom is of considerable importance, though, as Oppenheim maintains, Ortner's rule is liable to frequent exceptions.

Unilateral disturbances of sensation are less frequently met with than motor disturbances. This is easy to understand, considering the depressed state in which the mental functions are found, and on account of which it is seldom possible to determine accurately the state of sensibility. Unilateral disturbances of sensibility, anæsthesia, or even hyperæsthesia, are, however, very important signs if positively determined, as they point with considerable degree of certainty to posterior hæmatoma. Krönlein observed a number of such cases, in which contralateral disturbances of sensibility accompanied posterior hæmatoma.

A rare but extremely interesting symptom of localization is *aphasia*. The loss of consciousness, however, in most cases renders it impossible to determine this condition. But where this symptom is present, it is very valuable in locating the lesion. It is always produced by pressure on Broca's convolution, caused by an anterior hæmatoma or a very extensive middle hæmatoma on the left side.

An abnormal condition of the *pupils* is frequently found. Greisinger taught that in most cases of "hæmatoma of the dura mater" there was contraction of the pupils, and that as a rule the pupil of the opposite side was a little more dilated than that on the same side as the hemorrhage. On the other hand, experimental investigation of compression of the brain has demonstrated that at the beginning of pressure the pupil on the affected side was contracted; on increasing pressure and during the state of coma the pupils were dilated, the pupil on the side directly

The cardinal symptoms upon which a diagnosis of intracranial hemorrhage from rupture of the middle meningeal artery may be based are as follows:

1. The *free interval*, especially if it be of short duration, and regardless whether distinct concussion has preceded it or not. Depressed fractures produce pressure-symptoms immediately after injury, and can be easily discovered by palpation. If pressure-symptoms arise several days later, they may still be the result of hemorrhage; at the same time one suspects the presence of products of inflammation, and this is all the more probable the longer the time that has elapsed since the injury. Should there not have been an opportunity for observing the free interval, or if it cannot be positively confirmed by the history, the increase of pressure-symptoms permits the conclusion that hemorrhage is present.

2. The *pressure-pulse*, especially if it follows a slightly rapid and small pulse. If, again, a hard slow pulse be followed by marked increase in frequency, the terminal stage of vagus paralysis has set in, and there is imminent danger of a fatal termination.

3. *Stertorous respiration*, of great importance in differential diagnosis, as contrasted with the superficial respiration of cerebral concussion.

4. The *gradual development of hemiplegia*, especially if preceded by convulsions on the side of the body later paralyzed. Destruction of the cortical motor centres is also followed by contralateral paralyses; the latter, however, follow immediately after injury. Moderate contusions and irritation from penetrating fragments of bone produce convulsions of the opposite side in most cases.

If, in addition to these rational symptoms, there are local manifestations at the site of injury, either a compound or subcutaneous fracture, only a doughy swelling of the soft parts, or even only a slight abrasion of the skin, the diagnosis of rupture of the middle meningeal artery can be made with almost absolute certainty. Contralateral hemiplegia may aid in making the topical diagnosis in those cases in which there are evidences of external injury on the paralyzed side. One would assume that the artery had been injured by contrecoup and look for hemorrhage on the opposite side.

Aphasia and disturbances of sensibility may be important signs, the former pointing to anterior hæmatoma, the latter justifying the assumption of hemorrhage in the distribution of the posterior branch. Changes in the pupils and the fundus of the eye are frequently of help in making a diagnosis, as are also disturbances in the innervation of the muscles of the eye.

Unfortunately such a distinct and typical combination of symptoms is not always present; the picture may be obscured by many different factors, and the diagnosis in this way be rendered very difficult or even impossible.

Pure cerebral concussion is probably always distinguishable from possible cases of hemorrhage. Acute alcoholic intoxication and spontaneous apoplexy may cause doubt. Contusions of the brain and inflammatory manifestations—even simple active hyperæmia—may frequently obscure the picture to such an extent that the diagnosis cannot be made during life, or may approach so nearly the picture of hemorrhage that they become another source of error.

Among the affections to be considered in differential diagnosis particular attention is called to *secondary apoplexy* and *fat-embolism*. In the cases of secondary apoplexy published by Bollinger, a free interval of from twelve to twenty days or of several weeks was observed. Following is a brief clinical history of one of these cases:

A painter, twenty-six years old, received a wound 3 cm. long over the left parietal bone as the result of a blow with a bludgeon. The wound apparently healed well. After twenty days there were apathy and headache; after thirty days admitted to hospital; loss of intellectual powers; later deep unconsciousness; paralysis of left(!) side. Pulse 50, later rapid; still later paralysis on right side. Death on thirty-second day. Autopsy: traumatic secondary apoplexy of the walls of the fourth ventricle, capillary hemorrhage in the medulla oblongata, intermeningeal apoplexies over the left hemisphere.

The similarity to injury of the meningeal artery is unmistakable, even if the long duration of the free interval should cause the surgeon to hesitate.

The author is indebted to Krönlein for a report of a case of fat-embolism, a history of which is given for the sake of comparison:

A farmer, thirty-nine years old, fell down a cellar-stairs with a heavy barrel, in May, 1898, sustaining a subcutaneous fracture of the left leg. The injured man was unconscious for a little while, following which his mind was clear until the evening of the second day. Then occurred increasing stupor, stertorous respiration, paralysis of the right leg and arm, and the left facial. The ophthalmoscopic examination showed absolutely normal conditions. On the fifth day the patient was admitted to the canton hospital at Zürich. After trephining at the anterior and posterior site of election no supradural collection of blood could be discovered. After division of the dura considerable serous fluid was poured out. At both sites normal brain pulsation was present. Two days later increasing coma and death. The autopsy showed extensive fat-embolism of the cerebral vessels, which was confirmed by microscopical sections of fresh tissue. This condition had resulted from the subcutaneous fracture of the leg.

In *external hemorrhage* from the middle meningeal artery there is, besides the well-known danger from compound fractures of the skull, an additional danger through loss of blood, which may undoubtedly prove fatal in the absence of treatment or in consequence of improper treatment. In a case observed by v. Bergmann the artery, which had been injured by a blow with a hatchet, spurted fourteen hours afterward, and death took place from anæmia and exhaustion, although in the end ligation had been performed. The danger from hemorrhage is particularly serious in this injury owing to the fact, as pointed out by Tillaux, that this artery is located in the dura mater, and on account of its close attachment to this membrane the conditions favoring spontaneous arrest of hemorrhage—retraction of the vessel and diminution of its calibre—are absent, and hemorrhage is necessarily therefore particularly profuse and difficult to control.

Prognosis.—The prognosis of intracranial hemorrhage is in all cases grave, though not absolutely hopeless. Statistics compiled by the author, covering 143 cases receiving expectant treatment, show a mortality of over 90 per cent. Of 143 cases, 131 died and only 12 recovered. Even if these figures, taken alone, express only relative facts—for in the cases that recovered under expectant treatment, no proof of hemorrhage can be brought forward—the extreme danger of this injury is clearly demonstrated. This danger is best shown by the fact that of 167 fatal cases not less than 60—that is, more than one-third—died during the first twenty-four hours. Death rarely takes place within a few minutes, more frequently after a few hours. A survival for two or three days is not exceptional; a patient of Huguenin receiving expectant treatment survived his injury twenty-three days.

Most probably in the rapidly fatal cases death results from paralysis of the heart and respiratory centres in the medulla oblongata. In those cases dying after days or weeks v. Bergmann finds that the usual cause of death is progressive œdema of the brain or sudden and fatal increase of intracranial pressure, resulting either from secondary hemorrhage or congestive hyperæmia.

In many cases contusion of the brain accounts for death; but its significance must not be overestimated in considering the prognosis. On the other hand, the pernicious part played by aspiration pneumonia in many such cases must be pointed out. This is readily understood when one considers that patients in a deeply comatose state are very liable to swallow the wrong way, or that during the act of vomiting particles of food are aspirated. Aspiration pneumonia has frequently imperilled a patient after the dangers of intracranial pressure had been obviated by successful trephining. In one of Krönlein's cases, after trephining, on the third day consciousness became completely restored and paresis disappeared. Pneumonia manifested itself on the fifth day, leading to death on the seventh day.

Treatment.—Though formerly the treatment of rupture of the middle meningeal artery was a matter of much dispute, there is a unity of opinion at present.

Any method of interference must above all else fulfil two indications: the arrest of hemorrhage and the relief of compression of the brain.

In external hemorrhage, after the procedures indicated by fracture of the skull have been carried out: loose splinters of bone removed, depressed fragments elevated, sharp edges trimmed—in other words, the wound reduced to the simplest condition—the principal thing required is to meet the first indication (arrest of hemorrhage). It is hardly ever necessary to resort to actual trephining; one is usually able to proceed with roogeur forceps, sequestrum-forceps, and elevator; or possibly it may be necessary to employ chisel and mallet. If in the course of these manipulations the wound in the artery is discovered, the vessel should be ligated at the site of the lesion with some aseptic material, such as silk or catgut, whether at the given moment the vessel is bleeding or not. The peripheral end of the vessel should also be tied whenever possible, as Krönlein did in a case of comminuted fracture of the squamous portion of the temporal bone after he had removed the fragments of bone. The earliest ligation of the middle meningeal artery recorded in literature was performed by a Swiss physician, Thormann, at Chur, in the year 1828. He dissected out the artery for some distance with a bistoury, caught the vessel with hæmostatic forceps, and tied it; recovery ensued. It cannot be denied that the ligation of the artery, embedded as it is in the grooves of the bone, closely adherent to the dura, and possessing very thin walls, may be very difficult; it has, however, been successfully performed in a series of cases, especially in recent times. Ligation at the site of injury is naturally the sovereign method in those cases in which, after trephining and removal of blood-clots, the site of an existing hemorrhage is discovered. In a case trephined by Schlatter at the Zürich clinic the operator saw, by the aid of an electric lamp passed into the cavity of the wound, the spurting branch of the injured artery. He made a second trephine opening in order to reach the vessel, and tied it with catgut.

It is true that favorable conditions are necessary for the ligation of the artery in loco. When the difficulties are too great, especially when, although the artery is bleeding, the lesion cannot be discovered because it lies hidden behind the bone beyond the defect in the skull or the trephine-opening, it is best to make use of transfixion by the method suggested by Huter and Vogt. This method has also been successfully employed in a series of cases.

In the numerous cases in which it is impossible to discover the source of hemorrhage, it is proper to tampon, the best thing for this purpose being strips of iodoform gauze. It is nearly always possible to control hemorrhage in this way. It is seldom necessary to tampon a second time. Even if at the time of operation hemorrhage has ceased, it is a good plan to pack with iodoform gauze in order to prevent possible secondary hemorrhage.

The ligation in continuity of the arterial trunk at the site of election, following trephining, has little to recommend it. The ligation of the common and external carotid (Roser), especially endorsed by English and American authors, has until now produced few results, and is decidedly inferior to local hæmostasis. In a case reported by Symonds, in which hemorrhage continued after trephining, it ceased after digital compression had been made on the carotid for three hours; in another case the carotid was tied, with immediate result, but death took place twenty-four hours after injury, during deep coma. Ramschoff ligated the common carotid on account of secondary hemorrhage setting in twenty-four hours after trephining; on the sixteenth day death took place as a result of secondary hemorrhage at the site of ligation of the carotid.

The principal indication in treatment of rupture of the middle meningeal artery is to relieve the brain from pressure caused by the extravasation. This is particularly the case when the soft and bony coverings are either intact or only slightly injured. It is true that formerly, when the views in regard to trephining were different, cases were numerous in which under purely expectant treatment (rest in bed, application of cold, venesection, etc.) the patients recovered. There were, however, a great many more cases in which death took place on account of constantly increasing compression of the brain. Unfortunately such cases occur quite frequently at the present time, either because they receive no treatment or at least no operative treatment; or because when treatment is instituted hemorrhage is not discovered, and the indications are not fulfilled. At the same time special attention must be called to the fact that interference should not be postponed too long. Not only does the threatened paralysis of the respiratory and circulatory centres render the chances of success less favorable the longer treatment is delayed, but aspiration pneumonia also endangers the life of the patient, to which attention was particularly called by Gubler.

According to present views in regard to the whole question, active interference is indicated, consisting in a search for and arrest of the hemorrhage producing pressure.

It is difficult for the surgeon to decide, not whether, but how and when to act. Obviously, in case of an intact or only fissured skull, it is necessary to resect the latter, in order to gain access to the source of hemorrhage. Whether the classical trephine, a chisel, saw, etc., be used, whether an actual or only a temporary (osteoplastic) resection be performed, is irrelevant here. These questions will be discussed later.

Different authors have laid down exact rules in regard to the site of election—that is, where the opening should be placed—in case of the intact skull, for it only concerns the latter, as in punctured wounds, gunshot fractures, splintered and comminuted fractures, the injury will determine the location. Vogt advises that the point of the trephine be placed in the temporal fossa at the intersection of two lines, one horizontal, two fingers' breadth above the arch of the zygoma, the other vertical the breadth of the thumb, behind the sphenofrontal process of the malar bone. Of the other methods suggested only a description of the one advocated by Krönlein will be given. Krönlein describes an anterior and a posterior site of election, and determines them in the following way: A line is drawn through the supraorbital ridge, backward, parallel with the horizontal line of the skull (line through the external auditory opening and inferior orbital ridge). Both sites of election for trephining should lie on this line, the anterior one 3 to 4 cm. behind the zygomatic process of the frontal bone, the posterior point of election at the intersection of the given line with a vertical line passing immediately behind the mastoid process. By means of the first trephine-opening, diffuse as well as circumscribed frontotemporal and especially temporo-parietal hæmatomata are exposed; by means of the second, parieto-occipital hæmatomata are exposed. Krönlein advised that when a diagnosis of rupture of the middle meningeal artery and intracranial hemorrhage has been made, to trephine at the anterior site of election, and if no blood-clot be found here, to trephine at the posterior site of election. Krönlein himself departed from this rule in a case operated on in 1894, when, having made a positive diagnosis of posterior hæmatoma in a patient with intact skull, he trephined at the posterior site of election. The guide in this case was an ecchymosis, slightly sensitive to pressure, situated in the occipital region a little to the left of the median line; also the positive statement in the history that the patient had struck with the back of his head against a beer-barrel. Immediately after the disk of bone was removed extensive blood-clots poured out of the opening in the bone. The case possesses additional interest, as the hæmatoma had caused separation of the dura and transverse sinus to within 1½ cm. of the foramen magnum. As this extensive cavity could only be partially evacuated, stupor continued and the patient died from bronchopneumonia. Krönlein suggests that in such cases the posterior fossa be also trephined at some point behind the mastoid process, in the middle of the inferior semicircular line. Making two trephine-openings has the advantage in very extensive hæmatoma that evacuation can be most thoroughly performed and more favorable arrangements be made for drainage. In general, the operator, in choosing a method, in answering the question whether temporal, parietal, or occipital trephining should be performed, whether any one of these operations should be combined with another, and in what order they are to follow, must be guided by close observation at the bedside of the patient, and during the operation by careful consideration of all the circumstances.

Recently the temporary or osteoplastic trephining, the bone-flap method, has been proposed and practised for the purpose of exposing intracranial hemorrhage. Krause advised that the artery be exposed by the same incision that he proposed for intracranial resection of the (trigeminal) trifacial nerve. The pedicle of the flap, which includes skin, muscle, periosteum, and bone, lies over the zygoma. The incision begins just in front of the tragus, extends upward convex posteriorly, describes a semicircular line, becoming convex anteriorly, and returns to the zygoma. The base of this uterus-shaped flap measures about 3½ cm., its height about 6½ cm., its greatest width, situated superiorly, 5½ cm. Stenzel, Wölfler, and Nasse have successfully exposed and removed extradural hæmatoma according to the osteoplastic method described by Wagner.[1]

Trephining having been successfully performed, no matter by what method it is carried out, it is possible to solve the principal problem, which consists in the *removal of extravasated blood*. Under all circumstances this must be done; it must not be allowed to remain in the hope of spontaneous removal. Otherwise the actual indication, relieving the brain of dangerous pressure, is not fulfilled, and the blood-clots if allowed to remain, even with strict antisepsis or rather asepsis, have a decided tendency to become infected and the immediately favorable results of the operation rendered negative through a complicating meningitis or

[1] Recently Wiemann has reported several cases successfully operated upon.

encephalitis. For this purpose it is occasionally necessary to widen the original opening by means of a chisel or gouge-forceps.

The principal mass of blood-clots can be readily removed by the operator's finger. But blood-clots adhering to the bone and dura should be removed with appropriate instruments, a sharp spoon, small spatula, etc. In other words, the toilet of the dura should be carefully performed, and following this the cavity should be thoroughly disinfected. If it has been possible to carry out the operation under strict aseptic precautions, it is sufficient to irrigate the cavity with (physiological) normal salt solution.

Packing the cavity with iodoform gauze and the advisability of making a second trephine-opening for drainage were discussed above. The after-treatment consists in carrying out the general principles indicated in cranial injuries.

Frequently during evacuation the cavity is seen to become gradually smaller; the brain, relieved of pressure, unfolds itself under the eyes of the operator, pressing the dura before it, against the bone. In other cases, especially if pressure has continued for some time, the cavity persists. In a few days, however, the dura again comes in contact with the bone.

The immediate effect of a completely performed operation is frequently striking. The patient, who until this time has lain unconscious, may as soon perhaps as the disk of bone is removed, or immediately after the blood-clot has been evacuated, or in some cases after several hours, regain complete consciousness; the slow and hard pulse becomes rapid and soft; the extremities that until this time have been paralyzed can again be moved; the threatening symptoms have apparently been relieved. The result of an operation is not always so rapid and striking. At times the brain, after having been subjected to pressure, recovers more slowly, so that several days elapse before the patient recovers from his stupor and regains complete consciousness and the use of his limbs.

Finally, there are cases, unfortunately, in which the operation produces no change in the condition of the patient, and in which death takes place in a very short time. Cases in which hemorrhage was not discovered should not be included in considering the question of result. On the other hand, complicating brain lesions, extensive contusions, fractures of the base of the skull, and resulting meningo-encephalitis, or an existing aspiration pneumonia, may cause death of the patient when trephining was immediately successful.

The author is not of the opinion that contusion of the brain contraindicates search for and removal of coexisting extravasation of blood. In the first place, the surgeon rarely can obtain a clear idea of its extent in the beginning; in the second place, he has always to face the problem of combating at least one dangerous factor, namely, compression of the brain.

Statistics collated by the author, covering 110 cases treated by operation, show 74 recoveries and 36 deaths (67.27 and 32.27 per cent.), or a ratio of 2: 1. These figures alone, considering the hopelessness of expectant treatment, make active interference the imperative duty of the s The question of therapeutics would, however, be placed in a prop if statistics were collected covering as uniform a material as p cases of purely extradural hemorrhage which were exposed at the time and completely evacuated. Then trephining for rupture meningeal artery would be ranked with other life-saving operatior as tracheotomy, herniotomy, etc.

Obviously a rare complication of injury of the meningeal a the *development of aneurysm*. With the exception of a few anc of this artery that have developed spontaneously the author only of the one case reported by Gamgee.

Injuries of the Sinuses of the Dura Mater.—In this con only those blood-channels of the vault which are accessible to the will be considered: the superior longitudinal sinus, the lateral sin the junction of these two, the torcular Herophili. Of the sinuse: base, the sinus cavernosus, which is accessible to violence throt orbit, possesses special interest; it will be discussed in another c

The sinuses are distinguished from ordinary veins by the rig their walls and by their fixed position. The venules and the layer bring about a firm attachment to the walls of the skull sinuses run in depressions in the bone, which are shallow and nificant in the case of the longitudinal sinus, but very marked of the lateral sinus. If a transverse incision be made in the a sinus, it does not collapse—the blood channel remains wide Though these qualities favor the flow of venous blood from the cavity, they also predispose to hemorrhage in case of injury and its spontaneous arrest. The lack of elasticity and the firm attac especially of the lateral sinus, allow little opportunity of avoidin matism affecting the respective part of the skull. The longitudin: embedded in the falx cerebri, which is somewhat distensible, is in a somewhat more favorable position in this regard.

In regard to the topographical relations, the longitudinal sinus. from the glabella to the external occipital protuberance, occupying the median line. About 10 cm. from its origin at the crista g: lumen attains sufficient size to permit serious hemorrhage in injury. The junction of the sinuses (sinus confluens) corre: closely with the external occipital protuberance. The lateral extends from here forward, its direction being very nearly tha horizontal line passing through the zygomatic arch. Having r the posterior border of the mastoid process, the horizontal portion into the vertical portion.

The sinuses are injured in fracture of the skull by splinters o from the inner table, or they are traversed by foreign bodies, c are torn during sudden changes in form of the skull. The longit sinus is particularly exposed to penetration by splinters of bo: according to experience, the parietals are more frequently broke: any other bones of the vault, and it is particularly at this site as that fissures and splintering of the inner table extend for consid

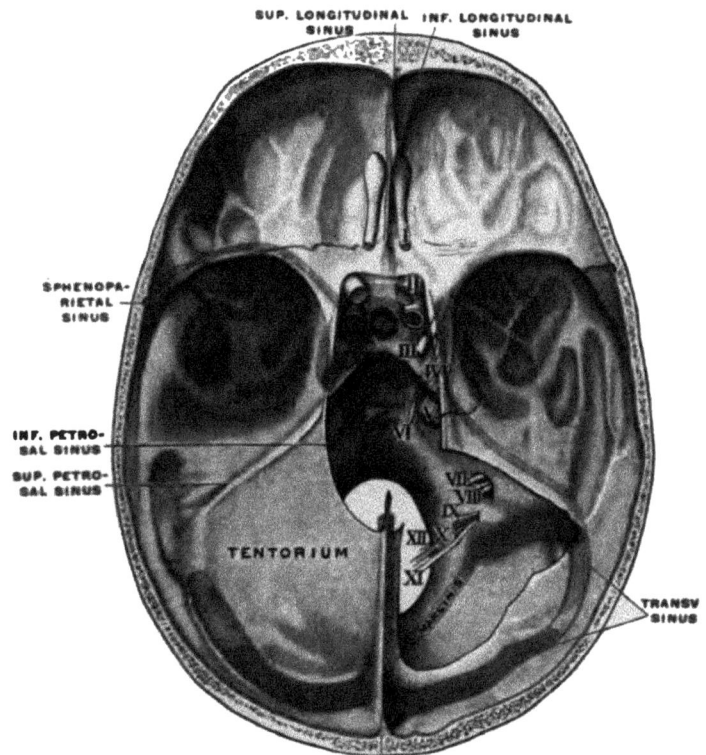

Interior of the Base of the Skull Covered by Dura, showing the Sinuses, Nerve Exits and Tentorium.   Cranial nerves
are numbered in Roman figures. (Merkel.)

distance. Puncturing by splinters occurs less frequently in case of the lateral sinus. On account of the greater thickness of the diploë in this region comminuted fractures occur less frequently than fissured fractures. Yet Chassaignac saw an injury of the torcular Herophili caused by a splinter of bone. By reason of the peculiar character of the walls, even small punctured wounds remain open and may give rise to considerable hemorrhage. On the other hand, splinters of bone may remain fast in the wound, filling it, so that hemorrhage does not take place until the piece of bone is removed. (Cases of Reid, Abel, Scholtz.) There is usually a compound fracture of the skull; injuries of the sinus from splinters of bone occur very rarely without coexisting wounds of the skin.

Instruments puncturing the skull from without usually perforate the sinus completely, and consequently produce more severe hemorrhage. Tension and fixation of the sinus naturally favor complete perforation. The object causing the injury may remain in the wound and close it, like a bone-splinter, so that hemorrhage does not take place until the foreign body is removed.

In gunshot-wounds the projectile may penetrate the sinus directly, or the sinus may be transfixed by a splinter of bone.

It may be mentioned that occasionally in trephining, a sinus may be lacerated by the teeth of the trephine; further, that for the purpose of removing tumors large portions of a sinus have been resected.

Ruptures of sinuses, besides those occurring through excessive displacement of the cranial bones along the sutures during birth, may be produced by stretching and twisting in case of fissured fractures, especially in the region of the lateral sinus. Violence by blunt objects causes the skull suddenly and momentarily to change its shape, as the result of which the bone and the sinus adhering to it may be torn. It happens very rarely, as in the case of the middle meningeal artery, that the bone remains intact, while the sinus itself is torn. Lacerations of the longitudinal sinus, as well as of the lateral sinus several centimetres long, have been observed.

In cases combined with external injuries, hemorrhage from a sinus is usually external; venous blood flows from the wound in a large stream; not infrequently the flow of blood is intermittent and synchronous with respiration.

After punctured wounds by splinters of bone blood may accumulate between skull and dura, causing the latter to be separated from the bone. In case of the longitudinal sinus, as a result of firm attachment, there occurs a bilateral accumulation along the suture-line, an extravasation straddling the sinus—"épanchement en dos d'âne." In case of rupture, extravasation may be extradural or intradural, or "en bouton de chemise," partly above and partly below the dura. Intracranial accumulation naturally always takes place in case of subcutaneous injury, but even in case of compound fracture the outward flow of blood may be prevented by the form of the wound and position of the bone fragments. Under such circumstances hemorrhage produces separation of the dura from

the bone, blood accumulating between the two. A large ex
hemorrhage weighing 180 grammes, the result of a lacerated tr
sinus, was observed by Parcels. Castan found in a case of long
fracture of the vault, in which the longitudinal sinus had been
large blood-clot, entirely intradural.

A three-lobed extravasation of blood has been observed.
year-old child fell into a paved court from out of the seco
window. An extravasation of blood was found beneath the per
of the occipital bone, communicating through a cleft in the bo
an extravasation between bone and dura, and through a tear in t
with an extravasation beneath the dura. The source of hemorrh
a tear in the lateral sinus. Several authenticated cases of injur
sinuses have been reported in which there was absence of app
hemorrhage.

Genzmer first described a very peculiar complication of sinn
—the possibility of air entering an opened sinus. During the
of a sarcoma of the dura mater by Volkmann the tumor was ra
and cut away from the falx, when suddenly, with a sucking n
entered the longitudinal sinus, followed by immediate collapse a
death. The case is certainly a rare one, for besides a case of
suffering perforation observed by P. Müller, and a similar obs
by v. Bergmann, in the case of a man with compound fractur
occiput, only one other case has so far been recorded. Kuhn
case of extirpation of a cholesteatoma of the middle ear, in whic
operation death took place as the result of air entering the sigmo
which had been injured. The hemorrhage that followed wa
worth mentioning. As there is usually positive pressure in the
extraordinary circumstances must be present to render the ent
air possible, such as a high degree of anæmia and extreme d
Genzmer advises that the field of operation be irrigated with som
fluid in order to prevent such an unfortunate occurrence.

Diagnosis.—The only sign of injury of a sinus combined with
wounds, but one that will positively confirm the diagnosis, is the
out of large quantities of venous blood at the site of injury. Th
toms of intracranial hemorrhage from a ruptured sinus are
progressively increasing compression of the brain, as described
in connection with the middle meningeal artery, the only differen
that the symptoms develop much more slowly, corresponding to t
blood-pressure in the sinus. At the same time absolutely a
conditions may develop, as the cases of Parcels and Holmes show
were diagnosticated as cases of rupture of the meningeal arter
in both there was laceration of the transverse sinus.

The conditions for a positive diagnosis are the characteristic sy
of intracranial hemorrhage, and, in addition, that its location
determined by the external examination. Cerebral symptom
permit an exact diagnosis of location are usually absent.

Prognosis.—In determining the prognosis, there must be con
besides the danger of hemorrhage—which should by no means be

estimated—and compression of the brain, progressive thrombosis and the decomposition of the thrombi, as well as accompanying complications, especially contusion of the brain. Schellman has demonstrated by experiments on dogs that sinus-wounds may heal without obliteration of the blood-channel. Experience has taught that narrowing and even obliteration of a large blood-channel may take place without disturbing the intracranial circulation.

Treatment.—It is hardly necessary at the present time to mention that in the treatment of sinus injuries complicated by external wounds a strict antiseptic technic is indicated, particularly on account of the danger of purulent phlebitis. Hemorrhage can usually be controlled by packing with iodoform gauze. Schwartz in elevating a depressed fracture made a tear in the lateral sinus 1 cm. long, which he closed with two silk sutures. Keer in a case of compound fracture of the skull, in which the longitudinal sinus was wounded in two places, closed the larger opening by means of a clamp left in place for two days and then packed the smaller one.

Whenever an intracranial accumulation of blood produces pressure-symptoms, and its diagnosis has been made, trephining and evacuation of blood-clots are positively indicated. In choosing a site for trephining one should be guided by the local conditions. According to the statistics of Luys, of 42 cases of sinus injury, 20 were saved by the surgical interference.

The swelling called by Stromeyer *sinus pericranii*[1] has already been mentioned. This is a tumor situated beneath the pericranium, containing venous blood, and which communicates more or less directly with a sinus by means of clefts in the vault of the skull. Its pathogenesis varies, but in several cases its traumatic origin—that is, its relation to sinus injury—has been clearly proved. In a case of Hutin, a splinter of bone, broken from the parietal bone by a blow from a sabre, had become reunited; forty years later, in falling and striking on the chin, it penetrated the longitudinal sinus and blood escaped through an unclosed cleft in the bone, penetrating to beneath the pericranium and forming the tumor. In a case of Percival Pott, a nine-year-old boy had received a blow with a stick on his head. Some time later a swelling the size of a walnut appeared in the region of the sagittal suture. On incision it was discovered that blood was escaping at a considerable depth, and that a splinter from the parietal bone had penetrated the longitudinal sinus. Either the swelling is noticeable in the erect posture or it appears on stooping over—in fact, under all circumstances that hinder venous return. The swelling is round or oval, soft, fluctuating; the skin over it is thin and transparently blue in color. Pressure upon the jugular veins causes the tumor to fill to its greatest extent, while compression of the veins of the scalp has no influence upon it.

"Sinus pericranii" has been observed most frequently on the forehead and in the occipital region, less frequently in the region of the sagittal and lambdoidal sutures. Subjective symptoms are generally insignifi-

---

[1] Synonyms: Fistule osteovasculaire (Dufour), varix spurius venæ diploeticæ (Becker), varix spurius traumaticus simplex (Bruns), varix spurius communicans (Heinecke).

of a cap applied to the surface of the brain. In many cases the extravasated blood remains more circumscribed, similar in form to that which is characteristic of supradural hemorrhage. Probably in these cases a flat-shaped extravasation took place in the beginning, which coagulated at the periphery, preventing diffuse spreading when hemorrhage took place later.

The conditions are more favorable for the absorption of subdural hemorrhage than for supradural hæmatoma, not only on account of the close relationship between the subdural space and the many lymph-spaces, especially at the base of the skull, but also on account of the mingling with cerebrospinal fluid, which is constantly being renewed and constantly in motion. If the patient survives, the coagulated blood disappears, though slowly, and only an extensive pigmentation on the inner surface of the dura remains as a trace of the extravasation. Occasionally cystic cavities develop. They are filled with serous fluid and may be the cause of later disturbances. The bearing of such traumatic extravasatious on pachymeningitis hemorrhagica may only be referred to here.

Symptoms.—A constant clinical picture of subdural hemorrhage cannot be described; for, in addition to the fact that it is usually combined with contusion of the brain, it presents great varieties as to size, form, and site of extravasation. To be sure, it presents the combination of symptoms characteristic of intracranial hemorrhage. The question, however, whether hemorrhage is extradural or intradural, can be decided from the symptoms only under particularly favorable circumstances. A prominent symptom is marked disturbance of consciousness; but even in regard to the free interval, opinions differ widely. While Jacobson and Allen Starr believe that a long-continued free interval points more to extradural than to intradural hemorrhage, other authors are of decidedly the opposite opinion. Leclerc found a free interval varying from several hours to two months in duration. According to Brion, there is as a rule a latent period of five, six, or seven days in cases of intradural hemorrhage; while as remarked, in extradural hemorrhage from the middle meningeal artery the free interval usually continues only several hours. On the whole, the course is apparently more protracted in subdural hemorrhage; though, on the other hand, very rapidly developing cases have been observed. Pressure-pulse and stertorous respiration are also usually present, accompanying these forms of extravasation. Starr assumes that in intradural hemorrhage there is an increase in frequency of the pulse from the beginning. Manifestations referable to localized pressure, contralateral hemiplegias, aphasia, etc., do occur in connection with intradural hemorrhage. Aphasia caused by pressure on Broca's convolution is by no means a rare occurrence—according to Brion, it occurs in one-third of the cases. On the other hand, monoplegias, or conditions affecting principally the lower extremities, have been observed, particularly in cases of intradural hemorrhage. This does not take place in typical cases of hemorrhage from the middle meningeal artery. The fact that the site of hemorrhage is much less constant than in hemorrhage resulting from rupture of the middle meningeal artery produces a variety

of local symptoms, which are of importance in differential (
Owing to the irregularity in outline of these hæmatomata, cen
widely separated may be affected at the same time, while th
vening may remain free. An important point bearing on the
of intradural hæmatoma is evidence of injury of the nerve-ro
base depending upon extension of extravasation to the base.

In a noteworthy case, operated upon by Henle, a diag
made of intradural hæmatoma in the region of the right
fossa of the skull and of the central convolutions. The ding
confirmed by the operation. The patient, who was thirty-one
had been thrown from a sleigh against the curbstone. There
mary loss of consciousness lasting twelve hours. In the cours
weeks he gradually developed paresis of the left leg and of 1
branch of the left facial, the left arm remaining free; there w
on the right side; bilateral choked disk, more marked on the r
marked amblyopia on the right side; anosmia on the right sid

Unilateral convulsions apparently occur more frequently in o
with intradural hemorrhage than with extradural.

The behavior of the pupils is as variable as in extradural hen
Rise of the body temperature is observed more frequently than
dural hemorrhage, and may *perhaps* be caused by the rapid al
of the extravasation.

Diagnosis.—From the above, it appears that in the case of
hemorrhage the diagnosis of intracranial hemorrhage can b
at with quite a degree of certainty, but that only under pa
characteristic circumstances can cases of intradural and e
hemorrhage be differentiated.

Prognosis.—Owing to the great variation of individual cases
have been observed, it is impossible to offer a general prog
intradural hemorrhage. It is obvious that in cases in which t
is practically floating in a pool of blood, cases that are classe
the severest cranial injuries, the prognosis is unfavorable f
beginning. On the other hand, after loss of consciousness fo
weeks there may be gradual absorption of the extravasation, ci
may be restored, and the cerebral cortex again react. Consci
dawning a little at first, gradually returns entirely, and complete
takes place.

The prognosis of intradural hemorrhage must not be viewed t
ably, for in addition to those cases in which through increased
pressure paralysis of the cardiac and respiratory centres take
there are others in which through long-continued pressure on the
centres there results a cortical atrophy, which is followed by d
tion of the lateral columns of the spinal cord.

Treatment.—The views in regard to treatment are undergoing a
While v. Bergmann in his teachings on cranial injuries occupie
conservative stand and advises purely expectant treatment, mar
have been reported in which active treatment was successful.
manifestations indicating the site of operation are absent, if onl

incised and the blood removed as completely as possible. A complicating contusion of the brain can only be favorably influenced by such a procedure, as the circulation will be improved. In 25 cases of intradural hemorrhage in which trephining was performed on account of threatened danger from compression of the brain, Brion observed 21 recoveries. Brion lays particular stress on the fact that just as puncture for extensive pleural exudates favors absorption of that portion of the exudate allowed to remain, so also the removal of only a part of the extravasated blood may favor the absorption of the blood allowed to remain.

Cases even with a protracted course, in which paralysis, aphasia, etc., had existed for weeks and months, showed good results after trephining. In Henle's case, previously mentioned, the constantly increasing amblyopia resulting from choked disk was the indication for trephining twenty-two days after injury, and the operation was successful from every point of view.

In regard to the choice of site for trephining, the same principles may be applied as were stated in the case of hemorrhage from the middle meningeal artery.

Injuries of the Cerebral Carotid.—The internal carotid has been found injured within the cranial cavity as the result of punctured wounds through the skull, and particularly through the orbit; also by projectiles from firearms and splinters of bone; further, in fractures of the base of the skull, particularly when they have resulted from severe lateral compression of the skull, the vessel being torn during the production of a widely gaping fissure. Both carotids have been found torn at the same time.

Intracranial lesions of the carotid are disproportionately less frequent than such injuries of the middle meningeal artery. This may be due partly to the peculiar arrangement of the sinus cavernosus, which, being placed between the artery and the bony wall, allows the artery a certain freedom of motion, permitting it to slip aside opposite fissures intersecting it. Whenever there is complete laceration blood probably pours out with so much force and in such large quantities that death takes place in a very short time. Marchant, however, cites a case in which during a duel a dragoon had his ophthalmic artery severed at its junction with the carotid by a sabre-blow, and lived for sixteen days.

Prompt ligation of the common carotid might prove successful if it were possible to make a diagnosis.

Exophthalmos Pulsans (Arterioaneurysm of the Inten
—Though the lesions of the above artery have hardly more
logical significance, the injuries of the carotid at the base
play an important part in the etiology of a condition know
thalmos pulsans. Travers recognized (1813) as its cause a
communication between the cerebral carotid and cavernous
plaining its occurrence through an aneurysm by anastomosis
The condition occurs both spontaneously and as the result
injury. Sattler, in his great treatise on exophthalmos pulsans
traumatic origin in 59 of 106 cases. Slomann estimated the
traumatic cases at 71 per cent. and found, as did other observi
f equent occurrence in males, in the ratio of 57 to 12. Cori
with this the average age in traumatic cases is considerably
years) than in those occurring spontaneously (37.7 years).
present time an injury of the internal carotid in the cavern
and the development of an arteriovenous aneurysm have been
confirmed by autopsy in at least 5 cases.

In a case of Nélaton (a man twenty-one years old) the pc
umbrella had been thrust through the right lower eyelid. W
months a distinct exophthalmos pulsans developed. The ca
been penetrated within the cavernous sinus and below the bo
sphenoid bone.

In cases caused by trauma there is usually violence of a na
likely to produce fracture of the base of the skull, as, for exi
falling and striking the head, or by contrecoup when landing or
through a blow on the top of the head, in the face, or the orbit
or through the head being caught and squeezed; further by dir
through puncture or blows in the region of the eye, gunshot-wor

Well-developed cases are characterized by marked protrusi
eyeball. The eyeball can be forced back into the orbital cavit
producing pain, but as soon as pressure is removed it retur
former position. The upper eyelid is swollen and tense, the cor
ecchymosed, and the bloodvessels traversing it are markedl
and deep red in color. The cornea is usually dull and lustr
pupil widely dilated and fixed. Vision is very much dimir
entirely lost, rarely unimpaired or only slightly affected. Op
scopic examination shows choked disk and retinal veins markedl
frequently also a venous pulse. In the later stages the papilla
atrophic. Motility of the eyeball and the eyelids is disturbed, u
connection with the swelling and protrusion. Schalkhauer espec
pointed out that abducens paresis is a pretty constant symptom
developed exophthalmos pulsans, being brought about by the
of the aneurysmal sac (Blutsach) on the abducens nerve within th
cavity. Abducens paresis is, however, pathognomonic only
develops in the course of the disease. In the histories of two ca
the Zürich clinic, placed at the author's disposal through the l
of Krönlein, the occurrence of abducens paresis was not noted i
third and fourth weeks, respectively. The pulsation of the e

particularly noticeable; a distinct whirring is detected if the hand be laid on the eyeball. Above and to the inner side of the eyeball a pulsating swelling is generally seen, varying in size from that of a bean to that of a filbert. With the stethoscope a loud blowing sound can be heard over the orbital region, at times over the entire head. This is synchronous with the radial pulse. The patients usually complain of more or less headache, of a painful pounding and buzzing in the head and ears. Pulsation and noise cease at once if the common carotid be compressed. Not infrequently there is profuse bleeding from the nose. In Nélaton's case blood escaped from the venous sinus into the cavities of the sphenoid and then into the nose.

Symptoms.—Occasionally the symptoms appear after twenty-four hours; usually, however, they appear after several days or weeks. so that it takes several months to a year for all of the symptoms to develop. The course is rarely more protracted. In a case observed by Poirier the symptoms of a right exophthalmos pulsans appeared fully eight years after a shot in the right parotid region from a revolver. Spontaneous subsidence of symptoms is rare, but may take place after years. More frequently death takes place suddenly, preceded now and then by paralysis and disturbance of speech.

Treatment.—In regard to treatment, the results with intermittent digital compression of the common carotid in traumatic cases are not good, as the walls of the injured vessel, except at the site of laceration, are healthy, the intima smooth and normal in character, and the conditions for coagulation of blood within the artery generally unfavorable. At the same time compression should be tried in every case before ligating. Acupuncture, galvanopuncture, injection of ergotin or coagulating fluids, are not only ineffectual, but decidedly dangerous. The best results have been obtained by ligation of the common carotid. Sattler found that of 56 cases of pure varicose aneurysm of the carotid sinus, in which ligation of the carotid had been performed, 37 recovered, in 11 the results were negative, and 8 died. In a case operated upon by Krönlein the symptoms remained unchanged after ligation of the one carotid, and it was only after the other carotid had been ligated that the symptoms gradually subsided.

INJURIES OF THE CRANIAL NERVES DURING THEIR COURSE IN AND THROUGH THE SKULL.

Injuries of the cranial nerves during their course within and through the skull are almost entirely of diagnostic significance. The cranial nerves may be divided, contused, or compressed by different kinds of violence, and in consequence their functions are partially or totally lost. Paralysis of the region supplied by the respective nerves is the direct result of such lesions. Some of these injuries are caused directly by penetrating, punctured, or gunshot-wounds; others occur in connection with fracture of the base of the skull. If the line of fracture involves

the foramen or canal through which the respective nerve l
cranial cavity, the nerve may be partially or completely torn
may be divided, contused, or compressed by a broken splinte
But even in the absence of fracture, nerves may be torn off in
way as has been observed in the case of the vessels of the pia
Finally, nerves may be injured by the pressure of blood esca
the bony canals from fissures in bones, also in extensive suprad
subdural extravasations the nerves suffer impairment of functi

FIG. 79.

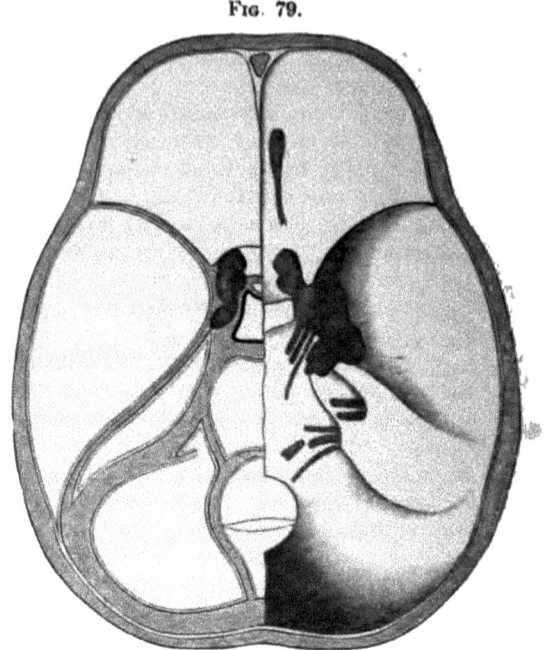

Intracranial venous sinuses on right side; cranial nerves as they pierce dura on l
(Amberger.)

Besides those paralyses of the cranial nerves following immed
soon after injury, there are paralyses which develop some ti
injury. These depend upon an inflammation progressing along t
of the nerve. This neuritis ascendens is a frequent cause o
meningitis. Conversely, an existing purulent inflammation at
of the brain may be followed by a neuritis descendens travelling
erally within the nerve-sheath, and which may be the cause of
developing later.

Isolated paralyses of cranial nerves are on the whole rare. Mc
several cranial nerves are injured at the same time. It is evid
from the existing paralyses one can draw conclusions regard
direction of a fracture of the base. As, however, injuries of the

centres, as well as of the ganglia of the trunks, etc., may be followed by paralyses of the cranial nerves, this subject offers a rich field for the exercise of diagnostic skill.

The prognosis of injuries of nerves depends upon the cause. After lacerations and extensive contusion paralysis is permanent; extravasations of blood producing pressure may be absorbed or may be removed by operative measures, following which function is gradually restored.

There is no treatment for the paralysis that can be seriously considered.

Olfactory Nerve.—One or both of the olfactory bulbs have been found injured by punctured wounds in the region of the nose as the result of gunshots and following violence with blunt objects. The latter may strike the frontal region directly; but more frequently injuries are produced by contrecoup from the occipital, temporal, or parietal regions. It is plausible that in fractures of the base extending to the anterior fossa of the skull the nerves traversing the horizontal plate of the ethmoid may be torn off at the moment that the edges of the fissures are forced apart, as this is analogous to the tearing off of the middle meningeal artery at the foramen spinosum. Frequently the frontal lobes of the hemispheres are crushed at the same time. Pressure from hemorrhage into the nerve-sheaths, also pressure from extensive extravasations into the anterior fossa of the skull, may cause anosmia. This must be assumed to be the cause when sooner or later the sense of smell is restored. In the case of Henle, mentioned in connection with intradural hemorrhage, there was anosmia on the right side in addition to other symptoms. Anosmia may be produced, however, by a deflected septum, and this should be considered whenever the sense of smell is tested. Whether after evacuation of the blood-clot, which was successful in all other respects, the sense of smell was also restored, is not mentioned in the history of the case. Paralysis of the olfactory nerve may exist alone—in fact, it may be the only disturbance following cranial injury, but more frequently it is combined with other forms of paralysis.

Optic Nerve.—Cases of injury of the optic nerve are numerous, but their detailed description is more properly a subject for a text-book on ophthalmology. Punctured and incised wounds of the optic nerve have been observed anywhere between the sclerotic and the base of the brain; also complete laceration close to the sclerotic, and shot injuries of one or both optic nerves. Heister observed that in gunshot-wounds of the temporal region both optic nerves may be injured without involvement of the eyeball. Rose was accustomed to mention in his lectures an observation of his own concerning a Russian student, who, in attempting to commit suicide, shot through the optic nerves at the chiasma, and naturally was totally blind.

Injuries of the optic nerve occur most frequently in connection with fracture of the base of the skull, especially fractures of the roof of the orbit. Fissures traversing the walls of the optic canal are particularly liable to injure the nerve, which in this situation is firmly attached to the bone. Hölder found in 86 cases of fracture of the base in which the anatomical relations were carefully investigated, that in 53 cases there

were injuries of the bones forming the ...
quences of such injuries are ...
the optic nerve. Distortion and ...
result. Transfixion or compression by ...
found here as well as more posteriorly.

Disturbances of vision observed after violence ...
with blunt objects are divided into those that ...
injury and are permanent; those that, developing ...
after injury, disappear in part or entirely after some ...
those which develop later. If actual destruction of the ...
optic nerve has taken place, the disturbance of vision ...
and permanent. If hemorrhage interferes with the ...
optic nerve, disturbance of vision also takes place ...
after injury. Under some circumstances this may be ...
a part of these injuries there is the chance that after the ...
absorbed and the nerve relieved a certain degree of ...
will be restored.

Hemorrhage into the sheath of the optic nerves has a ...
unfavorable prognosis than extravasation surrounding the ...
optic tract. Late-developing disturbances of vision ...
injuries are almost always referable to secondary ...
especially of the brain and meninges.

According to Leber, it can be determined by ophthalm...
amination whether the nerve-trunk is affected in front or b
entrance of the central artery of the retina; for if behind the
of the artery, the fundus appears normal at first, and only aft
weeks a discoloration of the papilla becomes noticeable; w
front of the entrance of the artery the vessels are hardly visi
embolism of the retina.

Oculomotor, Trochlear, and Abducens Nerves.—The thi
nerve has been injured many times in connection with puncture
penetrating the orbital roof. However, it is injured more ·f
in connection with severe cranial injuries, especially fractur
base. Pressure of an arteriovenous aneurysm in the carotid ·
particularly extensive extravasation, may be followed by o
paralysis. In regard to the latter accident, an extensive h
from the middle meningeal artery spreading down into the mi
of the skull may produce direct pressure on the nerve-trunk. H
assumed this to be the condition in a case of laceration of the r
artery in which the pupil of the same side was widely dila
remarks that not all fibres of the oculomotor nerve are equally
to pressure. As a matter of fact, dilatation of the pupil, and
also ptosis, are not infrequently found as the only signs of
this nerve. Also the cortical centres of the oculomotor nerve, a
situated in front of and below the arm centres, may be dist
contusion or localized pressure and produce paresis of the eye
In a case of total right-sided oculomotor paralysis combined
alysis of the left arm, which subsided to considerable degree in t

of six weeks, a diagnosis was made, according to Van Wess, of hemorrhage located at the right crus cerebri pressing upon the oculomotor trunk and the pyramidal fibres.

Trochlear paralysis seldom occurs alone, but is combined more frequently with paralyses of other muscles of the eye. In a case successfully trephined by Krönlein on account of hemorrhage from the left middle meningeal artery, there remained a left-sided trochlear paralysis after a right-sided cortical hemiplegia of the extremities and facial nerve had disappeared.

The *abducens nerve* seems to be the one oculomotor nerve particularly exposed to injury, owing to its long course within the skull and its relation to the apex of the petrous portion, which is frequently fractured. Indeed, some authors consider intracranial abducens paralysis a frequent occurrence, but Purtscher, Köhler, and Th. v. Schröder draw attention to the fact that it is by no means so frequent, even taking into account that in the presence of severe general disturbances following cranial injuries the possible existence of paralysis of the muscles of the eye might easily be overlooked.

Of 58 cases of traumatic abducens paralysis compiled from literature by v. Schröder, 12 were isolated unilateral and 8 bilateral. A case of nuclear bilateral combined with unilateral facial paralysis is reported by Van Wess. *Abducens* paralysis occurring in the course of an exophthalmos pulsans has been mentioned.

Trigeminal Nerve.—Isolated trigeminus paralysis is certainly a rare occurrence. Anæsthesia of the face has been found more frequently in combination with paralysis of other cranial nerves following fractures of the base. Dunn found paralysis of the fifth, sixth, and seventh cranial nerves on the right side six weeks after severe cranial injury. Regarding a case of multiple cranial nerve injury in which the trigeminal nerve was involved also, see below. Injury of single branches, either in the cranial cavity or in the bony canals, does occur. In one of Krönlein's cases, besides both abducens nerves, two branches of the fifth were injured; in one of Sonnenburg's cases there was present, in addition to abducens paresis, anæsthesia over the distribution of the first and second branches of the trigeminal nerve. Sonnenburg assumes that the trunk was injured above the Gasserian ganglion. The usual consequence of anæsthesia of the trigeminus following cranial injury is so-called keratitis neuroparalytica. In Krönlein's case mentioned above herpes developed at the sites of exit of the infraorbital and mental nerves soon after injury.

Facial Nerve.—It is the unanimous opinion of all observers that of all the cranial nerves the facial nerve is the one most frequently injured. The frequency of this occurrence is accounted for by the long course of the nerve through the Fallopian canal of the petrous portion of the temporal bone, the latter being frequently involved in fractures of the base of the skull. As the nerve gives off numerous branches in its course through the petrous portion, it is possible to determine more accurately the site of the nerve lesion and the course of fracture from

unimpaired. If the nerve is injured below the point at chorda tympanæ is given off in the lowest portion of the ca muscles of the face are paralyzed. The nerve has been fou close to the styloid foramen as the result of shots and kicks. injury above the chorda tympani and below the nerve to the there is, in addition to total facial paralysis, disturbance in tl of saliva and the sense of taste in the anterior half of the lesion below the geniculate ganglion and above the brancl nerve to the stapedius produced in addition disturbance of the form of the so-called hyperacusis. In case of an injury ir above the branching of the superficial petrosal nerve or at tl itself, there is added paralysis of the palatal muscles. Final situated centrally from the geniculated ganglion leave the ser intact, while all the other disturbances mentioned above are

In favor of a cortical lesion caused by pressure through h or by a contusion are (besides the frequent involvement o motor areas, particularly the arm centre) paralysis limited and buccal branches of the facial nerve, the frontal branch unaffected, and the fact that electrical excitability is pres case of a nuclear injury paralysis is also complete; peripher tion still excites reflex movements in the paralyzed area in les the nucleus.

A not infrequent cause of late-developing facial paralysis ascendens mentioned above, which is very liable to lead to fa meningitis.

Injury of the facial nerve is frequently combined with inj auditory nerve and of the abducens nerve.

Auditory Nerve.—Isolated injury of the eighth cranial rarely been observed, and would be difficult to diagnostica turbances of hearing following cranial injuries may be caused of the labyrinth or of the tympanic cavity. In most cases nerve of the same side is injured at the same time. This cc to the anatomical relations. A. Heer found this to be the in 6 of 9 cases. Bilateral lesions of the auditory nerve oc observed in symmetrical fractures of the base do not attract attention.

Regarding injuries of the ninth to the twelfth pairs of n observations have been made. They cause difficulty in swallc moving the tongue. They are almost always combined w nerve injuries. A case of fracture of the base with paraly; distribution of the tenth and twelfth nerves has been re; Stierlin. (Figs. 29 to 32.)

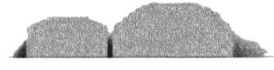

CONTUSIONS OF THE BRAIN.

By Prof. Dr. R. U. KRÖNLEIN.

External violence affecting the skull may be transmitted to the brain, producing in the latter injuries, of greater or less severity, which possess the anatomical character of a *solution of continuity of tissue*. Only these injuries will be discussed here. Simple functional and circulatory disturbances of the brain, even if caused by traumatism, will not be considered, as in them the anatomical changes found do not result in a solution of continuity of tissue. Such traumatic disturbances have been discussed in preceding chapters on cerebral concussion and compression of the brain.

Owing to the almost complete closure of the bony capsule of the skull in the adult, direct injury to the brain, in the sense of a solution of continuity of tissue as a result of external violence without injury of the skull at the same time seems hardly possible. The only place where the anatomical structures renders such direct injury of the brain possible is at the apex of the orbital cavity, where at the sphenoidal fissure there is an extensive opening, which occasionally allows the passage of small pointed instruments and projectiles to the middle fossa of the skull and the adjacent portions of the brain. Cases have been reported in which the point of a foil or the broken blade of a "schlager," or a grain of shot have found their way to the brain through the above-mentioned fissure. A patient in whom Zehender observed the latter condition expired instantly; the grain of shot had passed through the sphenoidal fissure to the posterior fossa of the skull.

Excluding such rare exceptions, traumatic solution of continuity of brain-tissue takes place indirectly through the medium of the bony capsule. This is brought about by external violence, whether such injury consists of a sudden change in the shape of the skull, the latter returning to its former shape immediately after injury, or in a fracture or wound of the bones. Injuries of the brain which are discussed below are frequently met with as complications of contusions and perforation of the skull.

In the great majority of cases the surgeon has to deal with brain injuries which are in the nature of contusions. This applies naturally to all those injuries that result from violence with blunt objects or from broad surfaces; but even in punctured and lacerated wounds of the skull, if they extend to the brain-substance, the lesion, as far as the brain is concerned, shows the character of a contusion more than that of a clean incised wound. In the first place, as a cause of this phenomenon it is found that penetrating instruments become blunted in traversing the bony capsule of the skull; and in the second place, that the soft consistency of the brain-substance, in accordance with hydrodynamic laws, easily transmits force in all directions, and therefore also in a direction perpendicular to that of the inflicted violence. At

all events, there is, anatomically considered, no wide difference l
the forms of traumatic brain injuries produced by different mech:
but only a gradual transition, which is manifested by the w
narrower zone of contusion surrounding the area of solution
tinuity: and for practical purposes it is sufficient to divide
matic injuries of the brain into two groups, contusions of the
and wounds of the brain, according to which we consider 'con
of the brain (*contusio cerebri*) a solution of continuity of tissu
is not exposed to the outer air, but covered by more superfici
uninjured layers of tissue, whether this latter is brain-tissue
meninges, or the bony or soft coverings of the skull. The term "
of the brain" is limited, on the other hand, to a solution of cor
of brain-tissue, which lies open and exposed, or which has bee
duced by external violence only after the latter has opened
from the surface of the head through the various coverings, no
what variation in direction and character this path may show.

Contusions of the brain show solutions of continuity and dest:
of brain-tissue which may present great differences as regards size
tion, and number. They may consist of small punctate areas
tusion, or they may be as large as a cherry or walnut or a goose
Frequently an entire lobe or several lobes may be crushed. A
ingly the anatomical picture varies. In their recent state inju
slight extent and degree present the appearance of hemorrhagic
as they are frequently found in cases of so-called spontaneous c
hemorrhage; surrounding a central blood-clot, possibly only a:
as a pin-head or a pea, there extends a zone of edematous brair
reminding one by its appearance of currant jelly, and in this ar
tered small deep-red specks of blood, so that the entire area of cor
looks speckled. Where contusion is more severe and extensive
may be a large pool of blood, the bed of which is formed of irre
torn brain-substance; further, areas of extravasations, between
the brain-substance appears frayed and deep red. Finally, an
brain area may be destroyed by violence and transformed into a
or reddish-brown mass, composed of blood and brain-pulp. Th
be removed in part by irrigating with a stream of water, leaving e:
a large brain defect of irregular outline, with walls full of clef
tags of tissue. When there is also present a comminuted fract
the skull, numerous large and small fragments of bone are foun
bedded in the pulp, or are driven still further into the walls of the
While in the injuries just described the appearance is more t
an actual crushing of the brain, there are rarer forms of brain con
in which the appearance found is decidedly different. More
extensive tears through the brain-substance are found. An
bursting of the brain takes place, which undoubtedly depends up
same mechanism for its production as does the so-called bursting fr
of the skull. Such ruptures of the brain have been observed p
larly in children. They occasionally extend through the entire la:
white medullary matter as far as the ventricle of the brain.

hydrodynamic laws, any violence affecting ▓▓▓▓▓
be transmitted in directions other than the ▓▓▓▓
tion of continuity of tissue. But according to ▓▓▓
observations on human beings do not bear out ▓▓▓
lesions of the fourth ventricle and of the aqu▓▓▓▓
occurrence; on the contrary, they are to be ▓▓▓▓
rare injuries. Relatively speaking, the walls of ▓▓ ▓
most frequently to be affected by areas of contusion ▓
of violence coincides with the major axis of these ca▓
most frequently therefore in connection with longitu▓
the base.

4. Where there are deep tears of brain-substance th▓
sidered, as previously mentioned, the result of a bur
of the brain—occurring like bursting fractures, in the
inflicting violence. Hydrocephalic brains in children, ▓
children in general, are apparently predisposing fact▓
rence of such ruptures of the brain.

Disregarding contusion of the brain, which, as has
most frequent, but not by any means a necessary compli
of the skull, attention must be drawn to *laceration* of ▓
hemorrhage into, between, and outside the brain-mem▓
of the dura mater is not infrequently found accompa▓
the skull. This is true also of lacerations of the pia m
to its source, hemorrhage at the surface of the brai▓
supradural, subdural, subarachnoidal, or subpial, vary
its extent. At the same time it is by no means limit
of the cortical contusion; it may extend over a larg
brain, the cerebral cortex being intact, while the are▓
situated in the subcortical layer or in the white med▓
These findings, however, indicate that meningeal hem▓
necessarily originate in the areas of brain contusion;
may in fact be considered an unusual one. More freq
which has spread between the meninges comes fro
meningeal vessels themselves, and the relation of the▓
to the contusions of the brain lies in the fact that the ▓
which in the course of a cranial injury produces lacerat
in the brain also brings about laceration of the menin
supradural hemorrhage the trunk and branches of the ▓
artery play the principal part: in subdural and int▓
veins emptying into the longitudinal sinus.

Course.—The course of *contusion of the brain* is deter
the fact that injuries of the brain not communicating
cannot be reached by any outside infection, and that ▓
through the circulation takes place only in exceptional c▓
is therefore, as a rule, unaccompanied by septic or sup

It is aseptic, analogous to that of subcutaneous injuries of other tissues and organs. Where, however, under exceptional circumstances septic or purulent processes take place in an area of contusion, the course and termination are similar to those in infected contused wounds of the brain. These will be discussed later. The pathological anatomical course in experimental contusions, according to E. Ziegler's description, is as follows: the area of contusion, in which the blood that has escaped from the lacerated vessels and the remains of destroyed brain-substance form a black or blackish-red soft or coagulated mass, first changes color, becomes more reddish-brown, while through diffusion of the blood-pigment the surrounding portions of the brain receive a yellow tinge. Blood and remains of brain-tissue are dissolved and absorbed in the course of time, following the appearance of fat and pigmented granular cells; and thus at the site of contusion, according to its location at the surface, in the cortex, or in the depths of the white medullary substance, there results a cleft, a defect, a valley, or a cavity, which gradually fills as the result of a process of inflammation and proliferation in the walls, and finally becomes transformed into a scar, which frequently appears for a long time yellow or brown in color owing to non-absorbed material, pigment-granules, especially hæmatoidin and hemosiderin. The course therefore corresponds in general to that of hemorrhagic softening in spontaneous cerebral hemorrhage.

The disputed question, which still engages pathological anatomists, involves particularly the origin of the scar—that is, the behavior, on the one hand, of the connective tissue and vessels, and, on the other hand, of the neuroglia-cells and ganglion-cells in the course of repair of brain defects. According to more recent investigations emanating from the institute of E. Ziegler, especially those of Tschistowitsch (1897), it appears conclusive that in this connection "the connective-tissue elements of the pia and the vessels play almost the only and at all events the principal part"; while the participation of the neuroglia is insignificant, a regeneration of nerve-cells must be entirely excluded and a regeneration of the nerve-fibres considered improbable. This much is absolutely certain, that extensive traumatic defects of the brain are not closed by a regeneration of brain-tissue, but by the development of a scar. This scar may be solid and firm, or may show a cystoid structure, the cavities of which are filled with a yellow fluid (cholesterin).

The course of *rupture of the brain*, already mentioned, still requires brief description. Regarding this, it was remarked that it apparently occurs only in children, and particularly in the hydrocephalic brain, as the result of injury. The author is forced, according to his observations, to assume positively that ruptures of the brain extending from the cerebral cortex into the ventricles may terminate in recovery and lead to the picture of so-called "porencephalia traumatica." In such a case observed and successfully operated upon by him, and which has been reported by Rahm, there extended from the meninges at the surface of the parietal lobe a bulging smooth-walled cavity through the cerebral cortex and white medullary substance to the lateral ventricle, with which it evi-

portions of the brain that require another explanation. Those processes are meant which in brain pathology are included under the term "secondary degeneration of the nervous elements," nerve-fibres as well as nerve-cells. These processes take place if at any point the continuity of these elements is destroyed. Since Türck, the teachings of secondary degeneration have been particularly promoted and broadened by v. Gudden's school, and the author elects to follow the description which one of its most celebrated representatives, v. Monakow, gave recently in his great work by quoting briefly the important features of this degenerative process. There is in this connection a retrograde change which possesses "the character either of an atrophy or of a gradually developing necrosis; both finally lead to death of the elements" (v. Monakow). This retrograde metamorphosis affects first the nerve-fibres, and consists of a fatty degeneration and an absorption of the medullary sheath, with which the development of the granular cells goes hand in hand. There are, further, atrophy and sclerosis of the axis-cylinder; the axis-cylinder may even disappear entirely. The same process may take place in the ganglion-cells (cellulipetal degeneration). Microscopically such a secondary degeneration of the collections of fibres and ganglion-cells may be evident as a distinct diminution in volume of those portions of the brain principally involved.

WOUNDS OF THE BRAIN.

Wounds of the brain may be divided according to the mechanism of their occurrence into *contused*, *punctured*, and *lacerated wounds*. In distinction to contusions of the brain, which have been discussed exclusively so far, they all possess one common feature, namely, that the inflicting violence has divided all the coverings of the head, the skull, and brain itself where they overlie the solution of continuity of brain-tissue, so that there is a path from the external surface of the body to the central organ, which is sufficiently wide to allow the escape of destroyed brain-substance, on the one hand, and the entrance of the atmospheric air and infectious germs, on the other. This exposure of the brain lesion is a factor of such great importance that a distinction between contusion and wound of the brain seems justifiable.

Wounds of the brain occur as the result of violence from blunt or sharp objects. Both mechanisms may occur at the same time; in fact, as a result of the cranial bones being involved in the injury, the original mechanism may be entirely altered in its transmission from without inward; so much so that violence from a blunt object may lead to a brain injury which possesses the character of a punctured or incised wound; while, on the other hand, violence from a sharp object may lead to a contused wound. The author must refer here to the laws of fractures of the skull, and for the purpose of illustrating the subject will refer to a case in which violence from a blunt object led to a compound comminuted fracture of the vault of the skull and a splinter of bone trans-

fixed the underlying brain, and
a knife had sharply divided the
duced splintering of the inner t
a contused wound of the cereb

Course.—The course of a wou
upon whether it bears the char
but much more upon the questi
place. If the micro-organisms
infectious wound diseases are i
the brain is the same as that of
is very different if a wound of
secondarily! The complication
such an infection will be discus

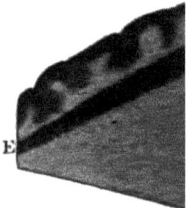

Bullet wound of brain by Flobert rifle
of softening. K. Original size

Contused Wounds.—Cont
quently found as complication
Circumscribed fractures of the
cated by wounds of the brain
the skull, and as the former o
the base, it is easy to explain
brain for the vault. Not inf
the brain complicated by fra
through the torn meninges d
applies particularly to a defini
namely, *gunshot-wounds*, whi
of the peculiarity of their m
The author has in view ex
the small-arm projectiles, for
guns, such as fragments of
different from those met with
drawn into moving machin
etc. Cases of crushing of the
hope for a favorable course

It has been remarked that anatomically the co
of the brain—and this applies particularly to
many cases identical with that of contusions.
not involve a vital centre; if other dangerous
flooding of the ventricles with blood or extei
intrameningeal hemorrhage remain absent; an
(shock, concussion of the brain) is not produced
the course terminated within a few hours or d
case, a contused wound may heal, leaving a co
quently pigmented and of a yellowish-brown aj
tinuous at the surface of the brain with the s(
and in this way may become attached to thei
addition to this superficial scar there is found in
of deeper contused wounds, a very delicate netw
of hollow spaces, frequently filled with a clear|
or only scattered and degenerated nervous eleﬂ
there is beyond the fibrous portion a broader
with degenerated and not infrequent calcareo|

The process of repair may run a very similaɪ
small fragments of bone have been carried iɪ
The foreign body is there surrounded by con
remain in position for years or for a lifetime witll
processes. The small projectiles of pocket rev(
in particular, may be encysted in this way.

Punctured Wounds.—Punctured wounds of
combined with fractures of the inner table, esp(
the instrument does not completely perforate tl
of the thickness of the diploë penetrates only ɪ
and the latter is broken off. Another reason f(
wounds is the fact that the instrument is freqɪ
the bone after having penetrated to the brain,
looked on superficial examination. In the ɡ
injuries, the so-called punctured fractures of t
pointed splinter of bone plays the part of a
piercing dura and pia, and remains embedded
Such were the conditions in a case published b
which an extremely pointed splinter of bone fɪ(
trated the posterior central convolution to a d(
being otherwise uninjured, and produced a com
could not have been more typical in an experiɪɪ
animal. Regarding the second group of stal
puncturing instrument breaks off at a level wiɪ
embedded, literature contains a series of strikiɪɪ
that under circumstances knife-blades, needlɛ‹
way become encysted and remain for years witll
tion.

In the year 1879, at the Giessen clinic, the
blade from the skull of a young farmer where ‖

is, paralysis affects, at the same time, two regions to a greater or less
extent, as, for example, *arm and leg* (brachiocrural   or *arm
and head* (brachiofacial monoplegia), but never the
crural monoplegia) without involvement of the arm, because the centres
of the leg and head are separated by the arm-centre; therefore a single
local cause cannot affect these two separated centres, and at the same
time leave the interposed area (arm-centre) intact. Among the pure
monoplegias there is *monoplegia of the leg, in lesions of* the *upper fourth
of the anterior central convolution and paracentral lobule*. In the case
of mechanical irritation caused, for example, by splinters, shot, etc., it
is accompanied by *monospasm*—i. e., an early contracture (paresis
combined with attacks of convulsions) of the affected leg. Further,
such a cortical lesion may become the starting-point of a Jacksonian
epilepsy.

Monoplegia of the arm has been found in lesions of the *middle two-
fourths of the central convolutions*, including the *cortex of the adjacent
sulci*. Here also following traumatism, monospasm, clonic convulsions
and transition into Jacksonian epilepsy are frequently observed.

The disturbances of sensibility develop more typically and regularly
in brachial monoplegia than in crural monoplegia; muscular sense
(stereoscopic sense) in particular is frequently unimpaired.

A pure or isolated cortical facial paralysis apparently never occurs
In case of localized injury in the head (facial and hypoglossal region)
there is either an associated faciobrachial or a faciolingual monoplegia.

In *faciobrachial* monoplegia, besides the oral branches of the facial
the forearm muscles are affected.

In so-called facial monoplegia the lower facial muscles are affected
the upper ones may possibly show slight paresis. The tongue points
toward the paralyzed side in faciolingual monoplegia. Frequently disturbances of consciousness are present at the same time.

Below are given two clinical histories from the author's observation
which will illustrate better than a general description the symptomatology
diagnosis, and course of circumscribed injury of the motor region:

I. *Punctured fracture in right parietal region; penetration of the right
posterior central convolution in its middle portion to the width and depth
of about 1 cm. Left faciobrachial monoplegia and monospasm. Trephining. Recovery.*—A twenty-six-year-old mason was injured in the
right parietal region by a sharp iron hook thrown at him on October
29, 1881. For the first moment there was a peculiar itching or burning
in all his limbs, particularly in the left arm. This was followed by loss
of consciousness lasting ten minutes; afterward he felt well subjectively,
had no headache, never vomited, but from the moment of injury suffered
loss of power in the left arm, which had not improved much when
patient walked into the clinic on the third day.

The patient was a strong man. His temperature was 36.8° C.
(98.6° F.), pulse 72. In the region of the right parietal bone, at a point
2 cm. behind a line drawn vertically from one external auditory meatus
across the top of the head to the external auditory meatus of the

of the left oral branch of the facial. Face red; headache; dizziness and nausea; pulse 84.

Operation at the clinic three hours after attack: disinfection; exposure of the bone, by an incision 8 cm. long, traversing the scab. Corresponding to the wound, the edges of which adhered, the external table of the parietal bone showed a four-sided, sharply defined, 1 cm. long, 4 to 5 mm. broad punctured wound of bone reaching to the diploë, without fissures or depression. In order to expose the probable fracture of the inner table the wound in the bone was enlarged with a chisel to about the size of a quarter dollar, whereupon the inner table was exposed and found to be comminuted. From a wound in the dura there projected a three-cornered plate of bone, 1 cm. long and 1 to 2 mm. broad, perpendicularly embedded in the cerebral cortex. After removal of all the splinters the dural wound was enlarged to the extent of the trephine-opening, exposing in the posterior central convolution a linear wound about 1 cm. wide and about 1 cm. deep. No other complications. The cutaneous wound was closed with sutures, antiseptic dressing.

Four hours after the operation there was another attack of clonic convulsions limited to the left arm, lasting twelve to fifteen minutes. On November 5th there was a third attack of clonic convulsions in the left arm and shooting pains in the left half of the face. Consciousness was unimpaired. On November 15th in the left forearm there was a feeling of weight and weakness. On November 18th the headaches were more severe; there were vomiting, apathy, photophobia; pulse 48 until November 27th, then rapid recovery and disappearance of all symptoms. By the middle of December the wound was firmly cicatrized.

Two months after injury there was no trace of functional disturbance of the eyes or their auxiliary apparatus. Still a trace of paralysis of the oral branch of the left facial. The gross motor strength of the left arm was markedly less than the right, showing particularly some uncertainty in carrying out finer complicated and combined movements. Temporary paræsthesia in the forearm and hands. Noticeable uncertainty in the localization and qualification of cutaneous stimuli on the dorsal surface of the left hand and forearm. No disturbances of muscular sense.

II. *Punctured fracture of the left parietal region; injury of the left central convolution in its middle portion. Right-sided faciobrachial monoplegia and monospasm. Trephining. Recovery.*—A fourteen-year-old schoolboy received a blow in the left parietal region with a pointed iron rod, thrown at him by a fellow-pupil, on October 23, 1897. The point entered his head. The small wound located on the left parietal eminence was washed out with water by the patient himself and caused no immediate manifestations. The patient walked home, where violent vomiting set in; from the beginning there were headache and considerable weakness of the right arm. On October 26th again vomiting, disturbance of consciousness, convulsions; pulse 48. No fever.

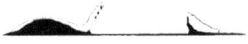

PLATE VI.

FIG. 1.

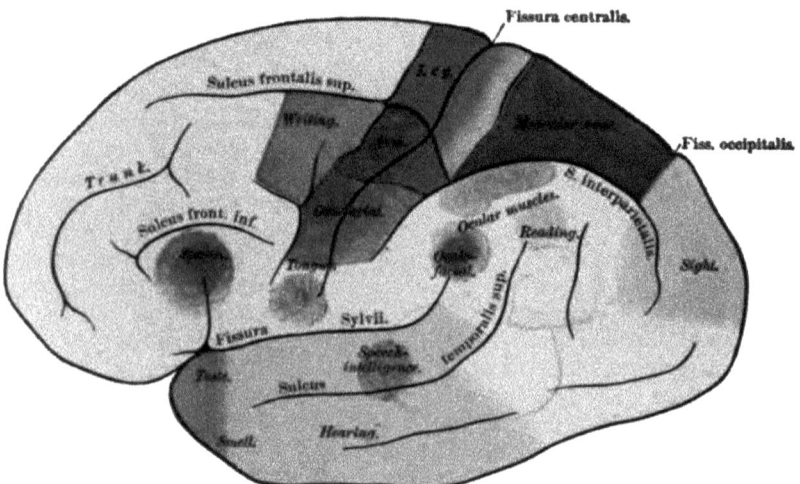

Topographical Anatomy of Cortex.   Localization of
Functions.   (Ziehen.)

FIG. 2.

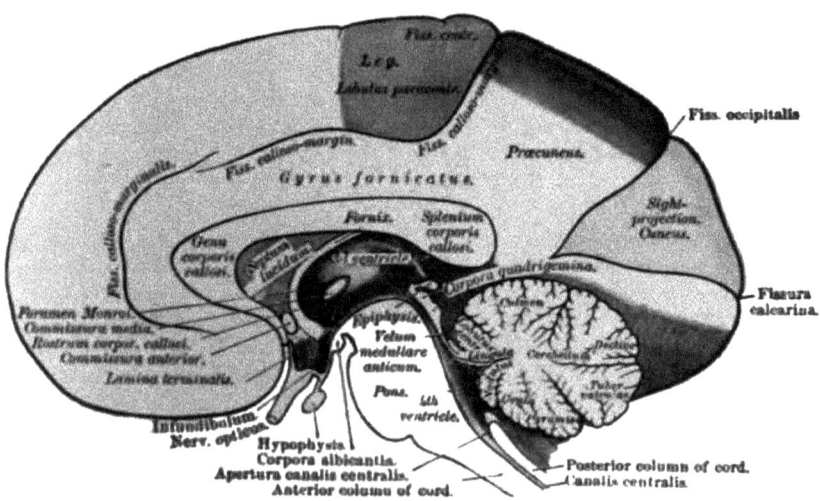

Topographical Anatomy of Inner Surface of Right Hemisphere. Localization of Functions. (Ziehen.)

n, October 28, 1897, the patient, a strong boy, showed
nce of general consciousness. Pulse 72. Speech, stam-
Pupils reacted slowly. Paresis of right arm. In the
ft parietal eminence, situated, topographically, over the
do, was a doughy cutaneous swelling the size of a walnut.
: of the swelling was a wound about 7 mm. long with
d edges glued together. The patient while being ex-
clinic was suddenly seized with clonic convulsions, be-
flexors of the fingers of the right hand and right flexor
ifter four minutes increasing intensity, with affection of
ight forearm, and gradually leading to affection of pecto-
en twitching of orbicularis oris muscle and the muscles
e right oral branch of the facial, and finally also in the
the right frontal branch of the facial. The twitching
n outlasted that in the distribution of the facial by about
es.

rephining, under extremely strict asepsis and ether anæs-
division of the scalp at the site of the small cutaneous
vas found in the external table a round defect 2 to 3 mm.
atted with hair. Escape of brain-substance. Removal
: with circular trephine, the wound in the bone as centre.
osed thereby was lacerated and soiled with hair. Six
me from the inner table were embedded in the bruised
r. Careful toilet of the wound; arrest of hemorrhage
n, which was considerable, by packing with iodoform
was introduced through the cutaneous wound. Sutures.
ig.

ion there was quiet sleep for three hours, patient awaken-
consciousness and undisturbed speech. Paresis of the
h less than before the operation. On October 29th right-
resis was distinctly noticeable. In the evening there were
ons over the entire distribution of the right facial of one
ion, while the right arm remained absolutely quiet. On
there were two similar attacks, the second lasting six
g which the pharyngeal muscles were apparently affected
ber 31st there was an attack of convulsions of long dura-
g in the distribution of the right facial, extending after
to the left half of the face; at the same time convulsions
m for two minutes. On November 2d there was a slight
ulsions in the distribution of the right facial in the face
x finger. Paresis of the right arm and right facial very
ble. On November 11th symptoms disappeared, wound
: reaction. Pulse which had varied between 48 and 60
to 70. On December 12th was discharged completely

rolutions.—The parietal convolutions include those con-
d the posterior central convolution, above and below the
ssure, the *superior parietal lobe* and the *inferior parietal*
17

lobe; the latter is again divided into the two inferior divisions, *g supramarginalis* and *gyrus angularis.*

Very little is definitely known regarding the physiological significa of this region. Flechsig locates his "posterior large association-cen in this region and ascribes to it a higher psychical function. Clin experience indicates that the muscular sense has its centre in the par lobe (Redlich). Accordingly, in case of extensive focal injuries of parietal lobes the muscular sense alone may be completely lost witl being accompanied by any important disturbances of motion.

Occipital Convolutions.—These include the entire occipital lobe its lateral and median surfaces, the region, therefore, of the *supι occipital gyrus,* the *middle* and *inferior occipital gyrus,* the *cuneus, lingual lobule,* and the *descending gyrus.*

The most important manifestation of paralysis in lesions of the oc tal lobe is so-called *hemianopsia*—that is, loss of power of vision in half of the visual field of each eye, caused by a focal lesion on one ι cases being exclusively those of so-called *bilateral homonymous hem opsia—i. e.,* affecting the *lateral (temporal) half of the visual field of one eye and the median (nasal) half of the visual field of the other.* paralytic manifestation, as is known, has an anatomical basis in *hemidecussation* of the optic nerve-trunk in the *chiasma.*

What portions of the cortex of the occipital lobe are especially sig cant in the production of hemianopsia is still a subject of investigat But the median cortical region of the calcarine fissure, the cuneus, lingual lobule, and the descending gyrus appear to be more intima related to the optic fibres than do the lateral regions of the three occip lobes. According to v. Monakow, however, in all lesions of the occip lobe leading to hemianopsia disease or loss of function of the optic fil is a necessary condition, and it is wrong therefore to consider it a pu cortical lesion.

Independent of complete hemianopsia cases of *incomplete* hemianoη occur, which, according to the loss or limitation of the function of vis have been described as *hemiamblyopia, hemiachromatopsia,* or *quadι hemianopsia.*

Finally, as the result of focal disease of both occipital lobes, the pic of *bilateral hemianopsia* may be produced with almost complete blindι (cortical blindness). In such cases, however, besides this marked turbance of vision there are peculiar psychical disturbances which h been included under the conception *soul-blindness,* and which pre various combinations of symptoms according to the location and ex of the lesion, and which have been described as *optic aphasia, al* and *asymbolia.*

The author must be content, however, simply to refer to these diffi provinces of brain pathology.

Frontal Convolutions.—"This region includes the entire and ι extensive surface of the convolutions stretching from the precen fissure to the frontal pole of the brain, including the cortex of the l as far as the fissure of Sylvius" (v. Monakow). They are the *supι *middle* and *inferior frontal convolutions* (*gyrus frontalis superior, medius,* and *inferior*). With the exception of those portions of the first and second frontal convolution bordering on the motor area, and the posterior half of the third frontal convolution, which we must consider part of the speech-centre, as will be discussed hereafter, knowledge of the special significance of the "frontal brain" is still very uncertain. It is only known that as regards localization (in the sense of a special sense-centre) it possesses no special significance (v. Monakow). Even extensive destruction of a frontal lobe may occur with complete absence of all symptoms, and even in bilateral lesions it is not exactly motility that is impaired. It appears more likely that the frontal brain is intrusted with higher nervous (psychical) accomplishments, as v. Monakow expresses it.

Finally, L. Bruns has pointed out a form of ataxia, a disturbance of power of equilibrium like that accompanying cerebellar lesions, which he has observed in cases of tumor of the frontal lobe.

Speech Region.—This includes the cortical area of all the convolutions entering into the formation of the fossa of Sylvius, as follows: the *posterior half of the third frontal convolution* (*Broca's convolution*), the entire island (Reil), the *first temporal convolution,* including the *cortex of the whole of the fissure of Sylvius as far as the gyrus supramarginalis* (v. Monakow).

Lesions in this region can all produce disturbances which are generally called *aphasia.* An extremely important fact has been elicited in this connection, that both hemispheres have not the same value; but on the contrary there is a distinct difference between them in so far as *right-handed individuals—i. e.,* those who in carrying out the operations of daily life (eating, working, writing) use the right hand by preference—will only become aphasic if the speech-centre of the left hemisphere (Broca's convolution) is injured; while on the other hand, *left-handed individuals* will behave just the reverse, their powers of speech remaining intact if the speech region of the left side is affected, while they become aphasic if the speech centre of the right side is affected.

As is known, brain pathology distinguished an expressive form of aphasic disturbance of speech, the so-called motor aphasia (word-dumbness), and implies under the term the inability to find an expression in speech for the most common things and objects or to repeat spoken words. In this condition therefore voluntary oral speech is either totally or partially inhibited.

This form of aphasia is undoubtedly caused by destruction in the region of the third (left) frontal convolution. This condition may be combined with *agraphia—i. e.,* the inability to write correctly.

Sensory aphasia (word-deafness) is different from motor aphasia (word-dumbness). It is the form of perceptive speech disorder which consists in the inability to understand spoken words. Disturbances in the region of the first temporal convolution (left) cause this form of aphasia. Alexia (the inability to understand written and printed words) frequently accompanies it.

Total aphasia occurs, then, when the two mentioned forms of apl motor and sensory, are combined.

It is easy to understand that frequently in extensive lesions of the *frontal convolution* the adjoining provinces of the *motor area*, particu the head region, also suffer. As a matter of fact, the picture of aphasia is not infrequently found combined with that of *faciolingu* even that of *faciobrachial monoplegia*. Indeed a *total right-sided plegia* may be combined with aphasia. If symptoms of irritation in connection with destruction, the picture of a Jacksonian epilepsy finally develop.

In focal lesions of the *upper temporal convolution* (including the s marginal gyrus), in addition to sensory aphasia, there may occur di ances of *sensibility* on the opposite side, particularly of the *mus sense*, if the lesion extend to the lower parietal lobule. Or the optic are involved as the result of a deep focal lesion of the temporal thus sensory aphasia may be combined with *hemianopsia*.

As far as the *island* is concerned, smaller lesions frequently see run their course without any symptoms whatsoever. More exte lesions can, however, if located on the left side, produce *aphasic dis ances;* according as to whether the focus is located more anterior more posteriorly, aphasia may be *motor* or *sensory*.

Internal Capsule.—"The term 'internal capsule' is applied t massive medullary layer interposed between the optic thalamus an lenticular nucleus on one side, and the corpus striatum and putame the other. The internal capsule is principally a point for the colle of projection-fibres, which are derived partly from different portio the cerebral cortex to be connected with peripheral parts, and part fibres originating in the deeper portions of the brain which lead t cerebrum" (v. Monakow). Lesions of the internal capsule are foll by different symptoms; therefore, according as to whether they destroyed the entire capsule or only a portion of it and interruptec course of the corresponding fibres. Complete hemiplegia, together hemianæsthesia, hemianopsia, or incomplete hemiplegia, with parti involvement of single tracts of fibres, such as facial and leg paralys facial and hypoglossal paralysis, or hemianæsthesia and hemiano etc., may thus determine the character of a clinical picture of a cap lesion. Pure monoplegias and monospasms, isolated facial paralysi isolated paralysis of other cranial nerves, on the other hand, have r been observed or, at any rate, never positively confirmed. This is to the fact that different tracts of fibres lie so close together.

We must be satisfied with these references for the reason that matic lesions of the internal capsule can hardly acquire practical si cance, and the combination of capsular symptoms can be important in the differential diagnosis of certain focal cortical diseases. Pure sular focal injuries are scarcely to be expected in traumatic lesions (injuries, contusions); the adjacent regions of the brain, optic thala and lenticular nucleus, corpus striatum and putamen, are almost al affected at the same time.

tracts for both halves of the body, as a result of which bilateral m
festations are easily produced; and the circumstance that the cortical
mid-brain tracts (fillet) are crossed by the cranial nerves of the s
side, usually motor and sensory. From this necessarily follows the
called alternating and other combined paralyses." For example: |
sided hemiplegia of the extremities with slight involvement of the
facial and tongue, and a right-sided total facial paralysis (hemipl
alternans inferior); or left-sided hemiplegia of the extremities and ri
sided abducens or trigeminus paralysis, etc.

But the roots or nuclei of single cranial nerves, originating in the |
may be affected by a lesion without being accompanied by moto
sensory disturbances of the extremities; this results in isolated or (
combined paralysis of single cranial nerves (for example, of the abduc
facial, hypoglossal).

A pons symptom considered extremely important by some autho
conjugate paralysis of the lateral recti of the eye—i. e., of the exte
rectus of one and the internal rectus of the other side.

Finally, in lesions of the pons there may be disturbances in the
tribution of the hypoglossal, leading to dysarthria and anarthria.

Cerebellum.—Probably the cerebellum exercises an important influe
upon the extremities in the sense of maintaining equilibrium, and |
sibly also upon the face and eyes in the sense of regulating force (
co-ordination. There are found in the cerebellum, "important c
ponents for maintaining equilibrium and for the proper application
force, as well as for the proper gradation of various muscular ac
(v. Monakow).

The principal cerebellar symptom of paralysis is so-called *cerebe
ataxia*, the swaying walk (Démarche d'ivresse), very similar to the |
of an intoxicated person. A symptom of irritation is *dizziness*. B
symptoms, confirmed at the same time, are of great diagnostic sigi
cance.

Certain focal lesions of the cerebellum may, of course, produce dist
effects, as a result of which the chiasma or medulla or the pons r
suffer. In this way may be explained certain symptoms occasion
observed in cerebellar lesions, such as disturbances of vision, vo
ing, difficulty in swallowing, diabetes mellitus and insipidus, etc.

Medalla Oblongata.—The not infrequent involvement of the med
oblongata in lesions affecting the skull and its contents makes it ju
liable to include under cerebral localization a brief discussion of bul
manifestations of focal injuries. Severe lesions of the bulb would, |
sumably, be rapidly fatal, in so far as the centres for respiration |
circulation are affected thereby. For the rest the picture of a bul
lesion depends upon how extensively the motor and sensory nerve-tr
of the extremities, as well as the nuclei and roots which lie within
bulb, are affected, particularly the nuclei and roots of the ninth to
twelfth cranial nerves—i. e., the glossopharyngeal, vagus, accessory, :
hypoglossal. Accordingly there may result a motor paralysis of
extremities, with the picture of a complete or incomplete paraplegia

hemiplegia of the extremities. Sensory disturbances of the extremities seem to occur but rarely. Besides the paralysis of the extremities the following bulbar symptoms may occur: anarthria, dysphagia, aphonia, singultus, disturbances of respiration and circulation, such as stertorous respiration, Cheyne-Stokes breathing, slowing of the pulse, and terminal pneumonia.

Finally, there should be borne in mind certain manifestations on the part of the urinary apparatus, such as glycosuria, polyuria, and albuminuria, which may occur in diseases of the floor of the fourth ventricle.

The Treatment of Recent Injuries of the Brain.—The treatment of a contusion of the brain presupposes its diagnosis. If this is impossible as is frequently the case, direct treatment of such a brain lesion is out of the question. In these cases our efforts at treatment must therefore frequently be limited to the injury of the skull and its covering. The injury may be a simple contusion, a wound of the soft parts, or a fracture of the skull. In some such cases it is only after years that the autopsy gives a clear idea of the former brain injury, the patient having died from some other cause. One then finds those anatomical changes described above in discussing the course of contusion foci in the brain. If, however, a diagnosis of a traumatic focus of the brain at a certain location be made from the primary symptoms—and in the majority of cases, under such circumstances, there is a lesion of the cerebral cortex within the motor area—it may always be firmly maintained that the brain injury itself did not justify active interference. What would be the purpose of active interference? The reparative processes which follow brain lesions are completed, as far as is possible, without assistance; and unfortunately more than repair is not to be hoped for.

Only two conditions indicate operative interference: First, the removal whenever possible of foreign bodies embedded in the brain, such as splinters of bone or objects which have penetrated the cranial cavity from without, as, for example, points of knife-blades, needles, rifle-bullets, etc. Second, to prevent threatened septic infection, or at least to cut short such a process during its early stages. Both of these indications may, of course, exist at the same time.

Regarding the first indication, the removal of a foreign body, the proof of such a complication may be very easy, very difficult, or impossible. It is easy when the character of the injury forces upon the surgeon the fact that a foreign body has been introduced. In this group are gunshot injuries, with simple wound of entrance of the skull and escape of brain matter; further, stab-wounds, in which the instrument (knife-blade, a nail, or a hook) remains deeply embedded in the bone of the skull; also compound comminuted fractures of the vault which permit of inspection and digital examination of the crushed cerebral cortex, the latter filled with fragments of bone. In all such cases the diagnosis of a foreign body embedded in the brain is based upon its direct detection by the senses—the determination of the gross local lesion, through the eye and the finger.

The diagnosis is more difficult and frequently is impossible when the presence of a foreign body in the brain can only be deduced from dis-

turbance of the brain functions which are referable to a foreign bo
For, just as a traumatic focus of the brain does not in itself necessar
cause manifestations of paralysis or irritation, so these symptoms
not necessarily produced by the presence of a foreign body. Whetl
a focal injury or a foreign body produces symptoms or not depends,
the first place, upon the localization of the injury, and, further, upon
degree of mechanical irritation which it produces upon the brain-su
stance; form, size, and weight may have some bearing. Frequently
symptoms are absent at first, and only after several days certain ma
festations of irritation set in which arouse suspicion of a foreign bo
at the site of the lesion. Of particular importance are certain manif
tations of irritation, which develop soon after the injury, associated w
paralytic symptoms occurring immediately after the trauma, and wh
possess the strict character of focal symptoms (thus, for example, mo
spasm following primary monoparesis, as in the cases referred to abo
observed by the author).

Finally, the importance of x-rays in determining the presence
foreign bodies in the brain—metallic ones especially—must be dw
upon. In spite of the wonderful discovery being a very recent o
extensive experience has shown that by means of the x-ray method
is possible to determine, for example, the position and size of p
jectiles in the brain. In fact, it is possible, as the result of such findin
to institute operative treatment.

No matter in what way the diagnosis of a foreign body in the br
may have been made, whether by direct inspection and palpation
the cranial wound, whether by deduction from the functional distu
ances of the central organ with the assistance of the clinical history,
finally, by means of the x-ray picture, there is no question that
ideal treatment consists in the removal of the foreign body fr
the brain, thus paving the way for the best possible recovery, f
from all early or late complications. For the foreign body allowed
remain is always a complication of a brain injury, and may hinder
local reparative processes. In some cases it may render repair i
possible. Even if under favorable circumstances it does become
cysted, as foreign bodies become encysted in other organs and tissu
it still remains an object of anxiety, and frequently after a longer
shorter latent period becomes the starting point of severe functional d
turbances of a general character or of local processes, which may res
in death after many years. Thus foreign bodies are met with in d
cussing the etiology of traumatic epilepsy, certain psychoses, trauma
late abscess, and meningitis. Of course, in endowing the foreign bo
remaining in the brain with this odium, it is proper to add that ev
simple brain lesions without the addition of a foreign body may oc
sionally lead to the same termination.

Of all foreign bodies in the brain, rifle-bullets have always excit
great surgical interest, and regarding the latter and their fate there exi
a special class of literature which has undergone considerable increa
during the last few years. It has been shown that particularly ama

calibre bullets, with slight penetrating power, such as Flobert bullets, revolver projectiles of 4, 5, or 7 mm. calibre, not infrequently become encysted in the brain. With these weapons, frequently very cheap, used occasionally by suicides, the effect of the shot often consists of only a small circular perforation of the cranial bone and a narrow blind bullet-track in the brain, without lateral action worth mentioning. The fragments of bone carried along are small in number and hemorrhage from the parts of the brain traversed is moderate. An x-ray picture shows the small projectile at the end of the shot-sinus as a small black spot. The author has had the opportunity to follow for years the course of several patients with encysted projectiles. The following is an example:

A girl was admitted to the clinic having received, about two hours before, an accidental shot in the right side of the skull, from a Flobert rifle, fired at a distance of 1½ metres. The diameter of the projectile was 6 mm. Immediately after the shot was fired the girl collapsed with a loud cry, was raised at once and carried to bed. The mother noticed then that she was totally paralyzed on the left side. The patient was never unconscious, but complained of severe headaches and vomited once, one and a half hours after the injury. Hemorrhage was insignificant; there was repeated vomiting. Under slight chloroform anæsthesia the entire head was shaved and the skin carefully disinfected. A cutaneous incision 6 cm. long was carried through the wound and deepened as far as the bone. After detaching the soft parts from the bone there was discovered in the parietal bone a circular defect 6 mm. in diameter, without fissures. At the bottom of the bone wound were several dark blood-clots; the escaping blood was distinctly pulsating. The wound in the bone was carefully enlarged with a chisel, and, after removal of a zone of the external table, there was found rather extensive splintering of the inner table. One such splinter lying flat and loose upon the dura was immediately removed. It was approximately triangular in shape, 11 to 12 mm. long and 9 mm. wide. Upon searching with a probe, an opening was discovered in the dura, and the probe entered the bullet-track. By means of the probe more splinters of bone from the inner table were discovered which had penetrated the dura n the cerebral cortex. It was possible to remove The largest was 18 mm. long and 8 mm. wide. about half as large; several blood-clots were removed with the splinters; there was no subsequent hemorrhage. No three in succession bullet could be discovered even after removal of the splinter. Antiseptic dressing. Recovery took place in a surprisingly short time, without further incident and with the disappearance of all paralytic manifestations. It was completed at the end of four weeks. Since then ten years have elapsed. The girl has developed to womanhood, and never up to the present time has there been a single manifestation of a somatic, intellectual, or psychical character to recall the former severe brain lesion.

This description suffices to show that the course of brain injuries complicated by foreign bodies may vary much, and although the author has pointed out that the removal of foreign bodies is ᵗʰᵃᵗ ᵃᵗ ᵃᵗ and to be sought for in the treatment of such injuries, ᵇᵘᵗ size the fact that there are certain limits for such ᵃᶜᵗᶦᵛᵉ which it is well to respect if the surgeon does not wish to ᵉˣᵖᵒˢᵉ ᵗʰᵉ life of the patient to a danger which is greater perhaps than might possibly arise from the presence of a foreign body. ᵀʰᵉ of the right path under such circumstances is at the ᵖʳᵉˢᵉⁿᵗ ᵗᶦᵐᵉ ᵃ of the difficult and not fully solved problems of operative brain ˢᵘʳᵍᵉ The proper course is clearly indicated in wounds of the cerebral complicated by compound comminuted fractures of the vault. If such cases splinters or other foreign bodies, such as hair, sand, pebble machine oil, etc., have been forced through the torn meninges into t brain-substance, the operation rendered necessary by the splinteri of the skull and which consists in the primary removal of splinters a cleansing of the cranial wound, is simply extended to the wound the brain, and is completed by the careful removal of all fragments bone and foreign bodies which might interfere with the process of repa including those situated in the brain itself. Loose fragments of br are best wiped with dry mull wipes, and hemorrhage from the brai substance should be arrested by pressure with iodoform gauze, whi should wherever possible be led out between the skin-flaps, the lat being then united. The earlier this important part in the primary ca of the wound is carried out, the more favorable is the prognosis. It surprising how smoothly and without any reaction the repair of even ve complicated wounds of the brain proceeds under favorable circumstance

In those cases in which there is not free access to the contusion foc or wound of the cerebral cortex, the choice of procedure is more diffict than in those wounds of the brain which are open and exposed, ev if there are grounds for suspecting that splinters or other foreign bodi complicate a cerebral injury. Splinters broken from the inner tab in fracture without fracture of the outer table, punctured wounds, at the numerous cases of gunshot fractures with blind bullet-track at small wound of entrance, come under consideration in this clas Whether, however, in these cases, the surgeon should proceed to open or not, depends very much upon what he may assume to be the charact of the wound or contusion of the brain situated beneath the bone lesio The author has already pointed out the difficulty in making such diagnosis. By employing the results of modern teaching in regard cerebral localization, we are, however, in a position in certain cases determine in all probability the presence of foreign bodies in the cerebi cortex. In most instances the surgeon will have to deal with injuri of the limited portion of the brain included within the motor ar Here the succession of certain symptoms of paralysis and irritation m make the diagnosis so positive that operative interference is not on justifiable, but actually imperative as well. The author refers to o two observations, which were recounted in the section on Cerebr Localization, and which he refers to as classical cases on the questic of operative interference.

There can be no question that at the moment the diagnosis of isolated fracture or punctured fracture of the inner table with penetration of the cerebral cortex by splinters is determined, it becomes the duty of the surgeon to expose the site of the brain lesion, and to remove the fragment which is irritating the central organ. Access is established by means of trephining, and it may be left to the discretion of the operator whether for this purpose he employs the classical trephine or the mallet and chisel. The author is accustomed to use either method, according to the local conditions of the wound, as the clinical histories formerly recounted show, and has always accomplished his purpose. A circular opening, 2 to 3 cm. in diameter, in the bone of the skull, whose centre corresponds to the point of impact, will usually suffice for the exploration of the cerebral cortex and the removal of any existing splinters, for the comminution of the inner table is always circumscribed in those forms of violence coming under consideration here, and at the same time the brain injury is usually limited to the cortex.

Conditions are not so simple in gunshot-wounds of the brain caused by rifle-bullets. If the projectile has gone completely through, or, in other words, if there is a perforating gunshot-wound of the brain with wound of entrance and exit in the skull, it is not justifiable to attempt operative interference simply for the purpose of removing from the bullet-track any particles of bone that have been carried along. The danger resulting from interference is too serious, and at the same time the result is very uncertain. In practice, however, these cases are hardly ever the object of such consideration, for the simple reason that a projectile which possesses sufficient penetrating power to produce such an injury would inflict such devastation, such destruction of the brain, such meningeal, cerebral, and ventricular hemorrhage, etc., that death would take place immediately or within a few hours without recovery of consciousness. How shall the surgeon act if there is a simple gunshot-wound of the head, with a bullet-track terminating blindly and the projectile embedded somewhere in the cranial cavity?

This question has been repeatedly discussed during the last few years, and is by no means settled at the present time. Owing to the difference in conditions, it would hardly appear justifiable to proceed in all cases according to a fixed rule. One must remember that the projectile, after having perforated the bone, may, according to the degree of velocity, follow a course of different length. It may be located behind the wound of entrance, upon or within the dura; it may be embedded within the cerebral cortex; it may have cut a short or a long channel through the brain-substance. Possibly it may have penetrated as far as the inner table of the opposite side and remained in this situation, or it may have rebounded from this point, as has been previously shown in connection with a case observed by the author, and have been driven through the brain in another direction. And even here the possible variety of cases is by no means exhausted. In many cases, death ensuing frees the patient from suffering and the surgeon from his predicament — operative interference cannot be considered; as has not to seek further for the projectile, nor to extract the same from the bottom of the shot-hole; frequently one should be satisfied with simply probing the wound of entrance, and, if the result is negative, proceed at once to apply an antiseptic dressing to the small cutaneous wound. The author has never seen harm result from such probing if carried out under strict antiseptic precaution and with a gentle hand. In many cases, on the other hand, he has obtained positive results which led him to take a step further and to enlarge the wound of entrance in the bone. This positive result obtained by probing is the detection of bone-splinters which lie within the wound of entrance in the skull, either to one side upon the dura, in the dura, or embedded deeper within the cerebral cortex. Occasionally the probe descends directly into the shot-sinus in the brain, and at a moderate depth meets with strong resistance, which may be caused either by a splinter or a bullet. In such a case the author has never regretted immediately enlarging the wound of the bone with a chisel or Luer's gouge-forceps and removing a foreign body rendered accessible by such an easy and safe procedure. In numerous cases the spent projectile lay upon the dura, in others the projectile was embedded in the cerebral cortex and could easily be removed together with bone splinters. Where, however, the projectile is deeply embedded within the brain, it is advisable, in view of the principle expressed above, not to attempt extraction, but to be satisfied with the removal of superficial bone-splinters. This procedure was followed in the case of gunshot-wound of the brain, recounted before; and who would question that by the removal of the large superficial splinters and the three splinters in the cerebral cortex, of which the largest was 18 mm. long and 8 mm. wide, the patient was done a great service, even if search was not made for the projectile in the depths of the brain and even if it was not extracted.

In concluding the discussion of recent gunshot-injuries of the brain and their treatment, attention is called to the recent attempts that have been made to search for and excise, a long time after injury, *projectiles encysted in the brain* under the guidance of an *x*-ray picture. Experience has so far shown that it is possible, by means of the *x*-ray process, to determine the site of a bullet in the brain with such exactness that in certain cases through the topical diagnosis it becomes accessible to operation. Experience has shown that in some cases this operation has accomplished its end and the patient recovered. E. Braatz, Kümmell, A. E. Barker, and others have described such successful operations. Undoubtedly such interference may be indicated by the severity of the symptoms, which must be referred to the continued presence of a foreign body. The careful surgeon will, however, do well to limit himself to such cases and to weigh carefully the danger of interference before taking up the knife and the saw. There exists, as it would appear to the author, more danger in doing too much than too little.

A second indication, which may lead the surgeon to operate immediately in wounds of the brain, and which has been previously mentioned, is the contamination of the wound with infectious material. At the same

time the author added that this indication usually existed with tha
removing larger foreign bodies that had been forced into the brain fr
the outside by the mechanism of the injury. These are the carrier:
infection. Primary extraction of splinters with careful cleansing of
vicinity of the wound, removal of blood-clots and brain fragmen
dividing the dura where retention of wound secretion is feared, trimm
the lacerated and contused wound-edges, carefully stopping all hem:
rhage, drying the entire wound with simple sterile mull wipes, a
finally, accurate filling the wound with iodoform gauze—these are
measures necessary in such cases. The earlier they are carried out,
more certainly do they promise that, in spite of evident contaminat
of the wound either with hair, sand, street dirt, etc., the process of wou
repair will go on smoothly and simply. Disinfection of wounds w
antiseptic irrigating fluids the author has not made use of during
past few years; the more energetically and fastidiously, however, I
he shaved the entire scalp and disinfected it according to Fürbringe
method with soap, alcohol, and (1 : 1000) sublimate solution bef
carrying out any of the above procedures.

TRAUMATIC MENINGITIS.

Simple injury of the dura mater or pia mater is unnoticed in the gre
of symptoms caused by injuries to the brain unless it is associated w
extensive hemorrhage from some of the meningeal vessels. This
already been spoken of. The condition is quite different if infect
is added to the injury within the skull. This unfortunate compli
tion is by no means a rare one, and is marked by symptoms due
the inflammation of the pia, which may be so prominent as to obse
all other symptoms. Contusions of the dura and the pia and tears
these membranes may heal and leave no trace except a more or l
marked cicatrix, provided there is no infection. If suppuration foll
injury, it has a tendency to spread rapidly within the membranes, as
mentioned in the description of encephalitis.

Etiology.—The etiology of traumatic meningitis, like that of trauma
encephalitis, is dependent upon the action of certain pathological mic
organisms. According to Macewen's examinations, the microbes m
often present are *Streptococcus pyogenes* and *Staphylococcus pyoge
aureus*, less often *Staphylococcus albus* and *citreus*. In the great majo
of cases these microbes are introduced from the surface of the sc
through the wound. Only in rare instances does bacterial infection co
through the bloodvessels. Even though the bacteria are introdu
through the blood, the traumatism is an essential factor in the infla
mation, since the injured portions of the meninges and the brain furn
a favorable soil for bacterial growth. Thus whatever the source of
infection, the localization of a traumatic meningitis is determined by
injury. Therefore the division of traumatic meningitis into basilar a
cortical is of significance merely as showing that certain injuries l

well to remember the point made by Billroth, that blood laden with the toxic products of suppuration may act directly upon the centres of the brain and tend to irritate or to paralyze them. Thus in most cases one should be content simply to say that a leptomeningitis exists without attempting to fix the extent of the suppurative inflammation.

Prognosis and Treatment.—Traumatic meningitis has a most unfavorable prognosis, as stated above. Treatment is generally prophylactic. Every open wound of the skull and every compound fracture of the skull should be made as aseptic as possible. One ought to keep in mind the risk of infectious meningitis under such circumstances. The success which attends such treatment in most cases is in striking contrast to the suppurative meningo-encephalitis which so often followed such injuries in the pre-antiseptic period.

If traumatic meningitis is not recognized until its symptoms are well marked, the outlook is most unfavorable. In many respects the meninges are similar to the membranes which line other large cavities, such as the peritoneum, pleura, or the synovial membranes of joints. This comparison is a superficial one, however, and when the pia mater becomes infected the differences due to its multilocular meshwork and its inclosure within the skull become prominent.

If there is an open fracture of the skull, and if in spite of cleansing of the wound and the extraction of splinters meningitis develops, the surgeon is justified in reopening the wound in the soft parts and in the skull, and dividing the dura and exposing the pia as far as possible. Even though the hope of eliminating the infection in this manner is a slim one, still further exit will be afforded the purulent secretion, any blood-clots present will be discovered and dislodged, and the intracranial pressure will be reduced. Whether osteoplastic craniotomy by exposing more widely the affected parts will yield better results than those obtained with the use of the smaller trephine-openings must be determined in the future.

HERNIA OF THE BRAIN.

The substance of the brain may flow or protrude from an open wound in the skull. Such a wound must of necessity extend through the scalp, skull, and both dura and pia mater. This symptom is usually observed in cases of severe compound fractures of the convexity; but it may also accompany narrow fissures, at least immediately after the injury. Sometimes this symptom is seen with compound fractures of the base, in which case the cerebral substance may appear in the orbit, or in the nose, or in one of the sinuses connected with the nose, or in the external auditory canal. A microscopical examination will remove any doubt as to the nature of grayish-white flakes and bits of soft material. Perhaps the most common cause of the protrusion of cerebral matter is a gun-shot-wound. The flow of semifluid cerebral substance may continue from such a wound for several hours.

Experience shows that recovery without appreciable loss of fui
may follow what at first appeared to be a very serious injury t
brain with loss of cerebral substance. Whether such a happy
will take place depends primarily upon the portion of the brain
is injured. Furthermore, the prognosis with reference to life de
primarily on the physiological importance of the portions of the
which have been injured or removed, and secondarily upon the ab
or development of infectious meningitis and encephalitis. If
complications arise, death will not be long delayed.

Besides this primary pouring out of the brain-substance, then
secondary protrusion which may occur in the first week after ii
or perhaps not until several weeks have passed. Such a protrus
properly termed a cerebral prolapse. A portion of the brain not
rated from the rest gradually protrudes through the rent in the
and skull caused by the injury. The pia may cover the prol
portion of the cortex completely, or, if it was destroyed by the tra
tism, the prolapse may take place without it. The protruding
first fills the gap in the skull and then slowly or more rapidly
above the level of the bones until it reaches the size of a waln
of an orange, or even of the fist. Usually the prolapsed brain s
distinctly the pulsation of the heart. This sign may be wantin
account of tension or irregularity in shape. In the beginning
surface of the prolapse may show the normal convolutions, color
consistence of the brain in so far as these have not been altere
the injury; but this normal appearance is gradually lost and the t
becomes livid or black from extravasations of blood, while its su
softens and becomes gangrenous. If the development of encep
meningitis does not produce speedy death, the necrotic portions o
brain will be cast off and the tumor will appear smaller and fii
Here and there grayish-red granulations appear, and owing to
traction the tumor may shrink within the skull and finally be
covered by the growth of the scalp. In this manner the wound
become completely cicatrized, but the pulsation of the brain bei
may be plainly felt through the scar. If the defect in the skin
soft parts is so large that the wound is not likely to heal from gi
at its edges, or because the granulating tumor is elevated above
surface, healing may be obtained by means of a plastic operatio
by the application of Thiersch skin-grafts. When the conditions pe
it is far better to cover the defect with an osteoplastic flap accordii
König's method.

Etiology.—The etiology of traumatic cerebral prolapse is at pro
well understood. The experience of the last few years has shown
prolapse after traumatism as well as after operation only occurs in
the intracranial pressure is abnormally high. This pressure ma
increased in a variety of ways. In one case mentioned by Bockelm
the cause in the case of a child was an almost constant scream
The cause after traumatism is usually the development of infect
processes in the meninges and brain, exudates in the meninges

ventricles, and abscesses in the cerebral substance. These processes cause an abnormal intracranial pressure, and may force the brain out through any rent in the dura and skull. The condition of cerebral prolapse was therefore much more frequently seen in the pre-antiseptic days. At present traumatic cerebral prolapse must be classed as one of the rarest occurrences in surgery.

Within the last ten years many cases have been reported in which following operations upon the brain serious prolapse has developed. This usually follows extensive exposure of the brain for the purpose of opening abscesses or extirpating tumors. On account of the high intracranial pressure existing at operation the brain projected either immediately upon incision of the dura, or later if the surgeon failed to find the abscess or tumor and relieve the increased intracranial pressure.

The conclusion which has been drawn from such unfortunate cases is to perform craniectomy as a palliative operation to relieve the pressure in the case of inoperable cerebral tumors. This advice should not be blindly followed, since v. Bergmann has shown that craniectomy under such circumstances may be followed by acute œdema of the brain. This may aggravate the prolapse already existing, or cause a fresh prolapse.

Prognosis.—The prognosis of prolapse following craniectomy is grave. It is seldom possible to prevent by bandages an increase in the size of the prolapse, while the risk of secondary infection cannot well be avoided.

There is another condition which may develop in an open wound of the skull, and which may easily be confounded with cerebral prolapse. Reference is made to hemorrhagic granuloma, which, starting in an ulceration of the surface of the brain, may grow like a fungus through the gap in the skull and spread over its surface until it reaches the size of a walnut or of a small apple. Such extensive granulation may be caused by the presence within the skull of some splinter of bone or very small foreign body which by its presence stimulates the abnormal growth. Such a tumor is soft, pulsating, livid, bleeds easily when touched, and often contains small abscesses. Careful examination of the tissue will show that it is not cerebral tissue but simply granulation-tissue. The removal of this granulation-tissue, together with any foreign body which may be present or any necrotic bone, or collection of pus, will usually change the wound into a healthy one. Such unhealthy granulations may be prevented by a proper treatment from the first of compound fractures of the skull and injuries of the brain.

ABSCESS OF THE BRAIN.

By PROF. DR. VON BERGMANN.

The subject of cerebral abscesses rests on a very definite etiology. There are acute and chronic abscesses. The former are due to infection through an open wound in the skull, the usual condition being cavities filled with a milky fluid, or pus may collect until the appearance is that of a well-encapsulated abscess. Wernicke and Hahn had the good fortune to recognize such a condition, and to operate upon it successfully. Without doubt many so-called idiopathic abscesses of the brain are really of a tuberculous character. Abscesses of the brain which are situated beneath portions of the skull which are affected with tuberculosis may be classed with cerebral abscess due to osteitis and caries of the skull.

Acute Traumatic Cerebral Abscess.—Acute´ abscess of the cortex due to traumatism develops in consequence of infection of the exposed and injured brain. If it is accompanied by an extensive purulent leptomeningitis, various symptoms which are due to the abscess are joined with those due to the meningitis. If it is limited to the spot

FIG. 84.

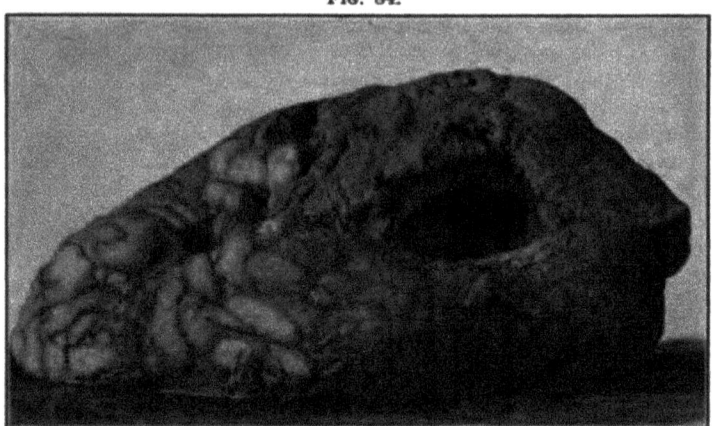

Large abscess in the inferior parietal region secondary to fracture of the skull. The thick capsule of the abscess can be seen. (Starr.)

in which there is a localized fracture of the skull and contusion of the brain, early opening will often prevent the development of a leptomeningitis spreading from the affected point. Beneath the pia which is infiltrated with pus will be found a flat collection of pus of moderate extent. The pia which covers it externally is stretched and often broken in pieces, and the base of the abscess is formed by a depression in the cortex which marks the extent of the contusion. There is a zone of red softening about the abscess, and further removed from it a zone of œdema. The abscess contains a brownish pus mixed with free fat and granular darker detritus. The borders of such an abscess are indistinct and its walls are ragged, a result, doubtless, of the rapid spread of the suppuration. If a diffuse meningitis does not develop and the pus is promptly evacuated, recovery may follow. Granulations spring from the margin about the purulent collection, and grow until they reach those from the opposite wall and cicatrization is completed

... usual manner. There will then be found in the site of the ... a shallow depression lined with scar-tissue. This depression be ... by cerebrospinal fluid, and oftentimes the lateral ventricl ... it is situated is correspondingly dilated.

An abscess of the cortex is a retention of pus whose outward ... by overlapping of the broken bone or by some other ... is marked by certain external signs other than those due to the o ... The wound becomes yellow and granulations that ... degenerate. There are redness and swelling immediately ... wound, and drops of pus well up from its depths. Such an a ... from a commencing, rapidly spreading leptomeningitis ... appearance—perhaps a week or ten days after the injury ... in the first few days. Both affections may be accompani ... of irritation and paralysis, but when these are due to a ... are not so sudden and severe as when due to meningitis.

Treatment.—If a retention of pus is suspected, the wound sho... ... be widely opened and the broken fragments of the skull ... If this action exposes a pia which is already widely infil ... purulent secretion, the operation should not be abandoned. ... has been saved from the fatal spread of suppurative meni ... operative treatment.

Chronic Traumatic Cerebral Abscess.—The chronic traumati ... differs from the acute in that it is not always an abscess of th... ... but arises more often in a deeper layer and works toward the su... ... in three forms. It may begin acutely, just as the acute co ... described above. If a portion of the pus is discharged an ... become firmly adherent to the skull around the dan ... the patient may escape extensive œdema of the brain as w... ... As long as pus flows from the depths to the surfac... ... in the cortex will become gradually larger. Even thoug... ... freely from a complicated fracture, there is danger that it... ... become obstructed by alterations in its channel. A second ... chronic cerebral abscess is the presence in the brain of small ... such as knife-blades or projectiles of small arms. It ... that the projectiles of small firearms may heal within a ... giving rise to any special disturbance. The metallic o ... not produce suppuration, but this is often caused by the ... which lie upon its surface or are carried in with it. ... give rise to deep abscesses more often relatively than do b... ... A third etiological factor is thrombosis, which in the ca... ... osteitis and osteomyelitis may begin outside of the skull ... through the sinuses into the base of the brain. It is ea... ... how a suppurating portion of the skull can lead to a brain ab... ... Thrombosis explains this process. Furthermore, ... for an abscess to form deep in the brain and separated ... the primary focuses of infection by a layer of normal brain-tissue. ... true that such a thrombosed vein extending from the surface ... the brain has not often been demonstrated.

All chronic abscesses, whether of traumatic or other origin, are characterized by the so-called abscess membrane, which is a smooth, yellowish-white, rather thick layer of connective tissue. Such an encapsulated abscess may remain stationary for a considerable time, but it is more likely to extend, not gradually, but in steps. Each step represents a new inflammation, and at autopsy one finds the traces of a recent red softening adjacent to some portion of an older abscess cavity. Both may be due in such cases to this new encephalitis, and not to the size of the abscess or to its rupture. In favorable cases the extension joins with the old abscess, and a new capsule is formed to include the whole suppurating area. If the margin of the abscess is not well defined and there is a diffuse infiltration of pus, the growth of the abscess will he rapid. Under such circumstances the abscess may break into the ventricle, or, reaching the surface, set up a diffuse meningitis which will cause the patient's death. Abscesses of the frontal and parietal lobes of the brain often reach the lateral ventricle, but seldom extend to the cortex. Meyes has estimated that it requires three weeks for encapsulation to make itself manifest, and that six weeks must elapse before the membrane is well developed.

An abscess is rarely smaller than a pigeon's egg, but may be so large that it involves both hemispheres.

An acute abscess of the brain does not last more than three to five weeks. If the duration exceeds this, it is properly called a chronic abscess. Such an abscess may exist for a long time on account of its slow growth, or because of its favorable situation, or for some other reason. It may last for months, and there are well-authenticated cases of cerebral abscess lasting for more than twenty years.

Cerebral pus has a greenish-yellow color, a consistence similar to synovial fluid, and an acid reaction. It is generally odorless and becomes fetid only if contaminated by necrosis of the bone or by the presence of foreign bodies.

Chronic cerebral abscess runs a characteristic course. Immediately after the injury there are cerebral symptoms which are called primary. Then there is a latent period in which the patient feels well. Following this period are the secondary symptoms. Such is the typical course of chronic abscess of the brain. In traumatic cases it is easy to understand this sequence of symptoms. The first acute stage is produced by the injury to the brain, which may be severe and associated with concussion, hemorrhage beneath and above the dura, and compression of the brain. As soon as these conditions quiet down recovery turns chiefly upon the situation around the abscess. It is well known that large portions of the brain may be destroyed without producing any apparent loss of its functions. The connections are only pushed aside and not destroyed. If the gray matter is preserved, an abscess may extend through the whole lobe or even throughout the cerebral hemisphere without producing symptoms which indicate the trouble.

Symptoms.—As has been stated, a chronic abscess of the brain advances by steps and remains quiet for a shorter or longer interval and then

since disappeared it suddenly leads to a suppurative inflammation of the diploë. At that time there will be two groups of symptoms which will point to a phlebitis. The symptoms of the first group will be those arising from the thrombosis of the particular sinus which is affected; while secondly there will be the pyæmia which so often follows sinus-thrombosis.

Diagnosis.—Repeated typical chills, with quick temperature elevations, suggest pyæmia, and the diagnosis will be strengthened by tenderness in the hepatic region, swelling of the joints, and pleuritic symptoms. If, therefore, a patient has many severe chills in the third or some succeeding week after an injury to the head, the diagnosis is probably pyæmia.

The temperature elevations are most significant when observed in the latent period. Renewed and increased fever points to the beginning of an unfavorable turn.

The most important clinical signs of cerebral abscess are well-marked symptoms of localization, provided they are accompanied with headache and fever. Sometimes there will be sudden spasms. Sometimes the new cerebral symptoms will be ushered in with a cry or a convulsive trembling in the whole body, or there may be an apoplectic attack which passes over, leaving the patient comfortable, but which is followed by other attacks until there is hemiplegia, unconsciousness, coma, and death.

If the unilateral paralysis of the side of the body opposite to the wound develops late after the symptoms of fever, headache, and convulsive attack, a brain abscess is probably present.

The condition of the wound may help in establishing the diagnosis. Its appearance will usually be altered. The granulations are swollen and the edges of the wound œdematous. Sometimes this œdema affects the surrounding scalp. The pressure of the pus may lift any loose fragments of bone which are lying in the bottom of the wound, or may push a loose splinter above the level of the granulations. A very important symptom is the flow of pus from the fissure in the skull or from between two fragments of the comminuted fracture.

Treatment.—Abscesses in the brain, whether traumatic or not, must be evacuated at any cost, since they cannot remain stationary or disappear by reabsorption or inspissation, but must increase in size, and sooner or later terminate the life of the patient. The evacuation of pus is the surest indication for trephining that can be had. Furthermore, the skull should be opene , or a compound fracture should be explored in those cases in which the diagnosis of abscess is merely probable. Delvoie cites 21 cases in which the skull was trephined for acute cortical abscess, with 15 recoveries; and 33 operations upon chronic deep traumatic cerebral abscesses with 19 recoveries.

If a removal of a portion of the skull which is already somewhat loosened is followed by a stream of pus from the depth of the wound, and the opening is sufficient to afford free drainage, it need not be enlarged. If the flow is obstructed or appears insufficient, the opening in the skull should be enlarged with cutting forceps. If the dura is found

float in the purulent discharge; (2) inflammation accompanied with the foul-smelling pus of necrotic bone; (3) recurring inflammation with acute or subacute attacks separated by long intervals; (4) an inflammation associated with the formation of polypoid-like granulations in the tympanic cavity and in the deeper portion of the external auditory canal; (5) that associated with a fine perforation in the upper portion of the tympanic membrane which affords insufficient drainage.

If the surgeon is able to locate the site of the primary suppuration in the petrous portion of the temporal bone he possesses a valuable guide to the site of the abscess in the brain. Körner has shown that otitic disease of the brain, of the membranes, and of the bloodvessels usually begins at the point in which the original suppuration in the temporal bone first reached the cranial cavity. As the attic of the tympanum (epitympanic recess) is the commonest seat of the carious process, the suppuration spreads from it either through the roof of the tympanic cavity or through the aditus (ad antrum) into the mastoid antrum. In the first case, that is to say, when there are osteitis and necrosis of the tegmen tympani, an epitympanic or extradural abscess will be formed, which will usually be in connection with the tympanic cavity or else a cerebral abscess will be formed which is separated from the tympanic cavity by a much discolored and degenerated dura. Both of these conditions may coexist, that is to say, there may be at the same time an extradural and an intradural abscess. Suppuration in the tympanic cavity which extends to the mastoid antrum leads to the collection of pus in the mastoid cells and possibly to an extension of the suppuration to their outer surface, or an extradural abscess in the lateral sinus between the bloodvessel and the bone. This suppuration may produce thrombosis of the vein or it may extend beneath the tentorium and produce an abscess in the cerebellum. In this manner, therefore, the situation of the suppuration in the ear determines whether an abscess shall be formed in the cerebrum or in the cerebellum. Cerebellar abscess may also follow suppuration in the labyrinth, according to Janses and Koch. Suppuration in the lateral sinus either with or without sinus-thrombosis leads to abscess in the lateral portion of the cerebellum, while suppuration in the labyrinth leads to abscess in the median lobe. Cerebellar abscess follows disease in the right ear oftener than disease in the left, perhaps because the transverse sinus presses closer to the base of the petrous portion on the right side than on the left.

Although it is important to know the seat of the suppuration which has spread to the cranial cavity, this is a point which it is often difficult to determine.

Diagnosis.—The diagnosis of an otitic cerebral abscess, like that of every other cerebral abscess, depends upon etiological factors. Three groups of symptoms are especially worthy of notice: First, the symptoms which are immediately dependent upon the suppuration; second, signs of increased intracranial pressure; and, third, disturbances of cerebral function, or signs of local irritation corresponding to the seat of the abscess. Temperature variations belong to the first group of symptoms. Marked

g in otitic abscess, so that t
00° F.). Macewen looks up
a sign of intracranial bot i
hich are almost always pres
ligestion, lack of appetite, c

Short acute attacks of l
r indicate an extension of
o the mastoid cells rather t

Headache increased tov
are belongs to the second g
invariably caused or incre
of the skull. By repeating
the other side of the skull
as may be made very valu
more-symptom that is al
the food taken, but is bro
nest or a change from a n
ness, sluggish mental proc
of these patients. The
arked. But the most vali
isk on the affected side.
isent to make a diagnosis
wanting when there is a

Furthermore, they ma
mation and sinus-thromb
s on the seat of the ab
are is situated in the temp
physiologists assign to
are of the corresponding
pands with this inasmuc
peech 23 times in 54 cas
of bearing in any case n
pative inflammation of

brens of the temporal re
symptoms, and is there
and paralysis of the fa
of the pupil on the affe
as in the petrous por

as difficult to diagnosti
pause likely to be obscu
affects and epidural sup
- - well-marked local syn
. as which are produ
. \ abscess, even thou
. moved. If present, t
. of the neck. Dizzin

in the beginning of the disease is more likely to be due to an affection of the labyrinth. The diagnosis of cerebellar abscess will usually not be made until the transverse sinus has been exposed and one has an opportunity to observe in which direction the suppuration has extended.

FIG. 85.

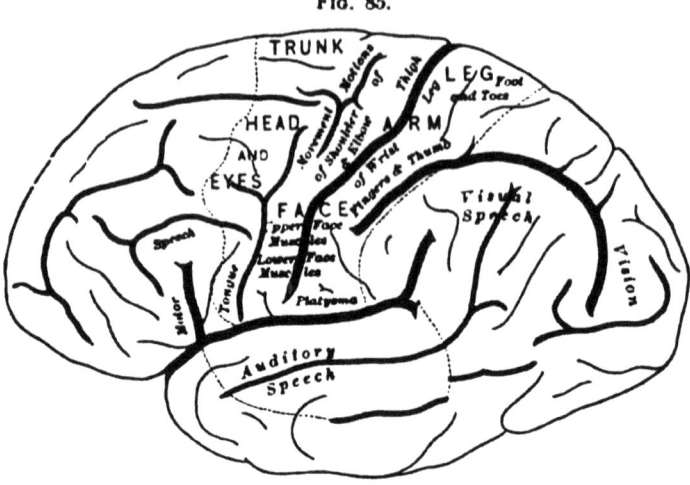

The functional areas of the cerebral cortex. Left hemisphere. (Starr.)

FIG. 86.

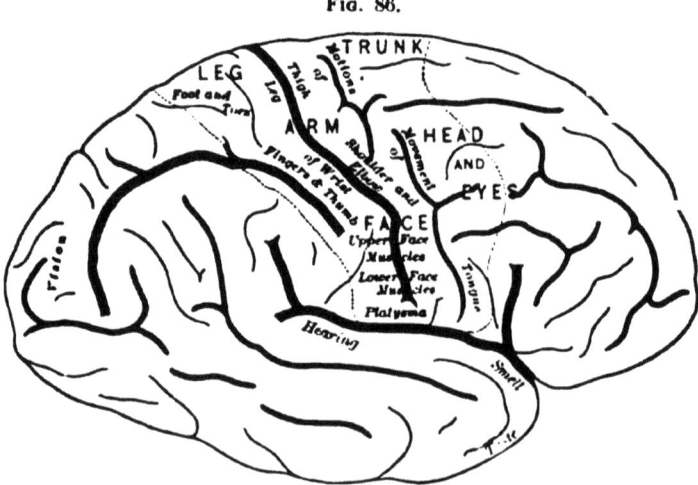

The functional areas of the cerebral cortex. Right hemisphere. (Starr.)

Before making a definite diagnosis of otitic abscess of the temporal lobe or of the cerebellum, one has to differentiate between this and a suppurative meningitis, an infectious sinus-thrombosis, an epidural

external surface of the squamous portion of the temporal is laid bare. In the anterior part of the wound the long root of the zygomatic process is plainly visible, and in the posterior part the junction of the serrated edge of the parietal bone with the squamous and mastoid portions of the temporal. The bone is chiselled or sawed through in a line which is drawn from this junction to the point where the incision began in front. Thus the middle fossa on the inner side of the skull is reached, where the anterosuperior surface of the pyramidal portion meets the squamous portion of the temporal bone at almost right angles. Two short cuts are next made through the squamous portion vertically upward from this horizontal bone incision, in the direction of the boundary-lines of the operative field. A rectangular piece of bone is finally detached by an incision in the squamous portion parallel to the lower one and corresponding nearly to the linea horizontalis supraorbitalis in Figs. 92 and 93, and a view is given into the interior of the skull. This piece of bone should not be replaced, since the operation is performed for a suppurative process. If the dura is lifted up by means of a broad elevator, the upper surface of the petrous portion as far as the prominence made by the superior semicircular canal and the region of the tegmen tympani will be exposed. This region is the usual site of an epidural as well as an intracerebral suppuration. If the surface of brain does not give evidence of the situation of the abscess within it, the third temporal convolution should be incised in its under surface.

This incision may be extended, if necessary, either forward or backward. If it is extended forward, it will expose the region of the Gasserian ganglion; and if it is extended backward, the groove will be exposed in which the transverse sinus lies. In this manner this sinus can be easily and thoroughly exposed. Through the same incision an otitic abscess of the cerebellum may be reached. This is of great advantage, since the diagnosis in such cases lies not only between that of a cerebral abscess and a sinus-thrombosis, but also between suppuration in the cerebrum and suppuration in the cerebellum.

If the abscess is opened and further drainage of the wound is required, the wound may be stretched by opening within it a closed pair of artery-forceps. Drainage may be secured by a tube or short strips of iodoform gauze. The wound should be kept open as long as it suppurates. The walls of the abscess cavity have a tendency to sink together and to close at the surface before healing takes place from the bottom. Often on the third day the drainage of pus through the tube ceases; at other times, on the third day or later, artery-forceps must be thrust into the brain to break up adhesions and to introduce anew the drainage-tube which has fallen out. Prolapse of the brain readily occurs during the period of after-treatment. This is often a sign of a new collection of pus deeper in the brain. If it is dependent on an increase of cerebrospinal fluid in a near-by ventricle, it can be relieved or completely reduced by lumbar puncture.

Cerebral Abscess of Nasal Origin.—Cerebral abscess of nasal origin may follow suppuration in the upper nasal passages and their associated

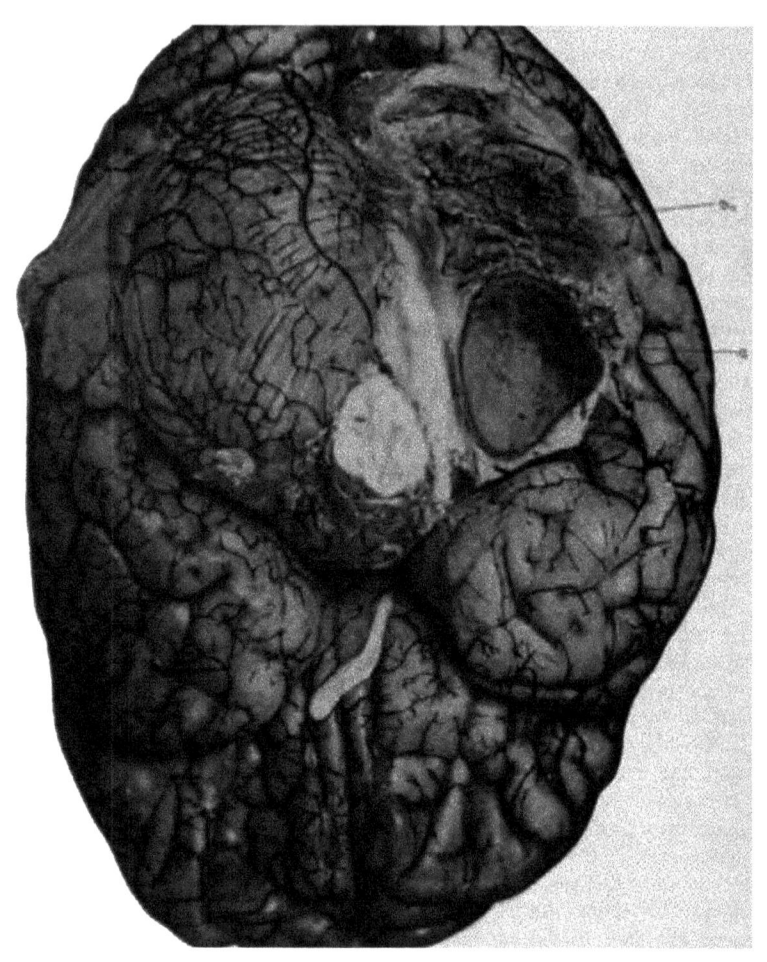

skull due to tuberculosis or syphilis may lead to cerebral abscess. The diagnosis of such an abscess can easily be made if the principles already spoken of are borne in mind.

Metastatic Cerebral Abscess.—In the last few years metastatic cerebral abscess has received considerable attention on account of certain operations which have succeeded in reaching and curing abscesses of this character. A metastatic abscess is secondary to suppurative processes elsewhere in the body, and especially in the thorax. Such abscesses are usually multiple, and this fact gives an unfavorable prognosis, since it is hardly possible to reach and drain all of the abscesses at one time. Martins, who collected reports of 22 metastatic cerebral abscesses, found that in 9 cases a single abscess existed. Gangrene of the lung, putrid bronchitis with ectasia, and long-standing empyema complicated with fistulæ, are the general sources of these abscesses. They are started by emboli, which are more likely to enter the left carotid than the right on account of its relation to the aorta. From this vessel they pass easily to the artery which lies in the fossa of Sylvius, just as non-infective emboli do. Eight of the 9 solitary abscesses mentioned by Martins were so situated. The branches to the ganglia at the base of the brain spring from this vessel at right angles, a position not favorable for the arrest of emboli, while the five terminal branches which go to the cortex are given off at an acute angle. It follows, therefore, that particles floating in the blood are more likely to pass into the terminal branches. If the abscess is a single one, it should therefore be looked for in this locality. If a great many abscesses coexist, of which there may perhaps be hundreds, they will be found in all portions of the brain. If the abscess is situated in the motor region of the cortex, there will be convulsions and paralysis of the opposite side of the body, which may serve for an exact localization of the abscess. Under such circumstances the operator may be able to expose and drain the abscess.

The author operated on such a case recently, in which an abscess was localized and opened, although the patient survived only a few hours.

THROMBOSIS OF THE INTRACRANIAL BLOOD-SINUSES.

By Dr. SCHLATTER.

Two very different kinds of thrombosis are recognized: primary, marasmic thrombosis, and secondary, infectious or inflammatory thrombosis.

Primary or Marasmic Sinus-thrombosis.—This condition will be only briefly described here, as surgically it possesses little interest. It is much rarer than the second form, or inflammatory thrombosis, and is most frequently situated in the longitudinal sinus. It has been observed in weak individuals and in those run down as the result of exhausting diseases, such as typhoid, carcinoma, pulmonary tuberculosis, particularly in childhood and old age.

and pharyngeal cavities. Thus anthrax of the lips, the mouth, the nasal and orbital cavities, periostitis of the jaw from caries of the teeth, inflammation of the tonsils, and retropharyngeal abscess have been described as etiological factors. But the most important starting point—according to Körner in nearly two-thirds of the cases of sinus-phlebitis—is the ear. Regarding the frequency of otitic cerebral diseases in general, the statistics of Pitt show that in 9000 successive autopsies in Guy's Hospital (in the years 1869–1888) there were 57 deaths from ear suppuration, or 1 in every 158 autopsies. Of these, 22 were cases of otitic sinus disease, 18 were cases of otitic cerebral abscess, and 15 were cases of pure otitic meningitis. Hessler has calculated the proportion of sinus-phlebitis and pyæmia to the number of cases of disease of the ear, with the following results: in 81,648 cases of disease of the ear, death took place 116 times as the result of complicating intracranial disease, according to the following table:

40 deaths	(34.5 per cent.)	. .	from meningitis.
28 "	(24.1 " ")	. :	" cerebral abscess.
48 "	(41.4 " ")	.	" sinus-phlebitis and pyæmia.

The difference in sex is rather noticeable as predisposing to this disease. The male sex is affected more than six times as frequently as the female by these complications of suppuration.

Like all otogenic cerebral diseases, sinus-phlebitis occurs more frequently on the right side than on the left. The right sigmoid fossa is generally broader and deeper; it also extends further out and forward than that of the opposite side. The greater flow of blood from the brain through the right sinus is looked upon as the cause of this condition, the longitudinal sinus generally emptying into the right transverse sinus. The emptying of the longitudinal sinus on the right side is again explained by the shorter and straighter course on the right side for the blood flowing through the sinus to the heart. The longitudinal sinus finds an easier outlet therefore on the right side.

The transverse sinus and the bulb of the jugular vein, like the sigmoid sinus, lie somewhat deeper in the bone on the right side than on the left for the same reasons.

In spite of an article questioning the accuracy of his investigations, Körner remains firm in his opinion that in brachycephalitics the danger of extension of suppuration from the temporal bone to the cranial contents is greater than in dolichocephalitics, because in the former the roof of the tympanic cavity is not only thinner and frequently shows openings, but the sigmoid fossa also penetrates more deeply into the bone than in the latter. According to Politzer and Hartman, small solid mastoid processes generally show a deep sigmoid fossa.

Starting at the primary focus of inflammation, development of sinus-thrombosis may proceed in two ways: either inflammation extends by continuity to the sinus and affects the wall of the latter, in consequence of which the blood within the sinus coagulates and there is formed a thrombus firmly attached to the wall—this mode of infection being called *thrombophlebitis;* or a vein within the diseased focus beco thrombosed, and this infectious thrombus extends to the sinus (o *phlebitis*). The first manner of extension of infection is much c frequent, particularly in otitic sinus thrombosis.

The site of the original disease is generally located in the ma: process and consists of a chronic suppuration. In nearly all case suppuration of the ear either pneumococci or streptococci, or more n staphylococci have been found. The primary disease is rarely a or accompanied by serous exudation. Inflammation progresses as as the sigmoid fossa, where direct contact between the diseased l and the sinus is established. Frequently openings in the bone facil: the spread of the suppuration. At times granulations shoot out fron wall of the sinus and the adjacent dura which may hinder the progre inflammation. Frequently extradural abscesses are formed. If pur infiltration and softening of the wall of the sinus increase, perforation t place. This may vary in size. Hemorrhage from the sinus is unu because as soon as the walls are attacked by a purulent process and endothelium is destroyed the contained blood coagulates. In a s time, however, as a result of the infectious process, purulent softe develops in the central portions of the thrombus. In the beginning outer layers of the thrombus may still be firmly adherent to the wall of the sinus; later the thrombus undergoes suppuration and tl creamy pus fills the sinus. Ichorous decomposition of the thrombus been observed, particularly in cholesteatoma of the middle ear. W the central portion of the thrombus undergoes purulent decomposi the upper and lower ends of the thrombus may form plugs tightly clo off the sinus. Hessler collected 15 cases in which there was almost obliteration of the sinus through the organization of a thrombus. rule, however, thrombosis and inflammation proceed in both direct with and against the blood-current.

The disease begins usually in the sigmoid sinus, owing to the proximity of the latter to the cavities of the middle ear; the thron frequently extends into the lateral sinus, which empties its blood the sigmoid sinus (rarely it extends as far as the longitudinal sinu: through the superior petrosal sinus forward to the cavernous sinu: possibly as far as the ophthalmic veins. At times primary throml occurs in the superior petrosal sinus and advances from this point t sigmoid sinus.

Not infrequently infections thrombosis proceeds with the blood-str as far as the internal jugular vein. Generally this affects only the u third; however, a thrombus may extend as far as the superior venn c The further embolic extension of infectious masses through the circ tion will be found discussed in the following section on symptomatol

Symptoms.—There are no distinct pathognomonic symptoms of in tions sinus-thrombosis. The general manifestations are those of pyæ in general. The local manifestations are the result of disturbed ci lation. Within the skull there is disturbance of the brain function, side the skull œdema. In many cases, however, these signs are suffici to make a diagnosis of thrombosis of an intracranial blood-sinus with some degree of positiveness.

Certain general manifestations are met with in all cases of infections thrombosis. The earliest of these is headache. This may be diffuse or limited to the region of the affected sinus. Very frequently vomiting and dizziness follow. The rapidly increasing body temperature shows marked remissions. In a few hours the temperature rises to 104° and 106° F., and almost immediately this is followed by a fall, sometimes to subnormal. The fall in temperature is usually accompanied by profuse perspiration. In rare cases, particularly in children, the fever has been found continuous and not remittent. Repeated chills, a further characteristic sign of pyæmia, are an important symptom. Either the first chill occurs at the same time as the first symptoms of cerebral irritation, such as headache, dizziness or vomiting; or, as is more frequently the case, one, two, or more days later. In most cases two to six chills have been observed. The pulse is subject to the same variations as the temperature. At the time of the chill it may exceed 100, reaching 120 to 140.

Metastatic abscess-formation causes slighter remissions of pulse and temperature. The tongue is very much coated and dry, particularly in the later stages; there is a tendency to diarrhœa, especially in chronic cases.

Jaundice is an accompanying symptom frequently observed, occurring in pure sinus-phlebitis three times as frequently as in the complicated form. In all cases it was accounted for by an enlargement of the liver, so that it must be considered of hepatogenous and not hæmatogenous origin. Swelling of the spleen is always found.

In pure sinus-phlebitis convulsions rarely occur. In the complicated form they occur three times as frequently, and most frequently when complicated by cerebral abscess. In marked contradistinction to cerebral abscess, the activity of the brain is not impaired in uncomplicated infectious thrombosis, the intelligence of the patient being retained almost to the end.

If fragments of necrotic thrombi enter the circulation, they may be scattered to all the different organs as emboli and there set up metastases. The lungs are most frequently affected, so much so that a pulmonary type of the disease has been suggested. The emboli are washed out of the affected sinuses, or even from the internal jugular vein, through the superior vena cava into the right heart, and from here they enter the pulmonary artery to be caught in the capillary network of the latter. Even with complete closure of the central end of the transverse sinus or the internal jugular vein by a closely fitting thrombus, in rare cases the formation of metastases may take place, emboli being carried through the sinuses of the healthy side from the peripheral end of the affected blood-channel. In case of the sinus transversus, for example, they may be carried through the superior and inferior petrosal sinus, and then through the cavernous sinus and sinus of Ridley, lying close to the sella turcica, into the venous system of the opposite side.

monary vessels. Not all pulmonary emboli are infectious. If pathogenic germs are absent, the only result may be the production of an infarction. As a rule, however, metastatic infarctions suppurate and become putrid and ichorous, with the production of pulmonary abscess or gangrene. In the majority of cases both lungs are affected by multiple, frequently innumerable metastases, particularly in the lower portions. Solitary abscesses are rarely found. Small disseminated abscesses are not easily discovered. Frequently the characteristic purulent sputum is absent. Should a metastatic pulmonary abscess break through into the pleura, a pyopneumothorax results, which may be the first evidence of a metastasis of the lungs. If, however, the abscess in the lung undergo decomposition, the "prune-juice" sputum soon appears; here and there coarse râles can be heard, which are soon followed by moist râles over large areas of the lungs. As a result of being mixed with pus, the sputum later assumes a brownish-gray color and disseminates a fetid odor which frequently renders isolation of the patient necessary.

What a favorite site for metastases the lungs may be, is shown by the statistics of Hessler, according to which in 130 cases of sinus-phlebitis with metastases the lungs were found unaffected only 14 times.

In rare cases small emboli may pass relatively wide pulmonary capillaries, and after being washed through the lungs be scattered throughout the other organs of the body. Thus metastases have been observed in the joints, synovial sacs, muscles, kidneys, spleen, and liver, even in the eye, and in one case in the aryepiglottic fold.

In otogenic sinus-thrombosis, metastatic abscesses have been observed even in the brain. In literature there are to be found 9 pure cases of this kind in which extension of suppuration from the petrous portion to the brain can be positively excluded. Even tuberculosis of the petrous portion may lead to a general infection of the organism by way of a sinus-phlebitis, producing metastases.

. **Course.**—This course of the disease, the so-called *pulmonary type*, must be retained as the principal type of thrombotic disease of the cerebral blood-channels. Besides this, there have been set up an abdominal or typhoid type and a meningeal type of the disease; both rarely occur alone, but generally combined with the pulmonary type or with each other.

ABDOMINAL TYPE.—If toxæmia is manifested more in the abdominal organs, a typhoid-like complex of symptoms is developed. The high temperatures do not show such marked remissions. Besides enlargement of the spleen and at times a roseola-like exanthem of the skin, the abdomen is tympanitic and painful; diarrhœa is present and frequently "pea-soup" stools.

MENINGEAL TYPE.—At times meningitis, originating in an infectious thrombus or developing directly from the primary focus of disease, masks or complicates the symptoms of sinus-thrombosis and leads to a rapid fatal termination.

Following this preliminary description of the clinical picture, the *external evidences of thrombosis* of the different sinuses will be discussed in the following sections.

Zanfal discovered another sign in the cadaver that may be of value in the diagnosis of thrombosis of the sigmoid sinus—a unilateral dilatation of the mastoid vein to the size of the jugular vein of the same side.

The nerves which leave the skull with the sigmoid sinus through the jugular foramen are the *vagus, spinal accessory*, and *glossopharyngeal*. The manifestations of compression and inflammation of the vagus that have been observed are hoarseness, dyspnœa, slowing of the pulse, and even death through respiratory paralysis. Spasms have been produced in the distribution of the spinal accessory (sternocleidomastoid and trapezius muscles). In one case dysphagia occurred through disease of the glossopharyngeal nerve; in another there was in all probability paralysis of the palatal muscles. Even the hypoglossal nerve, which emerges through the anterior condyloid foramen, has been affected by inflammation and become paralyzed.

Other accompanying manifestations, which are, however, not characteristic of sinus-thrombosis, may be *choked disk* and *optic neuritis*, also nystagmus. All these symptoms, even if only partially present, may facilitate the diagnosis of thrombophlebitis of the sigmoid sinus. Unfortunately they do not often occur, even in typical cases of the disease, and it is a fact which should be borne in mind that a thrombus of the sigmoid sinus may be present without being accompanied by any of these outward manifestations.

Thrombosis of one of the two petrosal sinuses causes no local manifestations. In most cases it coexists with inflammation of the sigmoid sinus, the cavernous sinus, or the bulb of the jugular vein, which may on their part manifest symptoms valuable in the diagnosis of the site of the disease.

Thrombosis of the superior longitudinal sinus is usually of marasmic origin. In rare cases violence, with comminution of the bones of the cranial vault or inflammatory processes in the scalp, as, for example, erysipelas, or purulent processes in the adjacent bone itself, may set up a phlebitis of the superficial veins. There are no pathognomonic symptoms of thrombosis of the longitudinal sinus. Convulsions and bleeding from the nose, caused by stasis in the superior cerebral veins and the veins of the foramen cæcum, have been considered characteristic of this form of sinus-thrombosis. Hessler did not find bleeding from the nose or convulsions mentioned in one case of otogenous thrombophlebitis of the superior longitudinal sinus. Œdema of the scalp and marked dilatation of the veins of the parietal, occipital, and at times the frontal region are supposed to be usual accompanying manifestations.

Isolated thrombosis of the cavernous sinus rarely occurs; usually it has extended from the sigmoid sinus, or a thrombus in one of the ophthalmic veins may be the starting point. A large number of symptoms have been classed as important signs of disease of the cavernous sinus. In the first place, one must remember that in more than half the cases the thrombus, formed in the sinus of one side, extends through the sinus of Ridley to the sinus of the opposite side. Manifestations may therefore occur on both sides; finally, the manifestations may be more marked on the

Further, manifestations of stasis in the region of the ophthalmic vein and injury of the nerves near the cavernous sinus.

The most important general symptoms are pyæmic fever with marked remissions and chills, enlargement of the spleen, and embolic metastases in the lungs, more rarely in the large glandular organs, in the brain, in the joints and muscles. Should all these manifestations occur in a patient suffering from acute middle-ear suppuration, a positive diagnosis can easily be made. The history and result of the aural examination will establish the local and etiological connection. Frequently, however, suppuration of the middle ear, having run a benign course for some time, escapes notice or its etiological bearing on other causal factors is not considered. If, then, the above-mentioned complex of symptoms be not complete or not well marked, if the typical remissions of fever and symptoms of metastases are absent, the diagnosis will be difficult. A confusion with typhoid fever, miliary tuberculosis, acute septic endocarditis, and malaria is very apt to occur.

One should not forget that cerebral abscess may have the same origin as sinus-thrombosis and may frequently occur at the same time as the latter. In most cases cerebral abscess develops later than sinus-thrombosis; at times the formation of an abscess takes place earlier. The manifestations of thrombosis generally mask the symptoms of abscess. The symptoms accompanying abscess may, however, mask the symptoms of infectious sinus-thrombosis. If in case of abscess there are no cerebral symptoms which would permit of a conclusion as to the site of the disease in some portion of the brain, the diagnosis of complicating sinus-thrombosis is generally impossible. If both diseases are diagnosticated at the same time, sinus-thrombosis must be considered the more important disease and the one first to demand interference. Operating for abscess alone could not bring about recovery.

The abdominal type of infectious sinus-thrombosis, particularly where cases are late in coming under observation, may easily lead to confusion with typhoid fever (typhus abdominalis). Otorrhœa may escape notice or be taken for an incidental complication. Unless they should have developed as a result of typhoid fever, middle-ear suppuration and the local symptoms are of great significance in the differential diagnosis. Where roseola is present, the exanthem of infectious thrombosis is characterized by the fact that it is not raised above the level of the skin, does not disappear on pressure, and does not occur in successive crops.

In addition, the Widal serum reaction characteristic of typhoid fever (typhus abdominalis), possibly also the examination of the stools for typhoid bacilli, would render a positive differential diagnosis possible.

The differential diagnosis between sinus-thrombosis and miliary tuberculosis may be difficult. In both diseases there are high irregular fever, chills, disturbance of consciousness, and in case cerebral or cranial nerve symptoms develop, a mistake is very possible. The discovery of tubercles of the choroid, as well as the bacteriological examination of the blood, would determine the diagnosis. In comparing the symptoms of both diseases the following characteristics must be considered important in

the differential diagnosis: for pyæmia, the chills, followedly
tion, and the metastases; for miliary tuberculosis, the high
and rapid respiration, with almost negative findings in the
Acute septic endocarditis may present a similar picture in
sinus-thrombosis. The manifestations are similarly stormy in
with chills, high temperatures, as well as rapid, marked remis
embolic manifestations are also diagnostically significant of a
carditis. The differential diagnosis may be very difficult if,
hand, there is an absence of clinical symptoms referable to
and, on the other hand, absence of local manifestations of si
bosis.

In malarial regions the pyæmic manifestations of sinus-
might during the first week render a mistake with this diseas
Irregularity of the chills would speak for pyæmia, while the
would offer positive evidence. The discovery of malaria pl
the blood and the effect of quinine would render the diagnosis
easy.

It is a proved fact that *infectious sinus-thrombosis* left unt
almost always take a fatal course, either through the gener
intoxication or the development of metastases or complicating
and cerebral abscess; in rare cases through hemorrhage from
through vagus paralysis.

Prognosis.—The duration of the disease depends entirely
severity of the infection and its complications. The averag
is from two to six weeks, but the disease may last for eight wee
longer. Cases are found, however, in literature that were
diagnosticated as sinus-thrombosis with general pyæmic man
and even with metastases of the lungs, which recovered spoi
The virulence of the infectious germs must have been so din
these cases and the inflammatory process progressed so slo
formative process in the thrombus could bring about occlusion
and finally lead to its obliteration. At no time, however, shou
cration of such an exceptionally favorable course prevent the
of energetic therapeutic measures.

The ophthalmoscopic findings are of little value in the progn
so are the course of the temperature and the state of con
The prognosis seems to be less favorable in proportion to
with which the temperature-curve loses its remissions and be
tened, and to the degree that consciousness is disturbed.

The prognosis depends largely upon the time that the di
made. The increasing certainty with which the diagnosis ca
permits of earlier operative treatment, and at the same time ai
ment in the results of treatment. Sinus-phlebitis must be opei
as soon as it is recognized. General meningitis, which frequen
panics sinus-phlebitis, is the only contraindication for surg
ference that can be considered. All other complicating second
tions, such as cerebral abscess, metastases in the lungs, py
thorax, and embolism of other organs, may considerably ob

prognosis; but in all these affections recovery is not excluded if treatment is instituted at the proper time.

Treatment.—Through the valuable services of Zanfal, surgeons are no longer helpless in treating sinus-thrombosis. In the year 1880, supported by clinical experience and the results obtained at autopsies, he showed that in sinus-phlebitis not only trephining of the mastoid process, but also ligation of the jugular vein, and possibly opening a portion of the sinus itself, might be beneficial. In 1884 he reported a case in which, after trephining the mastoid process, he irrigated and drained the sigmoid sinus, which had opened spontaneously as the result of necrosis. Unfortunately death took place as the result of metastases in the lungs. At that time Zanfal proposed his "ideal plan." Trephining of the mastoid process should first be carried out, and from this point the sinus exposed. If the sinus is closed at the jugular foramen by a firm thrombus, ligation of the jugular is not necessary; if this is not the case, the jugular should be ligated; and if the vein itself is occluded by thromboses, the ligature should be applied below the diseased portion. The thrombosed jugular vein should be opened above the ligature and cleansed of all infectious masses by disinfecting injections, the fluid flowing out through the trephine-opening. Zanfal recommended ligation of the jugular as the most effective protection against the danger of metastases.

Similar proposals were made by Horsley in the year 1886. The operation was carried out for the first time in 1888 by Lane. The necrotic thrombosed sinus was first opened in both directions, and following this the jugular was ligated. The patient was discharged cured.

In the year 1896 Hessler had collected 88 cases of otogenous sinus-phlebitis with direct treatment of the sinus and of the jugular vein. The lateral sinus was incised 76 times and the jugular tied 32 times. The results were 52 recoveries (59.1 per cent.) and 36 deaths (40.9 per cent.). Still more brilliant results are shown by the statistics of Macewen, who reports a fatal termination in only 8 cases out of 28 cases operated on.

For the operative treatment of infectious thrombosis of the sigmoid sinus, which must be considered first, three methods have been proposed. They are as follows: opening and evacuation of the sigmoid sinus alone; opening and evacuation of the sigmoid sinus and ligation of the jugular vein; ligation of the jugular vein alone to prevent absorption of parts of a thrombus.

The last method, ligation of the jugular vein alone, must be considered a therapeutic error, as it is contrary to the most elementary surgical rule which requires direct treatment of the source of infection itself. Of what use will be ligation of a drainage-channel if the primary focus threatens the organism in various other ways? In the first place, the pus focus must be removed from the brain-sinus. *Opening and evacuation of the sigmoid sinus is necessary in all cases.*

Operation.—Where sinus-thrombosis is suspected, exposure of the sinus had best follow an empyema operation of the mastoid process, or, generally speaking, the removal of the primary disease in the temporal bone. If the bone cavity in the mastoid process is exposed posteriorly, the sinus can easily be reached. The portion of bone between the sinus and antrum can readily be removed with a chisel mallet or bone-forceps. The use of the chisel should be avoided whenever possible. The blows with the mallet cause very perceptible concussion, with the danger that thrombophlebitic masses may be detached. An excellent instrument with which to open the mastoid process and the sigmoid fossa is Doyen's spherical burr. Its use considerably facilitates this operation.

According to Macewen, an incision is carried over the mastoid process about 6 mm. in front of its posterior border, extending from the posterior root of the zygomatic process nearly to the tip of the mastoid process. The soft parts and periosteum are reflected with an elevator. At the upper end of the incision the parieto-squamomastoid suture becomes visible; it is the most inferior point in the parietal notch of the temporal bone and can easily be found. A line drawn from this point to the tip of the mastoid process marks the course of the sigmoid sinus. A trephine opening which touches this line with its posterior border and which is at a level with the external auditory meatus will expose that portion of the sigmoid sinus which is most frequently affected. (The asterion, the posterior end of the above-mentioned suture, corresponds to the transition of the lateral sinus into the sigmoid sinus.)

The sinus must be exposed sufficiently to ascertain its condition and to determine the nature of further operative steps necessary. If the thrombus is not softened, the wall of the sinus may have preserved normal appearance. By *palpation of the sinus* evidence of thrombus of its contents should be sought for. If the results obtained by this method of examination are uncertain, it is best to make use of the more certain aid to diagnosis—*puncture of the sinus.* If this shows fluid blood, thrombosis is excluded; if puncture is negative, it is evidence of occlusion of the vein.

Does simple thrombosis indicate evacuation of a blood-sinus? The theoretical answer to this question varies. As spontaneous recovery from simple sinus-thrombosis has been observed, there is no imperative reason for immediate interference. One may wait until later control punctures of the sinus show a purulent softening of the thrombus. In practice this decision is in most cases more simple. Generally, if one does not find pus, there will at least be inflammatory changes in the walls of the vessels. Purulent softening will almost positively be present there. Puncture through an inflamed vessel wall may have caused the infection. Thus in most cases immediate evacuation of the sinus is indicated.

For the removal of a decomposing thrombus, the sinus should be freely exposed for at least 2 cm. in a vertical direction. The wall of the sinus is divided centrally and peripherally as far as is necessary for the evacuation of the decomposing contents. A small sharp spoon is the most convenient instrument for the removal of the products of decomposition. A firm thrombus can frequently be removed with forceps.

If during evacuation hemorrhage takes place from the distal end, it should be controlled by tamponing with iodoform gauze. If there is no occluding thrombus on the proximal side, blood will flow from the proximal end when the jugular vein is compressed in the neck below its junction with the common facial and lingual veins. If hemorrhage does not take place, there is closure by a thrombus. Such thrombi should be left undisturbed; they are a protection against the entrance of decomposed particles of thrombi into the circulation.

In these simple cases of thrombosis of the sigmoid sinus it is difficult to believe in the necessity of immediate ligation of the jugular vein, and the author is of the opinion that if thrombosis is limited to the sigmoid sinus, only the sigmoid sinus should be operated upon.

If, however, the central end of the sigmoid sinus is not firmly closed by a thrombus, or if during the further course chills and fever lead to the assumption of a subsequent decomposition of the central thrombus, ligation of the internal jugular vein is indicated. Only after such ligation of the jugular vein, which prevents embolism, should the remainder of the focus in the sigmoid sinus be evacuated.

Immediate ligation of the jugular vein is still a disputed point in the operative treatment of infectious sinus-thrombosis. A. af Forselles considers ligation of the jugular vein justifiable in all cases, and is of the opinion that even if in two-thirds of the cases the vessel was opened unnecessarily it would be better than omitting to do so in one-third of those cases in which opening of the vessel is absolutely indicated. Körner also considers it advisable in case of a decomposed thrombus to ligate the internal jugular below the thrombus before undertaking further manipulation.

A critical discussion of the value of ligation of the jugular vein should not leave out of consideration the fact that ligation of the jugular on one side does not afford absolute protection against embolism—*i. e.*, that although the jugular vein is the principal channel, it is not the only vein which carries blood from the sigmoid sinus to the heart. Infectious masses may be transported not only through the anterior and posterior condyloid emissary veins and the occipital sinus, but also through the drainage system of the opposite jugular vein. Thrombosis may extend to the opposite side, either posteriorly through the torcular Herophili or anteriorly through the circular sinus of Ridley which encircles the hypophysis. The possibility of infectious masses being transported by other drainage-channels has been expressed in figures by Hessler. In 11 cases (21 per cent.) metastases subsequently occurred in spite of immediate ligation of the jugular vein.

Regarding the practicability of combined ligation of the jugular vein, it is impossible to judge one way or the other. It depends entirely upon the individual case, upon the manner, the location and the progress of the inflammatory destructive process downward. If the infectious thrombus has become decomposed to such a degree on the proximal

side that the products of decomposition cannot be sufficiently
through the site of opening in the sigmoid sinus, there is ar
indication to provide means of drainage at a more central sit
is impossible to locate all these sites for drainage, it is impe:
close the principal highway which is accessible to ligation. I
same time there are signs of accompanying disease of the upper
of the jugular, ligation of the jugular is **absolutely** necessa
account of the infiltration in the region of **the neck, its** execut
in these very cases be very difficult, if not **impossible.** It nec
mentioned that the ligature must always be applied below the th
Even in the lower third of the neck ligation of the common jugu
is possible without occasioning any disturbance of circulation.

In general it can be said that in the majority of cases evacu
the upper two-thirds of the sigmoid sinus is sufficient to prevent i
of the entire organism.

A few brief remarks in regard to the method of operation in
of the jugular vein may be appropriate here. Unless one is ob
account of thrombosis to go still lower, ligation is best perfo
the level of the hyoid bone or from 1 to 2 cm. higher. Divi
vein between two ligatures is preferable to a single ligature, as it
of a more exact inspection of the interior of the vessel, and also
tion of the peripheral portion of the jugular vein if this shoul
necessary. The skin-incision should run along the anterior b
the sternocleidomastoid muscle. After dividing the platysma
and retracting the sternomastoid outward, the large vessels of t
will be seen beneath the deep layer of the fascia of the necl
jugular vein lies to the outer side of the pulsating carotid.

The treatment of thrombophlebitis of the petrosal sinus ι
cavernous sinus does not require lengthy discussion. Disease:
petrosal sinus are usually inflammatory processes that have e
from the sigmoid sinus and internal jugular vein; their treatme
cides therefore with that of the large drainage-channels.

The superior petrosal sinus extends from the cavernous sinu
point where the lateral sinus merges into the sigmoid sinus. Tl
site is marked on the surface of the skull by the asterion (see ο|
for exposing the sigmoid sinus). The sinus should be opened
point in case there are indications for the evacuation of a th
extending into the superior petrosal sinus from the sigmoid sinu

The cavernous sinus lying at the side of the sella turcica is
accessible to operative interference. In addition, thrombosis is
ally bilateral. The unfavorable and dangerous situation of thi
and the slight prospect of recovery in unilateral operation shoul
one from such a rash procedure, especially so as the operatiοr
rarely be carried out on the strength of a positive diagnosis. O
of the cavernous has been performed only once so far (v. Birch

The section on the treatment of infectious sinus-thrombosis cai
closed without a brief consideration of *prophylaxis.* The clinical
is developed from a primary focus of inflammation. Its seriou·

nosis urgently demands conscientious disinfection of wounds situated within the possible region of infection and especially the careful treatment of middle-ear inflammations.

EPILEPSY FOLLOWING HEAD INJURIES, AND THE SURGICAL TREATMENT OF EPILEPSY.

By Prof. Dr. von Bergmann.

The occurrence of *epilepsy following cranial* injury has been positively confirmed by a large number of cases. In 783 cases of epilepsy, Echeverria found traumatic origin 63 times, and of 167 cases of cranial injury during the American Civil War in men who were previously sound, the pension rolls show 23, or 13.7 per cent., epileptics. Twenty-five cases of traumatic epilepsy were noted in the German Sanitary Reports for 1870–'71 as occurring among 571 cases of shot injuries of the cranial bones, with recovery. This would show only 4.3 per cent. If to these are added 128 cases affected by epileptiform conditions, such as periodic attacks of dizziness, unconsciousness, trembling, and palpitation of the heart, following injuries of the vault, it would bring the number up to 26.7 per cent.

Cases of epilepsy following cranial injuries may be divided into three categories. To the first belong those cases in which a peripheral nerve lesion in the soft coverings, usually a scar in the latter, becomes the point of origin of an epileptic attack. To the second belong changes in the bones or dura, as, for example, hyperostosis at the site of a contusion or fracture of the skull or firm adhesions between the dura and bone. The third category includes actual brain injuries which are followed sooner or later by epilepsy; they always affect the cortex.

In order to form a conception as to the manner in which lesions of the soft parts, bones, and cerebral cortex bring about epilepsy, it is essential to keep in mind the present teachings in regard to epilepsy. These assume a certain change, a property of the brain, which causes the habitual recurrence of convulsions. Whether this irritable state is called "spasmophilia" according to Féré, or "convulsible brain" according to Unverricht, nothing is known regarding the gross or microscopical anatomical condition. At the same time it must be considered, for the causes of its occurrence and development are known. In the first place, there is heredity, which predominates the entire etiology of epilepsy, whether the victims are descendants of individuals affected with the same or different nervous diseases. Among the latter must be included dipsomania. The question has frequently been brought up whether besides this predisposition other diseases could bring about an epileptic tendency, or whether infectious diseases and intoxications, terror, and cranial injuries were not simply incidental causes in the occurrence of epilepsy in those predisposed, and whether they would not prove ineffectual in those not predisposed. Even careful investigation

Seeligmüller. The same curative effect was produced by excision of neuromata in cases in which epileptic seizures took place when these tumors were manipulated or in which they had been the point of origin of an aura. In the same way reflex epilepsy has not infrequently been cured by the extraction of foreign bodies, from the ear, for example, and by the successful treatment of mucous membrane affections of the nose, pharynx, and larynx, provided the attacks had resulted from such affections. The number of histories of such operations is large, and to these must be added circumcisions, clitoridectomies, castrations, etc. It is a question, however, to the author's mind, whether recovery following removal of the cause of such attacks is permanent. Failure is certainly not infrequent, an experience explained by the behavior of the brain as a whole. The latter must at the time of the attack necessarily suffer from an epileptic change, this change being inherited or acquired at the time of the first attack. If there is reason to exclude heredity, and consequently to assume that the condition is acquired, the latter may be permanent or transitory; in fact, it may disappear with cessation of the attack. Assuming the latter, the brain would remain sound, provided no further attacks followed. Everything depends upon whether the dreaded fresh attack sets in or remains absent. As the scar was the point of origin of the first attack, it might also become the starting point of a second and of all subsequent attacks, until finally the convulsive condition of the brain would become changed from a transitory to a permanent one. Excision of the scar before this condition has developed may prevent fresh and possibly serious attacks, and in this way preserve the brain in a sound condition. With excision of the scar the cause of the epileptic attacks would be removed. On the other hand, the operation would be ineffectual if carried out at a time when the supposed epileptic change had become permanent. The attacks are then repeated through slight, hardly recognizable causes, or apparently without cause. These are the teachings of Féré, Jolly, and Unverricht.

This conception, which ascribes so much to the unknown epileptic changes and so little to the exciting local causes, diminishes very much the hope of surgically removing the causative factor. All will depend upon the development and the degree of the disease of the brain. If the brain was altered from the beginning, a single attack will suffice to awaken the slumbering disease and to cause it to continue unabated. If the brain is sound and capable of offering resistance at the onset of the disease, many attacks, repeated in the course of years, may be required to produce a permanent condition in which the slightest degree of irritation travelling along paths that have gradually become more beaten, to use a metaphor of Unverricht, leads to a state in which seizure follows seizure. The tendency to convulsions will then be fixed.

Scars of the scalp have more frequently caused epilepsy than scars of the trunk and of the extremities. As a rule these scars were very painful, or they were the seat of neuralgic attacks before convulsions occurred. The author has dissected out an old sensitive scar, manipulation of which *during* examination was followed by an epileptic attack, and showed improvement the author cannot accept, for variations between periods of improvement and relapse—*i. e.*, times with frequent and violent convulsions and times with infrequent and slight attacks—occur in the life of every epileptic individual.

Epilepsy originating in a certain focus of the cerebral cortex, *so-called cortical epilepsy*, was considered the most promising field for operative treatment, not only because of the characteristic change in the respective portion of the cortex (sclerotic or cystic scar), but also because at that time, when operations were beginning to be more frequently performed, the significance of the cerebral cortex in the occurrence of all forms of epilepsy, including non-traumatic—that is, general epilepsy—was brought forward by Unverricht and by the observations and experiments of his pupils. Upon applying a strictly localized stimulus to a certain part of the motor region in experiments on animals, the convulsion which begins in the muscles innervated by this part travels in a definite and always typical manner; "like a tornado it rushes over the entire nervous system." Whenever Unverricht resected portions of the motor area of the cortex in his stimulation experiments, the character of the progress of the convulsion became changed. The groups of muscles whose centres had been removed no longer participated in the convulsions. At that time Horsley resected diseased portions of the brain at the site of old cortical wounds on account of epilepsy (1886), and urged for the cure of this form of epilepsy the removal of the cortical centre, the irritation of which formed the point of origin of the attack, even if it was not the seat of visible change. The author welcomed the proposal with great hopes, and on February 2, 1887, he extirpated the centre for the extensors of the hand in a case of traumatic epilepsy. On April 23, of the same year, Horsley excised the centre for the facial nerve in a case of non-traumatic Jacksonian epilepsy. Since then this extirpation has frequently been repeated, but by no operator with such brilliant results as Braun.

A man, twenty-four years old, had suffered severe injury on the right side of the vault of the skull when twelve years of age. This led to the development of epileptic convulsions four years later. The latter always began in the thumb of the left hand. The convulsions were associated with loss of consciousness and post-epileptic paralysis. At the same time the right half of the skull had become tender; particularly upon pressure, violent headaches occurred. Upon opening the skull at the point of most intense pain a cyst was found at the surface of the brain. This was emptied, as a result of which the headaches ceased; not so, however, the epileptic convulsions. On a second operation, which consisted in the removal of the thickened cranial vault over the centre for the movements of the upper extremity, the latter having been determined by faradic stimulation, the convulsions did not cease; on the contrary, they increased in violence. Only on a third operation, when the centre for the movements of the left hand were extirpated, did the convulsions cease, and that permanently (observation for six years).

reports on 19 cases, Braun the same number (including
of extirpation of the motor centre in the cerebr
to the limb in which the convulsive movemen
cases the operation had no influence on the cor
did not prevent their recurrence; in 3 cases the
was too short, so that there remain 6 ca
3 continued to remain well after one yea
years, six, and nine years, respective
was assumed to be cured after six y
epileptic. Rasumowski has just published 9
a collection of those of others.

standpoint of Féré, Jolly, and Unverricht
of epileptic or "spasmophilic" chang
failures following these operations should
a time when the predominating unknown c
stable can a scar of the finger, of the
with good result. Surgeons possess no
the first attack with a transitory el
which occurs after permanent chang
and for this reason the prognosis regar
always uncertain.

is the cure of cases in which op
of epileptic or epileptiform con
recent injuries of the cerebral corte
1870–71 contains a number of
injuries with distinct epileptic
splinters effected rapid and certa
of similar observations. He
belong here, but rather to the
epileptiform convulsions cau
With recovery or improvement
removal of the tumor they

is always the result of a cic
It occurs years, possibly twelve
Braun cited above. In such ca
(1) if the seizures are
time; (2) if they are mar
that is, if they begin in one
groups, from the thun
leg, and then to the o
travelling over the entire
loss of consciousness and
affected by convulsior
the skull are distinctly visi
its surface, whether the
the skull. In these d
and vaulted durir

attack, the author was able to bring about cessation of the convulsions in 4 cases by bony closure by the König-Müller method. Not every case of epilepsy following cranial injury begins with the complex of symptoms of a Jacksonian epilepsy. Many cases are general from the beginning. Even during the first attack of convulsions the patient falls as if struck by lightning, and there are clonic convulsions affecting at once all the muscles of the body.

Surgical treatment in this form of epilepsy by excision of cicatrized skin, bone, or portion of brain at the site of former injury should always be considered, but similar interference in non-traumatic genuine epilepsy is naturally out of the question. The problem here is to fulfil an *indicatio morbi*, not an *indicatio causalis*. It hardly seems possible to exert a favorable influence upon the assumed epileptic change in the brain by surgical means as long as the anatomical and physiological character of this change is not known. Notwithstanding this fact, such operations have been performed, principally because on account of Kocher's experiments and explanations it was assumed that an *increased intracranial tension* was the cause of the "epileptic change" or "disposition" significant in the occurrence of epilepsy. This increase of pressure has been confirmed during the time of the attack itself. Stadelmann has observed that during an attack it increased from 35 to 500 mm. of water. Kocher emphasized the fact that large cystic scars and a large amount of cerebrospinal fluid in one or both lateral ventricles are frequently found in connection with epilepsy following cranial injury. This finding would certainly permit the assumption that intracranial pressure was abnormally high. For this reason attempts have been made to reduce this supposed increased tension by surgical means. Kocher recommends lumbar puncture and puncture of the ventricles, also drainage of the ventricles and the establishment of large openings in the skull with movable coverings. For this purpose he reduced the size of the Wagner bone-flap, after it had been turned down, to such a degree that after being replaced there remained a permanent cleft in the skull about one finger's breadth wide, covered only by the soft parts. He ascribed to this operation the function of a safety-valve for the epileptic attacks, and claims to have cured more cases of epilepsy by his procedure than by any other method of operation. The author has mentioned above that he obtained particularly good results by closing existing defects or openings. This is apparently confirmed by Grekow's collection. The assumption that ligation of both vertebral arteries proposed by Alexander and Smith would have a similar action, is obviously erroneous. Diminution of blood-pressure in the cerebral arteries, if brought about by ligation, would, on the contrary, hinder the absorption of cerebrospinal fluid. A further reason for operation is based on the theory that epileptic attacks are due to vasomotor spasm; just as many drugs are recommended on the strength of the latter theory. Alexander suggested that in order to diminish the vasomotor nerve-supply the highest ganglion of the cervical sympathetic be resected on one or both sides. It has been claimed that experimental stimulation (of the cervical sympathetic)

produces anæmia of the brain and convulsions. This assertion has [
justly opposed (Kronecker). Regarding the success of this opera
opinions differ widely, although Janesco has endorsed it very war
According to him, failure was due to incompleteness of the operat
As resection of the superior ganglion destroyed the function of the v
motor nerves of the carotid region and resection of the inferior gang
destroyed that of the nerves in the region of the vertebral (artery
was necessary to remove both, or, better still, to excise the entire
vical sympathetic. Of 97 cases operated upon by this method, Jan
cured 12, which were subsequently observed for more than two y
Whether the *indicatio causalis* be satisfied by excision of a scar in
scalp, the skull, or cerebral cortex, or whether, according to Koche
Alexander, the *indicatio morbi* be satisfied, in no case should i
forgotten that, following extensive accidental or intentional wou
epileptic seizures may remain absent for a long time. Schröder
der Kolk noted such experiences in employing cutaneous stimuli
well as after extensive burns of the surface of the body. Mach
collected instances of cessation of epilepsy following severe injurie
the body. The author performed amputation on account of a crus
foot in a case of long-standing epilepsy in which attacks occurred
or three times a week. Upon looking up the .patient four months l
the author was told that since the amputation the patient had not
any epileptic seizures. The author knows of cases also in which, foll
ing bromide treatment, epilepsy ceased for two years, but return
Under these circumstances one can claim a permanent cure only a
observation for a number of years and is justified in greeting every
method with skepticism.

MENTAL DISEASES FOLLOWING CRANIAL INJURIES AND T SURGICAL TREATMENT OF MENTAL DISEASES.

Etiology.—Of 18,606 cases of insanity cranial injury was put d
as a cause in 480. Stölper's observations, made in a large numbe
cases of injury in the "Knappschaftslazareth" at Königshütt
upper Silesia, are still more valuable. Among 981 cases of cra
injury, there were 12 cases of mental disturbance, or 1.2 per c
Nearly all these cases—with one exception perhaps—were severe f
tures of the vault and base of the skull. If out of these 981 cases i
the very severe ones are considered—and these are put down as 13
there would be 11 (or 8 per cent.) cases with subsequent mental distu
ance.
Severe injuries may be inflicted upon the *head of the newborn* dui
parturition, as was noted on page 18 and the following Pages, if
maternal pelvis is contracted and the head is forcibly drawn through
pelvis by forceps, with an additional possibility of its being graspe
an unfavorable manner. Besides the bones being fractured, the br
suffers, being crushed, and its membranes and parenchyma filled w

extravasated blood. It is obvious that following such injuries the development of the brain may be retarded. Even large defects in porencephalic individuals have been referred to cranial injuries occurring during or soon after birth. At the same time the compensatory power of the growing brain is so marked that only a very small number of children at birth, in which change in the shape of the skull, visible impressions, and palpable lines of fracture betray the trace of cranial injury, subsequently become insane. If, however, they do become insane the *subsequent psychosis is always the same*, namely, a distinct idiocy, though of varying degree, a weak-mindedness showing the greatest difference in gradation. Under such circumstances there is a real, definite disease of the mind, *congenital idiocy following severe cranial injuries inflicted during birth or during the first year.*

Every congenital idiocy is not produced by this cause, as is shown by the history of chronic congenital and acquired hydrocephalus, early meningitis with recovery, congenital defects of the brain, microcephalus, etc. The prominent part played by impaired development of the mind as a result of injury of the head during birth is shown by Wulff's calculations, which determined this cause in 198, or 13.4 per cent., of the cases among 1436 idiots. Obviously this does not prove that injury during birth was the only cause of congenital idiocy in these 198 cases, as many of them—Wulff mentions 51 per cent.—presented other coincident etiological factors, such as hereditary affection or dipsomania on the part of parents.

If lack of development of the brain following cranial injury explains the constant psychical disturbances during early childhood, this cause of a definite clinical picture is absent in adults, in whom development of the brain has been completed. In the latter therefore there are different forms of insanity caused by trauma. These vary considerably in symptomatology, course, and termination, possessing in common only the same etiological factor.

Symptoms.—Two groups of insanity following cranial injury must be distinguished. In the first, the psychosis follows violence, immediately and directly; in the second, it takes place indirectly, after a longer or shorter time, preceded by a more or less easily recognized prodromal stage.

Cases belonging to the first group of insanity following cranial injury usually run a course that the author observed in 5 cases. Violence is followed immediately by loss of consciousness and a condition of stupor, just as in severe concussion of the brain. This continues for a longer or shorter time, sometimes only for a few hours, frequently for a week, before passing into a stage of intense excitement, insomnia and irritability, seizures of terror with hallucinations, alternating with a tendency to violence. This condition continues as a rule for from two to three weeks, whereupon the patients become more quiet, and a comparatively rapid convalescence follows. In 2 of the author's patients, he had an opportunity of convincing himself of their permanent recovery after three years or a still longer time. One might be led to suspect meningitis, especially if psychical disturbance following fracture of the base, with

hemorrhage from the ears and nose, does not set in until the fourth
fifth day. The absence of elevation of temperature should soon le
to a correct diagnosis.

The more typical the attacks of delirium, excitement, confusion, a
the earlier they set in after the cessation of the somnolent state, 1
more favorable is the prognosis according to the author's experien
for all 5 of his patients recovered. In only 1 case did these remair
defect of memory. At the same time there are observations of transiti
into permanent insanity and of incomplete recovery.

The worst cases are probably those in which weak-mindedness i
mediately follows the initial somnolent, irritable condition.   This
often followed rapidly by idiocy and paralytic dementia, as described
Huguenin· Or, as was observed in 2 cases by Landerer, a fall on 1
head may be followed at first by loss of consciousness, later by headac
childish behavior, rapid diminution of mental power, increasing idic
mania, with hallucinations and imperative ideas, with a transition in
extreme psychical weakness and paralytic manifestations setting
early; finally general paralysis with progressive course until death.

The usual findings at the autopsy in these cases are atrophy of the cor
and general atrophy of the brain, dilatation and marked engorgement
the ventricles, thickening and clouding of the pia mater, and also pael
meningitis; in other words, the autopsy findings of paralytic dement
Huguenin is inclined to seek the original disturbance in a chronic u
purulent meningitis which gradually brings about atrophy of the cort
In his autopsy case, the pia mater of the vault was thickened to a c
siderable degree, studded with a number of large and small grayish-wh
plaques, absolutely opaque, and firmly adherent to the surface of
brain, so that in stripping it off particles of the latter were torn aw
The author believes that wherever signs of moderate intracranial pre
ure, such as loss of consciousness, headache, and mental irritabili
continue to be present for some time, in all probability the cereb
cortex is primarily injured.   Its nutrition is impaired in these ca
through abundant intrameningeal extravasation, and corresponding
the slow absorption of the latter, it is impaired for a protracted peri
This leads to passive changes in the ganglion-cells, which have b
observed by nearly all authors who have investigated encephalitis.
these degenerations are capable of undergoing resolution, the patie
recover, become capable of receiving impressions, and finally capable
combining ideas.   If, however, degeneration progresses further a
becomes continuously more severe, the picture of paralytic dementia
developed.   Microscopical examinations have not been made of t
cortex during the early stages of the disease produced by violence; b
the frequent occurrence of an early fatal termination from pneumor
and œdema of the lungs will probably offer an opportunity for su
examinations.

The second category of psychical disturbances following cranial inju
includes those cases in which insanity does not immediately or direct
follow violence, but in which it follows after a longer or shorter space

time. To this class belong those cases, first, which are characterized by a peculiar prodromal stage. On diligent inquiry it can be ascertained that since the cranial injury a variety of disturbances have been noticed in the patient: disturbances of sensibility and mental activity, change in disposition, tendencies, and character, which are the consequences of the cranial injury, and which pass over into psychical disturbances. The most conspicuous feature is the change in character and habits during this prodromal stage in contrast with the previous behavior. Peaceful individuals become violent; those who were formerly abstemious and moderate commit excesses in drinking, etc.

Many of these cases terminate in paralytic dementia; according to Schüller, in 11 out of 48; according to Hartmann, 39 out of 138. In other cases, however, the character of secondary traumatic psychosis was not constant. Hartmann is of the opinion that if traumatic insanity is ushered in by a condition of melancholia, depression forms will afterward predominate; and if it begins with attacks of mania, exaltation forms will predomina$_{te}$.

If the characteristic prodromal stage during the time between the cranial injury and the outbreak of mental disturbance is distinctly manifested, or if it is combined with symptoms of paralysis following traumatic destruction of certain portions of the brain, such as monoplegia and contracture, the surgeon is amply justified in referring the psychosis to violence, even if the latter occurred in the past. The author's opinion is based upon autopsies, at which, it must be admitted, the greatest variety of changes in the brain have been noted, but only such as might result from an injury of the brain; as, for example, depressed fractures with cortical softening beneath them; adhesions between the pia mater and dura and with the brain; cystic degeneration or sclerotic scars in the cerebral cortex; pigmentation and discoloration of the brain, as the remains of former blood infiltration, etc.

In such cases the surgeon, who is to judge the claims of the patient or his family against a liability company, must refer the disease of the brain to the previous cranial injury. Quite otherwise, however, in those cases in which the previous cranial injury caused only a predisposition to insanity. In suffering traumatism the brain seems to become more vulnerable, so that any fresh influence (an exciting cause of any kind) calls forth a psychosis. Here the surgeon is far removed from any palpable connection; he can describe the condition, as is true in so many other psychical diseases, but he cannot explain it. According to Krafft-Ebing these individuals affected by trauma are more irritable, more sensitive, than others. They are more easily exhausted by mental work. They may become delirious, with slightly febrile disturbance, and they cannot tolerate alcohol, so that a very small quantity of wine causes them to become deeply intoxicated. Under favorable conditions of living they are spared more severe affliction. If, however, they indulge in drink, for example, these excesses act as occasional factors in the outbreak of the disease. There are developed mania with recurrences, melancholia with delusions of persecution; or, on the other hand, general paralysis.

The cases become still more doubtful if the autopsy disclose particular pathological changes in the brain or only such an appearance depend upon other than traumatic disturbances.

Owing to this uncertainty regarding cause and effect, the physician must exclude entirely cases belonging to this latter class, in relation disease of the mind to a previous injury of the skull. He may establish connection between a cranial injury and a mental disease only if able to prove that the sensory disturbances and the disturbance of sciousness which preceded the psychosis immediately followed the in of the skull.

This also applies to cases in which, previous to injury, other c of insanity have existed and acted, the cranial injury simply incre the action of these causes, and to those cases in which previous t injury psychical disturbance had existed and which recurred immedi after the injury.

Among diseases of the brain following cranial injuries must be incl *epileptic mental disorders*, if the epilepsy preceding these disorders the result of a cranial injury.

Treatment.—The operative treatment of diseases of the brain has attempted a number of times within recent years.

A few unquestionable results have been obtained in the provin psychical epilepsy, which is important, as this form of mental di not infrequently follows severe cranial injury. In 49 cases of traum epilepsy, Wagner found it occurring 9 times. Heidenhain repor collection of several cases successfully operated upon.

To this class belongs the celebrated case of F. König, who devise method of bony closure of defects of the skull by means of a skin-pe teum-bone-flap. A man, thirty years old, with a traumatic defect o skull in the left parietal region, complained of headache, dizziness, fusion, almost complete loss of memory, and gave the impression of h an individual impaired mentally to the worst degree, bordering on idi there were *numerous convulsive seizures of an epileptic character.* bony closure of the defect in the skull recovery took place within a w no mental disturbance could be discovered in the patient. The st individual had been transformed into a cheerfully disposed one of ap ently normal mind. The convulsions had remained absent when he examined five years later, and found to be in perfect health.

Next in order are operations for reflex psychoses. The latter previously reported by Pinel and fully described by Koeppe. Ko cured a soldier who suffered from maniacal attacks following se injury of the skull, by means of a crucial incision through the : Many of these reflex psychoses are evidently epileptic equivalents they alternate with convulsions; others, on the contrary, appare belong to the much discussed class of traumatic neuroses. Case *mental disturbance, with brain tumors,* usually cases of deep melanch are rare. If they do occur, it would certainly seem probable that the extirpation of the tumor the psychical disturbance would also appear.

If insanity follows cranial injury in patients who, with deep depressions or bone defects of the skull beneath adherent scars, the idea would present itself to aid the patient by removing the evident lesion. As a matter of fact, Wood operated successfully by removing a cyst of the brain, and Stetter and Molière by chiselling away hyperostoses, as well as depressed areas of the skull.

In most of the similar cases operation has produced no results; in some instances the mental condition of the patient operated upon was made worse, particularly when paralytic dementia was distinctly developed. The claims of improvement occasionally made have been of such a vague, doubtful, and transitory character, that they cannot be considered successful results. This is particularly true of operations for other than traumatic psychoses. Either the operators showed a lack of judgment or an excess of phantastic ideas, like Burckhardt, who, by means of grooves cut into the cerebral cortex, within the limits of the central convolutions, endeavored to produce inhibition between the motor and sensory regions, which, according to his assumptions, was lacking in attacks of mania.

Also the *operation for idiocy in microcephalics*, introduced by Lannelongue, received the consideration of surgeons for a short time only. This consisted in sawing out strips of bone along the sutures, or forcibly breaking apart both halves of the skull, in order to provide space for the growing brain.

THE SURGICAL TREATMENT OF BRAIN TUMORS.

The fact that in a series of cases brain tumors, concealed within the skull, have been successfully located and removed is sufficient to turn the attention of practical surgeons to a province from which they have hitherto been barred. For a long time it was known that large portions of the skull which were the site of tumors could be successfully removed, this being true also of fungi which had grown through the bone from the dura, even if in this operation portions of the brain's surface had to be removed at the same time. Subsequently a tumor of the anterior fossa of the skull growing into the orbital cavity was removed by Durante. This operation was successfully terminated, in spite of its magnitude. But it was the work of Godlee to remove for the first time from an unaltered skull a brain tumor whose pressure was betrayed not by any visible signs, but only by the brain symptoms.

The operation is at the present time still a serious and dangerous one. For this reason the proposal to attempt exploratory craniotomy in all doubtful cases, claiming that the latter involves no more risk than an exploratory laparotomy, is to be condemned. Since an experienced neurologist may mistake a cerebellar tumor for a tumor of the frontal lobe, surgeons would like to see the diagnosis of a disease that can only be removed by a dangerous operation more perfect than it is at present. At the same time they are in a position to set up fairly safe indications

for operation, with the risk, however, of leaving unoperated ·uɟ
number of tumors that are operable but regarding which a po
diagnosis is not possible.

Except in certain cases, regarding which the surgeon must arri
an agreement with the neurologist and medical clinician, the a'
believes it is proper to limit the operation for the present to tum(
the motor region, and to those portions of the brain adjoining the l
Cases in which tumors of the motor region have been removed st
mortality of 19 per cent.; those of the cerebellum, 50 per cent.; thi
the frontal lobe, 40 per cent. These figures speak for themselves.
great majority of all tumors successfully located were situated i
central convolutions, as is indicated above; while those tumor
located are assumed to be situated in the remaining portions
brain. The author would presuppose further that of general brain s
toms caused by intracranial tumors, headache, at least, if not c
disk, be present. Finally, the local or regional symptoms correspoɪ
to irritation and subsequent destruction of portions of the motor
must be distinctly developed. Even with these premises operative
ference might still be justified in spite of an uncertain diagnosis, bec
by hesitating too long, a patient might be deprived of the advan
resulting from the fact that a tumor is of small size at the onset
development.

A complete discussion of the diagnosis of brain tumors is not in
here, for only a very small number of them can be reached by the
geon's knife. Oppenheim's analysis of 23 cases observed by
verified by autopsies is of the greatest value. Of these, only 1 could
been removed by operation.

The clinical symptoms of tumors of the central convolutions ma
divided into: (1) general brain symptoms, or, more correctly, symp
due to compression of the brain; and (2) local or focal symptoms.
most regular and constant general symptom is *headache.* Deep,
and boring in character, it is similar to that of migraine, particularly
is usually accompanied by nausea and vomiting. Everything prodt
either active or passive hyperæmia will increase it. In other won
behaves like the headache accompanying intracranial pressure, l
brought about by the same cause as the latter. *Vomiting* generally oɪ
without gagging, and with an empty stomach, which fact has cans
to be familiarly known as meningeal vomiting. The most importa
all the severe symptoms of compression of the brain is *choked disk.*
author refers to the statements made in this respect in the sectio
Intracranial Pressure. The increased tension of the cerebrospinal
which prevents the flow of venous blood from the skull, hinders still ɪ
its entrance into the cranial cavity. For this reason stasis of the vi
veins in the fundus of the eye is so marked. From the account of thɪ
bosis of the cavernous sinus it is known further how such stasis ma
brought about by obstruction of the large venous trunks. A tu
affecting and obstructing the latter, besides causing other symptoɪ
compression of the brain, will bring about unilateral or bilateral chɪ

disk. In fact, as a result of rapid and excessive compression of a si
it may cause extravasation of blood into the retina. V. Bramann
shown how much this action depends upon the site and extent of
tumor. Tumors of the frontal lobe, for example, produce unilateral
very distinct choked disk, associated with extravasations in the fu
of the eye, because they directly compress veins emptying into the
emous sinus. Tumors of the motor region exercise no such direct ac
they bring about choked disk only after they have attained a comp
tively large size. For this reason, in nearly 40 per cent. of tumors in
about the central fissure, these changes in the fundus of the eye
absent. A well-marked unilateral choked disk and headache, as the
symptoms during the first stage, followed later by disturbances of sp
and twitchings in the distribution of the facial nerve, show that a fr
tumor had advanced from the frontal lobe to the speech or motor reg

Focal symptoms of tumors of the central convolutions are characte
by the fact that they follow an extraordinarily uniform course, not
in the beginning, but also during their further development. Refe
to the scholarly descriptions by Oppenheim and L. Bruns, the au
will give here simply a description of the type which has enabled surg
to make the diagnosis in cases successfully operated upon, and w
has often made possible the recognition of tumors in the central co
lutions that were hardly the size of a hazelnut. The first sympton
a tumor are *strictly localized convulsions*, identical with those in J
sonian epilepsy, these having been preceded by disturbances of s
bility, such as numbness and formication or disturbances in the musi
sense. The clonic convulsions begin in a small but very definite g
of muscles; for example, not throughout the entire innervation of
facial nerve, but only in the eyelids or the angles of the mouth.
second sign is the manner of extension of the convulsions. This a
is identical with the course in Jacksonian epilepsy. The cortical
which lies adjacent to the one first irritated is the next to be affe
At first only the eyelids twitch, then the entire half of the face; fur
the hand and arm; finally the foot and leg of the same side of the b
Just as in cortical epilepsy, the convulsions, after having affected one
of the body, may travel to the other side from below upward, retur
to the face, thus in a manner encircling the entire body. But su
distribution is found only when the disease has advanced consideri
In the beginning convulsions are limited to a part of the face, or c
extremity, to the angles of the mouth, to a thumb, the large toe,
For a certain time they are repeated in these parts only. *Consciou*
is generally retained when the seizures are limited, but the more
quently the latter are repeated and the more extensively they travel
greater will be the disturbance on the part of the general senses.
alyses follow convulsions sooner or later, and as a rule they affect t
muscles which were first to twitch at the onset of the seizures. At
these paralyses pass off, like the post-epileptic paralyses, but they
become permanent. Even then, however, the affected muscles tv
distinctly during the convulsive seizures. Monoplegia is more certa

a guide in diagnosis of the site of the tumor than monospasm. The cause of the latter (monospasm) may be found in those portions of the cortex bordering on the edge of the tumor; the former (monoplegia), on the other hand, is always the result of destruction of a cortical area brought about directly by the tumor. The distribution of paralysis follows the topical arrangement of the motor centres, just as the convulsions did. Thus monoplegia develops into hemiplegia. The fibres from the cortex of the motor region lead fairly directly to the pyramidal tracts. This has been taught by secondary degenerations following destruction of definite portions of the cortex. Thus the pyramidal tracts are the next to undergo degeneration, and therefore contractures of the paralyzed muscles take place early. *Disturbance of speech* is occasionally associated

Fig. 89.

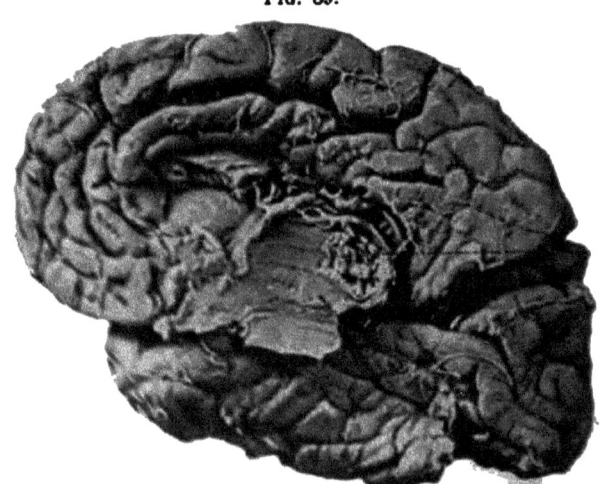

.... optic thalamus.   Tubercular meningitis of the median surface of the hemisphere.   (Starr.)

with .... muscles supplied by the facial nerve. Usually this is the result of an extension of the new growth from the centres for the facial to that for speech.

In order to pronounce a tumor operable, even if located in the motor region, which is the most accessible, the surgeon must be able to determine the boundaries to judge as to whether it is encapsulated or diffuse, and especially he must usually to decide as to its *location*, whether it lies near the surface or deeper down in the white matter. There are here several other important relations. If a tumor is situated over some higher above of the cerebral cortex, the skull overlying it is generally tender. The patients shrink from blows, and complaints about the pain, while at a corresponding point on the other side of the skull the blows are hardly noticed. The larger the tumor, the more likely will be choked disk. Encapsulated tumors require a long time to develop a complete clinical picture, while diffuse tumors require a shorter time. Finally it is the experience of surgeons that patients suffering from diffuse tumors appear very sick.

Three diseases regularly enter into the *differential diagnosis* of tumors of the central convolutions: conglomerated tubercle of the surface of the brain, circumscribed syphiloma, and circumscribed encephalitis. Obviously a collection of tuberculous or gummatous nodules can produce

Fig. 90.

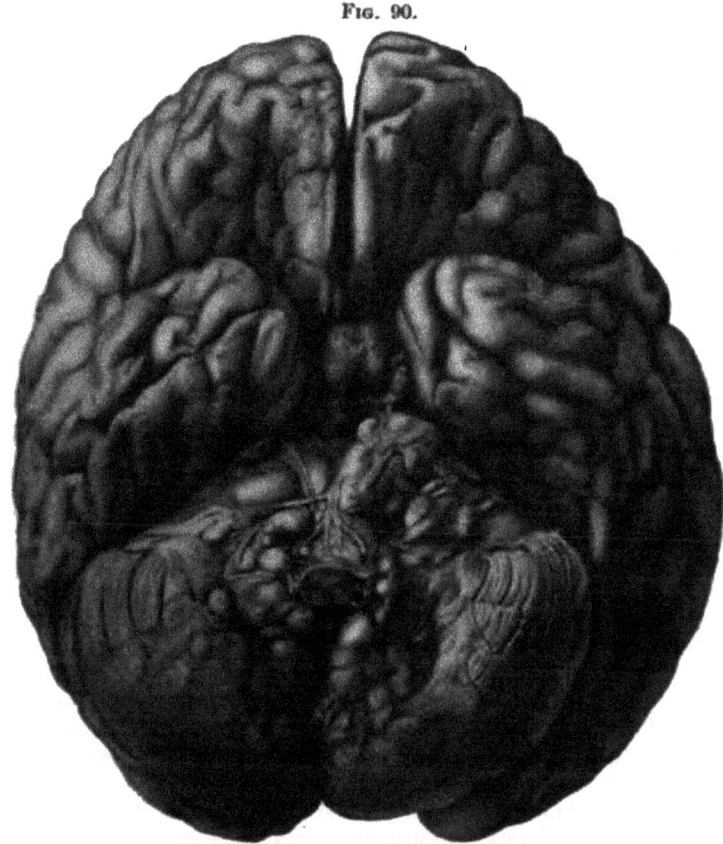

Multiple gummata upon the base of the brain and about the cerebellum. (Starr.)

the same symptoms as a tumor. In a number of instances only an anatomical-histological examination of the excised nodule has determined the fact that instead of a glioma or sarcoma, a conglomerate of tubercles was present. Without entering into the question as to whether operation for tubercle, especially in the cerebellum, should be undertaken, the author would advise the removal of every tumor-like tubercle at the surface of the brain whenever such a growth is exposed, under the

operating if he suspects a tumor in some other portion of the brain which does not offer such characteristic symptoms of irritation and paralysis as do the central convolutions. This explains the comparatively large number of operations in the presence of an uncertain diagnosis. In this border-land between surgery and internal medicine or neurology it is only by co-operation that the number of results will be increased and new fields for operation be opened. Thus in recent times operations for tumors of the base of the skull and the under surface of the brain have been attempted. The results up to the present time are not encouraging. However, the increase in the number of successfully located cerebellar tumors will not allow the ardor of the neurologist, combined with that of the surgeon, to become cooled. Tumors are frequently situated in the cerebellum whose presence is not betrayed by a single symptom. Cerebellar tumors combined with ataxia disturbances and paralysis of single cranial nerves do not produce these symptoms through the fact that a definite portion of the brain is destroyed, but because of a displacement of larger portions of the cerebellum; in other words, as a result of action upon adjacent or distant parts. In a certain way it is true also of basal tumors of the middle fossa of the skull whose encroachment has two actions: first, obstruction of the communication between the ventricles with unilateral effusion of the ventricles; and further, a distant action in the medulla. It would overstep the bounds of a handbook on practical surgery to enter into the diagnosis of these and other brain tumors. The books of Oppenheim, Auvray, and L. Bruns include all that is necessary in this respect. The author will refer to these works, as well as to his recent preparation of the respective chapter, in the third edition of his *Surgical Treatment of Diseases of the Brain.*

If modern teachings in regard to localization of the cerebral functions, together with the teachings in regard to compression of the brain, have made possible the diagnosis of tumors concealed within the skull, a practicable method for their operative removal was first found in Wagner's *osteoplastic resection.* Its execution, in the sense of a hemicraniotomy, will be described in the next chapter. Osteoplastic resection allows inspection of a more extensive portion of the brain, and spares the surgeon the necessity of determining with painful exactness the part of the cortex corresponding to the supposed tumor. At present, if the surgeon suspect a tumor of the facial centre, he freely exposes the entire motor area, and in this way not only more easily discovers the tumor itself, but also determines its boundaries; in short, he produces the same favorable conditions for possible removal as are found at the surface of the body. There is some advantage in Horsley's suggestion of operating in two stages: first performing hemicraniotomy and after several days proceeding to division of the dura and removal of the tumor.

No matter how much one might wish for better results from removal of brain tumors than are obtained at present, it must be borne in mind now and in the future that surgical treatment is the only treatment that can save the patient from an otherwise incurable disease. Even the most benign tumor within the skull will be fatal through its growth and on

account of the space it occupies. Without operation there
termination—death. In addition there is the suffering ca
growth of a tumor: the headache, blindness, paralyses, etc.
there is a desire on the part of surgeons to aid the patients
palliative operations in cases in which operation cannot be
owing to the location, the size, and uncertain boundaries
cerebral tumor. Operations performed for such purpose a
the skull, puncture of the ventricles, and lumbar punctur
operations for relieving compression of the brain. In the I
national Congress Horsley endorsed palliative trephining.
in a case of cerebellar tumor he obtained marked improve
forced movements (rotation about the axis of the body) an
aches disappeared for six months. Improvement was obtai
Beck by puncturing the lateral ventricles three times in su
case of cerebellar tumor; and by Broca by drainage of the
a case of tumor of the chiasma of the optic nerve. Lumb
has also been employed very frequently in these cases, but
some danger. The rapid evacuation of cerebrospinal fluie
brought hemorrhage in vascular tumors, for several patien
suddenly after this minor operation.

THE TECHNIC OF TREPHINING, RESECTION, CRA1 AND OSTEOPLASTIC RESECTION.

By Prof. Dr. R. U. KRÖNLEIN.

The surgeon is generally led to perform the surgical ope
skull in order to gain access to its contents at a certain situ
operation upon the bones is therefore only a means to an e
the end itself. The sound, healthy bones are only perfora
the contents of the skull would otherwise not be directly access
less infrequently division and removal of a portion of the
are the real and only object of the operation. Here are inclue
and secondary extraction of splinters in fractures of the skull
tion of the skull for tumors of the bones, tuberculosis, act
syphilis, etc.
While in the presence of these indications a permanent de
is an unavoidable result of operation, modern surgery has
to provide a method of entering the cranial cavity for the
performing intracranial operations without sacrificing any c
portion of the skull. This problem has been satisfactoril;
applying the principle of so-called *temporary* or *osteoplastic*
bones in general to the bones of the skull. W. Wagner (König
attempted this method, and demonstrated that it is possibl
by incision large portions of the bony skull in connection wit
lying skin and soft parts, to fold them back like a door, and
pleting the intracranial operation to fit them back again into

in the skull, allowing them to become reunited. The possibility of extending this operation over the area of an entire cerebral hemisphere has recently been realized by Doyen, with his bold operation of "hemicraniotomy."

By whatever method one may proceed, a general requirement in all these operations is, above all, the most careful *disinfection of the entire field of operation.* In order to accomplish this purpose, it is absolutely necessary to shave the entire scalp, and the surgeon should never allow himself to be forced into compromising with the patient. In other respects, the author retains the Fürbringer method of skin disinfection, and accordingly scrubs the scalp thoroughly with warm water, soap, and a brush, following this with alcohol and ether, and finally with a sublimate solution (1: 1000). As this whole operation requires a great deal of time, it is of advantage to have it performed the evening before the day set for operation. The head should then be covered by a moist antiseptic dressing, and the process of disinfection repeated immediately before the operation. Subsequent operations are carried out under the strictest aseptic precautions. Here, as elsewhere, the author decidedly prefers the dry method of asepsis.

As far as anæsthesia is concerned, the author has found it of advantage to use mixed morphine and ether anæsthesia in adults, and pure ether anæsthesia in children. Horsley prefers chloroform in brain operations, because it causes less excitation than ether. The author recommends, moreover, an ether mask that can be sterilized *in toto* immediately before the operation.

Methods of Operation.—Technically considered, the various operations for opening the skull may be divided into the following groups:

1. Simply drilling through the skull.
2. Simple resection of the skull.
   a. Classical trephining with an annular saw (trepan, trephine).
   b. Resection with the chisel.
3. Osteoplastic resection of the skull.
   a. The method of Wagner.
   b. The method of Doyen.
   c. The method of Toison and Obalinski.

1. **Simply drilling through the bony roof of the skull** may be indicated for two reasons: First, for the purpose of evacuating abnormally large quantities of fluid in the ventricles existing under high tension, either by *puncture* or by *drainage.* Secondly, for the purpose of injecting medicated fluids into the cavities of the ventricles (intracerebral injection). The last-mentioned method of application is limited exclusively to-day to *tetanus antitoxin,* and is based upon the experiments of Roux and Borrel, who were able by this means to keep alive guinea-pigs that had been tetanized. Puncture and drainage for effusion of the ventricles have been sufficiently discussed (see page 177). The technic of these operations is very simple. After the field of operation has been sufficiently prepared, the skin and soft parts are divided by a small incision as far as the bone at a point corresponding to the anterior or inferior

single incision. After control of hemorrhage the periosteum, together with the overlying coverings, is dissected back as one layer, with an elevator, until sufficient area for the trephine has been provided. The trephine is then applied. The projecting pyramidal point prevents slipping during the first few turns of the instrument. As soon as a circular cut has been made through the outer table the pyramidal point is withdrawn and sawing is continued, care being exercised, and the depth of the cut made by the saw frequently controlled until the disk of bone can be removed with an elevator. Auxiliary apparatus formerly in use, such as perforating trephine, crown-holder, quill, and brush, are dispensed with. Injury of the dura is easily avoided if the operation is carefully conducted.

RESECTION WITH CHISEL.—What is accomplished by the trephine, as has been described above, can unquestionably be accomplished with chisel and mallet also, namely, making a limited opening in the closed skull. As a matter of fact, many surgeons prefer the chisel to the trephine. It may be claimed for the chisel that it is possible to adopt the form and size of the opening to the peculiarities of a given case more easily than can be done with the trephine. More important than this is the fact that by gradually removing the bone in flakes with chisel and mallet injury to the dura can always be avoided. In addition the instrumentarium is the simplest imaginable. But opposed to these advantages are the facts that the operation requires more time than trephining, especially in thick and compact skulls, and owing to the numerous blows with the mallet it must be considered the more violent of the two, even admitting, as experience shows, that this operation does not actually lead to a "pounding of the brain," in the sense of the cerebral concussion experiments of Koch and Filehne. Both operations, however, accomplish their purpose, and a surgeon ought never allow himself to become so dependent upon his instrumentarium as to proclaim himself capable of working only with either a trephine or with the chisel.

When it is necessary subsequently to enlarge existing openings in the skull, to smooth off the edges of bone, to trim away the edges of clefts (as, for example, in cases of foreign bodies, knife-blades, nails, etc., which have remained embedded in or broken off at the level of the bone), the chisel is an excellent instrument. As auxiliary instruments may be employed: Luer's gouge-forceps, Collin's bone-cutting forceps, Langenbeck's fine elevators, and Horsley's flexible spatula, the latter being employed for the purpose of separating the dura from the bone and at the same time protecting it.

3. Osteoplastic Resection of the Skull.—An entirely different method of operation is employed when it is intended to provide free access to the cranial cavity for the purpose of performing an operation upon the brain. The principal operations of this kind known to modern surgery are: the localization and evacuation of cerebral abscesses, the removal of brain tumors, the localization and extraction of encysted projectiles, and the exposure and possibly the excision of epileptogenous zones in the cerebral cortex. As emphasized above, all these problems in brain surgery, as

far as technic is concerned, were satisfactorily solved for ...
by the method of Wagner. Therefore Wagner's method of ...
resection of the skull (1889) signifies a great and important pro
this province.

WAGNER'S METHOD.—W. Wagner described his method as
"The soft parts of the respective portions are divided as fa:
periosteum by an incision outlining the Greek letter omega (
soon as the flap has retracted, it is pressed down firmly upon t
and an incision is made through the periosteum along its edg
incision usually falls 0.5 to 1 cm. within the first. The bon
completely cut through with a chisel along the bow of this inner
At the two legs of the omega, however, only a groove is cut
becomes deeper from without inward. Two narrow chisels are
into the latter, and without injuring the overlying soft parts th
of bone is chiselled through subcutaneously.

"The area of bone bounded by the bow of the omega, togetl
the soft parts, can now be pried out with narrow elevators an(
back parallel with the two legs of the omega. Between the la:
bone-flap with all the soft parts covering it remains attached to
of the scalp by a pedicle at least 3 cm. wide."

This fundamental operation of Wagner was subsequently mo(
various ways, and to great advantage. In these modifications t
cipal idea was to shorten and simplify the tedious and blood
operation by employing bone-cutting forceps or bone-saws.

Thus Dahlgren (1896) recommended for this purpose his (
craniotome, with which the cranial bones were cut through step
starting from a small trephine-opening. This excellent instrumen
without doubt have come into more general use had it not alread
a rival in the revolving circular saw, which excels it in effect
Since Salzer (1889) recommended this saw it has been genera
ployed. On account of its high velocity the entire attention of the
must be directed toward preventing it from suddenly penetrat
deeply into and beyond the dura. It goes without saying that t
drilling machines of dentists, after White's system, are not suffi
powerful to overcome the resistance met by the circular saw in
through the skull. It is therefore recommended to substitute fc
hand-power or foot-power apparatus heavier ones propelled by
motor power.

DOYEN'S METHOD.—Such an electromotor apparatus is emplc
E. Doyen in performing his "hemicraniectomy temporaire," wl
first recommended in the year 1895. His method is a real perfec
osteoplastic resection of the skull. The soft parts as well as the
teum are first divided by an incision corresponding to the size an
of the flap to be folded back. Following this the bone correspon(
the above line is perforated at regular intervals at four or more
with a "fraise spherique," suggested by Doyen. This is a spheric
provided with laterally projecting cutting ribs. There is no dan
the dura being injured by this procedure. Through these small pe

tions and with a grooved director the dura is loosened from the inner surface of the skull and the bone between each opening rapidly sawn through. For this purpose Doyen employs his "Scie à curseur," a very ingeniously constructed circular saw, which bears a contrivance—a guide —which is inserted through the drill-hole between the skull and dura. This covers and protects the dura as the saw advances and divides the bone from without inward. The bone-flap, having been formed in this way as far as the bridge, the latter is chiselled through, as was described by Wagner. The whole flap is then folded back on its base. By this method Doyen is able to perform his craniotomy in an extraordinarily short time.

Though technically Doyen's method of operation is perfect, it requires great electromotive force to drive the drill and saw, and this is not at the service of every surgeon.

METHOD OF TOISON AND OBALINSKI.—Toison, in Lille (1891), first suggested and repeatedly employed the method of dividing the bone between a number of trephine-openings, from within outward, by means of wire saws. The latter were passed through the drill-holes, under the bone, between the dura and inner table. His "Scie linéaire" is a thin, flexible saw-blade, trapezoid on cross-section, armed with teeth. This is essentially different from the wire saw which was offered as an important addition to the surgical armamentarium by Gigli, of Florence, in the year 1894. The latter instrument at once took the place of Toison's saw, for Gigli's serrated wire, as cheap as it is simple, will divide the hardest bones in what one might call an ideal manner. The idea readily occurred of carrying out Toison's method, not with the author's own saw, but with Gigli's wire saw. Obalinski was the first (1897) to employ this idea, and thus decidedly improved upon Toison's operation. It is of no great significance whether the osteoplastic flap be made four-sided, as Toison does, or tongue-shaped, as Obalinski advised, or whether four, five, or seven drill-holes be made. This depends principally upon the extent and location of the field of operation.

In spite of the short time that has elapsed since Obalinski's suggestion, the method of dividing the cranial bones from within outward by means of Gigli's wire saw has been modified several times by v. Braatz, Lauenstein, and by Gigli himself. The modifications relate principally to a more practical method of leading the wire saw from one trephine-opening to the other, between the bone and the dura. Braatz, Gigli, and recently H. Gross recommend special cranial probes for this purpose. Lauenstein and A. Podrez recommend a specially constructed elastic watchspring. More experience is necessary to determine the value of these minor suggestions. P. Sudeck (1900) described and recommended under the name of "trephine drill" a new, simple, and extremely practical instrument. This is particularly true if it is propelled by an electric motor. It seems destined to replace all other bone-saws for craniectomy. This small instrument, a slender steel rod, is provided at its lower end with four spiral cutting blades wound about its axis, and in order to protect the dura is provided with a lens-shaped tip. By means of the

drill-tube of the electric motor it is rapidly rotated about its axis.
the skull has been perforated at one point with a Doyen spi
burr this instrument is inserted through the hole as far as the
pressed sideways against the edge of the opening, and thus pas
the direction of the line to be cut through the bone.   In this we
possible to cut rapidly and safely a Wagner resection-flap accord
any desired form.   A very similar trephine-burr, which has bee
for two years in Kraske's clinic, was recently described by P. }
(1900).   Furthermore, in the catalogue for 1899 of the S. S.
Dental Manufacturing Co., Philadelphia, there is recommende
illustrated an instrument for craniectomy which is identical with Su
burr.   It is called a *spiral osteotome.*

Fig. 91.

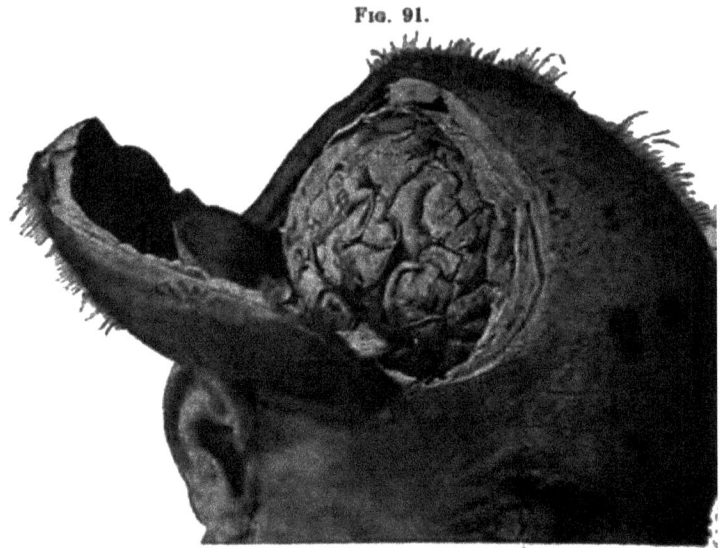

Extensive osteoplastic craniectomy. Bone divided by Sudeck's "trephine drill."

In concluding the discussion of the technic of resection of the
there remains to be described the method of *bringing about bony* a
of traumatic defects of the skullcap.
The old opinion still holds that the power of regeneration in the c
bones of the skull following loss of substance is small, and that c
quently defects of any extent are only filled with connective tissue
not with bone.   In certain cases such defects have recently been obs
to close through regeneration of bone.   These are, however, conspic
exceptions, and as such they only confirm the rule.   Experience s
that the connective-tissue scar, which usually closes small defects o
cranial bones, may be so firm and dense as to lead one to believe
a production of new bone has taken place.   The conditions are ent
different in case of more extensive defects of the skull which are

covered by skin and scar-tissue. Such patients are considered not only extraordinarily vulnerable as regards any violence affecting the skull, but their infirmity frequently manifests itself in an entirely different manner. This is very clearly shown by an observation recently communicated by König. König's patient had an extensive traumatic defect in the left parietal region. He "manifested a degree of weak-mindedness bordering on idiocy, terrible to contemplate, and suffered from epileptiform attacks." All these severe disturbances, which König very correctly, no doubt, referred to the displacement and distortion at the surface of the brain in the region of the defect, disappeared as soon as König successfully brought about bony closure of the defect.

Based upon such experiences it is altogether justifiable to demand that extensive and permanent defects of bones should be avoided from the beginning in case of operations upon the brain, and that existing defects should be closed secondarily whenever possible as soon as serious brain symptoms set in. The former indication is met by the osteoplastic resection of the skull described above, and does not require further comment; the latter, however, demands special discussion.

König (1890) was the first, in the case referred to above, to close the hole in the bone with a pedicle-flap composed of skin, periosteum, and bone, from the immediate vicinity. In this instance he used a superficial shell of bone to cover the defect (including the outer table and diploë), and not the entire thickness of the bone. A short time previously (1890) W. Müller, in Aix-la-Chapelle, had recommended this method in place of Wagner's osteoplastic resection of the skull. The author is of the same opinion as in König, that this König-Müller method of partial resection should not enter into competition with Wagner's method, but that it should only be employed where the object is to effect bony closure of existing defects of the skull, whether such defects be the result of accidental injury or of an operation where extensive removal of bone is unavoidable (as, for example, in case of tumors of the bones, tuberculosis, etc.). How effectual the Müller-König method is, is demonstrated by the history of the patient upon whom König performed the operation for the first time. The tongue-shaped bone-flap is best separated with a knife-edged chisel or cut out with a very narrow, pointed, flexible saw (Wölfler). In general one should follow the rules of osteoplastic surgery.

This method of "organic restitution" of lost portions of the cranial bones may be called "autoplastic," and must be considered the normal method. It deserves to take precedence over those methods which are included under the term "heteroplastic" operations. The latter possess this in common, that hard materials, having no connection with the edges of bone, are placed in the defects in the skull, with the hope and intention that they may become solidly united.

If the history of trephining be traced to remote times, it will be discovered that all those attempts made with so much zeal by numerous investigators during recent years have had their precedents. Thus, according to McGee, there is found in the collection of Incas skulls of Muñiz a skull in which a silver plate had been let into a large defect in

the frontal and parietal bones, and judging from the condition
edges of the bone this must have been worn for some time duri
life of the subject. There is also a communication, dated from the
teenth century (1670), by Job van Meek'ren, respecting a Rus
whom the cranial bone of a dog was grafted into a defect in the
but which was removed after a time, as otherwise the patient wou
suffered excommunication. The attempt was repeatedly made
the last century to reinsert the button of bone after completion of t
ing and allowing it to become reunited, by Phil. von Walther
Rossheim (1830), Wedemeyer (1842), and by others. In connecti
these earlier attempts, a number of surgeons have in recent times e
ored to close defects in the skull by heteroplastic means. It n
conceded that the results obtained during the antiseptic and asep
were better than those of former times. Below is given a con
review regarding newer methods.

1. Reimplantation of a button of bone obtained by trephining i
opening in the bone (Phil. von Walther, 1820).

2. Reimplantation of a previously broken-up fragment of sk
the trephine-opening (Macewen, 1888; W. Keen).

3. Grafting decalcified bone (Senn, 1890; Kümmell, 1891).

4. Grafting calcined bone-substance (Barth, 1895; Landerer,

5. Grafting boiled bone (Westerman, 1898).

6. Grafting fragments of bone from the inner surface of the i
the patient (Seydel, 1889; Sennander, 1890; Czerny, 1893).

7. Grafting a piece of the parietal of a young dog into the de
the skull (Macewen, 1882); a piece of the femur of a dog (Ricard
Succhi, 1894); cranial bone of a goose (v. Jaksch, 1889).

8. Implanting metal plates, aluminum (Booth and Curtis, 189

9. Implanting celluloid plates (Alex. Fränkel, 1890; Hinters
1891; v. Eiselberg, 1891; Berger, 1891; Postempski, 1892).

10. Implanting filagree nets (O. Witzel, 1900; Gleich, 1900).

A conclusive opinion regarding the value of these different m
cannot be given at the present time. In a certain number of c
was possible to bring about firm union of these foreign bodies, fo
they must be considered, even the buttons of bone from trephinir
the broken-up fragments of bones of the skull that had been rer
and it was also possible to confirm these good results for years afte
But opposed to these noteworthy results are a considerable num
failures. Either union failed from the beginning or a plate
become united had to be removed subsequently. Regarding some
vations in which implantation was successful there is no later
regarding the permanent result.

It is repeated, therefore, what was emphasized above, that the n
method of closing defects of the skull is the osteoplastic coverin
living bone-flaps according to the method of Müller and König. Y
however, this cannot be carried out (owing to abnormal thinness
surrounding cranial bones, lack of diploë, etc.), an attempt at h
plastic operation is permissible. Under such circumstances, as a

of present experience, the author would prefer the transpla:
ods of Westerman and Leydel (see above under 5 and 6).
be taken to freshen the entire edge of the defect, and to
that the transplanted bone fits as tightly as possible int
further, that blood and secretions do not collect beneath t
The latter indication can be most simply fulfilled by fashi
openings at the edge of the defect.

CRANIOCEREBRAL TOPOGRAPHY.

To determine the topical relations between the surface
and the skullcap, and to express by means of simple topog;
the relative position of the most practically important region:
constitute so-called "craniocerebral topography." Unfor
relative position is not absolutely constant, but varies withii
wide limits according to age, size, sex, and race of the indi
outcome of this is that every such topographical rule for tl
tion of one or another point on the surface of the brain
mathematically accurate in the concrete case; moreover, th;
should be satisfied if a rule applies generally and the play
variations does not exceed certain limits. For the practical
of the surgeon it is sufficient if such rules apply relatively.
ress in the technic of surgical operations upon the brain
years consists principally in the fact that surgeons have le
expose only small areas of the surface of the brain, but to p
to large and extensive regions of the cortex, so that they ma
with the eyes and fingers. One has only to consider Do
craniectomie temporaire!" In almost every instance the t
those portions of the brain to which access has been provide
sive that any individual variation falls well within these
necessity of exposing the greatest possible area of brain s
outset of every operation carries with it the further adva
enables the surgeon to proceed with few topographical rul
Having exposed an extensive region of the brain with t
of the latter, the next problem is to determine the more exac
of one or another cortical centre in the portion of the brain
exposed. How exactly under circumstances these sites n
mined has been shown by the investigations and observatio
regarding the motor region in the cerebral cortex, in apes
the human species. Armed with the special knowledge of t!
Waldeyer has recently subjected this entire region to a tho
research, and he arrives at the conclusion that of the many
lein's construction is evidently the best, as "it accomplishe
the simplest way." The author will discuss this constructic
below.
Among the few topographical determinations which c;
pensed with, and which are the only ones practically necess;

rules according to which are located on the surface of the skull direction and position of the *central fissure* (sulcus centralis, a. Rola and the *fissure of Sylvius*. Knowing the position of these, and location of their upper and lower ends, one can find the locatio those regions of the cerebral cortex which are most important in tical surgery, including the regions of both central convolutions, operculum, frontal, temporal, and parietal lobes of the cerebrum. are many rules for the topographical determination of these two im tant sulci of the brain. German, French, English, and American i tigators have endeavored to construct such, and whoever is interest the details will find in Chipault's large work an exhaustive compili and illustrated description of the various devices.

The results of these rules vary widely. Most of them are open t objection that in determining the location of craniocerebral landm absolute values (linear and angular measurements) have been These may coincide in certain cases, but do not take into accoun different size and shape of different types of skulls and brains. A author remarked recently on another occasion the point to be aim in all such topographical rules should be the "elimination of all absolute values and their replacement by relative values, which a proportion to the size of the skull and of the brain, and which accordingly in the individual case."

A. Froriep has subjected the relative position of points on the cerel and roof of the skull to a thorough investigation, and has presente results in an excellent atlas. Based upon the material containe Froriep's work, the author has endeavored to construct a simple for the topographical determination of the central sulcus and the fis of Sylvius without employing absolute values. A further claim may be made for this construction is the fact that it makes use of that are generally known and acknowledged in rules for the measurei of the skull, and that at the same time it includes the rules give v. Bergmann for resection of the skull, in locating otitic abscesses o temporal lobe, and by the author for the evacuation of different f of hæmatoma of the middle meningeal artery.

In referring to the accompanying illustration, the author will be designate the lines which enter into its construction:

1. The base-line, German horizontal line, auricular orbital line, horizontalis auriculo-orbitalis.

. The superior horizontal line, linea horizontalis supraorbitalis.

. The anterior vertical line, linea verticalis zygomatica.

. The middle vertical line, linea verticalis articularis.

. The posterior vertical line, linea verticalis retromastoidea.

₇. The line of Rolando (obliqua).

8. The line of Sylvius (obliqua).

The landmarks for the projection of lines 1 to 5 are easily determi as follows:

1. The base-line passes through the infraorbital ridge and the su rior border of the auditory meatus.

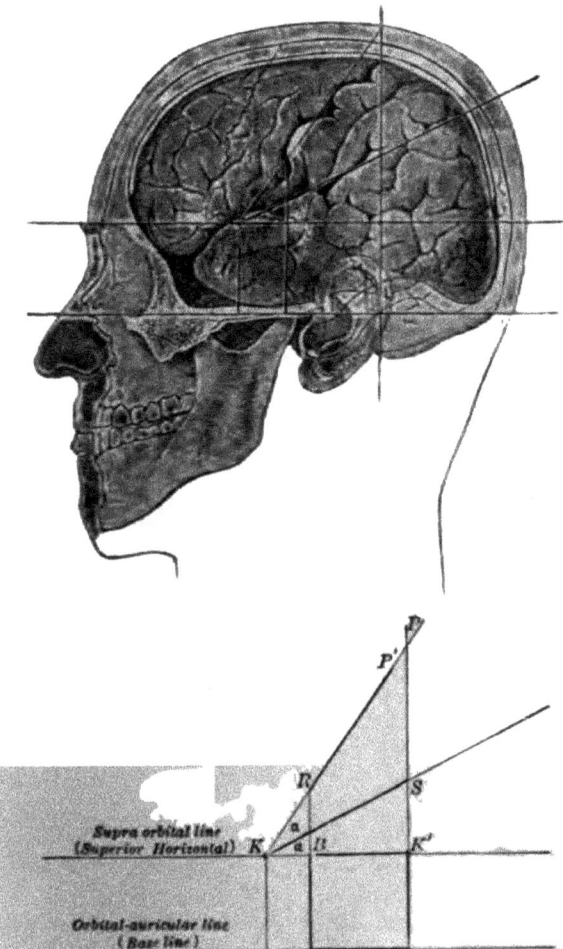

Supra orbital line
(Superior Horizontal) K

Orbital-auricular line
(Base line)

The two oblique lines are constructed secondarily; they are dr
follows:

6. The line of Rolando, the point of intersection of the anterior
and superior horizontal lines, is connected with a point where th
terior vertical line passes over the summit of the head.

7. The line of Sylvius, by bisecting the angle formed between t
of Rolando and the superior horizontal line and prolonging the
bisection posteriorly until it crosses the posterior vertical line.

FIG. 93.

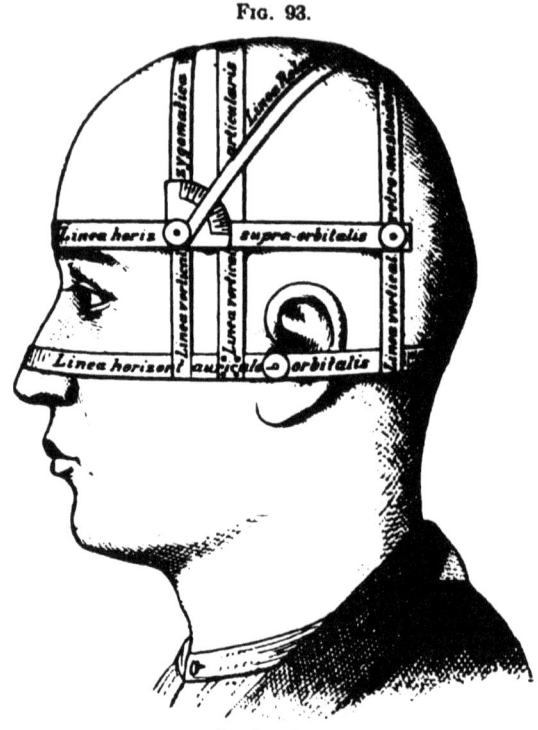

Craniometer.

In this construction therefore K = the point of bifurcation
fissure of Sylvius, S = upper end of the fissure of Sylvius, R =
end of the fissure of Sylvius, P' = upper end of the sulcus of R(
K and K' = Krönlein's two sites for trephining, $A B K' M$ = v.
mann's sites for resecting the skull (a rectangle).

Although in a given case this construction may be carried out
head of the patient without special apparatus immediately befo
operation, it can be done more easily and more exactly with the b
a craniometer, which the author has briefly described and illustra
the two drawings. (Figs. 93 and 94.) This instrument is nothing

Craniometer.

quainted with the former. The two illustrations show the apparatus as it is applied to the head of the patient.

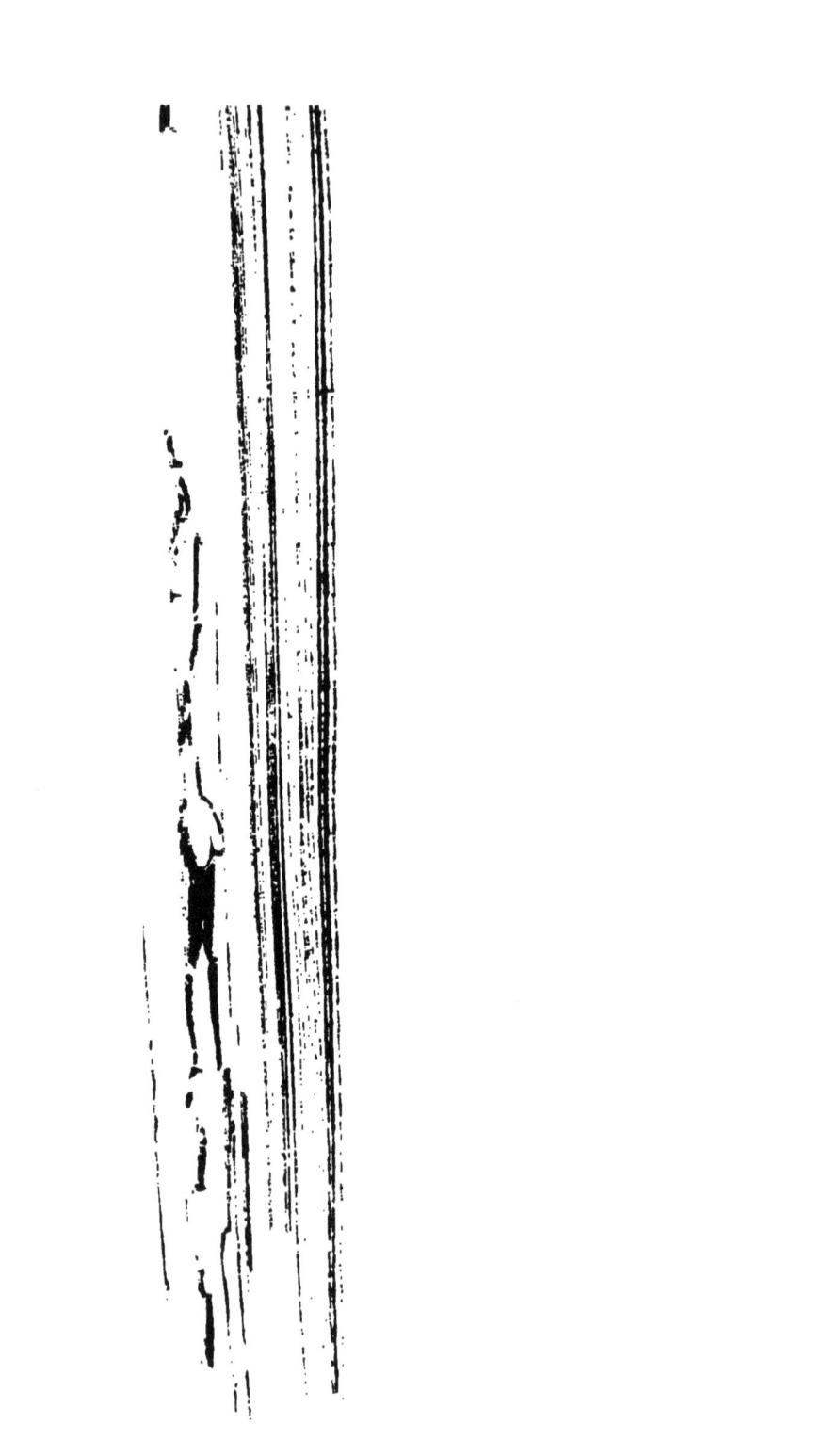

MALFORMATIONS, INJURIES, AND DISEASES OF THE EAR.

By Prof. W. KÜMMEL.

Preliminary Remarks.—The diseases of the ear in this article, according to the general plan of the work, can be treated only in so far as they present particular interest for the surgeon. Although no complete work on otiatrics is to be given, still a few hints on the anatomy and the technic of examination seem to be in place.

The outer opening of the auditory canal is concealed in most individuals by the tragus, which extends valve-like in front of it. Mesially opposite the tragus the anterior border of the ear cartilage projects sharply into the auditory meatus. At this point there is a bend at almost right angles between the hollow of the concha and its continuation, the external auditory canal. By pulling the pinna away from the head and somewhat backward, in the majority of cases this bend can be almost completely removed. At the junction of the membranous and bony part the canal shows a wider, but not always well-marked bend in the form of an obtuse angle open anteriorly and inferiorly. This can also be almost completely removed by pulling on the pinna. The canal thus stretched runs somewhat less than 65 degrees to the median plane in an almost horizontal direction. The canal is narrowest at the junction of the cartilaginous and bony portions.

The anteroinferior part of the wall of the canal is the longest on account of the inclination of the plane of the drum-membrane; therefore there is a somewhat roomy fossa in front of the anteroinferior pole of the drum-membrane.

The drum-membrane is inclined at an acute angle to the sagittal as well as to the horizontal plane, and shows besides a funnel-shaped depression, convex mesially and of varying depth.

During life, on account of the constant direction of the bony part of the auditory canal, the drum-membrane and other structures of the middle ear are always seen from behind and somewhat from above. For this reason they do not appear as they are generally presented in anatomical illustrations, side by side in the same plane, but behind one another, foreshortened and in perspective; a difference the author has tried to present in Figs. 95 and 96.

At birth and in young children only the cartilaginous part of the canal is developed. It is very narrow and completely filled with masses of

(339)

epithelium. An exact examination is therefore possible only a painstaking cleansing. Even then it is difficult, as the drum at th has a more horizontal position, so that the line of vision almost coi with the plane of the drum-membrane. Drawing the lobe of t downward and forward aids the examination.

To gain a free view into the auditory canal, as a rule it is nec to separate the tragus from the posterior wall of the auditory can to push aside the hairs at the meatus. A funnel-shaped specul used for this purpose. Of the many varieties, the author prefe

FIG. 95.   FIG. 96.

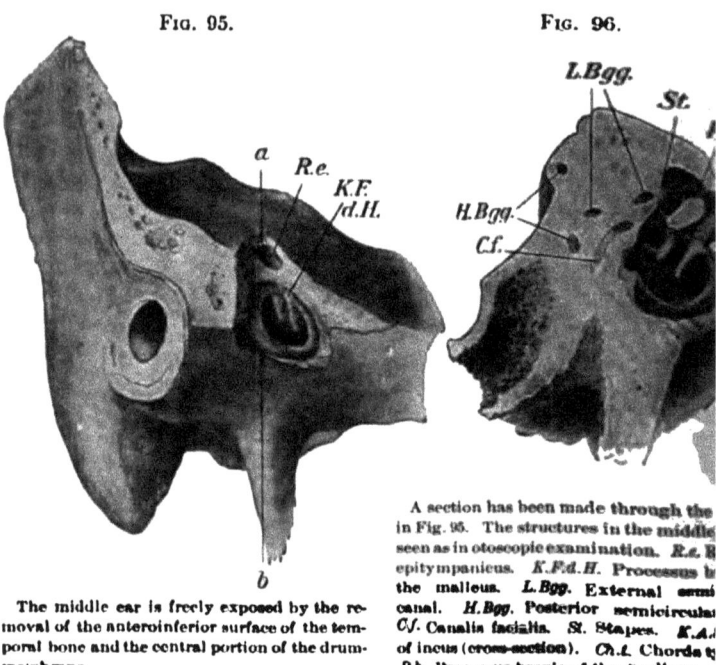

The middle ear is freely exposed by the removal of the anteroinferior surface of the temporal bone and the central portion of the drum-membrane.

A section has been made through the in Fig. 95. The structures in the middle seen as in otoscopic examination. *R.e.* epitympanicus. *K.Fd.H.* Processus b the malleus. *L.Bgg.* External semi canal. *H.Bgg.* Posterior semicircula *Cf.* Canalis facialis. *St.* Stapes. *K.A.* of incus (cross-section). *Ch.t.* Chorda ty *P.b.* Processus brevis of the malleus.

of Tröltsch with a flaring outer end. The speculum should not be to enlarge the opening; for this reason the bivalved instrumen rightly been abandoned. (Figs. 97 and 98.)

Owing to the narrowness of the passage, direct light can be emp in favorable cases only. In most instances reflected light, artifi daylight (but not sunlight), is necessary (concave mirror with c aperture, introduced by v. Tröltsch).

If the auditory canal is stretched and then illuminated in this the tympanic membrane can be seen at the bottom of the passage nearly oval surface of a pearly-gray transparent appearance, under mal conditions, showing in its anterior and inferior portion a fui shaped retraction which produces a triangular reflection of light. serce of the latter is not of significance, however. Owing to the obli position and retraction of the membrane, its posterosuperior portion is situated more in the line of vision, while the anteroinferior portion is placed more perpendicularly to the latter. The manubrium and short process of the malleus are embedded in the membrane, with their broad surfaces somewhat turned to view. (Fig. 96.) When the tympanic membrane is very transparent, a portion of the long process of the incus and possibly the head of the stapes can be seen, as in Fig. 96. Above the short process of the malleus is situated the flaccid portion of the tympanic membrane, Shrapnell's membrane, which forms a portion of the floor of the epitympanic space. Only a small portion of the malleus and incus lie in the principal part of the tympanic cavity, which is bounded externally by the tympanic membrane. The greater portions of these bones are situated in the epitympanic space (Kuppelraum, H. Hartmann), attic. According to the usual manner of inspecting the auditory canal, this cavity is placed with its long axis in the line of vision; a part of its floor is formed by the innermost portion of the superior wall of the auditory canal, also by Shrapnell's membrane; and beyond this it communicates with the middle ear (mesotympanum). One can distinguish an anterolateral and a posteromedian portion which are separated by the

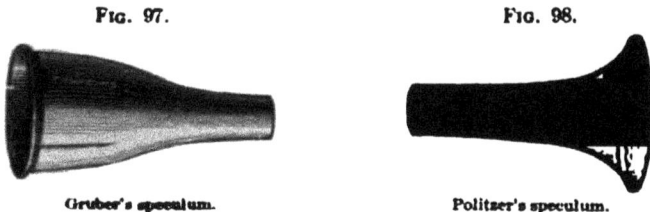

FIG. 97. FIG. 98.

Gruber's speculum. Politzer's speculum.

bodies and suspensory ligaments of the malleus and incus. The smaller lateral portion borders on Shrapnell's membrane and is provided with a small, narrow opening toward the mesotympanum. The posteromedian portion is somewhat larger, and communicates freely with the mesotympanum behind and to the inner side of the long process of the incus and the manubrium of the malleus. It extends above the roof of the auditory canal a little more laterally and posteriorly—*i. e.*, in the usual direction of the line of vision—and in this portion contains the short process of the incus. In the same direction it is continuous with the mastoid antrum, the floor of which lies about at the same level as that of the epitympanic recess and which, in respect to the observer, lies nearer the surface of the temporal bone. Beginning at the mastoid antrum, a large number of air-cells extend radially into the squamous portion, petrous portion, and the mastoid process. They vary in the degree of development in different individuals, and are lined with the same delicate mucous membrane as the antrum. They are called, according to situation, squamous cells, petrosal cells, or mastoid cells. The inferior mastoid cells are usually most developed. In exceptional cases these cavities may extend throughout the entire petrous portion as

far as its apex, posteriorly as far as the occipital bone,
far into the squamous portion of the temporal bone.

Beneath the mesotympanum there is also a recess, whi
shallower, however, than the epitympanic recess or attic. Tl
called recessus hypotympanicus by Kretschmann, or cellar (
by Grunert. At the floor of this hypotympanum, which lies
bulb of the jugular vein, are situated a large number of bon
covered with mucous membrane,which give it a honeycombed s

Regarding the topographical relations of the labyrinth, the
only remark here that at the anteroinferior portion of its inr
mesotympanum communicates with the scala tympani throug
tra rotunda and at the superoposterior portion with the vestib
the fenestra ovalis. Immediately above the fenestra ovalis
the posterior peripheral turning point of the facial nerve,
makes a distinct curve, and immediately above the latter t
semicircular canal forms a low swelling on the inner wall of
and the epitympanic recess (attic), as in Fig. 96. The post
circular canal lies parallel with the posterior surface of t
portion immediately above the sigmoid fossa and a little to
the internal auditory meatus.

CHAPTER VII.

MALFORMATIONS OF THE EAR.

MALFORMATIONS of the external ear and the auditory meatus are rare, and in the severe forms are usually associated with impaired development of the tympanic cavity, and occasionally also with that of the labyrinth. Marked impairment of hearing or absolute deafness does not necessarily follow, however.

Congenital fissures in an otherwise normal external ear are rare, but are relatively most frequent in the lobe of the ear (coloboma lobuli). They usually extend close beneath the tail of the helix, obliquely from above and in front, backward and downward. Schwartze has depicted one running in the opposite direction. Fistulæ are found more frequently than complete fissures, usually in front of and above the tragus, less

FIG. 99.

FIG. 100

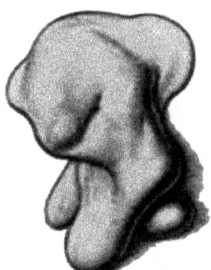

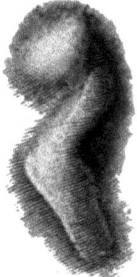

Fistulæ auris congenitalis. (Grunert.)　　　　Deformities of the concha.

frequently in the concha of the ear; and have been distinguished by Grunert as "fistulæ auriculæ" from the above-mentioned "fistulæ auris." They are found most frequently when the external ear is otherwise deformed, particularly in its lower portion. Both forms of fistula are usually shallow grooves, 1 mm. deep at the most. Occasionally, especially the deeper ones, they secrete a serous, frequently somewhat sticky fluid; occasionally also small cystic dilatations occur. The secreted fluid may occasionally cause an obstinate eczema in the neighborhood of the fistulous opening. According to recent investigations, none of these fistulæ corresponds to the first branchial cleft, to which Hinsinger previously referred their origin; more probably all such depressions, fistulæ, and fissures must be referred to absence of union between the swellings and prominences from which the external ear is derived. A fistula of the

(343)

first external branchial cleft must necessarily lie and open in
and below the auditory canal in a line between the auditory mea
the lesser cornua of the hyoid bone. Such fistulæ rarely occu
Vol. II., page 17.) Cysts of this cleft are more frequent and ma
to the lobe of the ear.

Auricular appendages, rather improperly called polyotia, pro
disturbance besides the deformity, which is usually of slight degre
occur with a normal ear as frequently as with a deformed exte
and are always situated on a line extending from the tragus to t
of the mouth, corresponding to one of the transverse facial clefts.
sionally one finds a chain of them. These formations consist of
cartilage covered with fat and epidermis; they vary much in for
be shaped like a leaf or horn, frequently bifurcated, occasionally
siderable size. At times they have attached to them fibres of the
of the face, and, in consequence of contractions of the latter, m

FIG. 101.

FIG. 102

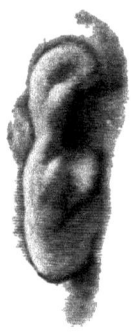

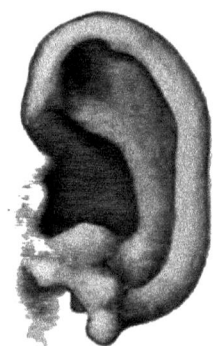

Deformity following perichondritis.   Malformation of the ear lobe.

very comical motions. Where such appendages are considerabl
oped, the rest of the external ear is placed with its inferior ex
pushed forward, so that it occupies a more horizontal position.
103 and 104.)

By "crippling" of the pinna of the ear, the author means a de
as a result of which the auricle markedly differs from the nor
respect to form and size. Thus there are "macrotia" and "mic
without other important disfigurement of the pinna; more fre
there are found abnormally small ears, more rarely abnormall
ears, which show marked deformity.

The milder grades of congenital deformity have recently attrac
attention of anthropologists and psychiatrists. On the one han
have been brought forward in connection with the phylogenetic de
ment of the pinna; on the other hand, they have been conside
stigmata of degeneration in connection with hereditary taint. (See
of Lombroso, Gradenigo, and others.)

On account of more serious disfigurer
development of larger portions of the
surgical assistance necessary, particul
marked degree, and for this reason th
by the manner of dressing the hair. 1
the helix, the ear appearing shortened f
ally, as in a case noted by Stetter, the
a kind of valve and bearing impaire
disease of the ear may be rendered vei
Extensive defects of the pinna with
portions are rare. Most frequently thei
ment of the lobe of the ear. Schwartz
contrary, the lobe of the ear was the or
methods for the plastic repair of such a

FIG. 103.

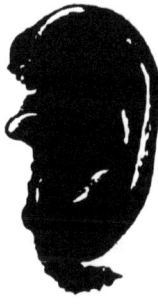

Auricular appendages.

been theoretically suggested, as, for a
Dieffenbach, and others. A good co:
employing a reduplicated flap from the
process. The flap may also be forme
the pinna and the resulting defect cove
by a Kraus skin-graft.
Rolling in of the helix most frequentl
treatment. It may occasionally be rem
of the pinna further upward or backwa
of skin. In one case Stetter undermine
which extended as far as the pinna. T
verse fold and made the resulting shor
mattress suture. The result was that
was raised and broadened. Incision a:

tion of the cartilage of the ear often facilitate very much the c
of such curvature. Ears that simply project may be impaved
manner of their attachment by corresponding excision of the ;
order to remove the deformity caused by a very large ear, the c
tion of a number of cuneiform excisions can be employed, pai
by the method suggested by Trendelenburg.

Clefts of the external ear should be closed by plastic operat
the case of harelip. Disfiguring auricular appendages can be
without difficulty. One should, however, not cut too deeply,
sionally they are very close to one of the larger branches of 1
nerve. If it should happen that there are defects of the pinn
same time, they may be employed to repair the latter. It is 1
impossible to give definite rules for a single case.

The only malformation of the *auditory meatus* observed is ;
absence—"atresia antis." This very rarely affects only the carti
portion, but more frequently the bony portion also. At the sa;
in most cases the mastoid process is poorly developed. Frequ
pinna is markedly deformed and frequently also displaced
and downward. At the site of the cartilaginous canal there is fo
connective tissue. At the site of the bony canal is solid bon
frequently there are present also, fistulous tracts, mentioned ab(
ticularly in front of the rudimentary pinna, and these are n
quently mistaken for a rudimentary auditory canal by parent:
as by the attending physician, attempts being made to dilate t
naturally to no purpose. A normal tympanic membrane is us
present in such cases, and therefore nothing can be hoped for thr
construction of an artificial auditory canal. Even if the tympan
is developed, it is very doubtful whether improvement in hearin
obtained by constructing an artificial fistula toward the antrum
all attempts have failed.

In regard to congenital exostoses of the auditory canal, see Ch;

CHAPTER VIII.

INJURIES OF THE EAR.

WOUNDS OF THE PINNA; OTHÆMATOMA.

On account of its exposed position the external ear is very liable to be injured. This occurs more frequently as the result of violence with blunt objects than with sharp weapons.

Incised and *lacerated wounds* are most frequently caused by "schlager-" and sabre-blows. These may completely cut off pieces of the ear, transversely or parallel with its flat surface, or produce extensive laceration. Portions of or the entire auricle may be torn or crushed off, as by the bite of a horse. The loss of either large portions or of the entire auricle results in serious deformity. Hearing is impaired if the injury is followed by narrowing of the auditory canal. The entire ear is never cut off completely unless the cutting or tearing instrument follows an unusual direction; as a rule greater or smaller portions of the cartilage of the concha are preserved, especially those parts in the vicinity of the auditory canal. They may possibly be used later for plastic purposes or for the attachment of artificial contrivances.

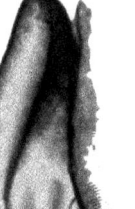

Fig. 105.

Perichondritis of the concha. (Biehl.)

Fortunately the auricle possesses great vitality Primary union frequently takes place even if the edges of the wounds are contused; and it is even possible that after having been completely severed the auricle may grow on if carefully sutured. In order to produce this result hemorrhage should be carefully controlled; at the same time care must be taken to prevent foreign bodies—i. e., ligatures—from remaining in the wound. It is better to transfix a spurting artery in the vicinity of a wound than to apply even a very fine ligature within the wound itself. A great deal depends upon exact coaptation of the wound-edges; in order to accomplish this it may be necessary to trim the surfaces of the wound when these are irregular. When such severed portions grow on, partial gangrene occasionally occurs. As a rule this affects only the most superficial layers and thus produces little damage; but the respective portion will have a cicatricial appearance. Care must be taken, particularly in the edge of the helix, to preserve even very small pieces that have been cut off. Very small defects may produce disfigurement and attract attention unpleasantly.

(347)

Minor injuries which divide the pinna in an oblique direc
.... In such case it may be difficult to fit togethe
the edges of the wound in such a way as to obtain a satisfacto
effect. The edges of the wound should be brought togethe
heavy sutures and fine silk or wire sutures carefully appl
...... the deep temporary sutures may be removed.

Injuries of the ear inflicted with blunt objects, such as ca
...... objects, may appear very much like incised wounds
on the lateral surface of the auricle is very thin and rather fin
and therefore presents sharp edges when torn.' But even
must be quite forcible and struck with a narrow edge, as the
auricle possesses considerable elasticity and ...ature of the
more apt to occur than laceration of the skin. Such frac
cartilage and severe contusions of the auricle as a whole are
othæmatoma if the skin remains untorn.

The cause of othæmatoma has until recently been a questio
among psychiatrists. According to these communications,
that this affection occurs more frequently among insane
particularly those suffering from paralytic dementia, ... i
are mentally sound. Virchow, L. Meyer, Parrelik, ...
discovered in the ears of such patients changes similar to
in the auricular and costal cartilages of old men—fibrous tra
and focal softening. Although it must be assumed that there
predisposition in such individuals, trauma is probably neces
production of othæmatoma. The degree of trauma necess
very slight. Sometimes it is impossible to obtain any inform
respect, even in those who are mentally sound (Schwartze .

Occasionally othæmatoma has been observed in carpente
carried a beam on their shoulder, which suddenly turned, so
the ear with its edge; also where the auricle has been roll
hand, as practised by schoolmasters, and which is also a favo
among rough boys. In such instances hæmatoma is prob:
fracture of the cartilage and usually of moderate extent.

The most extensive hæmatoma is found on the side of
toward the head, where the skin is comparatively loosely atta
however, this surface possesses a comparatively rich lymph-su
is absorbed in a relatively short time. There are hardly ever
turbances. On the outer surface of the pinna, cartilage, peri
and subcutaneous tissues insensibly merge into each othe
small pieces of cartilage, together with the perichondrium, are
torn off by extravasated blood. Blood tumors do not devel
great size as on the other surface, but on account of the sm
of lymph vessels extravasated blood is slowly absorbed from
taneous tissues, and as a result the cartilage is frequently
chronic inflammation which may lead to thickening and fina
tricial contraction of the latter. Whether infection of the ex
blood necessarily occurs remains doubtful. Owing to the thin
epidermis, this might possibly occur without solution of

Bloch has noted that ears thus affected become hyperæsthetic. Fresh injury may escape notice, and as a result of being frequently repeated chronic perichondritis can occur without infection. If, however, infection perichondritis occurs and an abscess forms, with necrosis of portions of cartilage, deformity may be still more severe. Cicatricial contraction takes place in such a manner that the helix is rolled in and turned down, and the auditory canal may become contracted. In the severest forms the auricle becomes transformed into a shapeless mass in which hardly a trace of its original form can be recognized. This conspicuous deformity is depicted in old Greek statues of prize-fighters. It is very probable that their opponents, whose fists were armed with the cæstus, frequently inflicted such injuries. Virchow found a similar condition in Japanese pugilists. Very probably this condition will soon be recognized as an occupation affection among professional boxers, as Bloch observed it in acrobats who were engaged in "saltomortale" performances.

Fortunately such severe disfigurement does not necessarily take place. If a hæmatoma is protected from infection and further injury, perichondritis may not occur. Infection is frequently unavoidable if the skin of the auricle is so severely crushed that nutrition is impaired and infectious germs can pass through the thin, necrotic tissue. Or at the moment of injury micro-organisms may lodge in small tears of the skin, which quickly heal, and thus infection take place. If the latter occurs, incision should be promptly performed at the first signs of inflammation. If an extravasation is not infected, it is unwise to empty it by incision even with all antiseptic precautions. Incision does not, moreover, accomplish much, for, as has been observed a number of times, extravasation may reaccumulate in a very short time. Evacuation by means of puncture with a Pravaz aspirating-needle is less dangerous; but even then extravasation may reaccumulate within a few hours after evacuation in spite of a well-applied compress, as the author can testify. Massage seems more useful in such cases. The fact that these portions of the skin are poorly supplied with bloodvessels and lymphatics would be in favor of this method of treatment. A compression-bandage does not accomplish much. Painting thickly with collodion may produce considerable pressure. In one case in which the author employed it, it almost produced gangrene of the pinna. The principal remedy is the protection of the ear from additional injury.

BURNS, FROSTBITE, AND INJURIES OF THE EXTERNAL EAR CAUSED BY CAUSTICS.

Burns of the pinna of moderate extent caused by contact of hot fluids or caustic substances, more frequently by live steam, are rather rare and without much significance, unless at the same time the lining of the auditory canal and the drum-membrane are injured.

The pinna is very liable to be frostbitten, as it is situated at the periphery of the body, and therefore, like other projecting organs, is not

well nourished (v. Recklinghausen). In severe cases involving
followed by perichondritis, with the same termination as in t
by other causes; also by partial or complete gangrene of th
also calcification or ossification of the cartilage of the pinna.

If the external auditory canal be injured at the same ti
injuries acquire serious significance.

INJURIES OF THE EXTERNAL AUDITORY CANAL.

The external auditory canal is occasionally injured at the sa
as the auricle, either by sharp instruments or through violence w
objects. Care should be taken to avoid contraction of the cai
cicatricial folds by firmly packing with iodoform gauze, or by
a suitable piece of glass or lead tubing or celluloid catheter.
of necessity a piece of beeswax will answer the purpose. Inser
rubber drain is not recommended. It always leads to the forn
areas of ulceration or even extensive gangrene of the auditor
especially if there is suppuration from the latter. Suppuratior
liable to be caused by defects in the wall of the auditory canal
beyond the site of stenosis. The drainage of secretions arising fr
defects may be seriously hindered by stenosis. Under such circui
they frequently cause the formation of polypoid granulations a
plete obstruction of the small opening. These conditions ma\
lowed by perichondritis and periostitis of the auditory canal, ci
possibly with rupture of the pus into the loose connective tissue st
ing the auditory canal and the formation of peri-auricular pl
In the event of such a rare occurrence, it might be difficult to di
whether as a result of injury there was inflammation of the
canal, of the middle ear, or possibly some complication of the
the form of mastoid disease. It may be necessary to remove the
in order to clear up the diagnosis. Thus, in a case of the ar
which the auricle of a young child was injured by a kick from
only after the resulting stenosis had been treated for three mor
it possible to discover that the sole source of the rather profuse a
smelling pus was a small defect of the skin, with exuberant gran
situated in the deeper portions of the auditory canal.

If stenosis has actually developed, hearing may be impaired;
atresia is not complete, the slightest accumulation of wax, or
swelling of the walls of the auditory canal accompanying otitis
will prevent the entrance of sound. In addition, the treatmei
incidental otitis media may be rendered difficult; therefore steno
frequently be removed. In doing this one is frequently limited to
or excision of the stenosis with subsequent mechanical dilatati
obstinate cases, one might expose the auditory canal behind b\
of an incision and proceed according to the methods employed in
plasty; but the author has never attempted this operation
Ostmann has recommended electrolysis, and it has apparently

service. After being destroyed by electrolysis the scars at the site of stenosis are so rapidly covered with epidermis that subsequent cicatricial contraction is slight. If stenosis involves the bony portions, the best plan is to abstain from all other methods and to proceed as in Körner's plastic operation on the auditory canal. (See page 406.)

There are still to be considered *fractures* and *fissures* of the antero-inferior bony wall of the auditory canal as the result of falls or blows on the chin. They are occasionally combined with other fractures of the petrous portion, but in most instances they occur alone. In addition to hemorrhage from the ear through laceration of the lining of the canal, there may occur exostoses of the respective portions of bone as a result of poor union or excessive callus; otherwise these injuries produce no effect.

Injuries of the external auditory canal as a result of accidental splashing with hot fluids or caustics are as a rule prevented by the position of the tragus in front of the external auditory meatus. If, however, the individual is lying on his side and such fluids are deliberately poured into the ear, as is sometimes done by rough individuals in order to wake up suddenly a sleeping fellow-workman, severe injuries may follow. These may even endanger life on account of the proximity of the meninges and the cavities of the labyrinth. When the fluids are sufficiently hot, as in the case of molten lead, death might take place immediately. The auditory canal tolerates superficial momentary action of strong caustic substances relatively well; even subsequent cicatricial stenosis is rare, as its lining is held rather tense by the cartilaginous ring. The drum-membrane, however, may be completely destroyed as a result of such action, with resulting long-continued suppuration.

If lead or other fluid metal is poured into the auditory canal, the treatment may occasionally be rendered difficult on account of the complete filling of the lumen with the hardened metal. Such metal-castings can, as a rule, be removed only by being broken up. As a result of such burns otitis externa generally occurs. Tenderness is in most instances very great, even if the mildest measures are used. The treatment of such injuries frequently requires general anæsthesia, and even under such conditions may be very difficult if some of the metal has reached the accessory spaces of the tympanic cavity. In such cases opening freely the cavities of the middle ear is indicated, the more so as on account of the injury hearing is generally destroyed and need not be considered.

FOREIGN BODIES IN THE EXTERNAL AUDITORY CANAL.

Foreign bodies frequently enter the external ear accidentally or are deliberately placed there. The majority of them are found in children; sometimes the latter insert them through playfulness; at times itching, occurring particularly in eczema of the auditory canal, may be responsible for these manipulations. Foreign bodies of all kinds are employed —buttons, pieces of toothpicks and matches; most frequently, cherry-

stones, peas, beans, glass-beads, small stones, and other ▓▓▓▓
In adults the foreign bodies are usually broken-off pieces ▓▓ ▓
inaptly employed for the removal of wax; plugs of cotton ▓▓▓
quently left in the ear. In addition, insects are found. The ▓
the so-called ear-wigs (*Forficula*) enter the ear is unforquded.

Most foreign bodies, especially in children, remain in the ▓
of the auditory canal immediately behind the projecting ▓▓▓
If they are found further inward, this is generally the result ▓
and persistent attempts at removal made either by the patie
selves or by relatives. Even physicians occasionally make ▓
attempting such removal, especially as to choice of instru
is stated in all text-books that forceps or bullet-forceps are lea:
for the removal of foreign bodies from the auditory canal, p
firm and smooth objects. But in spite of this, one of these in
is always the first to be employed. If it slips, as it usually
foreign body naturally advances deeper, and if the attempt a
is persisted in sufficiently long, it will reach that narrow port
boundary between the cartilaginous and the bony portion of
from which it is still more difficult to dislodge it. The forei
then very liable to reach the recess which is formed at the
anteroinferior portion of the auditory canal, where it is almo
sible. Small foreign bodies, such as minute insects, may be
concealed in this recess.

Treatment.—As long as a foreign body is situated in the ca
portion of the auditory canal it can usually be easily removed b
a forcible stream of water, with a syringe, into the auditory
latter being well retracted and stretched as in making exa
This method is usually successful unless sharp projections on t
body cause it to be caught in the wall of the auditory cana
stream of water is not successful and the patient is quiet
foreign body can be seen with the aid of light and mirror, a
may be made to pass a probe bent at right angles, or a sr
rounded hook, past the foreign body, and to withdraw
with the hook. Sharp hooks, which are frequently employed
adapted to the removal of soft bodies, particularly swollen
fruit-stones; but even in these cases care should be exercis
sharp book may penetrate the substance of the foreign body an
injure the walls of the auditory canal during the act of rem
in most cases surgeons have to do with children, and as the l
become restless if attempts at removal are not immediately s
such cases are best treated under general anæsthesia. It is
to be guided by the fact that most foreign bodies, as fi
danger of infection is concerned, may remain in the auditory
a long time without producing the slightest injury, and that, i
removal frequently becomes much easier after the lapse of so

---

[1] Living insects should be previously killed by dropping in alcohol, carbolised
simply oil, etc., in order that they may not be able to retain their hold.

There is only a minimal degree of reaction following the entrance of a foreign body unless the auditory canal has been injured as a result of unsuccessful attempts at removal, and unless at the same time infection of the wall of the auditory canal has occurred. And even if slight inflammation does occur, it may be successfully treated by the application of cold and antiseptic substances (iodoform-glycerin, carbolic acid glycerin, etc.). The swelling accompanying such inflammations is the greatest obstacle to removal, rendering the insertion of any instrument very painful, the narrowing of the canal making inspection impossible.

It is difficult to realize what a number of accidental injuries are produced by attempts to remove foreign bodies from the auditory canal, even by physicians. These injuries are most severe if a foreign body is only suspected to be present; and particularly when, as a matter of fact, none was inserted, or, as occasionally happens, where it was inserted only a short distance and has fallen out. That in such cases the drum-membrane should have been perforated with instruments employed in the removal of foreign bodies is excusable. Repeatedly, however, the malleus and even the incus and stapes have been extracted in place of a foreign body that never existed. Even more serious injuries have been reported—penetration of the promontory by the extraction instrument, perforation of the tegmen tympani, and other unfortunate occurrences. Recently in such a case a lawsuit resulted in the conviction of a practitioner for malpractice. Naturally, all surgical attempts do not terminate so seriously, but extensive laceration of the auditory canal, accidental perforation of the drum-membrane, etc., are frequently seen at the present day in spite of many warnings. It may be noted here that the danger of seeds swelling in consequence of irrigation is overestimated. If the object is not removed by irrigating, it may swell; but if attempts at irrigation fail, softening may be waited for, and then with proper instruments and further irrigation the body may be broken up and removed. Swelling may be combated by injecting a syringeful of alcohol. At the same time alcohol is an excellent substance with which to treat the otitis media which may follow such attempts at removal; to it may be added also 0.1 per cent. corrosive sublimate.

All forcible attempts at removal should be omitted unless rendered necessary by a very painful otitis externa caused by the foreign body or by attempts at its removal, or by other severe, especially cerebral manifestations. If in such urgent cases one has to deal with an inaccessible foreign body, one that has penetrated to the tympanic cavity and that cannot be detected on inspection, or if under anæsthesia it is impossible to insert a blunt hook behind the foreign body without inflicting injury, or if the auditory canal is so narrow that it seems impossible to pass the foreign body through it, it is better, instead of further attempts at extraction, to make a curved incision as far as the bone, behind the auricle, and to incise the posterosuperior wall of the auditory canal in a longitudinal direction as far as possible, using a grooved director in the auditory canal as a guide. By means of this wide incision removal can usually be easily effected. Occasionally it may be necessary to open the bony canal at its posterosuperior aspect with a chisel, the wound behind the auricle, and after control of hemorrhage if drum-membrane can be inspected, provided the longitudinal in the membranous canal is carried as near as possible to the dru brane and joined externally by two transverse incisions, so that t tory canal can be unfolded in two flaps. After the operation the wound can be sutured. During the after-treatment care must cised to prevent stenosis of the auditory canal. This is best plished by firmly packing with iodoform gauze.

INJURIES OF THE DRUM-MEMBRANE.

Etiology.—Injuries of the drum-membrane are divided in caused by direct and those by indirect violence. Those ca indirect violence are by far the most frequent, and are most c result of variations of air-pressure.

A normal drum-membrane is not very liable to injury from increase or decrease of air-pressure. Sudden variations in pres more readily overcome its power of resistance. Most drum-mei in which such injuries are observed were evidently previously dis the result of calcareous deposits, atrophy, or other changes. Dist of hearing does not necessarily accompany such changes. Fre however, the latter has existed, but was only noted after trau Objectively, the existence of such changes can only be determine: days after injury when the accompanying hemorrhage has subs Most injuries of the drum-membrane occur through increase ure. Rarefaction of the air in the auditory canal may, howe produce rupture, though this is usually insignificant. Mild de rarefaction may be sufficient, such as a kiss on the ear or sudd drawal of the finger placed in the ear. These ruptures are o analogous to those produced by increased air-pressure. Even com of air need not be very great in order to burst the drum-memt blow on the ear producing such an injury need not necessarily ha very severe. It is not so much the absolute degree of pressure suddenness of its development. Explosions in the vicinity of the the next most frequent cause of injury of the drum-membrane. C rupture or loss of substance of the membrane does not alway: more frequently there is found only a hæmatoma or a small extra: of blood. Increase of air-pressure in the Eustachian tubes, anc quently in the middle ear, is rarely an etiological factor. This h observed in players on wind-instruments; it occurs also after sneezing, but usually in cases in which the drum-membrane v normal. Rupture is occasionally caused by therapeutic measures on the part of the physician or the patient, in forcing air into the ear by means of a catheter, Politzer's method, etc. In these cas the surgeon has to deal with drum-membranes that have been pre diseased.

A special form of injury of the drum-membrane occurs during and after diving. In ordinary diving (without apparatus) the drum-membrane, with the rest of the body, is subjected to the full weight of the overlying column of water, as far as this weight is not balanced by increased air-pressure in the mouth and nasopharynx when the nose is closed. In most instances, however, this balance is not complete even if the nose be closed by a special clamp. For this reason rupture of the membrane frequently occurs in ordinary diving. Hemorrhage from the ear has come to be considered a sign of special proficiency in the art, as among the Greek sponge-divers. As rupture is regularly followed by entrance of considerable water into the middle ear, inflammation is developed, and if, as is usually the case, the act is repeated, serious injury of the drum-membrane may be produced.

In the case of divers who are provided with helmets or who work under compressed air in a diver's bell, the drum-membrane is subjected to severe pressure, particularly when at great depths; this is equalized, however, by breathing air that is under the same degree of atmospheric pressure, and by opening the Eustachian tubes, voluntarily or automatically by swallowing, in order to allow compressed air to enter them. (See A. Hartmann, *Investigations of the Pneumatic Cabinet.*) The entrance of compressed air may be prevented by pathological change in the nasopharynx (enlargement of the pharyngeal tonsil, stenosis of the tubes, etc.), or from lack of skill, or through emotional disturbance, and in such cases rupture of the drum-membrane may occur. Most divers, even those who use the helmet, suffer sooner or later from impairment of hearing.

It may be noted here that more severe disturbances of another character may occur as a result of rapid lowering of air-pressure. Under normal conditions variations of pressure on the drum-membrane act externally and internally at the same time. Changes in the tube may prevent this equalization, but ruptures of the membrane occur rarely even then. As a rule only small extravasations of blood have been found. Serious results follow from the fact that under higher pressure the blood absorbs more oxygen, which is rapidly given off under lower pressure. At the same time there occur extravasation and laceration in the vicinity of the vessels. The principal effect under these circumstances is manifested in the labyrinth, and not in the middle ear; the former, like the spinal cord and delicate nervous organs, may suffer considerable injury by the escape of bubbles of air. (See investigations of Alt and P. Koch.)

Injuries of the drum-membrane in case of fracture of the base (see page 88) are most frequently caused by indirect violence. Fissures of the base of the skull frequently traverse the tegmen tympani and the annulus tympanicus or its vicinity. The drum-membrane may then be torn by the sudden displacement of the edges of the fracture. Lacerations may be situated in a variety of different places, but most frequently occur at the borders of the membrane, and frequently extend to the wall of the auditory canal. Otherwise they possess the same character as all other traumatic perforations. They acquire special significance through

the fact that a tear of the dura may occur at the same time. Hem
which is at first profuse, is then followed by a flow of cerebrospi
and by the same path that the latter finds an outlet infectiou
may enter the cranial cavity.

Injuries of the drum-membrane and the tympanic cavity
direct violence occur far less frequently, but are often followed b
results. As a rule it happens that while an individual is prod
ear with a toothpick he suddenly moves his head or is knocked
and forces the instrument through his drum-membrane. Inju
caused by penetration of straws and branches of trees and by
attempts at removing actual or suspected foreign bodies. In sucl
the inflicting object may, according to its direction, penetra
as the wall of the tympanic cavity or through the latter, especially
the fenestra ovalis, into the labyrinth; or, on the other hand,
the tegmen tympani into the cavity of the skull. If the labyr

Fig. 106.

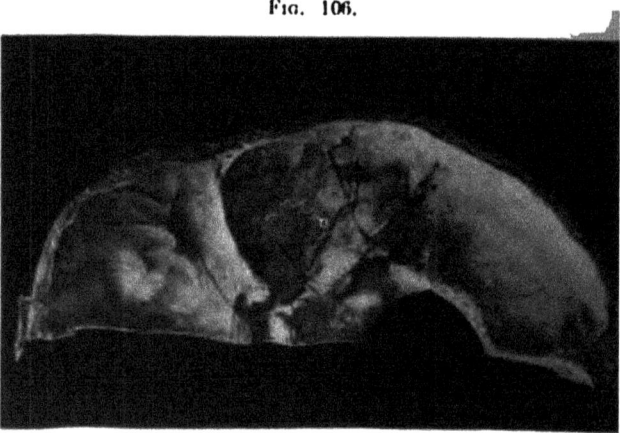

been injured, there are sudden and severe attacks of dizziness,
and at the same time severe subjective auditory impression
patients fall down unless they can grasp some object, and may b
to stand or sit for weeks. After some days or from two to fou
the symptoms subside, and usually it is only then that loss of
hearing is discovered. This is as a rule complete. If at the sa
the labyrinth or the tympanic cavity is infected, or if otitis m
previously existed, labyrinthitis may be brought about, and fr
infection may travel through the internal auditory meatus or th
ductus vestibuli to the meninges. Such infections may run a
course and terminate fatally within a few days. As a rule they
weeks and months, recovery finally taking place; but usually ther
permanent and complete deafness in the affected ear. Injuries
from direct violence usually affect the vestibule; those caused by
of the base, generally the semicircular canals, especially the extern

circular canal. Less frequently the bony capsule of the cochlea is injured, but hemorrhage into the canals of the cochlea as well as into the semicircular canals frequently occurs. Owing to the delicate character of the nerve-endings in the labyrinth such hemorrhage generally causes complete destruction of nerve-substance.

Diagnosis.—The diagnosis of rupture of the drum-membrane is difficult when due to direct as well as to indirect violence. If the patient is seen soon after injury, the auditory canal is as a rule filled with coagulated blood, or at least the site of rupture is covered with a blood-clot. Cleansing of the auditory canal is possible by the aid of irrigation; this

Fig. 107.

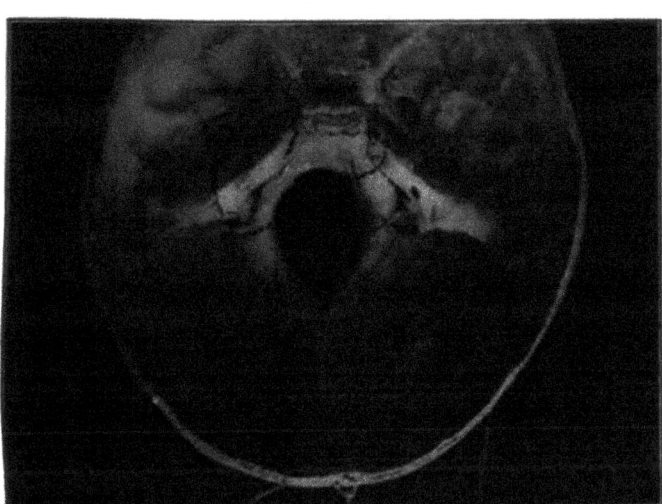

should, however, never be attempted. In case of such recent injury the determination of its extent and localization is of little significance; one should be content with the fact that considerable hemorrhage rarely follows injury of the wall of the auditory canal, and that when such hemorrhage is present, injury of the drum-membrane is very probable. If the determination of the site of perforation is desirable, attempts may be made to swab it out carefully with cotton. Generally, however, this is not necessary. If a view of the site of injury should be obtained shortly after its occurrence, only an irregular shaped dark spot or stripe is seen as a rule; surrounding this the drum-membrane may be markedly discolored by hemorrhage, while at a distance it appears more or less normal. The majority of ruptures, excepting those occurring in fracture of the base, are situated in the intermediary zone, about midway between the handle of the mallens and the annulus tympanicus; they occur, however, frequently in other parts of the drum-membrane. They vary greatly in size. The borders are usually irregularly serrated, corresponding to

the natural tendency would be to refer such complications to these irrigations. However, meningitis can occur without irrigations. This danger is especially great if suppuration of the ear has existed before injury; infectious germs may then reach the meninges through fissures. Under such circumstances these secretions must be rendered harmless by opening the cells and the antrum, and possibly, also, by seeking the site through which infection has reached the cavity of the skull. Fatal meningitis can be prevented, as was discussed in detail on page 106 and in subsequent pages of this volume.

INJURIES OF THE TYMPANIC CAVITY.

These injuries have in part been mentioned above. It may be noted here that occasionally, though rarely, there occurs fracture of the malleus, usually at the middle of the manubrium, more rarely fractures of the long process of incus. Such fractures sometimes unite with marked displacement of fragments, as a result of which the power of vibration of the ossicles may be seriously impaired. Also the adhesions between such injured bones and the surrounding mucous membrane which frequently occur after such injuries, particularly if they are situated in the vicinity of the stapes, may produce considerable impairment of hearing. It is hardly possible to prevent displacement during the process of repair; ankyloses and adhesions can be prevented by mechanical measures—passive motion of the drum-membrane, by increasing and diminishing air-pressure, either in the Eustachian tube or in the external auditory canal.

GUNSHOT INJURIES OF THE EAR.

Injuries resulting from firearms deserve special discussion, for, though they are rarely observed in the ear, they possess certain peculiarities. Occasionally the auricle or auditory canal is injured by a projectile, in most cases as a result of a glancing shot, or the projectile passes through the auricle and then penetrates the bone somewhere in the vicinity. By particular coincidence a projectile may strike exactly in the auditory canal. Under such circumstances, in case of older types of firearms and small revolvers, it usually remains embedded in the bony portion of the auditory canal and completely closes the latter. In this way it causes the drum-membrane and chain of ossicles to be forcibly driven inward. Frequently this results in severe concussion of the labyrinth; even complete inhibition of hearing may result, which may disappear after several weeks or a few days. Occasionally this may remain permanently. With modern firearms the projectile may by the same path penetrate deeper into the tympanic cavity and labyrinth. In the cases reported the projectile has generally passed through the mastoid cells, especially where these are well developed, or has come through the mouth from the opposite side of the body. In such instances there resulted as a rule extensive fracture and comminution of the temporal

NS OF THE EAR.

al Ear.—Etiology.—It was noted above
...e of chronic chondritis and perichon-
It is doubtful whether such processes
...y usually run their course without caus-
...produce an annoying sensation of tension
markedly swollen, the skin is reddened
...h processes generally affect the lateral
...xisted for some time, recovery generally
...catricial contraction.
...t, as has been observed particularly after
...and also after general infections (as
...frequently radiating pain. Swelling and
...distinct, and suppuration usually occurs
...le of the ear is more frequently involved,
...face also is affected. After spontaneous
...recovery takes place with the formation
...made early results in severe deformity.
...treatment be confined to "antiphlogistic"
...tion is suspected incision should be made

...ns a similar though more chronic course,
...ge, tumor-like swellings before suppura-
...e occasionally affects apparently healthy
...occur.
...by gouty nodules. Pain is not so severe
...rge toe. As soon as a tophus has fully
...ppear.
...urs frequently in the pinna. It is caused
...*Pediculosis capitis*, also by various chemical,

frequent and produce less disturbance, especially no pain. Th
panying itching may lead to manipulation of the auditory cana
latter be followed by a painful otitis externa. Many other skii
which are occasionally found on the external ear, as well as
parts of the face, and which present the same appearance an
same course as elsewhere, need no discussion.

Furuncles rarely occur, as the skin of the pinna possesses
downy hairs. Similar, however, are inflamed sebaceous gl
comedones. Especially in the concha these may attain conside
and form thin-walled abscesses as large as a pea or a bean.
directions for their diagnosis and treatment are unnecessary.

Inflammations of the auditory canal possess more interest.
and a circumscribed form are distinguished. The diffuse for
from the action of pus flowing out of the ear, more rarely throug
substances or irritating preparations, such as carbolic acid or i
It usually causes a painful swelling of the walls of the auditoi
which may lead to narrowing or even complete closure of the

The various forms of diseases due to moulds are peculiar,
become rare. A great variety of moulds (see Siebenmann)
formation of soft, crumbling membranes which can easily be
mechanically, but which readily form again. They may cover t
auditory canal, especially its deeper portions, and may even
tympanic membrane. The wall of the passage beneath the m
is intensely red and markedly swollen. In most cases there is
pain, frequently also slight fever. The mould-crusts may lea
being mistaken for a diphtheritic membrane or slough due to
these are distinguished, however, by the fact that they are thickly
all over or in certain portions with the various colored spor
particular kind of mould. If the membranes that have been wi
or removed by other means be treated with potassium hydroxide
the mycelia and possibly also the spores can be readily demo
These mycoses require the use of disinfecting solutions, such as
acid glycerin (10 per cent.), or alcoholic solution of salicylic ac
cent.), pure alcohol, etc.; untreated the disease may continue f
time.

Diagnosis and Treatment.—In general the diagnosis and trea
diffuse otitis externa are the same as those of the circumscrib
which is of more frequent occurrence. The latter (furuncles) a
gous to those of the integument, but the necrotic plug is small
easily recognizable, so that frequently only a cone-shaped sw
found in the auditory canal. Swelling of the adjacent portions i
considerable, and may often completely obscure the primary
affection. In most instances furuncles are caused by prodding
the canal with various instruments; men usually employ per
lead-pencils, toothpicks, and matches; women almost always u
pins and knitting-needles. Infection is especially liable to occur
purulent secretion from the tympanic cavity in the auditory
Clinically furuncles of the external auditory canal run the same

as in other portions of the integument, and after spontaneous or surgical evacuation they heal rapidly. As a rule a number of furuncles appear in succession, for on account of the narrowness of the passage new areas are readily infected.

As in diabetes diffuse and circumscribed otitis externa occur frequently even during the early stage of the disease, examination of the urine should never be omitted.

The diagnosis of otitis externa is usually easy. Where, however, the auditory canal is much swollen it is occasionally impossible to insert even the smallest size speculum and distend the canal in order to inspect the drum-membrane. It is thus impossible to exclude otitis media. If in such cases there is considerable swelling of the surrounding soft parts, particularly in the region of the mastoid process, it may be difficult to decide whether this is the result of an otitis externa or of an accompanying inflammation of the middle ear. While in the former "periauricular" inflammation as a rule recedes, and while in these cases delay is of no consequence, in periostitis of the mastoid process operative interference is urgently indicated. The differential diagnosis is therefore important.

Above all, it should be noted that marked disturbance of the sense of hearing occurs in otitis externa only when there is complete closure of the auditory canal. This may frequently be relieved by passing a small speculum, or by cleansing the passage; if deafness disappears, the diagnosis is cleared up, for even slight inflammation of the middle ear produces distinct impairment of hearing.

Further points are: The localization of the swelling. The lymphatics of the external ear empty for the most part into the preauricular lymphglands very constantly present in the fossa between the tragus and the cheeks. The lymphatics of the middle ear, on the other hand, usually empty into the glands situated along the squamomastoid suture, which are almost as constant in their presence. Swelling of the latter would therefore point to disease of the middle ear. During later stages the skin of the respective regions becomes swollen; if, particularly, the furrow between the tragus and the cheek is obliterated, it is to be concluded that otitis externa is present, without, however, being able to exclude inflammation of the middle ear. If, however, this region is relatively normal, while the skin over the mastoid process is considerably swollen, one would, on the contrary, conclude that disease of the middle ear and its accessory cavities was present.

Finally, in otitis externa the swelling is usually superficial, localized above the periosteum of the auditory canal and the mastoid process. It frequently advances in the subcutaneous tissue to the surface of the pinna toward the head, or possibly also to its lateral surface, obliterating the retroauricular furrow. In otitis media the swelling over the mastoid process is due to the accompanying inflammation of the mastoid cells, and is therefore at first situated beneath the periosteum, so that the furrow between the pinna and mastoid process is preserved. In the latter case the pinna as a whole is forced away from the head.

All these points will, however, be valueless as soon as the external and

III.

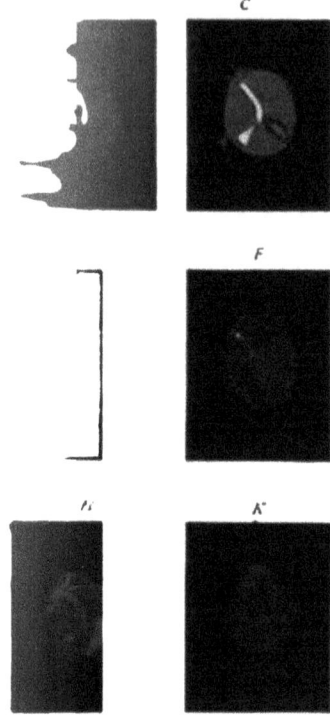

of the faucial tonsils. Various diseases of the nasopharynx, as, for example, nasal and pharyngeal polyps, swelling of the posterior extremity of the turbinated bones, also chronic pharyngeal catarrh, particularly inflammation of the " recessus pharyngei " (see Diseases of the Pharynx); less frequently chronic diseases of the nose, as, for example, atrophic rhinitis, empyema of the accessory cavities, are the immediate cause. With all these an acute irritation may become the direct exciting cause. Frequently also external irritation, such as irrigation of the nose, gargling with inappropriate substances, also cold applications producing an acute inflammation of the nose, chemical irritation of the nasal and pharyngeal mucous membrane, as the influence of vitiated air or noxious gases. Cold, particularly after previous overheating, certainly plays an important etiological part. As a rule, however, these act only by causing a catarrhal inflammation of the nasal and pharyngeal mucous membrane. The action of cold air or entrance of cold water into the ear, and similar injurious factors may, by simple thermal injury of the middle ear through the drum-membrane, bring about a mild otitis media. If, however, as is seldom the case, the inflammation becomes more severe, it may be assumed that the micro-organisms normally present in the healthy tube can, as a result of the inflammation, find conditions in the tympanic cavity more favorable for invasion and propagation, and by their proliferation increase the inflammation.

Where it is possible to observe middle-ear inflammation early, the manifestations of a "tubal catarrh" are first present. Swelling of the mucous membrane of the tubes produces a narrowing of the lumen of the tubes, and thus the tympanic cavity is shut off from the pharynx; air, not being renewed, is soon absorbed, as in every other cavity of the body, and the atmospheric pressure forces the drum-membrane inward, so that the normal central retraction becomes increased. On inspection the drum-membrane appears more retracted, and as a rule distinctly glistening. If the condition has existed for some time, there is more injection of the drum-membrane, causing the latter to assume a deeper, more violet color. The vessels behind the manubrium of the malleus and the fine radiating vessels are engorged. The vacuum in the tympanic cavity is not completely balanced by the change in position of the drum membrane; and as a result of the latter being subjected to less pressure passive hyperæmia of the mucous membrane of the tympanic cavity is produced, and according to most authors there occurs serous effusion, "hydrops ex vacuo." Whether, however, this is not the product of a mild inflammation, cannot be decided at present. Be that as it may, if the process is not terminated during this stage, distinct manifestations occur within a short time. Injection of the drum-membrane is increased; the exudate contains more albumin, as a result of which it becomes amber-yellow in color, which can at times be appreciated through the drum-membrane if the latter is transparent. Frequently, however, the boundary between the yellow and the more grayish portion of the drum-membrane can be appreciated only as a black or glistening line (so-called "*exudate line*"). Occasionally the exudate shows a certain mobility when the position of the head is changed. As on account of ca attraction in the abnormally narrow tympanic cavity, the line ; follows an irregular curve, deception is very liable to occur. the line is so delicate and sharp that it may be mistaken for a ha attempts made to wipe it off.

If the inflammatory manifestations increase, the injection of the membrane becomes more marked; the color, which at first was becomes more purely red, finally becoming a brilliant scarlet or ass the color of a dull copper plate. On account of the pressure increased quantity of exudate the drum-membrane becomes fla throughout its extent or bulges forward in circumscribed portions cause of the circumscribed bulging is to be sought for in the f mucous membrane and bands traversing the tympanic cavity, parti in the posterior and superior portions of the tympanic cavity. The many such folds of mucous membrane between the manubrium malleus, long process of the incus, stapes, and the region of the f ovalis. It happens, therefore, when they swell as a result of inflammation, that the respective portion of the drum-membrane i pletely closed off. Such a bulging in the superior posterior quad at first flatly spherical. If, as a result of inflammation, the drum brane at certain portions loses its power of resistance, it may h conical or sacculated, overlapping a large part of the underlying p and thus produce the appearance of a granulation polyp. More there is analogous bulging of Shrapnell's membrane, which cove short process of the malleus. This condition points to involv primarily of the anterior lateral region of the epitympanic recess.

If circumscribed bulging is not produced, the drum-membrane u perforates in its inferior portion after inflammation has continuec number of days. This results from lack of nutrition of the mem caused by inflammation and stretching. These perforations occasi produce very small openings, as if the membrane had been pun by a needle. In case of more severe inflammation these hole become as large as the head of a pin or a pea. In very severe which follow general infectious diseases, the entire drum-membran be destroyed, the manubrium of the mallens being as it were left dis out. In case of circumscribed bulging perforation ultimately take also, but as a rule only at the most projecting point, where it is sul to the greatest degree of pressure by the exudate. The exudate, e under considerable tension, is evacuated and the sac collapses account of the valve-like closing of the tear further evacuation take only when pressure again reaches a certain height, and in this w process may continue for weeks, while after perforation of the portion of the drum-membrane, which is as a rule more extensive, i mation rapidly subsides.

SYMPTOMS.—The most prominent symptom of the disease, c cases of mild inflammation, is pain. In most instances it sets in sn and soon becomes severe. It is as a rule described as boring, pou and stabbing in character, frequently radiating to the regions surrot

the ear, to the temporal bone, and particularly to the mastoid process
In the beginning spontaneous pain predominates, but later there is distinct tenderness on pressure throughout the whole region surrounding
the ear, especially over the mastoid process. In children simply touching
the external ear causes violent crying; on being washed they protest
vigorously. Following this the root of the mastoid process and the lymph-
gland, mentioned above as situated here, begin to be tender on pressure
and frequently remain sensitive throughout the entire course. Later,
however, the principal pain is situated in the tip of the mastoid process,
particularly in its posterior portion, where a large air-space is situated.
The localization of tenderness depends very much upon the well-known
variation in the character of the air-spaces, but in some inflammation
there is always some localized point of tenderness over the bone. Even
if the process does not go beyond that of a serous catarrh, adults at any
rate generally complain of a sensation of pressure and fulness, as if a
foreign body were present; children also complain of pain, which generally comes on in successive attacks.

After pain the most noticeable symptoms are subjective auditory perceptions, which are as a rule pulsating in character, frequently also
ringing and hissing; in milder cases there are humming noises. More
rarely there is increased resonance of the patient's own voice ("auto-
phonia"). As inflammatory manifestations increase, impairment of
hearing and at the same time the pain become more prominent, sounds
and speech are perceived as coming from a distance. Acuteness of hearing rapidly diminishes to almost complete loss of perceptions of sounds
transmitted by air. Tuning-forks placed on the bone are, however, more
distinctly heard by the diseased ear.

In milder forms of inflammation the general condition of the patient
is little, or not at all, impaired. Frequently the symptoms due to the
ear trouble are obscured by the symptoms of the primary causative disease. Headache, sensation of pressure in the ears and in the head, slight
febrile movement, disturbance of appetite, etc., are sufficiently explained
by an existing coryza, influenza, or other sickness. As the inflammatory
manifestations increase distinct signs of severe infection are developed.
The temperature frequently rises suddenly, but is irregular, with marked
variations and distinct evening exacerbations; in young individuals it
may reach 104° F., or even 106° F. Marked remissions occur, even to
subnormal, particularly in the morning, so that one is liable to make the
mistake of concluding that the disease has terminated. But the subjective symptoms do not subside. The general disturbance is most severe
in children, the more severe the younger they are. There are violent
headaches, marked stupor, and drowsiness. Even complete temporary
loss of consciousness or general convulsions are not rare in very young
children. Frequently meningitis or typhoid is wrongly suspected, and
it is surprising what a great change in the condition of these little patients
is produced by paracentesis of the drum-membrane. But in the most
severe forms of inflammation adults also suffer very much; besides the
fever there is great lassitude, and there may be complete loss of sleep

and appetite. After perforation the subjective symptoms subside и
... there is free evacuation of the exudate. If, however, th
... is situated at the apex of a cone-shaped projection, or if
complications are present, there is only an abatement of the sub‹
symptoms, or frequently sudden variations in their severity, and it і
after some time, frequently only after surgical interference, th
symptoms permanently disappear.

During the further course, instead of the profuse thin, almost ·
pus, there is after a few hours a more consistent, more mucous
in the course of a few days this diminishes in quantity, becomes
and sticky, and finally only a small quantity of glairy mucus is |
out. After complete cessation of the secretion the site of the perfoi
remains visible for a short time, then becomes closed, its edges, f‹
white wheals, approach each other and become united. Repaii
the production of distinct granulation, is found only in case of
extensive defects. After the site of perforation has become clo‹
abnormal retraction of the drum-membrane frequently continues
time until, as the result of a spontaneous opening up of the tube
inflation of air, the tympanic cavity again becomes filled. Not unt
is the acuteness of hearing restored. In the normal course the la
not materially impaired, even after extensive perforation and prot
course.

The duration of inflammation of the middle ear varies betweer
limits. If suppuration does not take place, if the drum-mem
remains uninjured, the whole course may be completed in a we
case of children possibly within two to three days. Those cases in v
without inflammatory manifestations, the exudate does not disa
the so-called chronic secreting middle-ear inflammations, need i
discussed here, as they are of exclusively otological interest. In c
rapid recovery without perforation it is to be assumed that evaci
of the exudate takes place through the tube, which has become o
up in some way. If perforation has taken place, it is rare in adu
recovery to be completed in less than three to four weeks, and
unfavorable position of the perforation a duration of from six to
weeks is not unusual and in itself of no unfavorable significance.
certain that acute suppuration may run into a chronic one, pro
every chronic otitis not caused by any specific disease or diathesis
in this way. The author has never been able to observe such a c
and other observers have had the same experience. It may be ass
therefore, that the occurrence of chronic suppuration without ᵴ
complication can only take place as a result of failure or lack of
ment. In view of the large number of cases of chronic otitis which
physician has an opportunity of observing, this fact deserves
specially emphasized.

COMPLICATIONS.—Acute middle-ear inflammation may be follow
severe involvement of the accessory air-spaces, the epitympanic
(attic), and the hypotympanic recess, and particularly the antrui
the mastoid cells; ulceration of the bony walls of the tympanic

or exposure of single portions of or complete exposure of the auditory ossicles, with subsequent periostitis or necrosis; extension of inflammation to the labyrinth; disease of the veins adjacent to the temporal bone; disease of the brain and the meninges.

Inflammation of the Accessory Air-spaces.—As was noted before, in every case of severe acute otitis media the lining of the epitympanic recess, the mastoid antrum, and cells are affected. The network of bands in the region of the incus and malleus, which bounds these spaces from the mesotympanum, prevents the entrance into these spaces of any large number of infectious micro-organisms when infection travels from the tube, except under unfavorable circumstances. As a rule therefore such affections are always mild in character.

What unfavorable circumstances may act as injurious factors are not exactly known. One of the most important of them is large size of the accessory cavities. Whenever it becomes necessary in cases of acute otitis to open the bone, the mastoid process is almost sure to contain large air-spaces; or an unusually wide communication exists between the tympanic cavity and the antrum; or a special arrangement of the bands situated near its boundary may come into consideration. Under certain circumstances the latter may produce a valve-like action, allowing the entrance of infectious agents, but preventing the escape of inflammatory secretion so that a good culture-medium for infectious micro-organisms is accumulated. General constitutional condition must also be considered. In diabetes otitis frequently involves the mastoid process. Influenza, which usually affects the general condition of the patient to a considerable degree, acts in a similar manner; also other infectious diseases, like typhoid fever.

Occasionally infection does not proceed from the middle ear, but both regions are infected at the same time through the circulation. In other cases again one must assume the occurrence of primary "osteomyelitis petrosa." The occurrence of the latter is difficult to prove, as it must necessarily soon lead to infection of the tympanic cavity, and it will then be impossible to determine where the primary focus was situated. Autopsies in which only the mastoid process was affected have not been reported so far. Clinically, however, it has been possible to elicit marked tenderness of the mastoid process some time before inflammation of the drum-membrane was manifested. One could not properly consider the middle-ear disease secondary and that of the bone primary. In diabetes primary disease of the mastoid process has been positively confirmed in a number of instances (Körner).

The most important way in which the accessory cavities become diseased is that evacuation of pus is prevented. By prompt treatment this can undoubtedly and should be avoided. Where the drum-membrane is intact, and where the middle ear is filled with an accumulation of pus that can only incompletely drain through the tube, pressure soon increases sufficiently to force the secretion into the accessory cavities, so that the mucous membrane of the latter is bathed by a considerable number of infectious organisms and severely infected.

As soou as a periosteal abscess has been formed, it may spontaneously rupture externally—mastoid fistula. At the same time more severe inflammatory symptoms usually subside. Recovery only takes place, however, if a large deep sequestrum is formed and thrown off, producing a large opening leading to the antrum. In most instances this does not occur, and while exuberant granulations vainly attempt to throw off the sequestrum, they only bring about extensive destruction of other portions of the temporal bone, which may reach the tegmen tympani or the posterior fossa of the skull.

Not infrequently inflammation of the mastoid process breaks through on the inner surface into the digastric fossa. This occurs less frequently, however, than external rupture. In order that it may occur, there must be present a large cell on the inner side of the mastoid process. The anatomical relations present in this form of rupture have been carefully studied by Bezold. If rupture takes place in this way, pus reaches the deep layers of cervical connective tissue and produces an abscess of the latter. Very frequently there is also extensive suppuration of the glands accompanied by severe septic symptoms. Under such circumstances inflammatory swelling in this situation might be mistaken for manifestations accompanying phlebitis of the jugular vein.

Like the mastoid process, the roof of the auditory canal may in portions undergo necrosis and be destroyed. In this way disease of the antrum may in rare cases be followed by recovery. An attempt is made to imitate this process in the method of complete operation, to be described later, just as external rupture serves as a reason for simple surgical opening of the antrum.

The most unfavorable termination is that pus or granulation-tissue confined within the mastoid process burrows toward the dura or into the labyrinth. These perforations may take place in a similar manner to those finding their way toward the external surface of the mastoid process, perhaps as the result of simple ulceration through pressure of the swollen mucous membrane ("granulations") confined within the bone. Rupture takes place either through the tegmen tympani into the middle fossa of the skull, or through the posterior mastoid cells into the sigmoid fossa or the region of the latter. In acute otitis the latter seems to be of more frequent occurrence, possible because in the most posterior, distant cells drainage is most likely to be impeded sufficiently to produce high pressure and consequent destruction of the bone-lamellæ. This results in what is called extradural abscess.

In the course of middle-ear inflammation rupture into the labyrinth may occur through one of the fenestræ. Not infrequently it follows chronic disease of the temporal bone through erosion or necrosis of that portion of the external semicircular canal which forms the median wall of the antrum near its floor. Inflammation may frequently be limited to the semicircular canal for some time and produce new symptoms, but sooner or later it may extend through the perilymphatic spaces to the vestibule, and possibly through the aqueducts or the sheath of the auditory nerve to the arachnoid space. Labyrinth disease is manifested clin-

membrane of the cells is usually markedly injected, but only slightly thickened; the contained pus is thick and creamy, and of a yellow color. In these forms the process frequently becomes chronic, the mucous membrane of the cells becoming pale, but remaining somewhat thickened and secreting permanently a slightly purulent fluid containing much mucous, which continues to flow out through the persistent opening in the drum-membrane. After weeks, months, or years conditions frequently become worse. There is a sudden rise in temperature, occasionally accompanied by a chill, and periostitis of the mastoid process or some intracranial complication develops. The usual cause of these exacerbations is an acute lighting-up of the inflammation in the mesotympanus. Sometimes this is due to fresh infection (influenza, coryza, etc.), sometimes to external irritation of various kinds, most frequently to stopping of the flow of pus (granulations, etc.). Such cases may be called acute or chronic empyema of the air-cells, even if they are decidedly different from cases of empyema of the pleura, for example.

b. Inflammatory infiltration of the lining of the cavities of the temporal bone.—Exuberant "proliferation of granulations"—*i. e.*, marked swelling of the mucous membrane lining the cells, frequently associated with extensive softening or destruction of the bone, or with cortical and deep necrosis of bone—is frequently found in cases of otitis which run a very acute course and which continue to exhibit very severe symptoms, especially cases of influenza otitis. This form preferably affects bones with large air-spaces. On opening the mastoid process in such cases no pus is found, or only a few drops, within the spaces, which are completely filled by proliferation of the mucous membrane. In the antrum also there is frequently very little pus; on the other hand, it frequently happens that a large abscess situated either within the bone or extradurally is opened. In this form the clinical manifestations are usually severe; as a rule there are severe pain and rather high fever which frequently shows only slight remissions. Complications generally develop rapidly in the course of the first two or three weeks following the onset of acute otitis.

c. Ostitis of the temporal bone.—Occasionally it happens that most of the cavities of the bone show not the slightest sign of inflammation; that, however, single cells are diseased alone, either those at the apex, or sometimes those at the posterior edge of the mastoid process. The remaining cavities in the bone are lined with pale thin mucous membrane. In most instances a number of inflammatory foci are present; the bone surrounding them is usually markedly injected and somewhat softened, occasionally small sequestra are present. These forms the author would, with some degree of probability, accept as being due to primary disease of the bone (see above).

In nearly every case of mastoid disease the termination of otitis media is considerably retarded; only very rarely is it possible to operate sufficiently early to avoid this. Especially the protracted forms just described may pursue their course for a long time without causing great disturbance, so that it is difficult to decide upon an operation. But they bring about a condition of chronic suppuration and sooner or l render operation necessary. The other forms are more liable to b about periostitic manifestations or severe complications, and for reason they are generally operated upon sooner. If this is not done, if the patient does not succumb to complications, there results rup externally, with the formation of fistula; whereupon the process continue for a long time, and after existing for a longer or shorter leads to disastrous consequences.

Clinical Manifestations.—The clinical manifestations are insignifi in the protracted form; in the other forms pain is usually not so se as in the beginning of an otitis, but sufficiently severe to disturb condition of the patient. Subjective pains are described as boring tearing in character, referred to the depth of the ears, and frequi also to the temporal bone. They frequently show irregular remiss in severity. Pain caused by pressure is much more severe. As a the most sensitive portion is near the base. Where single cells are principal seat of disease the corresponding portion of the exte surface is found to be tender on pressure. Pain is most sevei periostitis has set in.

The character of the fever is similar to that of otitis itself—*i. e.*, ' irregular, frequently remitting very much in the course of a day, t followed by a rapid rise. Rapid or continuous rise of temperatui always suspicious of extension of the disease and demands energ treatment. Fever is seldom entirely absent; still at times days may j with none or only very little rise of temperature. If other complicat set in, the temperature-curve undergoes a corresponding change.

The remaining disturbances, loss of appetite and sleep, lassitude, (are in most instances marked, particularly in children. The r severe disturbances are present during the development of perios or extradural abscess.

Diagnosis.—The diagnosis of mastoid disease is frequently difficult at its onset. Tenderness over the bone, as was mentio several times, occurs in nearly every case of severe acute otitis me Whether the manifestations are those of a simple otitis media or symptoms of an accumulation of pus in the bone is frequently diffi to decide. At all events, tenderness on pressure is one of the n important points upon which to base a diagnosis. Especially if an of tenderness, originally limited to a definite point, spreads rapidly, can conclude that disease of the bone exists. More positive points the occurrence of circumscribed or diffuse periostitic swelling. Du the earliest stage of the latter it is frequently found at the poste surface of the mastoid process. Actual purulent perforation and swell immediately preceding the latter are more frequently localised at rest of the process. Comparing both sides of the body does not alw offer positive results, as frequently both mastoid processes vary in tl degree of development.

Errors in diagnosis are very liable to be made as a result of p auricular phlegmon following simple otitis externa. This is frequen situated, as was mentioned above, in the soft parts overlying the mastoid process, not infrequently also in the skin of the neck below the external auditory meatus, and at times also in the region of the parotid. The author has offered a number of important points in differential diagnosis on page 363; in general if otitis media is positively known to be present, it would be more natural to assume the presence of mastoid disease than purely periauricular inflammation. In the worst case, if diagnosis is uncertain, incision of a phlegmon cannot but help the patient, while failure to operate in mastoid disease may lead to serious consequences. In order to determine whether operative interference is necessary or not, it is important to compare the temperature-curve with the conditions found in the ear, the tenderness on pressure over the bones, and with any possible manifestations of importance. If, for instance, the temperature rises without important changes in the appearance of the drum-membrane, or if marked variations in temperature continue for several weeks after perforation took place, it would point to suppuration within the bone, particularly when perforation of the drum-membrane occurred late, as mentioned above, in the superior posterior quadrant. If there is also tenderness on pressure at the posterior surface or base of the mastoid process for a long time, while the site of perforation remains open and the appearance of the drum-membrane shows abatement of the inflammatory symptoms, one can pretty positively assume the presence of pus in the bone. Still more in favor of the latter would be the continued secretion of pus from an opening situated in the superior posterior opening, accompanied by some, if only slight, pain in the bone. Profuse suppuration is by no means a sign that perforation is free. In the conical bulging there is considerable retention, and profuse suppuration is quite analogous to "ischuria paradoxa."

Objective methods of determining the presence of pus in the mastoid process have been employed. Körner, v. Wild, and others recommend percussion of the mastoid process. If the latter is filled with pus, the percussion-note will be duller than that on the other side. The note is, however, influenced by many outward relations (shutting and opening the mouth and nose, difference in number of air-cells, etc., further by swelling of the soft parts). If these sources of error be considered, the method may produce good results, especially in primary disease of the bone, and the slow secondary forms which run their course with few stormy manifestations. Whether examination with *x*-rays can be employed for diagnostic purposes is at present unknown.

Prognosis.—The prognosis of mastoid disease depends very much upon the promptness with which operation is performed. If operation is carried out at the proper time, severe complications can always be avoided except in cases of particularly severe inflammation.

In other cases complications may continue absent so long that death may occur from some other cause before recovery takes place. Spontaneous recovery from mastoiditis can be expected only in cases of mild inflammation during the onset of an acute otitis. The above-mentioned instances of spontaneous recovery through throwing off of large portions

of bone are extremely rare. After completion of the operation, a
the mastoid process be freely opened, recovery takes place within
to six weeks, but considerably longer time may be required. Rec
from such operations is often unsatisfactory, especially in tuberc
and diabetic subjects.

*Ulceration of the Bony Walls of the Tympanic Cavity and Au
Ossicles.*—The exposure of portions of the wall of the tympanum
probably also the removal of small cortical sequestra, very frequ
follow otitis media, but do not often occupy a very prominent po
in the clinical picture. Retarded cases of otitis, especially those
nixed too late or those which have been improperly treated, accom
ing severe infectious diseases, particularly scarlet fever, frequently
extensive necrosis, affecting particularly the auditory ossicles. Ne
bone may be transported into the auditory canal by granulation a
removed from here by pus, irrigations, or with instruments.

Owing to its slender form, the malleus is more readily throw
spontaneously, the incus only after extensive loss of substance,
occurs frequently, especially in the body and long process, or the nc
bone remains in the tympanic cavity, acting like a foreign bod
keeping up suppuration until it is removed surgically. The stapes
undergoes necrosis, and then usually in cases of otitis from scarlet
which run an unfavorable course. Infection of the contents of the
rinth is always to be expected under such circumstances.

Of the walls of the tympanic cavity, the annulus tympanicus ar
vicinity, as well as the portions adjoining the cochlea, are most frequ
affected by small or large cortical sequestra. Also the median po
of the roof of the auditory canal, described as "pars epitympanicu
occasionally thrown off either as a whole or in separate portions.
crosis also occurs in the recessus hypotympanicus, affecting the tra
lar bony processes. In a number of cases the entire cochlea, or po
of the latter, were thrown off; more rarely the semicircular canals
similarly affected.

Labyrinth Disease.—Besides the erosions of the external semicir
canal (see above), the labyrinth may also be infected if the inflamm
of the mucous membrane of the tympanum destroys the membran
the fenestræ and infectious organisms find entrance to the perilympl
fluid. Habermann and Scheibe, as well as others, have proved tha
bones of the labyrinth capsule, as well as other portions of the temp
bone, are affected by osteomyelitis, and that from this point the sp
of the labyrinth may be infected. This apparently occurs more
frequently than has generally been supposed.

Infection of the Sinus and the Bulb of the Jugular Vein.—The sinu
especially the sigmoid sinus, are involved in otitis media through
medium of the mastoid cells. More rarely phlebitis of the small ve
originating in the mucous membrane and emptying into the sinus, dire
causes infection of the contents of the latter. Still more freque
an extradural abscess in the sigmoid fossa infects the wall of the si
through direct contact. The other sinuses usually become invol

through an infectious sinus-thrombosis travelling along the transverse sinus. The bulb of the jugular vein may be infected in a similar way through the floor of the tympanic cavity, if separated from the latter by only a thin plate of bone. Thrombosis originating in this way is usually attached to the walls of the sinus. In a similar manner the carotid sinus surrounding the carotid artery may be infected also, and infection be carried along in the cavernous sinus.

Infection within the Skull.—Extradural abscesses, situated between the dura and bone, are quite frequent in connection with otitis media, especially in the sigmoid fossa, but less frequently above the tegmen tympani. Either the cranial cavity is directly opened through destruction of bone or infected bloodvessels and lymphatics serve to transport infectious agents from the mucous membrane of the tympanic cavity. The latter is more liable to occur in the tegmen, occasionally also through the medium of the connective-tissue strands which extend from the antrum, beneath the superior semicircular canal to the hiatus subarcuatus, the remains of a fetal process of the dura found in the subarcuate canal. Extradural abscesses may produce other intracranial complications, the most frequent of which is leptomeningitis. The latter may also be caused by inflammation of the labyrinth, more rarely through involvement of the facial canal. The bony wall of the latter frequently presents openings in the region of its lateral curve; also if inflammation of the mucous membrane is acute, inflammation may travel through the small opening in the eminentia pyramidalis, along the tendon of the stapes, into the canal. Neuritis of the facial occurs in both events, but does not seem absolutely necessary for transportation of inflammation. Finally, if air-cells reach as far as the apex of the petrous portion, infection may extend to the cavum Meckelii and meningitis be thus brought about. Cerebral abscess in the course of acute otitis are rare. In such cases the surgeon may assume that infection has reached the brain at once by travelling along one of the mentioned routes, or that he has to deal with less violent infections of the dura in the course of which adhesions have formed between the latter and the brain-surface, following which infection of the brain-substance itself takes place. (See page 282 and following.)

TREATMENT OF ACUTE OTITIS MEDIA.—According to the stage and severity of acute otitis media the physician must vary his treatment. In mild, so-called catarrhal forms which follow their course without important febrile movement, without disturbance of the general condition, and without severe pain, one may wait. But at the same time it is wise to remove as rapidly as possible any existing inflammatory conditions of the nose and epipharynx (only mild astringents). If pain is more severe, if infection of the drum-membrane is more marked, without bulging, however, being noticeable, one may still wait and apply antiphlogistic measures as long as fever is not high and there is no tenderness on pressure over the mastoid process. The entire region of the ear is sensitive to cold; the long-continued application of ice-bags in many patients increases the pain, and may even cause freezing of the auricle.

For this reason ice-bags should not be applied for longer than one h
and the auricle be protected by an interposed layer of flannel.
author finds that cloths cooled by laying on a block of ice and well wr
out act better. The entrance of cold water into the auditory canal sh
be absolutely prevented. Leiter's cooling apparatus, or an improv
coil of rubber tubing, acts well and is without danger.

Where there is tenderness on pressure over the mastoid pro
leeches applied to the mastoid process or to the tragus, painting
iodine or placing a vesicating plaster behind the ear are recommen
All these may act well, but a leech-bite causes almost as much pai
paracentesis and is certainly less efficacious. If suppuration takes pl
the wounds are nearly always infected, and sometimes render subseq
treatment difficult. Painting with iodine is followed by pain and swe
of the respective portion of the skin, and it is impossible to decide
critical moment whether this is due to disease of the bone or to
iodine. This applies even more to the vesicating plaster.

In all such cases paracentesis is a great deal more efficacious.
should always be carried out early where there is distinct tenderne:
the mastoid, especially where there is any considerable rise of tem
ature, even if the latter occurs only in the evening. One need hav
fear about performing this small and only slightly painful opera
unnecessarily when the diagnosis is doubtful. Where one can see
drum-membrane at all, paracentesis is rarely difficult, even in un
children, provided one has manual dexterity. Frequently, it is t
when the drum-membrane is markedly injected the boundary betw
the latter and the auditory canal is difficult to determine. One she
therefore always use the short process of the malleus as a guide. T
can almost always be distinguished as a white or yellow spot. P:
centesis should, of course, provide free and thorough evacuation of
exudate; too long an incision rarely does harm, and one less ski
usually makes the incision shorter than intended on account of the c
cavity of the drum-membrane. If the drum-membrane is unifor
bulged out, an incision situated anteroinferiorly would be most fav
able for drainage, and a radial incision theoretically the best, as,
account of the direction of the fibres of the drum-membrane, it wo
not stand open too far. In unruly patients it is frequently difficult
make this incision anteroinferiorly, and for this reason, following
suggestion of Schwartze, a horizontal incision near the inferior mar
of the membrane is to be recommended for those who are not skil
In case of circumscribed bulging posterosuperiorly paracentesis sho
be made parallel to and behind the manubrium of the malleus; in su
cases prompt incision is important, and may in many cases render op
ing of the mastoid process unnecessary.

In regard to the treatment of acute otitis media, it may be mentior
that the application of a 5, 10, or even 20 per cent. carbolic acid solut
in glycerin undoubtedly diminishes the painfulness of the drum-me
brane, and may even diminish that of a subsequent paracentesis.
cases of milder inflammation the actual course of disease seems to

favorably influenced by this treatment even after paracentesis or spontaneous rupture. Carbolic acid and glycerin seem to exert a good influence as long as severe inflammatory manifestations continue present. The solution may be simply dropped into the auditory canal, or pieces of cotton saturated with it may be inserted into the auditory canal as far as the drum-membrane. It should not be used for too long a time, as otherwise, even where the skin is little sensitive, eczema or a painful condition of the walls of the auditory canal may be produced. If after perforation has taken place there is much secretion, care should be taken to cleanse the ear. Recently much stress has been laid by many on the value of purely aseptic treatment, loosely packing the auditory canal with sterile gauze, and applying a complete antiseptic dressing. This seems to the author unnecessarily cumbersome. He cannot see either why irrigation of the ear should be rejected where suppuration is profuse. Irrigation of the auditory canal filled with pus is entirely different from irrigation of an incised abscess cavity; the surgeon is simply applying a cleansing measure and cannot expect it to be more than that. Certainly by using such irrigations, the patient is less dependent upon the surgeon than under the aseptic dry method of treatment. In very obstinate and profuse suppuration irrigation through the Eustachian tube by means of a catheter may be indicated. It was formerly practised more than at present, but is decidedly useful in some cases. Where suppuration is not so profuse, careful swabbing with clean pieces of cotton, aided by forceps, is certainly to be preferred, whether or not it is followed by the application of a proper medicating fluid. It must be frequently repeated, however, in order that the vicinity of the ear may not be bathed in pus, the skin macerated, and eczema produced. If secretion diminishes and the perforation opening is free, the further treatment is limited to cleansing the auditory canal or applying 10 per cent. boric acid glycerin, weak solutions of zinc sulphate or hydrogen peroxide, according to personal preference. If, however, in spite of free perforation, secretion does not cease, the safest method to bring about rapid recovery of the disease is the insufflation of powdered boric acid (Bezold), according to the author's experience and that of many others, in spite of all the agitation against this method. It has been asserted that boric acid combines with secretion to form hard lumps, which prevent drainage and may thereby lead to serious complications. This objection does not apply to the method, but to its incorrect application. Insufflated in small quantities, boric acid is dissolved by the secretion and is easily evacuated with the latter. The principal condition for its application is free perforation. It is surprising with what rapidity suppuration which has previously resisted all other methods subsides after a few insufflations of this substance.

If there are present those signs described under the head of diagnosis, which would justify one in assuming the presence of a more intense form of disease of the temporal bone, one may first enlarge the opening of perforation unless high fever or intense tenderness on pressure over the bone, or cerebral or pyæmic manifestations, force one to open the mastoid process. For the purpose of enlarging the opening one can either make

... probe to which is fused a small quan...
... The ... method causes very little pain and is...
... it is especially recommendable in...
... If, however, drainage is free and...
... process do not subside, one...
... for frequently hours are pr...
... spontaneously and in a surprisingly...
... of the antrum.

... Middle Ear.—At the outset of the ...
... of the middle ear the author wishes t...
... acute otitis media completely re...
... occurred early enough, either spontan...
... predisposing general disease do...
... tuberculosis, for example, te...
... and that 3) no general condition of d...
... would hinder recovery from inflammati...
... for example, diabetes. Undoubtedly a transition from...
... inflammation is rather frequent. If, however, none ...
... exists in, it is usually due to insufficient ...
... of treatment. Thus, according to the author's conceptio...
... suppuration are in a way only complications of an a...
... an entirely different character when it is protr...
... It is therefore justifiable to discuss chronic inflamm...
... as a special form of disease.

... causes and treatment of chronic middle-ear inflamma...
... form, and character of the ... in the drum-memb...
... All the possible occurrences cannot, of cou...
... but a number of types may be mentioned which...

... may be extensive destruction of the drum-membrane,...
... from the exposed mucous membrane. This form...
... frequently found after severe or very much neglected case...
... from scarlet fever or diphtheria. The form and si...
... vary; sometimes the drum-membrane is comple...
... except for a small remnant bounding the annulus tympani...
... of the malleus projects from the margin of the form...
... is either uninjured or only slightly eroded at its lower extrem...
... other cases extensive portions of the drum-membrane in the vici...
... of the malleus are preserved. These parts of...
... drum-membrane are better nourished. Owing to the projection of...
... of the malleus the gap becomes heart- or kidney-sha...
... other cases again there are large oval or round perforations, wh...
... the anteroinferior or both inferior quadrants. The size of...
... perforation plays a part in determining the chronic character, as ...
... mentioned above; also certain relations in the position of the dru...
... membrane; thus, for example, marked cicatricial retraction of the m...
... of the malleus may cause a portion of the tympanic cavity to...
... closed off, particularly the superoposterior portion, and thus br...

etention of the secretion, the latter then causing continuation
nflammation.

e may be oval or slit-like perforations varying in size, which in-
1e superoposterior quadrant of the drum-membrane and some-
xpose the articulation between the incus and the stapes. These
lions indicate disease of the system of bands mentioned a number
1, which lie between the malleus and the incus, and which divide
essory cavities from the mesotympanum; also disease of the
membrane covering these bands, frequently also disease of the
1anic recess and the mastoid antrum.

e may be small perforations lying superiorly and at the same
mediately in front of or behind the short process of the malleus.
1erforations are frequently observed with scars or sclerotic changes
lrum-membrane, where the rest of the drum-membrane is either
1r a solution of continuity has been restored. In such cases there
1bably only a mild form of inflammation in the mesotympanum
ubsided, while at the same time unfavorable circumstances in the
aused more severe inflammation and suppuration. In such per-
1s pus generally originates in the recess or in the antrum.
1rations may be more or less obstructed by exuberant granula-
The perforations usually possess the character described under
preceding forms. These exuberant granulations generally orig-
om the edge of the perforation, its vicinity, or the wall of the
ic cavity lying opposite. The many causes which may produce
ill be discussed later.

1haracter of suppuration varies very much in such cases of otitis.
rge perforations, described under the first type, the surgeon usually
eal with rather profuse or possibly diminishing secretion of glairy
or slightly tinged pus. This is sometimes the case with larger
1ions of the second type. The smaller openings of various forms
empty a somewhat thicker and more deeply colored pus, which
ently mixed with crumbly or cheesy masses, in which are found
pidermis cells, cholesterin, and fatty acid crystals. Frequently
imparts a disagreeable rancid odor, which is the result of decom-
1 of its fatty elements. Frequently it offends the olfactory organ
1 various other qualities, which are worse accordingly as the pus
1 thick and crumbly. If irrigation is regularly performed, the
1appears, provided that in irrigating the source of pus is reached.

1osis.—The prognosis of chronic suppuration of the ear is
able in so far as it is frequently followed by fatal complications,
often only after having existed for a long time. Location plays
1rtant part here. Suppuration from the anterior portion of the
1anic recess not infrequently causes abscess of the temporal lobe.
suppuration originates in the antrum, the semicircular canal or
1r fossa is frequently eroded (sinus-phlebitis, cerebellar abscess).
labyrinth is involved, there is danger of meningitis. Further,
1r suppuration continues for any length of time it produces cica-
1ontraction, and the more extensive the disease the more seriously

tion with a syringe will not suffice in such cases; it is necessary to use specially curved tubes, so-called middle-ear tubes, which direct a stream of water directly into the position required. This must obviously be done under inspection, and may under circumstances be one of the most difficult performances of special technic. Frequently free access must be provided by removing granulations or by enlarging the perforation with a knife or caustics. The details can be obtained from works on otology. More difficult than cleansing by irrigation is that of dry swabbing or wiping. Under any circumstances it is necessary to exercise not only patience and care, but also to possess accurate knowledge of the anatomical relations of the tympanic cavities.

Annoying exuberant granulations frequently require removal. For this purpose a very fine wire loop, sharp curette, or a sharp spoon, or in other cases caustics, may be employed. For the latter purpose small quantities of the caustic material can be fused to a fine silver probe. The substances principally used are silver nitrate, trichloracetic or chromic acid. The author has found the last named to be the most satisfactory, as its action can be most easily controlled and it causes the least amount of pain. Many prefer a very fine galvanocautery to caustics. The author has never been able to persuade himself of its practicability on account of the intense pain it causes, though it is true that this soon subsides.

Another frequent hinderance to evacuation of pus, as well as to mechanical cleansing, is the presence of the ossicles or their remains. If the epitympanic recess, or even the antrum, is the principal seat of the suppurative process, the resulting secretion can only flow around the head of the malleus or the body of the incus, and occasionally drainage may be considerably facilitated if these obstacles are removed. With proper selection of cases excellent results can be obtained by this operation, regardless of whether the ossicles be affected by caries or not.

After mechanical cleansing the most important point in the treatment of chronic middle-ear suppuration is the drying of the cavities. This can be accomplished by simple, frequent swabbing out; in most instances, however, it will be more successful if desiccating substances are employed. For this purpose boric acid is highly recommended. In proper cases this may cause the secretion to be absorbed immediately, besides producing an astringent action. Where it cannot properly be applied, other astringents in common use can be employed—solutions of zinc sulphate, lead acetate, alum, silver nitrate, etc. The strength of these solutions must be adapted to the conditions present in each case. Silver nitrate solutions occupy a peculiar position in so far as their application may produce acute irritation of the mucous membrane, which can be employed, according to the suggestion by Schwartze, in a similar manner as it is employed by ophthalmologists to remove torpid chronic inflammatory conditions.

Alcohol has an astringent and at the same time a dehydrating action, and was first introduced as a means of treatment by Politzer. If, however, it is desired to produce an active dehydration with this solution, it is necessary first to carry out thorough mechanical cleansing, subsequent drying, and then to apply large quantities of alcohol. several portions of alcohol may be successively dropped in, or, to the very commendable suggestion of Körner, a large quantity of hol may be employed for a single irrigation by means of a tube. Attacks of dizziness sometimes occur from its use and necessitate the abandonment of this treatment.

It would not be proper to enter upon all the special disposal of otologists in the treatment of such cases of mation. In the same way the author can only sum up tions for possible operations. At present surgeons are the "radical operation," described later, to cure every middle-ear suppuration that does not rest on some diathesis. It is necessary to perform this operation if signs of the mastoid process or of intracranial complications become able. These may occur at any time in the course of chronic midd suppuration, and in a similar manner as in acute. Regardless of complications, which render operation necessary, operative interfe is indicated to prevent these complications. There is danger in a suppuration of the superior accessory spaces of the tympanic c particularly in otitis desquamativa, especially so if the labyrinth i eased; also if a true pearl tumor (cholesteatoma) is the cause of si ration. In all such cases radical operation is indicated when ra and carefully carried out special treatment cannot bring about ces of suppuration; above all, if in spite of this treatment suppuration tinues to be foul-smelling, a sign that the actual focus is not reach therapeutic measures employed. Another indication for radical o tion is marked narrowing of the auditory canal, as it occurs th cicatricial contraction or inflammatory hyperostosis in all varieti cases of chronic middle-ear suppuration; on account of the na auditory canal rational treatment is rendered impossible.

Tuberculosis.—Lupoid changes in the skin occur in the ext ear, and may extend to the auditory canal. Tuberculous perichon has occasionally been observed. There is a very rare form produ tumors, seen especially in the lobe of the ear, which may cause deformity.

The middle ear is frequently diseased in all stages of pulmonary t culosis; pure and mixed infections have been observed. Most frequ there is found rapidly progressing destruction of the mucous memb of the drum-membrane and the tympanic cavity, combined with se functional disturbance, but without marked inflammatory manifestati particularly without pain. Rapid destruction of bone frequently l to facial paralysis and labyrinth disease. Tuberculous foci of the dr membrane have repeatedly been seen, even without suppuration. A forms with rapid destruction of tissue and exuberant granulation more rare. The various intracranial complications do not, of cou occur very frequently in these cases. The complicating diseases are regularly of a specific tuberculous nature.

Prognosis.—Complete recovery does not often take place, but has been positively observed in a number of cases with and without treatment, even in cases of advanced phthisis.

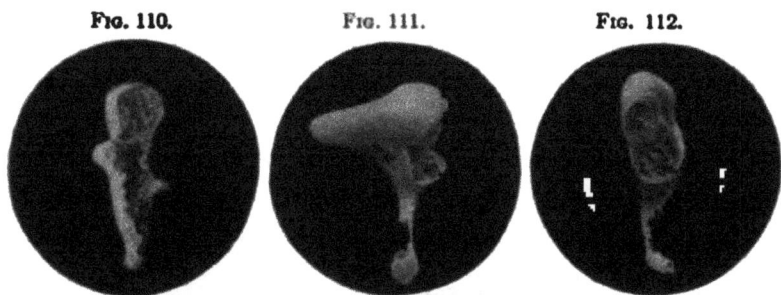

FIG. 110.   FIG. 111.   FIG. 112.

Tuberculous caries of malleus.   Tuberculous caries of incus.

FIG. 113.

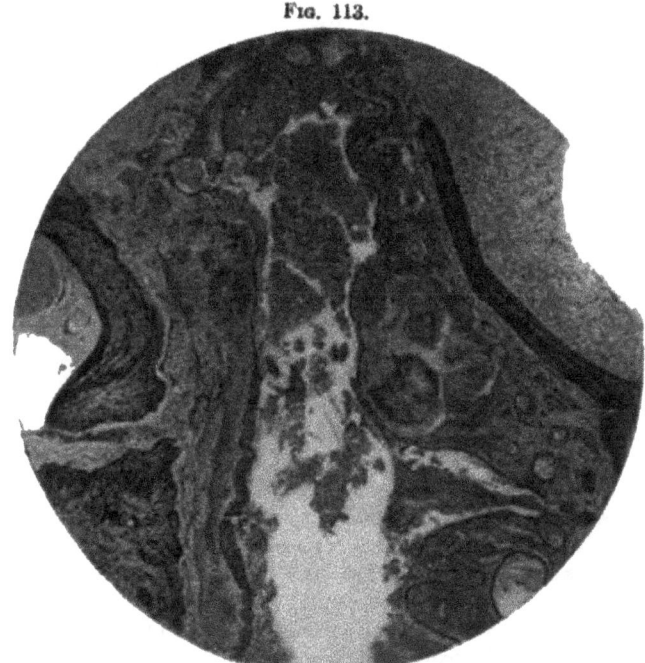

Tuberculous infiltrated mucous membrane of ear.

Treatment.—Besides the general treatment, local therapeutic measures must be considered, especially where there are profuse suppuration and granulation. Where cases are not altogether unfavorable, operative treatment by the so-called radical operation may achieve good results.

large polyps are so tough as not to be torn. Small granulomata can frequently be removed with a sharp spoon or curette. Such operations should, however, never be performed unless guided by inspection, as otherwise injury of the facial nerve or labyrinth may result.

Fibroma.—Real fibromata rarely occur of sufficient size on the ear to render removal necessary on account of deformity; for this reason probably few cases have been reported. The small projections in the region of the tragus are not true fibromata, but the cartilaginous congenital auricular appendages already described.

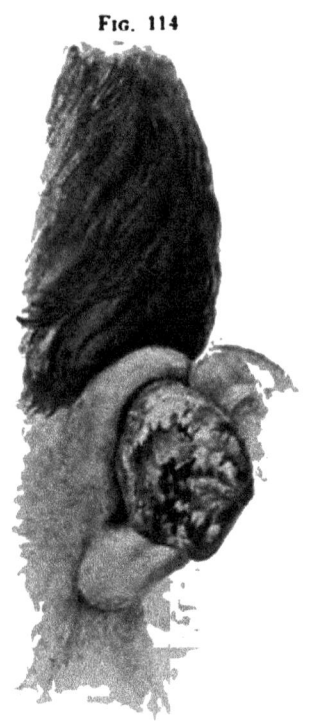

Fig. 114

According to Billroth, the term *keloid* may be applied to a class of tumors, usually called hard fibroma, which develop in the puncture designed for ear-rings, and which are consequently more frequent in the female sex. They are more frequent in the colored race. Cheap earrings, particularly of the base metals, are supposed to favor the development of these tumors. They may attain considerable size, transforming the lobe into a shapeless mass reaching to the shoulder, and thus produce great deformity. Histologically they are composed of a dense connective tissue, poor in cells; they are not very sharply circumscribed from the surrounding tissue, so that in dissecting them portions are liable to remain and cause recurrence. Scars following dissection of keloids are very liable to develop keloids. These tumors are rather rare in Germany.

Fibroma of the external ear in a boy aged seventeen years.

Treatment.—The treatment consists in their excision. Recurrence is frequent, however, as was mentioned, and is best prevented by obtaining the most perfect primary union.

In the external auditory canal, usually in its lateral portion and as far as the tragus, partially pedunculated, dense fibromata have been observed in several cases. These tumors were removed without difficulty.

In the temporal bone, as in other bones, fibroma is observed. The so-called fibroma of the auditory nerve always shows the presence of nervous or sarcomatous tissue, and should therefore be discussed separately.

Tumors of the tympanic cavity described as fibromata have probably always been cases of granuloma which have undergone connective-tissue transformation.

Angioma.—Angioma is found on the auricle, especially in cl……… involving also the neighboring region of the cheek. It is of congenital origin. When situated in the region of the tragu……… a plexiform angioma, a telangiectasis, while if situated ……… portions of the auricle it is more frequently caver……… character. The latter form may attain great size and extend auditory canal, or even to the drum-membrane.

Plexiform angioma is frequently considered malignant on acc the presence of a large amount of young connective tissue (or fa……… correctly put down as angiosarcoma. This is readily conceiv……… these tumors proliferate extensively and often very rapidly into t……… rounding tissues, and frequently after incomplete dissection they……… occur.

One of the favorite sites for cirsoid aneurysm (pes anastomo……… the auricle and its vicinity, particularly the tissues between the lov and the mastoid process. From this point it commonly extend……… large areas of the scalp, not infrequently also to the neighboring ……… membrane and into the bone. The usual point of origin is the p……… auricular artery.

Diagnosis.—Angioma possesses considerable clinical significa……… account of liability of hemorrhage, particularly in the case of cirsoid……… rysm, and in many instances death has taken place in spite of ever……… extensive operations as ligation of the common carotid, etc.

In cases of arterial tumors of the auricular region very seve……… annoying pulsating sounds in the ear are frequently the principal……… tom: they may be very annoying even in small aneurysms (case of……… Occasionally these vascular sounds can be suppressed by press……… certain portions of the mastoid process. This fact in itself ma……… to a correct diagnosis. If after extirpation of a cirsoid aneurysm……… sounds do not completely disappear, as occasionally happens, it i……… assumed that somewhere there is present a sufficient portion of th……… volution to produce the same disturbance that was caused by the……… tumor.

Treatment.—In angioma simplex extending over the region of t……… aneurism, dissection is not to be recommended on account of the d……… of injuring the facial nerve. Multiple galvanopuncture is prefe……… The latter is, however, frequently followed by recurrence, but the……… easily be removed in the same way. If the angioma extends rather ……… toward the temporal bone into the tissues of the parotid and alo……… base of the skull (Turnbull), dissection may be so dangerous that li……… of the afferent vessels would be more practicable.

Intratympanal angioma, unless it is really granuloma, rarely oc……

Cartilaginous Tumors.—Cartilaginous tumors in the region ……… auricle and bony portion of the auditory canal have frequently……… described. These cases are, however, either examples of auricula……… pendages, previously discussed, or cartilaginous mixed tumors ……… parotid region that have extended into the auditory canal. True ……… droma (Wallicsek) is extremely rare. Spine-shaped ecchondros……

observed in one case by G. Politzer, proceeding from the anterior wall of the auditory canal, are closely related to *tumors of the bone*. All forms of the latter have been observed in the auditory canal.

Bone Tumors.—*Ecchondrosis ossificans* (*exostosis cartilaginea*) is completely analogous to exostosis of the epiphyseal boundaries in youthful individuals, and like the latter may be very extensive. It occurs in the form of conical or spinous projections, covered on the surface by cartilage, which may project the full width of the auditory canal and conceal large portions of the drum-membrane.

Exostosis eburnea and *spongiosa* occurs in the form of single or multiple tumors. The ivory forms are more frequently flatly spherical, the spongy forms generally more conical, though the latter may occur as partially pedunculated, almost polypoid tumors, containing large medullary spaces, so that they can easily be snared with a wire loop. They have been supposed to originate from granulomata, but there is no proof of this mode of origin. In a case of this kind recently operated upon by the author there was absolutely no ground for this assumption.

Hyperostosis of the auditory canal possesses least of all the character of a neoplasm. As a rule it extends as a uniform thickening of bone, presenting an irregular surface and covering large areas, particularly on the anterior and inferior wall of the auditory canal, frequently closing the lumen to a small slit.

Diagnosis.—Clinically, exostoses frequently cause impairment of hearing, or deafness, owing to the fact that they obstruct the auditory canal or leave only such a small slit that it is easily obstructed by wax. More infrequently they cause neuralgic pains which disappear with the removal of the exostosis. All exostoses are, as a matter of fact, extremely sensitive to touch. Finally, the presence of exostoses renders difficult the diagnosis and treatment of inflammations of the middle ear and the auditory canal, and in this way unpleasant complications may occur.

Treatment.—The removal of such exostoses can easily be accomplished only in the very soft spongy forms. In removing the other forms, a moderate-sized gouge is recommended. The latter should be handled with great caution, as otherwise there is danger, after tedious removal of an ivory-like mass of bone, of suddenly passing through the drum-membrane or even further. If it is necessary to operate in the presence of middle-ear suppuration, infection of the wound occurs, and the recovery of what would otherwise have been a trivial injury is complicated by granulation with subsequent cicatricial stenosis, etc. Some authors have recommended for this purpose burrs driven by dental drills. They may be practicable in some cases, but require great skill and a good view of the auditory canal.

Osteoma.—Finally, there occurs, though rarely, true osteoma. This regularly occurs as a sharply circumscribed rounded mass of bone of an ivory-like consistence, situated in the cavities of the mastoid process, causing the posterior wall of the auditory canal to bulge forward. It may reach the size of a filbert or walnut. It is analogous to osteoma of the ethmoidal and frontal sinuses, and, if opening of the mastoid pro becomes necessary, may occasion great difficulty in technic.

Lipoma.—The only cases of lipoma are one each of Walli (auricle) and Ole Bull (auditory canal).

Myxoma.—Myxoma of the tympanic cavity has been frequ described, but in all cases in which careful histological examina was made they might more properly have been interpreted as uloma with "œdematous degeneration," and occasionally deposit mnem.

Warts.—Real warts are rare in the ear. In several instances a p lary granuloma has been described as such. The latter may als mistaken for carcinoma, but can be readily distinguished by its cli course (Kühn).

Adenoma.—True adenoma originating in the sebaceous glands of auricle (Klingel) is an extremely rare tumor and without clinical si cance. Granuloma with glandular formation has frequently been scribed as adenofibroma of the tympanic cavity. A case of true ade of the tympanic cavity is represented by a small intratympanal t operated upon by Jansen.

Sebaceous Cysts.—Sebaceous cysts have frequently been obse on the auricle and in its immediate vicinity, particularly on its co surface and in the fossa of the helix. They rarely grow larger th filbert, but may become as large as a hen's egg, as in one of Gru cases. They present no special peculiarities. In several cases obse by the author he was surprised at the thinness of the walls, which dered dissection very difficult.

Dermoid Cysts.—It appears doubtful whether true dermoid occur on the auricle itself. In genuine cases they have been eithe front of the auricle on the tragus, or on the mastoid process in a de sion of the latter. They may be considered in part derived from first branchial cleft, and in part from epithelial cells which were displ during the development of the auricle.

Cholesteatoma.—Pearl tumors, which are of great clinical importa bear a certain relation to dermoid cysts.

These formations constitute one of the most discussed subject otology. While Cruveilhier, J. Müller, and Virchow consider them tumors of heterotopic epidermoidal formation, v. Tröltsch consid them masses of epidermal scales which have collected about a cen mass composed of cheesy pus. The latter interpretation has recei such strong support from a large number of otologists that the occurre of true pearl tumors is at present disputed on many sides. Such tun certainly do occur; they are well circumscribed rounded tumors, bedded in smooth-walled cavities in the bone, frequently also provi with long processes and enclosed in a delicate membrane. As a re of their onion-like stratification, they have a distinct pearly lus In most cases such tumors are associated with suppuration of the mid ear, but it is hardly conceivable that as a result of such inflammat processes such enormous masses of epidermis could accumulate even the course of years. Those rare cases in which suppuration was absent deserve special consideration (Lucae, Schwartze).

Clinically such tumors are only seen after they have attained considerable size. During recent years the author has operated in a number of cases in which they were the size of a pigeon's or hen's egg. Unless they have become softened by inflammatory processes, they may be bluntly dissected out and enucleated *in toto*. Smaller pearl tumors are observed in the epitympanic recess and antrum. They usually break off in fragments, accompanied by suppuration, through a perforation of the drum-membrane or wall of the auditory canal, following which in rare cases spontaneous recovery takes place.

An entirely different class of tumor, frequently described as cholesteatoma, are masses of epidermis sometimes distinctly stratified, which are found in the antrum or the recess in the presence of chronic suppuration of the middle ear. These are as a rule of a semisolid consistency, uniformly saturated with pus, can never be enucleated *in toto* with the delicate, enclosure membrane. It is very difficult to remove their cortical layers from the cavities containing them. If bluntly dissected, there always remains a comparatively thick membrane of epidermoidal appearance adherent to the bone, which can only be removed with some force, leaving a more or less rough surface of bone. The surgeon has to deal here with the products of otitis chronica desquamativa (see above). As most cases of cholesteatoma, if situated in the middle ear, sooner or later set up otitis media, it is occasionally impossible to decide upon one cause or the other as the active agent in producing the disease. It would, however, be incorrect on that account to question the occurrence of true pearl tumors.

The origin of pearl tumors has generally been referred to the inclusion of epidermoidal cells within the cavities of the temporal bone during development of the ear (Mikulicz). Inclusion may, however, result from trauma; for instance, in chiselling a mastoid process containing a fistula lined with epidermis (Leutert). These cases are analogous to traumatic epithelial cysts of the fingers in the vicinity of ingrowing nails, etc. It is difficult to state whether they occur frequently or not.

The origin of cholesteatoma in endothelial clefts has been maintained on several sides (Wendt, Gläser), but is more than doubtful. The separation of true pearl tumors from desquamative otitis is proper, for the reason that the treatment of the two diseases is necessarily different.

Prognosis.—Both diseases differ as to prognosis. The extensive destruction of bone caused by a true pearl tumor may expose the fossæ of the skull, and, if the former are the seat of inflammation, may lead indirectly to intracranial complications. A large number of diseases of the brain and sinuses following after otitis are due to pearl tumors. Desquamative otitis may lead to ulceration of bone and, under certain circumstances, even to the above-mentioned complications. This is more infrequent, however, than in true cholesteatoma.

Treatment.—Most of the tumors must be removed by operation as a rule by the "radical operation," to be described below, though true

deafness. The latter shows in its later stages the character of a nerve deafness. Facial paralysis may offer information as to the point of origin of carcinoma (Steinbrügge). Otherwise this is frequently very difficult. These cases of carcinoma show such a tendency to become necrotic, as compared with actual formation of tumors, that the affected parts soon entirely disappear, and in advanced cases characteristic tumor-tissue can with difficulty be found. This necrosis is especially apt to occur if, as is true in most cases, the tumor has ruptured through the skin over the mastoid process. Carcinoma also frequently advances toward the lower jaw, destroying the articular fossa, causing pain on chewing and later displacement of the jaw. Rupture through the base of the skull frequently occurs, but meningitis and particularly cerebral abscess rarely occur in these cases. Thrombosis of the sigmoid sinus is more frequent, but also rather rare. The internal carotid is frequently exposed by cancerous ulceration, and it is remarkable that severe hemorrhage does not usually occur owing to obliteration of the vessel. The tumor may extend along the base of the skull, as well as to the upper jaw and deep into the neck and suboccipital region. Paralyses of cranial nerves (abducens, oculomotor, optic, trigeminal) may then occur, also rupture into the retronasal space and affection of the atlanto-occipital articulation. Finally, even more severe destruction may be produced.

Prognosis.—Death usually results from marasmus, more rarely from complicating diseases of the brain or lungs. Metastases are rather rare, even in the regional lymph-glands.

Sarcoma.—According to the compilation of P. Asch, sarcoma occurs more frequently than carcinoma. The various portions of the auricle are all equally frequently the seat of the disease, the auditory canal seldom so, the middle ear more frequently. In the latter instance it is difficult to distinguish these tumors from those of the temporal bone. Among the latter undoubtedly belong those very rare bilateral, metastatic tumors, chloroma and lymphosarcoma. Sarcoma of the inner ear is usually benign in character. It always originates in the region of the auditory nerve, and is at first situated intracranially, reaching the labyrinth subsequently, and eventually advancing into the tympanic cavity. On the other hand, the auditory nerve and its origin in the brain are so completely involved in the tumor mass that the latter sometimes cannot be determined.

Symptoms.—The symptoms of sarcoma are similar to those of carcinoma, but the course of the disease is on the whole more rapid and irregular, corresponding to the greater difference in points of origin. The manifestations are most interesting in sarcoma of the auditory nerve; according to the direction in which the new growth advances, it produces the greatest variety of cerebral, cerebellar, and basal symptoms. The most characteristic feature is deafness, with the character of a nerve disturbance of hearing; then paralysis of the facial nerve. But in addition there occur paralysis of the muscles of the eye, changes in the optic nerve, trigeminal neuralgia, or anæsthesia. General symptoms of compression of the brain usually close the scene unless some intercur-

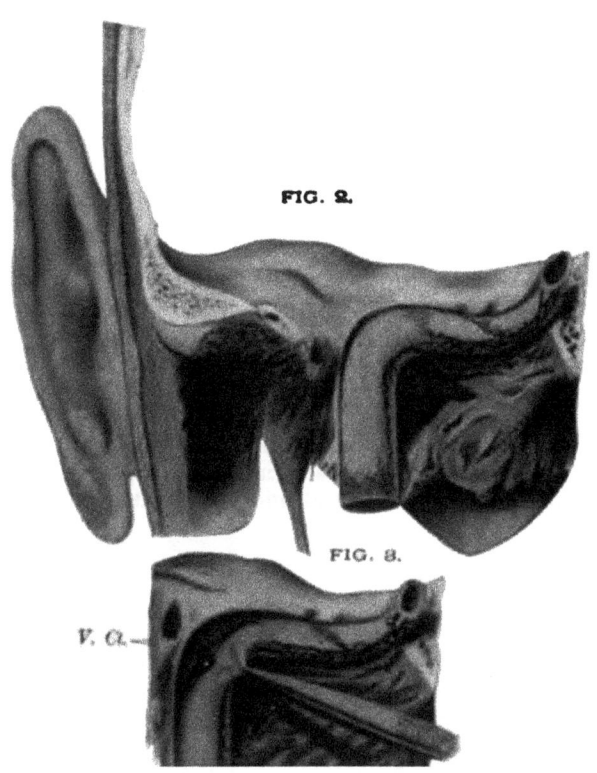

FIG. 2.

FIG. 3.

V. a.—

The differential diagnosis between carcinoma and sarcoma is based rincipally upon the fact that in the latter the tumor growth is the most rominent feature, while in the former destruction of tumor is the most rominent feature. This does not, however, always apply. The differntiation of sarcoma and carcinoma is of as little clinical importance, s, on account of the slower growth and the fact of their being fairly ell circumscribed, there is more chance of recovery by operating early i carcinoma than there is in sarcoma—the more so as in the former :vere symptoms, particularly pain, set in relatively earlier, causing the atient to consult a physician sooner. Obviously, operation involves the anger of opening the skull, and above all that of hemorrhage from 1e carotid.

Prognosis.—If promptly operated upon, endothelioma does not offer very unfavorable prognosis. It is liable to recur locally; general metasises have never been observed and infection of glands very rarely. Vithout operation the prognosis is identical with that of other malignant 1mors.

OPERATIVE EXPOSURE OF THE MASTOID CELLS.

In opening the mastoid antrum and other air-cells of the mastoid rocess a number of structures are endangered. For this reason attempts ave been made to determine positive landmarks on the surface of the one corresponding to their position.

The dura of the middle fossa of the skull lies above the antrum, in a orizontal plane, passing through the temporal line (the prolongation f the superior border of the zygoma) to the mastoid process (Schwartze). horizontal plane corresponding to the floor of the mastoid antrum, nd which corresponds also to the situation of the peripheral posterior end of the facial nerve, is placed about at the level of the highest point f the bony portion of the auditory canal, and would intersect the external urface of the bone at a point marked by a very constant process of bone, 1e suprameatal spine, "spina supra meatum" (Henle). The anterior rall of the posterior fossa of the skull has no landmarks; in respect to 1e latter as well as the region of the facial nerve, dependence must be laced upon careful chiselling. Simple exposure of the dura does no arm as a rule; its accidental surgical opening is more dangerous, while eliberate opening after thorough cleansing of the surface is less alarm1g. More frequently, however, there is produced a laceration of the rall of the sigmoid sinus, which frequently extends within a few milli1etrea of the mastoid cells. The dangers of hemorrhage, except in eneral hemorrhagic conditions, and the danger of septic infection of 1ntents of the sinus are not very great, but the flooding of the field of peration with blood is so serious that further procedures must be abanoned and hemorrhage controlled by packing. If, as occasionally occurs, 1ere is only about a space 1 cm. wide between the anterior wall of the inns and the posterior wall of the auditory canal, it is extremely difficult

ts short process upon the innermost portion of the bony auditory canal, und the facial nerves situated further inward and forward at the site of he bend, previously mentioned. The situation of these structures is

FIG. 118

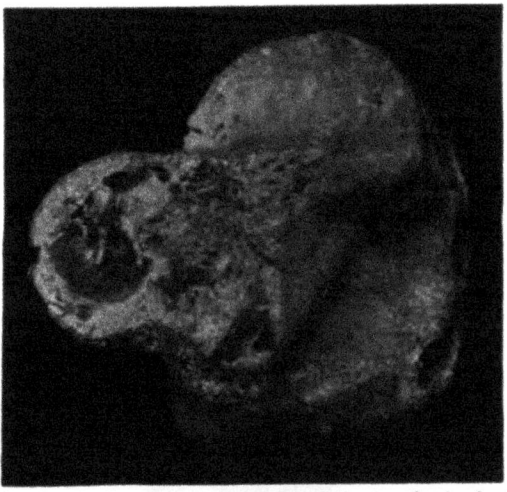

section of bone showing the inner or mucous surface of the drumhead; also the articulation of the head of the malleus with the body of the incus contained within the attic. (Bacon.)

FIG. 119.

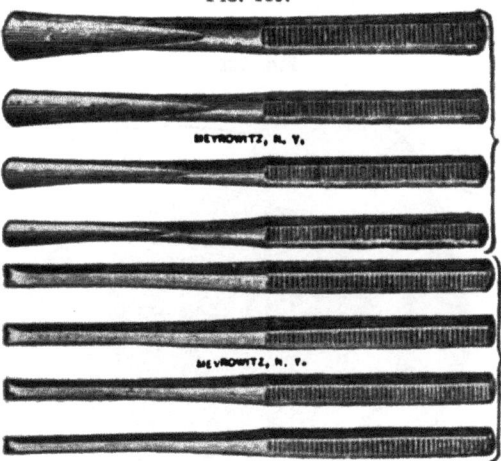

Chisels and gouges. (Schwartse's.)

shown in Fig. 116. In order to appreciate those intricate relations frequent practice on the cadaver is absolutely necessary.

Opening the Cells and the Mastoid Antrum.—In order to evacuate accumulations of pus which might endanger life or produce protracted

ackward. By such an incision even the sigmoid fossa and the transerse sulcus can be exposed if necessary.

FIG. 120.

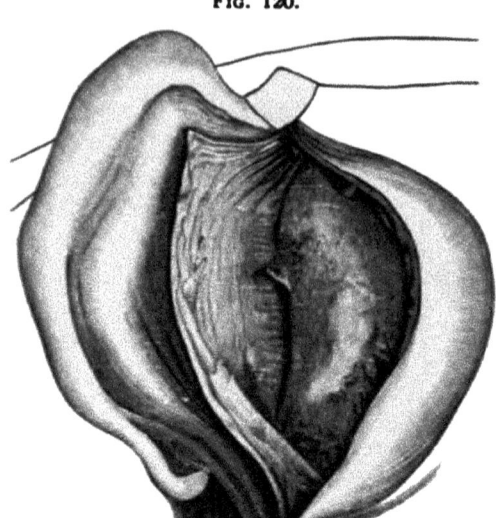

Outer surface of mastoid process after division of skin and retraction of periosteum.

FIG. 121.

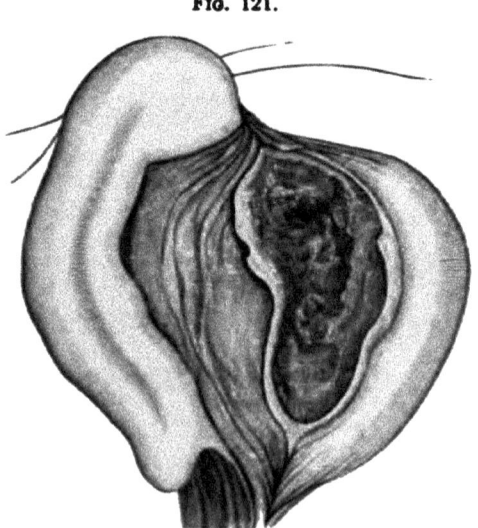

Same preparation as Fig. 120 after fully opening the mastoid process.

place in the deeper portions of the bone-wound or antrum itself, and this is best prevented by carefully continuing to pack the wound.

Recovery may be disturbed by subsequent necrosis of bone or the gradual expulsion of splinters caused by the chisel, and which were allowed to remain. The latter occurrence is quite frequent. It can, however, readily be avoided by carefully wiping out the cavity during operation. Subsequent bone necrosis is most frequently observed in disease of the mastoid process following acute general infectious dis-

Fig. 124.

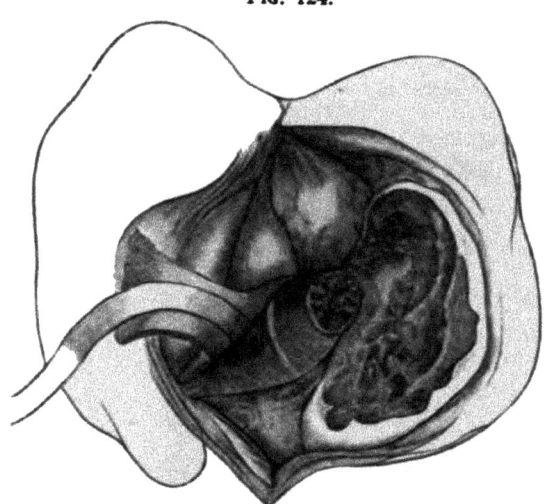

Same preparation after complete radical operation, the metal protector removed.

eases or in cases of diabetes. Frequently it also results from the chisel only partially removing portions of bone, which thus suffer impaired nutrition.

Opening all the Spaces of the Middle Ear (*"So-called Radical Operation" for Chronic Suppuration of the Middle Ear and Cholesteatoma*).—According to the method recommended by Zaufal, the typical operation of opening the mastoid antrum is first performed as described above; at the same time attempts should be made from the outset to obtain as large a funnel-shaped wound as possible by removing also the posterosuperior portion of the bony auditory canal. This is not difficult provided the soft parts including the periosteum are dissected back with the aid of a raspatorium from the mastoid process well into the bony auditory canal, and the membranous auditory canal is separated from the posterior wall with a blunt narrow elevator. After the antrum has in this way been opened a probe may be passed from it into the epitympanic recess, and beyond the latter into the tympanic cavity, and in this way it can be ascertained how much of the posterosuperior wall of the auditory canal may or should be removed: only so much should be

erve ascends along the posterior wall of the
ing in a flat curve inward and forward, behind
:ra ovalis in the median wall of the tympanic
s bend there is great danger of injuring the
of too broad a chisel or striking too forcibly
;uarded against, as otherwise there is danger
h may extend into the canal. The prominence
r canal, situated immediately above the facial
iner side, is not exposed quite so much. As
:es, so far as is known, always show a constant
: readily be avoided unless the existing disease
ceed regardless of damage produced. Just at
:nd the facial canal frequently shows gaps in

Fig. 127.

toid cells. *c.* External osseous meatus. (Bacon.)

injury of the nerve may be brought about by
i blunt instruments (forceps, probe) or throngh

lical operation is more difficult than that of
toid antrum, for the reason that in most cases
rers are removed there are not found cavities
ions through which one can gradually proceed,
k through apparently healthy sound bone. In
he wound it is therefore necessary to keep close
ill of the auditory canal, and first dissect out
osterosuperior portion is chiselled away as far
he remaining portions of the drum-membrane,
mpanic cavity, and the remains of the auditory

cavity. For the removal of this particular portion Zaufal especially recommends a small pair of gouge-forceps somewhat curved, as by employing the latter injury of the facial canal or the semicircular can best be avoided.

Stacke proceeds somewhat differently. He first shells out the entire membranous auditory canal with a fine elevator and draws out the tube of the auditory canal in connection with the auricle, thus exposing the bottom of the canal and the drum-membrane. He then chisels away sufficient of the posterior wall of the auditory canal to obtain a good view of the tympanic cavity. Then if necessary he removes the postero-superior portion of the drum-membrane, or, if the latter is destroyed, passes through the opening into the recess a so-called stapes protector. This instrument consists of a flat probe, bent at right angles near its tip, and provided with a handle. It protects the facial canal and the stapes, and the surrounding bone is chiselled away until it can be withdrawn without being caught by the edges of the latter. In this way these structures can be protected from injury provided they are not injured by the instrument itself. After having accomplished what in Zaufal's operation is the last and most difficult step, the mastoid cavities can be thoroughly exposed without running risk of injuring the facial nerve. With this advantage, the Stacke operation has the drawback that during the most difficult step in the operation the field of operation is narrow and the structures difficult to recognize unless one is absolutely sure of the anatomical relations. In spite of Stacke's objections, the author believes that Zaufal's method receives more support from surgeons than Stacke's. The principle of freely opening up all diseased or suspected portions of the mastoid process and temporal bone and bringing them into free communication with the auditory canal can be carried out by both methods.

There may still be mentioned certain minor technical steps which facilitate this rather difficult operation. Much depends upon a careful arrest of hemorrhage. If blood obscures the field of operation, small details, which ought to be noted, will be obscured, and accidental injuries are apt to follow. The sponges usually employed in surgical operations are too large. It is advisable to use small sponges held by anatomical forceps. Spurting arteries of the bone may be very annoying. If they are not too small, a fine silver wire may be pressed into their lumen and in this way hemorrhage be arrested. It is more convenient to use a strong blunt instrument and simply press upon the site of hemorrhage for a short time. Small projections of bone interfere with sponging, as the sponges are continually being caught. The projecting bone can be cut off with gouge forceps as soon as discovered. In cases of obstinate parenchymatous hemorrhage gauze wrung out in hydrogen peroxide is frequently of great service.

After the antrum and tympanic cavity have been cleaned out, and it is necessary to chisel away still more bone, these cavities should first be filled with a small sponge, otherwise splinters of bone may find their way into them, and it is difficult to remove them later. Besides, this com-the bony wall of the operation-wound and might possibly even reach into the antrum.

Finally one can proceed by making a longitudinal incision in the middle of the posterior circumference of the auditory canal, and at the outer extremity of the latter making a transverse incision so that the entire incision forms a T. It is possible in this way to cover the superior and inferior border of the wound in the bone. It is to be admitted, however, that the terminal portions of the flap are situated at the narrowest part of the opening in the bone, and that if exuberant granulations develop the after-treatment may be rendered difficult.

It is useful in all these plastic operations to remove as much of the cartilaginous substance from these flaps as possible, as this renders the latter more easily applicable to the bony surfaces, and causes them to become more readily united.

The choice of these plastic operations is a matter of taste. The author would recommend complete removal of the posterior wall of the membranous auditory canal only if the latter is extensively destroyed, and it is therefore unsuitable for plastic purposes. Otherwise the author employs Körner's operation in the majority of cases, without, however, being willing to name it as the only method. If carefully carried out, it provides a great deal of material, and renders it possible, if the bone operation has established sufficiently free communication between the mastoid process and the auditory canal, to shorten considerably the duration of after-treatment. This plastic operation has been advised against in cases in which the cavities in the bone were very large; but, on the contrary, the author has really obtained the best results in very large cavities which had resulted from very extensive cholesteatoma.

Where it is intended from the outset to allow the "retroauricular opening" to remain, in order to be able to inspect permanently the mastoid cavities through the former, a Thiersch graft may be employed either primarily or secondarily, as has been advised by many; though as a rule these grafts become only partially united and are liable to break down. The different plastic methods furnish a more durable material. Those of Stacke and Passow are to be recommended.

Stacke dissects from the mastoid process a blunt triangular flap consisting only of skin. This is placed with its base uppermost. Beneath this he dissects a second flap, with its base downward, consisting only of periosteum. Both are applied to the interior of the cavity by tamponing. The unprotected portions of the periosteal flap can then be covered by a Thiersch graft. These flaps can also be fashioned with their bases reversed.

Passow carries a skin-incision obliquely from in front above the auricle downward and behind the tip of the mastoid process, and from the lower portion of the anterior border he forms a quadrangular flap with its smaller side in front along the auricle. This covers in the posterior and lower portion of the cavity of the bone. The upper portion is covered by a flap formed from the skin of the auditory canal, its broad base being placed uppermost. Thiersch grafts may be employed in addition.

... operations can be found in the respec

... part in the operation is the after

... wound is allowed to remain open o

... simple during the first eight to fourteen

... with iodoform gauze after operation in orde

... drainage and to hold the plastic flaps in place

... wound is hardly attainable, it would not be

... the wound with sterile gauze. Nor is the autho

... the iodoform. Of these nosophen has been

... for this purpose. The first packing should

... in place as long as possible; occasionally one

... before removing it; sometimes it is necessary

... this. This is avoided if the packing is not a

... simply removed gradually as it becomes loosen

... firmly embedded, the author attempts to work

... with boric acid or similar solution. After the fi

... removed, it is only necessary to repack the wour

... dressing the entire wound cavity should be insp

... for exuberant granulations or supp

... and in doing this the probe should always be emp

... granulations are discovered they should

... quantity of chromic acid fused to the tip of a

... were not noticed during their development and

... size, they should be removed with a lo

... Suppuration of the recess rarely occurs pro

... carefully performed. It occurs very freque

... communication between the auditory canal and tl

... of the prominence of the facial nerve was

... of injuring the latter. It may frequently

... chromic acid at each dressing. It may also hap

... been formed, and the latter does not extend f

... sufficiently backward and outward by ta

... adherent to the opposite edges of tl

... and there forms a bridge-shaped proje

... canal and the antrum, which covers tl

... cavity. Technical errors and want of ca

... in this way during the after-treatment,

... considerably prolonged. This has led to th

... should be allowed to remain. It is

... carefully carried out and after-t

... auditory canal, to exercise as good c

... If the latter is insufficiently att

... result as in conducting the after-t

... cause a great deal of annoyanc

... becoming embedded in granulations. V

... occurrence is characterized by prol

... of the granulations, and the p

frequently changed at once, cicatrization often following with amazing rapidity if such a foreign body is removed.

For this reason the author has for some time employed in packing these wounds iodoform gauze strips about 1 cm. wide with woven uncut edges, and he cannot therefore be favorably impressed with Stacke's proposal. Stacke employs single pieces of about 1 to 2 square centimetres in area, with which he fills the wound. Every cut edge is liable to cause fraying, and after two weeks a wound treated in this way frequently appears covered with threads. In removing tampons threads are particularly liable to be caught by the edges of bone corresponding to the superior and inferior border of the wound of the auditory canal. At these sites the formation of exuberant granulations is especially annoying. Careful packing under guidance of inspection can be carried out with one or two long strips, provided these are sufficiently narrow. If the entire cavity of the wound is granulating in a healthy manner, the author generally abstains from packing. If necessary, he thoroughly packs the outer portion of the auditory canal in order to keep this widely open, filling the rest of the wound with boric acid or with a mixture of the latter with iodoform or airol. He has found that cicatrization proceeds more rapidly by this treatment than when tamponing is continued to the last. The secretion from the wound rapidly diminishes and loses the very unpleasant odor which it usually has. From time to time the masses of powder should be removed by washing through a tympanum-tube, and the cavity after having been thoroughly dried should be carefully inspected. The process of healing is only completed when the entire bone cavity is lined with a firm, glistening but dry epidermis. It frequently requires some time before this is completed at the orifice of the tube. Mucopus is sometimes secreted here for months.

MALFORMATIONS, INJURIES, AND DISEASES OF THE FACE. PLASTIC OPERATIONS.

By Privat-Docent Dr. E. LEXER.

CHAPTER X.

MALFORMATIONS OF THE FACE.

CLEFT FORMATIONS.

Origin.—The formation of clefts occurring during the normal development of the face offers the key to the understanding of the frequent as well as the rare forms of deformities. These deformities must be referred to disturbances in development in early fetal life. The normal development of the face, so far as it is concerned in the origin of malformations, occurs in the following manner: The frontal process growing downward approaches the rudimentary first branchial arches growing in from the sides. These arches join in the fourth week to form the lower jaw (mandibula). At the same time a process from their upper border, the processus maxillaris, pushes itself in toward the centre from the two sides between the mandibula and the frontal process (processus nasalis). This frontal process is divided by the two nasal grooves into a central part (processus nasalis medius) and two lateral parts (processus nasalis lateralis). Two lateral processes (processus globularis) divided by an incisure project outward from the central process. (Fig. 129.)

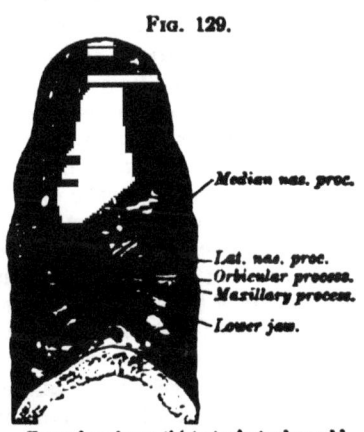

FIG. 129.

Median nas. proc.

Lat. nas. proc.
Orbicular process.
Maxillary process.

Lower jaw.

Face of embryo, thirty to forty days old.

The complicated interdigitation of the processes and clefts may be represented in a simple manner if one considers the central nasal process as bounded laterally by two Y-shaped systems of clefts (Merkel). The lower single limb of the Y extends into the cavity of the mouth between the superior maxillary process and the processus globularis, the latter being a portion of the processus nasalis medialis. Of the two upper limbs, the median passes between the middle and lateral nasal process

(411)

(for example, a frontal encephalocele causing an oblique cleft of the face), in like manner the influence of other congenital tumors should be regarded; for example, teratomata. Thus Broca found a tumor of the base of the skull as the cause of a complicated harelip; Lannelongue, a tumor of the tongue together with a cleft palate. The abnormal widening of the primitive cranial base has also been brought forward as an explanation, so that the superior maxillary processes could not join with the frontal flaps, while, according to Biondi, the possibility of a primary atrophy of the edges of the cleft through inflammatory processes should be kept in mind in these cases. Opposed to the assumption of a force working from within outward, which hinders the junction of the various processes at the right time, is the influence of an abnormally formed amnion working from without, which can make itself felt in various ways. Indeed, from Panum's investigations it seems probable that amniotic folds and bands are the cause of the cleft formation by the mechanical interposition of abnormal parts. The influence of adhesions of the amnion with single points of the skin in the region of the clefts is more pronounced. They occur in deficient liquor amnii, and lead to formation of the so-called bands of Simonast, and they appear to work by binding down the parts, thus holding clefts gaping and giving a changed direction to the development of the processes. Broad adhesions between the face and the membranes are found in conjunction with the most severe malformations of the face (Ziegler's *Allg. Path.*, 1895). However, a traction toward both sides, which influences the union of the clefts, can also occur from small narrow adhesions. Fronhöfer, among others, brought forward examples of this from the clinic of v. Bergmann; other abuormalities point to the influence exerted by the amnion, for the flattening of half the face, club-feet, etc., besides various cutaneous appendages—the remains of amniotic adhesions. These occur on both eyes and ears, and are said to be the point of origin of the tractions which cause the clefts of the upper lip. Through such observations it is evident that the abnormal behavior of the amnion has great etiological significance for the origin of the arrests of development; still it does not give an explanation for everything, as, for example, for the marked preponderance of left-sided labial clefts, the occurrence of which exceeds the right by almost 2 to 1.

A series of cleft formations can only be explained partially or not at all by the remaining open of fetal clefts. The cause of the fissures is not typical here; that is to say, it does not correspond to the latter. Such forms find their explanation in this fact, that the separation of a piece has been caused by means of an amniotic hand stretching across the portion of the face involved subsequent to the more or less complete union of the processes. The disastrous action of such bands is best demonstrated by the fact that they can by means of their tension amputate *in utero* limbs which are already completely formed. Such mutilations are often found simultaneously with malformations of the face, whereby the etiological connection of the combined anomalies with the adhesions and bands of the membranes can be readily inferred. With the large number of possible causes it is plain that the correct exp............ of a cleft formation, especially an unusual form, must at times .... great difficulties not simply on account of the complicated embryol.......... relationship.

Individual Cleft Formations.—According to Trendelenburg's ...., the disturbances in development occur in the region o........ frontal process and in the ar........ the first branchial arch. Me............ schematic representation, in w........ however, only the most impo........ forms are shown (Fig. 130), gi............ general survey of the embry........ clefts.

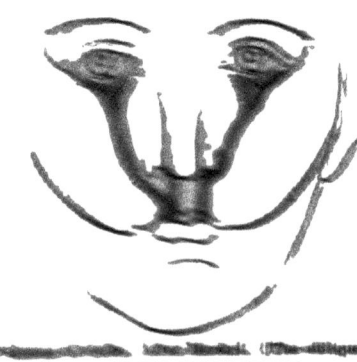

The **lateral** nasal cleft is d........ **between the middle** and l........ **frontal process,** the lateral cle............ **the upper lip lateral** to the phil.......... which, according as one cons............ that the apex of the external .... process reaches down to the l........ ..., has its position between .... and the philtrum—that is, bet.......... the two intermaxillaries (Albrecht) or between the superior maxi........ process and the philtrum (Th. Kölliker). The oblique cleft of the .... or coloboma of the lower eyelid, is situated between .... superior maxillary and lateral frontal process, and the transverse .... of the cheek between the former and the first branchial arch.

Clefts of the Upper Lip.—The median cleft of the upper lip, w........ arises through failure of union of the median side of the two proce........ globular and corresponds exactly to the split lip of the hare, does .... occur. The least degree of the cleft is represented here as well ...... other cleft formations by a slight incurving of the border of ...... If the cleft involves only the soft parts, it reaches more or .... nasal septum (M. B. Smith); if the jaw is also divided, ... lies in the centre between the two intermaxillaries (Lannelongu........ which describes the most severe form, in which cases the median c............ extends up even into the nasal septum. An apparent median clef........ ...., in addition, by the complete absence of the middle piece (p........ ...... and intermaxillaries) in double harelip and cleft palate, especially w........ the cleft borders of the lip do not stand far from one another. (Fig. 13......

The most usual form of the cleft formation of the upper lip is ...., the so-called harelip (labium leporinum), which occurs in ...., one-sided and two-sided, simple and complicated with cl........ ...... A small indentation of the border of the lip lateral to the pl........ ...... i.e., the intermaxillary lip formed out of the middle nasal proc............ represents the slightest grade of the partial form. At times a narrow ...... shining strip of the skin is continued from this indentation to .... (Fig. 132.) This is usually considered a strip of scar-tissue, a........

this formation is looked on as a subsequent intrauterine healing of the cleft. However, as no scar-tissue has been found on histological investigation of the supposed scar, and no remains of mucous membrane within the strip, there can be no question of either a cicatrization or a subsequent union of the fissure. But a delayed union, or according to Trendelenburg a union incomplete but occurring at the proper time, can be assumed, in which situation there always remains a slight change in the skin, as, for example, in the raphé of the scrotum and perineum. These so-called strips of scar-tissue, which are always considered as the slightest disturbance in the normal processes of development, are found in the region of all the facial clefts as well as in the mucous membrane in the position of clefts of the hard and soft palate.

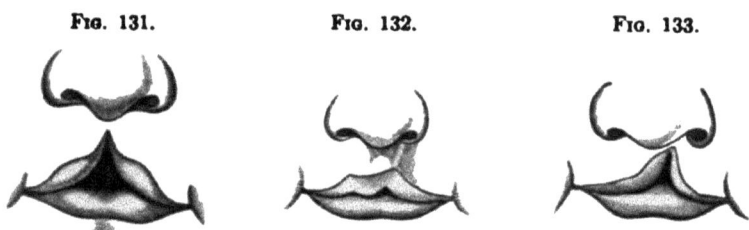

Fig. 131.   Fig. 132.   Fig. 133.

Median cleft of upper lip.   Partial lateral harelip.

As a rule the one-sided partial harelip is in the form of a cleft, which is directed toward the nostril and extends more or less to it, so that only a small bridge of skin of the upper lip remains. The borders of the cleft, which are always covered with mucous membrane, are furthest apart at the level of the normal vermilion border, especially by the distortion outward of the outer border, and come together in an acute angle toward the nose. If the cleft is continued into the nostril, it lacks a posterior border and appears widened, and the alæ nasi flare outward, so that often the outer border of this complete lateral fissure, which in most cases is thin, passes directly into the ala nasi.

In double harelip one fissure is usually total, the other partial if the alveolar arch is not cleft or only so on one side. Between the two fissures stands the philtrum bordered with mucous membrane, which is well formed, in contradistinction to cases with simultaneous cleft of the jaw, while the nasal septum retains almost completely its form. In double complete cleft of the jaw the cleft of the lip is also a total one on both sides.

The majority of the total single and double harelips are accompanied with cleft formation of the jaw, which then forms the direct continuation of the cleft of the lip, but it can also occur without this. Of all these varieties, the double total harelip and cleft palate represent the highest degree of cleft formation which can occur on account of the failure of union of the lateral borders of the entire central frontal process with its surroundings.

... ording to the old cor
... ated by Th. Köll
... between the inter
... and supports the tw
... which is provi
... e superior maxillary
... ght forward in 1
... intermaxilla—th
... this theory the late
... kes part in the forn
... mation of an exter:
... of the cleft must
... view, the outer incis
... anomalies of the te
... and form, and exte
... characteristic marl
... inion often very diffic
... teeth are present in t
... cleft—while the later
... a third incisor, is in
... one depends on atavi
... veen the assumed me
... the other hand, consi
... ted in the superior ma
... as incisivo-maxillary.
... f Th. Kölliker concer
... ws are shared also by 1
... es in which the lateral
... as the first tooth of the
... intermaxilla are situate
... er a critical examinatio
... nclusion " that the later
... s entirely shut out from
... ss." Whether in path
... process grows down to
... for the normal, howev
... rable to Albrecht. In
... ich the cleft passes betw
... side, and consequent
... one does not, as Merke
... assumption of anomalies
... findings do Broca and Kin
...

... he views concerning the qu
... Indeed, according to Biond

... man. The middle one on both sides.
... cleft palate. Benno Sachs considere
... splitting of the dental bud.

intermaxilla is developed in two portions on each side, but the external does not arise in the lateral nasal process, but originates out of the processus maxillares. Trendelenburg is inclined to consider the lateral os incisivum of Albrecht as a Wormian bone, which has arisen the same as the supernumerary teeth from fetal overproduction in the origin of

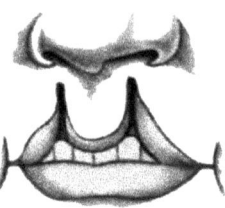
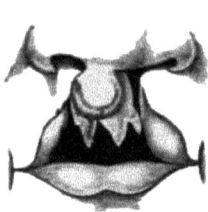

Complete lateral harelip.   Double harelip.

the cleft borders. (See the report of Biondi, and the interesting discussion following it, in the *Verhandlungen des XV. Chirurgen-Congresses*, 1886, i. p. 44.)

By the continuation of the labial cleft into the jaw, and further into the palate, the deformities are as a rule apparently much more considerable. When the total labial cleft of a one-sided or double harelip is combined with a lateral fissure of the jaw, the intermaxilla can project very far toward the side which is not cleft. As in such cases especially the lateral support to the vomer on the border of the cleft is wanting, it develops here further forward, whereby an oblique position of the intermaxilla occurs, so that the median border of the cleft projects far ante-

FIG. 137.   FIG. 138.

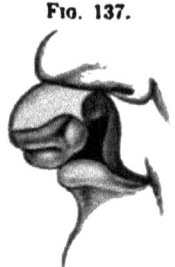
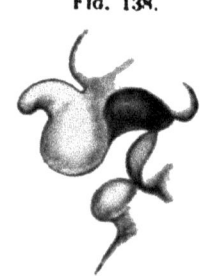

Total labial cleft, one-sided, combined with fissure of the jaw, showing prominent intermaxillary bone.   Double harelip with prominent intermaxillary bone.

riorly beyond the normal line of the alveolar arch. The apex of the nose and the septum, together with the intermaxilla, is thereby displaced toward the side, while the ala nasi of the cleft side spans over the cleft broad and flat, especially if the superior maxilla has here been deficient in development. The projection of the intermaxilla is made still more

still other facial clefts is similar. In the child of Landow there was found, in the position of the left half of the nose, between the root of the nose and the eye, beneath the skin, a body in the shape of a proboscis, consisting of mucous membrane and cartilage. In a case of Nash the eye was wanting on the cleft side.

In regard to the explanation of lateral nasal clefts, which are very interesting embryologically, the views differ. According to Trendelenburg, with whom Merkel also agrees, this cleft formation is to be considered as a continuation of the lateral labial cleft, whereby the middle nasal process is separated from the lateral in its entire length (Merkel). Landow has objected to this on the ground that in very marked clefts the end of this lies far above the nose, so that this cannot correspond to any fetal cleft; he assumes for this only mechanical agents through disturbances in the amnion, which in the peculiar process of folding can very easily give cause for secondary cleft formations.

The complete absence of nose, very seldom observed, has slight surgical interest on account of the other severe malformations which are present at the same time.

THE OBLIQUE FACIAL CLEFT (*Meloschisis*).—The malformation known under this name belongs indeed to the rarities; in consequence of anomalies of the brain, which in most cases are present at the same time (acrania, anencephalus, hemicrania, hydrocephalus, cephalocele), most of the cases are stillborn or soon die. In general the oblique facial cleft indicates a fissure passing from the upper lip to the eye and beyond, which penetrates either the soft parts only or the bone as well, and can occur in varying degree completely or incompletely, one- or two-sided. A simple indentation of the upper lip on the side of the harelip simultaneously with a wedge-shaped defect (colobom) of the lower eyelid or a gaping inner angle of the lids, both joined by a strip of scar-tissue, represent the mildest form of malformation (Morian): in this case the opening between the eyelids is often obliquely placed, the inner angle of the eye markedly lower than the outer. If the cleft involves the

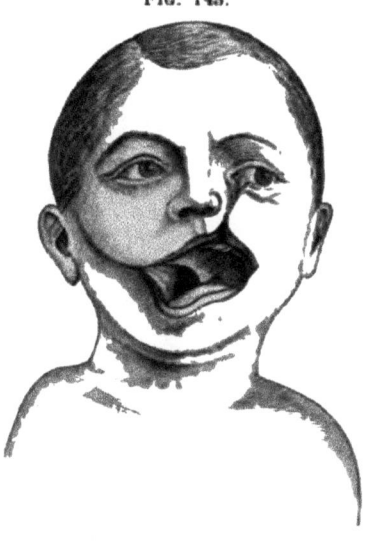

FIG. 143.

Oblique and transverse facial cleft.

bone also, it is, especially if either partial or total defects exist on the bones along the border of the cleft, very broad and deep, and is always in the severe cases continued into a cleft of the maxillary palate.

The discussion concerning the intermaxilla is also touched on by

this malformation, which v. Bruns has designated "an unheard
degree of a single or double cleft of the lip," the more so as the cat
of the cleft is not always the same in spite of the fact that certa
typical lines indicate it. Morian, who has collected the cases, a
increased them by description of preparations from the clinic of
Bergmann, has been able to distinguish several varieties in the arrang
ment of the course of this cleft formation. The first begins as a harel
the cleft passes into the nose lateral to the philtrum, then goes furth
around the ala nasi between the nose and cheek through the inner an
of the eye or the under lid to the slit of the lids, and then through t
outer angle of the eye obliquely upward to the forehead. The seco
form, beginning in the same way on the site of the harelip, does not p
into the nasal cavity, but lateral to the ala nasi through the inner canth
or the under lid into the slit of the lids, and then through the ou
canthus or the upper lids to the forehead. (Fig. 143.) In the bone tl
fissure runs between the outer intermaxilla and the superior maxil
inward from the foramen infraorbitalis to the orbit.

FIG. 144.

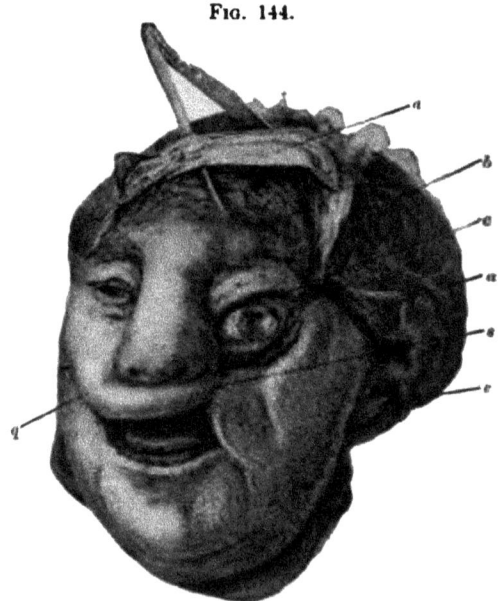

Oblique facial cleft. *a a.* Amniotic bands. *b.* Encephalocele. *c.* Left external canthus.
q. Right transverse facial cleft. *s.* Left oblique facial cleft.

These two forms can be explained as arrested development in embryonal clefts, not, however, uniformly, but only with the aid of the
various theories. The first variety is explained by the observation that the
external nasal process does not take part in the formation of the lip and
alveolar arch (Th. Kölliker); or also by the view of Biondi, according
to which the external intermaxilla is approximated to the superior maxil-

lary process; accordingly the cleft in the alveolar arch has its position between the superior maxilla and the os intermaxillare or between the inner and outer intermaxilla. The second variety, which passes lateral to the nasal opening, corresponds to the stomato-orbital groove of Albrecht between the external nasal process and the superior maxilla.

The third variety of Morian is where the cleft of the soft parts begins at the angle of the mouth and that of the bone external to the canine tooth, and passes to the orbital cavity in the region of the infraorbital canal. It is in this variety alone that the mechanical disturbance must have had as the result a splitting off of the median portion of the superior maxillary flap, apparently through the pressure of an amniotic band stretching over it. On this account this variety has been considered as an atypical cleft formation.

The Transverse Facial Clefts, Cheer Clefts (*Makrostoma*).— A cleft formation under this name is observed more frequently than the foregoing, which corresponds to the embryonal cleft existing between the superior maxillary process and the first branchial arch. The union of the two portions for the formation of the cheek remains undeveloped; the mouth opening is thus continued for a' distance into the cheek (makrostoma); or, in other words, a more or less wide cleft, edged with a vermilion border, begins in the angle of the mouth and passes transversely through the cheek, where it frequently ends at the masseter. This formation occurs on both sides. The mildest degree is a lengthening of the angle of the mouth outward, from which at times a strip of scar-tissue passes outward as far as in front of the ear, as evidence of the disturbed union. The further course of the fissure is not constant. The typical groove ends in front of the tragus; there are, in addition, clefts which divide the malar bone and pass to the temporal or proceed obliquely downward toward the angle of the inferior maxilla. In our case (Fig. 143) the arch of the palatoglossus on the right side is indeed pulled inward into the transverse facial cleft by a firm scar.

Amniotic adhesions in the region of the inferior maxilla and superior maxillary process can together with the traction, which disturbs the union of the two portions, produce through pressure and expansion a grooving in this superior maxilla and first branchial arch, sometimes in one more than the other, whereby the course of the transverse facial clefts can assume the atypical varieties mentioned, or hinder the growth of the neighboring parts; thus there are cases known with the inferior maxilla rudimentarily developed, or with deformities of the external ear. Through the analogy in development those varieties, which are associated with oblique facial clefts or other cleft formations of the opposite side, are easily explained.

A beautiful example of the origin of the atypical cleft formations is described by Chavane. Here a broad amniotic hand, joined with the meninges, passes to both sides of the face into the mouth and grooves the halves of the face as a tightly drawn line. On the left side the cleft, beginning in the upper lip near the angle of the mouth and in the alveolar arch between the canine and first premolar, approaches the third variety

sidered are the bleeding, wound infection, and narcosis. On this account anæsthesia is not employed in the newborn by the majority of operators, and yet in general it is well borne by children. The occurrence of wound infection in aseptic operations is to be feared less in the first weeks and months of life than in older children, in whom a chronic catarrh of the mucous membrane must sometimes be made responsible for the tearing out and suppuration of the sutures, also for the severe inflammations and erysipelas. Furthermore, the bleeding in a well-conducted operation is so slight that it needs consideration only with very weak, anæmic children. The flowing of blood and saliva into the air-passages may be avoided, even if one does not operate with the head hanging down, by means of immediate compression of the wounds and sponging out of the cheek pockets with stick sponges; the same is true of the swallowing of blood, to which has been ascribed the occurrence of intestinal catarrh. The author, with the majority of surgeons, on this account prefers to operate on harelip in strong, healthy children with simple or complicated clefts even within the first days, or better in the second to fourth week, in order to protect them, by means of closure of the lip, against the obvious dangers. If, however, diseases of the mucous membrane of the buccal cavity or of the respiratory and intestinal tracts are present, if it is a question of weak and sickly children, the outlook for the operation is indeed poor, especially if the clefts are extensive and penetrate jaw and palate; here an early operation is a venture, the success of which can on the whole mean the rescue of a child otherwise doomed. Still, general rules cannot well be given. Hence in the individual case the dangers of the early operation and of the expectant treatment are to be weighed exactly according to the extensiveness of the cleft formation, the general condition of the child, and the diseases present.

An attempt has been made by means of statistics to determine the mortality in children operated on early. It is well known that the mortality in children operated on increases with the severity of the deformity and decreases with increasing age. This last fact, however, cannot be a guide to early operation, because, in the first place, in older children the greater power of resistance must be considered, and, furthermore, it is self-evident that in the calculations the number of children who have died in early life unoperated on is wanting. And this number is considerable. According to Abel, by far the greatest number of harelip children die in the first month.

Operations for Cleft Formations.—OPERATIONS FOR CLEFT OF UPPER LIP.—*Preparation for the Operation.*—The young patient may be held immovable by an assistant who sits opposite to the operator, or a bandage may be employed as is done, for example, in the clinic of v. Bergmann, by means of which the child can be firmly fastened to the high-placed head-piece of an operating-table. The assistant, whose duty it is to control bleeding by compression, can hold the head at the same time when necessary. With a view to prevent eczema from too energetic cleansing of the tender skin, it is best to wash with soap and water only. Elastic clamps can be placed in the angle of the mouth to compress the

...it is advisable to ...the gum and the cheek, which will abso... ...the cavity of the mouth. With such prec... ...perate with the hand pendant. Usuall... ...mother continue to care for the child, as ... ...desirable for the general condition of the child. ...incisions give a smooth wound-surfa... ...lip is stretched while making the incisio... ...arrested carefully by means of forceps a... ...a narrow or lancet-shaped knife. Small ... ...improving the border of the wound by the r... ...attempt to make the wound-border as ... ...by passing the knife through the ... ...and it is immaterial whether more ...membrane or from the skin.

...methods of suture has narrowed down ...with silk or fine silver wire. The ... ...three or four comparatively strong sutur... ...limited to the mucous membran... ...sutures are placed in the mucous mem... ...lip in the region of the vermilion b... ...perforating the skin only, appro... ...wound. Sometimes it is advisable to pl... ...suture of stronger silk (Simon), by whi... ...from the border of the wound.

Fig. 146.

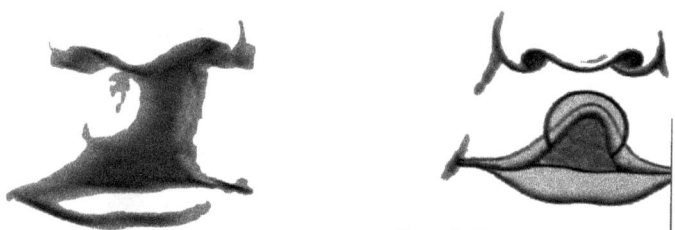

...uncomplicated cleft lip is concerne... ...of which single types are depicte... ...difficulties to be overcome, give... ...cleft or a narrow complete fissur... ...borders of the lip pass at a right angl... ...is also rare to have the cleft bord... ...cleft borders are more or less obli... ...border at an obtuse angle. On ac... ...the oldest method, in which the bo... ...must leave, after union takes ...

if indeed this occurs at all, a notching of the edge of the lip. Gräfe (1825) tried to overcome this disadvantage by curving his freshening incision. (Figs. 145 and 146.) The concave borders of the wound are straightened by the suture, and thereby the upper lip is lengthened. The shorter border of the cleft in incomplete harelip can be made to equal the longer border by shifting the uppermost angle of the wound to the side of the longer border; or, according to v. Bruns, the curved incision can be used for the shorter limb only, in order to make it the same length as the longer limb which was freshened in a straight line.

FIG. 147.　　　　　　　FIG. 148.

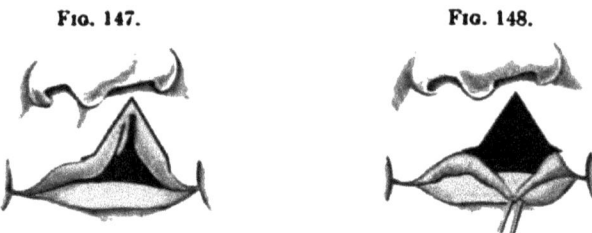

Line of incision of Malgaigne, according to v. Bruns.

The lengthening of the cleft borders is accomplished still better by making an angular incision, whereby the border of the cleft, which was formerly cut away, is partially made use of in the union. The borders are freshened in such a manner that the detached edge of mucous membrane together with the true vermilion border remains attached at the point of transition between the two. The small flaps, which are formed in this manner, are folded down, and cut to correspond to one another in such a way that after their union a small prominence, like a proboscis, projects on the border of the lip and prevents an indentation, and can

FIG. 149.　　　　　　　FIG. 150.

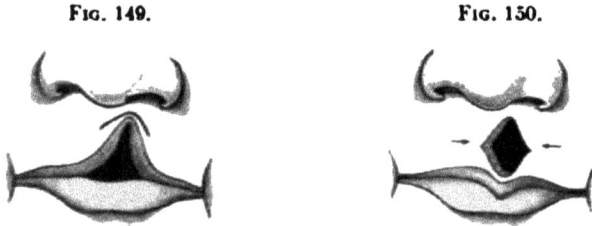

Line of incision, according to Nélaton.

be removed later in case it has not shrunken enough. This method, first described by Malgaigne in 1844, practised before that time, however, by Clemat, can be adapted by means of a series of smaller modifications to the numerous varieties of single complete or incomplete clefts. V. Bruns has lengthened the freshening incision so that the base of the small flap is formed by the true vermilion border. (Figs. 147 and 148.) The method of Nélaton, which is only applicable to small defects or

æral border of the cleft a longer—and on this account movable—flap is formed. The median, on the contrary, ısary, ao that by drawing over the lateral flap the line ı the centre line, where a small prominence is formed ıation of the vermilion border of each apex with sutures.

153   Fıo. 154.

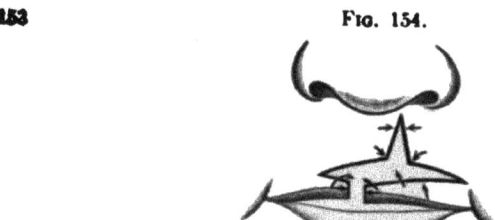

Line of Incision, according to König.

advocated the drawing over of the edge of the lip for rovement of a healed harelip, in the same manner as ırily in the above method, and was first done by v. emedying a defect of the lower lip by the aid of the ɾes a more normal shape to the lip by detaching the and then by suturing in the correct manner. Later ıd was also recommended for larger clefts. (Figs. 155 ıuture, however, has to sustain a rather strong pull ıs is evidenced from the illustration.

ı. 155.   Fıı. 156.

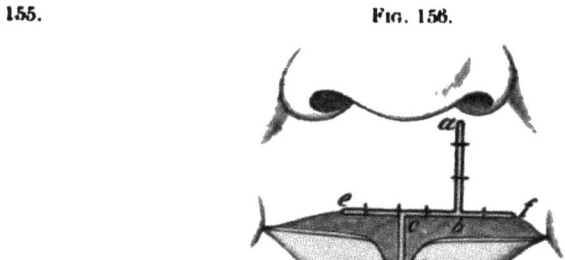

Langenbeck's operation, according to Wolf.

König has been modified by Hagedorn (1884) in order position of the suture where the corners of the freshened er. Hagedorn's incision gives a so-called zigzag suture. ı.) A narrow knife is inserted at 1 and 1_1, and the ı 1_1-2_1 are first made along the boundary-line of the , As the border of the wound should be as broad as ly in an atrophic lip, the incision is not made perpen- iquely; that is to say, in such a manner that somewhat mhrane is removed than skin. The detached border of to hang down. Then follows incision 3–4 on the lateral

uble harelip, naturally can only give good results
philtrum is of sufficient length.

m quite a different standpoint, also modified the old
double harelip. Here also he completely sacrifices
edge of the cleft and forms flaps 7 to 8 mm. wide
ailion border. He obtains these flaps on each side
sion 1 to 1½ cm. long parallel to the border of the
illustrated in Figs. 164 and 165. The method of
r.

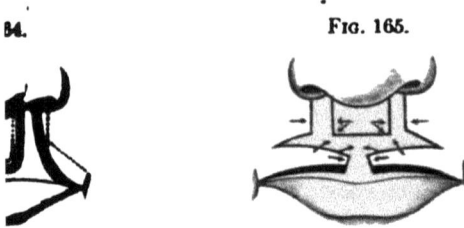

34. FIG. 165.

König incision and suture.

mplicated method of Hagedorn is modelled after
lengthening of the cleft borders, after the formation
membrane, is obtained by means of a small notch-
ision is placed in a manner corresponding to the
eral border of the cleft in one-sided cases. The
eued to fit. The borders of the wound come well
tures. (Figs. 166 to 168.)

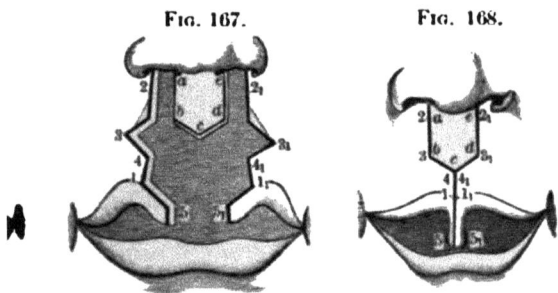

FIG. 167. FIG. 168.

ncision and suture, according to Hagedorn.

ry broad, one side only can be closed first, in order
incisions, and to lessen also the danger and duration
Later the other side can be closed and the result
subsequent operations.

nt methods have been introduced in order to bring
ouble harelip with projecting intermaxilla.

f the cleft borders appears impossible on account of
ting intermaxilla, the oldest method can be followed,

ons (A. Broca and le Dentu) prefer the bony suture
rönlein pushes the intermaxilla back after the man-
ı and holds the freshened intermaxilla in place by
te, which passes from the region of the nasolabial
behind the philtrum. In older children or adults
to obtain by this method a bony union between the
solar arch. On the other hand, this favorable result
ng children. This may be due partly to deep-seated
involves the bone, partly to the injury to the
:th caused by the lateral freshening (v. Esmarch).

169.   Fig. 170.

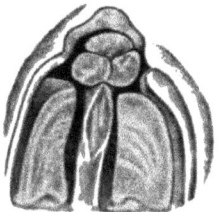

ent of the intermaxilla, according to v. Bardeleben.

e placed on a firm union between the portions of
pushed by one another after the method of v. Bar-
ne mucoperiosteal flaps of v. Langenbeck will give
'or a firm union. On the other hand, experience
rmaxilla, which is pushed back, is sufficiently fixed
abial clefts, which is immediately undertaken, espe-
illa fits at all into the cleft of the jaw. From these
er firm connective-tissue union between the inter-
ft border of the jaw. On this account König and
in most cases that the pushing back of the inter-
o v. Bardeleben, be followed by the union of the

narrowed in the centre is halved, and the halves reunited by sev
rubber band 1½ cm. long between them. The two portions of ad
plaster are fastened to the cheeks, while the elastic centre port
rubber exercises a continuous pressure on the intermaxilla. V. Esi
utilized the elastic pressure of this so-called "Thiersch butterfly" t
in place the intermaxilla, after it had been pushed back after the m
of v. Bardeleben. The children wear a night-cap, on which a be
rubber is fastened in such a way that it lies against the snout. Acco
to Albert's experience, this pushing back without immediate sutu
the cleft has a favorable influence on the poorly developed se
cutaneum, which is better developed even in a few weeks.

The effort to push back the intermaxilla by gradual pressure
the foundation of Simon's method. This method, however, has
few adherents on account of the
that in forming the flaps the soft
of the face are wounded. Even I
the method of v. Bardeleben was k
Simon tried to make movable fla
encircling the ala nasi with incision
then by pushing over these flaps to
them below with the snout which
been freshened. After these flaps
a gradual recession of the interm
occurs. This is brought about b
tension which these flaps exert on the intermaxilla. Later, whe
recession is complete, that portion of the lip which is deficient
centre is completed.

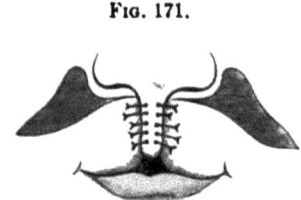

Fig. 171.

Nostril flaps, according to Simon.

When the intermaxilla projects very markedly, the flap, former
Simon's method, can be tried first on one side, and after several
on the other. The intermaxilla then grows obliquely, inclining t
the side which is united, on account of the traction exerted by th
Later, however, it is again pulled straight to the middle line l
closure of the labial defect on the other side. An upper lip can be f
in this manner even when the centre-piece is entirely lacking o
poorly developed and the cleft is a broad one.

Wolff has tried to make use of this method, and to push back
ually the intermaxilla of a three-day-old child. He did this in s
sittings, first suturing one side and then four weeks later the othe
order to beautify the lip he did two subsequent operations six
later.

Although Wolff considers the main advantage of this gradua
cedure to be that the intermaxilla is not deprived of nutrition i
way by the spontaneous recession, and that it is important to
making the incisions of Simon for cosmetic reasons, still the
method is hardly in the position to take the place of v. Bardele
simple method of reposition, which interferes with the nutrition o
intermaxilla to an insignificant degree, and which can be followed a
same sitting by a complete union of the upper lip. By this method

as good results can be obtained without subjecting the children to several operations.

All attempts to preserve the intermaxilla are justified by the hope that the patient will not present the peculiar profile characteristic of the removal of the centre-piece. On the other hand, too much concerning the function must not be expected, for, as has been mentioned, the inter- maxilla remains movable in most cases and is characterized by very faulty dental conditions; with a markedly retracted upper lip a cosmetic improvement can be obtained by removing a wedge from the under lip (Simon). In spite of all this, preservation of the intermaxilla is not recommended in all cases in which it is prominent; often it is so poorly developed that it can be of no cosmetic use. It may be added that, according to observations of Gotthelf, Partsch, and others, although in many cases the middle piece was removed, no marked deformity occurred later, and the teeth of the upper jaw articulated well with those of the lower.

Choice of Incision.—A surgeon of experience will not use one method for all harelips nor regularly make it his choice; for experience teaches to choose certain definite methods for certain forms. From the rich material afforded by the clinic of v. Bergmann the author has formulated the following rules:

In One-sided Harelip.—1. For incomplete and complete clefts, operate according to Mirault—v. Bruns. (Figs. 151 and 152.) For pushing back of intermaxilla, operate according to König's method.

2. For the subsequent operation for indentations or small colobomata, adopt v. Langenbeck's method of drawing over the edge of the lip accord- ing to Wolff. (Figs. 155 and 156.)

In Double Harelip.—1. In uneven or complete double clefts with large philtrum, proceed according to Mirault. (Figs. 162 and 163.)

2. In uneven or complete double clefts with small philtrum, proceed according to Hagedorn. (Figs. 166 to 168.) For pushing back of the intermaxilla, proceed according to v. Bardeleben. (Figs. 169 and 170.)

Subsequent Treatment and Subsequent Operations for Harelip.—The general condition of the child is to be considered most in the after- treatment. As experience shows that the swallowing of blood leads to digestive disturbances, it is often advised to free the stomach and intes- tines from the swallowed material by the administration of a mild laxa- tive. The breathing of the child should be especially watched after operation. Cases of suffocation may occur in the following manner: the narrowed nasal openings become occluded and the children, as Busch remarks, do not instinctively open the mouth. Immediate opening of the mouth removes the danger. It is self-evident that the nourishment of the child should remain as nearly as possible the same as before the closure of the labial cleft.

The question as to the best manner of protecting the wound or the suture against external insults and infections has been answered quite dif- ferently according to the experience of different operators. The greatest factor in the healing of this suture, which in most cases is under tension,

is rest. This is obtained not only by trying to obviate the greatest dai
namely, the continuous crying of the child, but also by omitting all su
fluous manipulations. The first indication may be met by the gre
possible quiet, or by the administration of a drop of tincture of op
or wrapping the hands in cotton-wool and binding them to the sid
the bed or to the thorax, and by administering fluid nourishmer
carefully as possible; the second may be obtained by the physician o
ting completely, at least during the first three or four days, clean
and examination of the line of suture.

A satisfactory relaxation in the line of suture is obtained by band
and strips of adhesive plaster. A lasting effect by these measure
however, uncertain, as the apparatus must fit very well (for exampl
Bruns' bandage-clasps). V. Bruns tried to avoid the pressure of rela
strips of adhesive plaster by fastening small wedge-shaped pads on
cheeks. Every movement of the dressing, however, has an injur
effect on the wound and necessitates a new adjustment, whereby
child's restlessness is increased. Often a strip of gauze smeared '
an ointment is attached without tension on the upper lip by mean
adhesive plaster. This small dressing, however, must be renewec
least daily or even more frequently, as particles of food, saliva, n
mucus, and dirt collect beneath the adhesive plaster. On the o
hand, if the suture is left entirely uncovered and is smeared witl
ointment immediately after the operation, and is protected from
hands of the child, and the cleansing of the face and the feedin
done with care, a scab firmly adherent to the suture, which one ⟨
well to leave, soon forms, undisturbed during the first days,
vided the nostrils do not become occluded. This scab not only
tects the suture-line from dirt, but efforts to remove it cause ⟨
lessness of the child, which has an even more unfavorable effect f
the tension caused by crying than a superficial inflammation or supp
tion of a stitch-hole. On the fourth or fifth day the scab is remove⟨
smearing with boric acid or zinc ointment, and with care the rem
of the sutures is begun, during which restless children should be a⟨
thetized slightly. Those sutures are to be removed first which hav
inflamed appearance. When possible, the larger sutures are left a co
of days longer, so that in the course of a week all the sutures are remo

Many authors try to guard the young scar after removal of the sut
against breaking open, by relaxing with strips of adhesive plaster. '
is recommended when the scar begins to give way in any spot.

Usually the surgeon should be content, especially in children a
weeks old, if he has obtained by the first operation a closure of the le
defect without undue tension and notching. On the other hand, s
notches or irregularities of the vermilion border may be left for su
quent treatment. Since after six months or a year a larger opera
field is offered, surgical procedures for cosmetic effect can be carried
much more easily and satisfactorily at this time or even later tha
possible on the small lips of a very young child. (Compare Al
cheiloplastic.)

If the entire suture gives way, it is best to wait until the freshened cleft borders have completely healed. A closure of the gaping wound is almost never obtained by a secondary suture. If a small bridge of skin is all that remains after the first operation, it must be sacrificed as a rule at the second operation in order to obtain a broad denudation of the cleft borders.

Improvements in the shape of the nose are often necessary also. For example, when a poorly developed septum cutaneum is distorted downward by union of the philtrum with the borders of the cleft, an improvement in the profile may be obtained by the formation of a small skin-flap formed out of the philtrum and the septum. The apex of this flap is directed forward, and it is pushed backward and downward and a Y-shaped line of union results (Le Dentu). A concave indentation in the ala nasi on the side of the cleft can be remedied by cutting out a small wedge.

Concerning the further complications of harelip, see the chapter dealing with cleft palate and its operations.

OPERATIONS FOR OTHER CLEFT FORMATIONS.—Isolated cases of other facial clefts have been healed by fortunate operations. These operations, however, belong to the rarities and lack any typical mode of procedure on account of the great diversity of the individual forms. They are regulated in general by the fundamental rules of plastic surgery.

Small colobomata, as they occur on the upper lip and lower eyelid as the slightest degree of oblique facial cleft, are closed without special difficulties by denudation, undermining the surrounding area, and suture. Small notches or defects of the ala nasi may be remedied by plastic methods with equally good results. On the other hand, complete closure of an extensive cleft formation is a difficult task on account of distortion of the soft portions of the face and abnormalities of the bones. The oblique facial clefts operated on by Hasselmann best illustrate these difficulties.

For good cosmetic result the median nasal cleft presents the most unfavorable conditions, and this is on account of the increase in width of the face, which cannot be altered, and on account of the alæ nasi being widely separated from one another.

In the case of Nasse the author replaced the missing nasal bones in the following manner: he formed small plates of bone from the broad flat frontal processes of the superior maxilla, after having denuded the entire rim on each side of the wound, and laid them on one another. These flaps included the soft parts also, which were moved over with the bones. The diverging cartilaginous plates of the septum were joined. A case of Kredel and a second case reported by the author were more difficult to operate on. In an incomplete lateral nasal cleft Kredel filled out the groove in the ala nasi by means of a small wedge-shaped piece from the cartilage of the ear; this was pushed beneath the loosened skin and healed there.

A median cleft formation of the under jaw has been operated on by Wölffler. The edges of the cleft were denuded, and the separated ends

of the inferior maxilla were sutured with s
were approximated also, and the cleft in t
Mirault's method.

ABNORMALITIES IN THE REGION Ol

Malformations of the face are also of sur
has occurred to an abnormal degree, and is
in the size of or complete closure of the
cases are very rare. Such disturbances as
clefts and the nostrils, also synchilia or atre
observed. Furthermore an abnormal degr
cleft is the cause of the deformity designat
been described by Ammon, and in connectio
of the first branchial arch by Ahlfeldt.

Fig. 172.

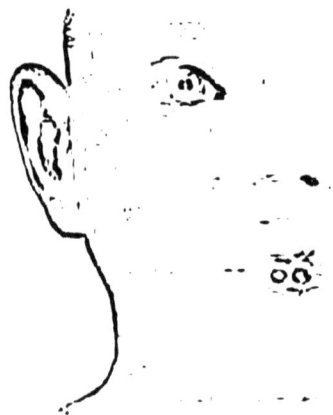

Congenital fistula of the lower lip of a

Remarkable forms arise about the cl
intrauterine union of a harelip. If i
occurred with a short philtrum, a mark
lip is the result (v. Bruns). V. Bruns
right- and left-sided cleft of the mouth
the angle of the cleft of a one-sided har
should be mentioned, namely, that a
upper lip may also be caused by a fren
far down.

In addition to an atresia of the nostri
on a complete defect of the nose, the ph
even cutaneous surface. Defective f

colobomata, according to Manz and others, cannot be viewed as formations due to arrested development, as the lids are formed homogeneously without the formation of clefts. A series of defects of the upper and lower lid may be explained by the action of an amniotic band. This band is closely adherent to the cornea of the eye, which in the early stages projects prominently, and is stretched over the lids, which in development become more movable and leave behind a hole. On the other

FIG. 173.

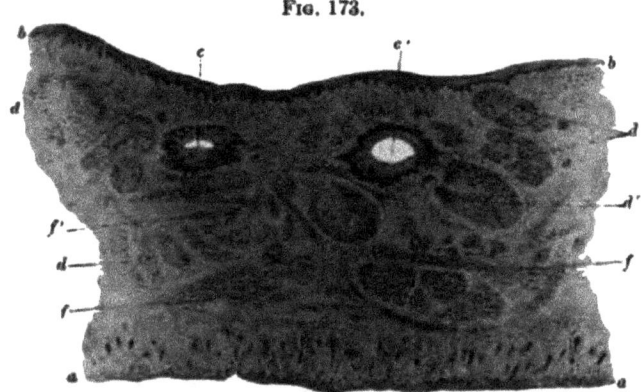

Horizontal section of lower lip of same child. *a.* External skin. *b.* Mucous membrane. *c, c'.* Sections of fistulæ 4½ mm. from their openings. *d, d'.* Mucous glands. *f, f'.* Muscle fibres.

hand, however, colobomata of the lower lid have been found more than once in connection with anomalies of the tear-sacs, as the results of an oblique facial cleft. Such defects apparently, according to Fr. Schanz, are only connected with the lower lid; for they have arisen as portions of oblique facial clefts not in this, but in the inner angle of the lid out of the orbital nasal border, and have come to lie more externally (laterally) on account of the unequal development of the frontal and superior maxilla process. Thus it is true that the under lid appears in part to be lacking, but, as Schanz showed, the defect is characterized as a coloboma of the inner angle, for the puncta lacrymalia are situated on its two corners.

FIG. 174.

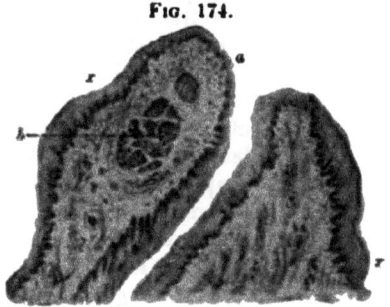

Sagittal section through the papilla on right side, containing fistulous opening. *a.* Lumen of fistula. *b.* Muscle fibres. *x x.* Marks the origin of papilla from mucous membrane.

Congenital fistulæ and dermoids (see these) have a certain relation to fetal clefts. On this account both have been considered ('Trendelenburg, v. Bramann) as the least degree of incomplete union of such a fissure. The fistulæ are rare, much rarer indeed than the fistulous for-

mations on the neck, which are in connect
it is interesting, however, that up to the p
corresponding to almost all the fetal clefts
upper lip, for example, Feurer described s
situated on the right side of the philtrun
vermilion border. The course of the fistul
the right nostril. Here the blind end was
tion of the labial mucous membrane. In
had been formed, which was lined above ɩ
brane.

It is more difficult to explain a fistula o
this has been observed associated with otl
and has not been situated in the median
sponding to the median clefts of the under
but the openings of the double fistulæ
one another laterally from the median li
projected like a proboscis (Rose, Fritsc
Miller). The secretion of a fluid resembl
opinion that there was present an abnor
This view, however, was disproved by M
the canals were shown to be lined with n
parallel or slightly converging and end
fistulæ can be explained in a similar mai
as arrests in development, caused by inco
tion with the lateral divisions of the lip; t
embryological discovery of a central piec
inences (Dursy). (Figs. 172, 173 and 17ɩ

Fistulous formations are likewise found
the median and lateral fissures. They are i
on the bridge of the nose a canal with a fi
epidermis. A similar formation can occu
cyst, which was originally present and t
distinguished from that of a congenital fis
The tract in such cases still contains rem
characteristic of a dermoid. The author
has operated on them. V. Mangoldt foui
the centre of a trough-shaped bridge of th
of the nose. In the centre of an abu naɪ
lateral fissure—he saw in a girl fourteen
shaped retraction of the skin, beneath wl
few millimetres and ended blindly.

The transverse cleft of the cheek has b
fistula in a single case (Trendelenburgɩ.

In the region of the oblique clefts of ɩ
by Lannelongue and by Kraske. The ɩ
found at the frenulum; the tract had a lɩ
in the direction of a strip of scar whicɩ.
lower eyelid.

through the jaw and lip. (Fig. 178.) If a double harelip is also present, the labial maxillary cleft is complete only on the side of the cleft palate. On the side of the cleft the palate plate is present only as a narrow ledge, which has a horizontal direction; the upper jaw is deficient in its development, so that the alveolar arch has a position posterior to its normal curve. The latter appearance is made still more pronounced by the projection of the intermaxilla, which is joined with the other side ; it is due to this that deformities of the nose occur, as have been pictured under complicated harelip. The processus palatinus in many cases merges abruptly above into the vomer, with which it is joined.

The partial cleft, the uranocolobom of the hard palate, is subject to the most numerous variations and in most cases it is in conjunction with a simple or double harelip and median cleft of the soft palate. The anterior uranocolobom, single or double, according to the relation between the palate plate and the vomer, represents nothing more than the continuation into the hard palate of the single or double alveolar cleft. Sometimes a cleft of the soft palate is associated with this cleft in its anterior portion, while the greater part of the hard palate is closed. The uranocolobom in the posterior portion of the hard palate is combined with the cleft soft palate. The cleft here usually involves only the palate bone; less often it extends through the palatine processes up to the normally formed alveolar arch, in which case the vomer lies exposed so the cleft is a double one. The rarest of all, according to v. Langenbeck, is where the cleft is present between the palatine processes of the superior maxilla only, while the horizontal processes of the palate bones, the velum, and the alveolar arch are normally developed. If such a cleft is one-sided, the defect can apparently lie in the centre of one of the palate processes on account of the marked development of the lower border of the vomer (O. Weber). The slightest grade of anterior uranocolobom is the abnormal widening of the canalis incisivus, which is considered by v. Langenbeck as a partial cleft.

The cleft of the soft palate in most cases is associated with the various forms of cleft of the hard palate; still it may exist independently of the latter, and then shows slight nickings in the centre of the uvula up to complete clefts, which extend up into the horizontal processes of palate bones.

Cases of so-called intrauterine healed cleft palate represent, so to speak, the slightest grade of cleft palate. This is due either to a delayed union or to one which occurs not quite completely. Beneath the mucous membrane which is joined everywhere, a cleft-like defect in the bone can sometimes be felt; if the velum is too short in this case, the speech has a strong nasal twang similar to that in real clefts.

The disadvantages which are connected with the congenital cleft of the palate have been partly spoken of above under complicated harelip. The deficient partition between the buccal and nasal cavities has dependent upon it disturbances which in the first place are concerned in the act of sucking and swallowing and later of phonation, and in the second

place those which are caused by all ki...
membranes. The latter aris... only ...
the open cavity of the nasopharv...
severe catarrh of the mucous mem...
of the lymphatic tissue of th... ph...
the tube (Eustachian), and in ...
widely cleft there is added... ...
mation of the mucous membr...
difficulty in swallowing food, the
and the constant escape through th...
cases in which no harelip is pres...
noticed by the mothers. Feeding...
children, offers very great diffic ulties
spoon or a tube to the poster... ...
lowing possible. A certain ...
quence of the difficulties in g...
quence of the inflammation of the ...
associated with severe intestinal di...
decomposed masses of secr... ...
These inflammations also fa...
monia. That all these facto...
greatest extent in cases of ext...
harelip is apparent without fur...
absent and the cleft of the pal...
ing nourishment are often slight, ...
tongue the cleft in the palate ...
has been made under operat... ...
labial cleft not only can the ...
the inflammation of the muc... ...
that gradually a narrowing ...
lips. In later life the difficul...
of the tendency to catarrh ...
in swallowing, which by ...
in phonation is the most ...
for there exists, quite indep... ...
free communication betwe... ...
nouncing certain sounds.

These changes in phonation
accurately determined, especi...
tigations of W. Gutzmann. ...
sonants, with the exception ...
through the buccal cavity; with ...
passes through the nose. If the ...
the nasal cavity does not occur,
useless. The degree of "nasal"
and e, and is most marked with ...
of the nasopharynx is necessary ...
conditions this closure occurs ...

... during narcosis is ...
... method of operating wi...
... anatomy and the tampon...
... the pauses which must occur
... are of great advantage
... compression. The use of
... the exact placing of the
... placing and tying of the
... at the head of the patient.
... is washed with soap and
... other operations, and the
... or a sterile bandage; then
... The most widely used mouth-
... In using the latter, care must
... the tongue is not pressed too
... tion. On this account the
... and an attempt is made
... which presses it down,
... The lower jaw during the
... the assistant who supports
... instrument, which rests
... and is in the way in cleft
... bending.
... to-day differs only in several
... of v. Langenbeck, who

... complete clefts of the soft
... apex of which is seized with
... A fine-pointed knife is
... forceps, so that the border
... motion in such a way that a
... possible for union. This is
... more of the mucous mem-
... the other side by holding the
... separated first from the hard
... uvula with a pair of scissors.
... occurs without difficulty is
... the forceps and knife can
... of the patient may be made
... the right hand also. A stout
... freshening of the cleft border
... the edge of this knife curved
... The mucous membrane and
... from the cleft border. This
... somewhat beyond the anterior
... in the so-called one-sided cleft
... with the vomer, merges into this
... the bone is made along the line

... on both sides, and are carried through mucous membrane
... with the same knife as was used in freshening the cleft
... of the ... hard palate. They begin in the region of the hamular
... passing close along the row of teeth terminate, according
... Langenbeck's rule, anteriorly in double clefts between the two
... teeth of the side involved, in single clefts between the canine and
... molar tooth. In no case should the bridge which joins the flaps
... anteriorly be too narrow, for it is here that in loosening from the bone
... readily tear still further. If the line of incision passes near the row
... teeth, and slipping of the knife is prevented by firm support of the
... and the arteria palatina will not be injured, and can remain as a
... nutrient vessel for the detached palate flap. Although it has been proved
... that the injury to this vessel does not seriously interfere with the nour-
... ishment of the flap, still it is just as well to avoid dividing the vessel;
... or although the bleeding can as a rule be readily controlled by com-
... pression, secondary hemorrhages are possible, and these may become
... dangerous, as a case which was operated on outside and brought into
... Bergmann's clinic proves. At first the bleeding, even without injury
... of the artery, after completion of the lateral incisions is usually rather
... profuse. The following procedure has given the author the best results.
... After the periosteum has been divided on any side the flap is immediately
... raised from the palate by an elevator, rapidly even if incompletely, and
... the pocket thus formed is packed firmly with gauze. After this the
... lateral incision on the other side can be made without trouble, and when
... the packing has been done here after detaching the flap the bleeding on
... the first side has ceased for the most part and it is possible to proceed
... further. The lateral incisions are not always necessary on both sides.
... Langenbeck omitted this incision on the half of the palate which
... extends perpendicularly into the vomer and the nasal septum, and
... with a curved elevator accomplishes the detachment of the flaps
... from the palate through the incision which runs along the edge of the
... palate mucous membrane. The flap after being detached from the
... palate lies horizontal and forms a kind of curtain, and when in double

swan's neck; the cleft border must be pierced from behind forward, as pointed out by König, that is to say, from the side of the nasal mucous membrane, and each end of the suture must be provided with a needle. The most difficult point to suture is the anterior angle of the cleft. Just here, and for the entire suture as well, the author has obtained very good service from the Langenbeck holder. The needles with handles appear to be simple and sufficient. They possess anteriorly a curve similar to the Deschamp needles, or are bent at a right angle for certain places. Trélat also uses needles with similar handles and a hook-shaped curve. The suturing, for which most surgeons use only fine silk, commences in every method at the uvula. The sutures are not immediately tied, the end being caught in artery-forceps, so that the entire cleft remains open during the suturing until all the through-and-through sutures are placed; when all these sutures have been tied, several superficial sutures with the very finest intestinal silk are necessary in many

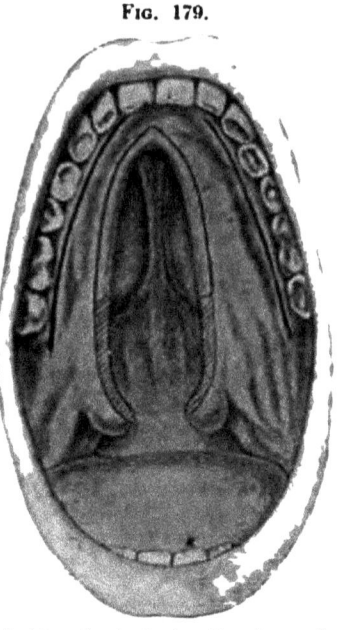

Fig. 179.

Incisions for freshening the edges and freeing the flaps.

places for the better union of the border of the mucous membrane. These are also placed on the posterior surface of the uvula, as far upward on this as it is possible to reach. The author has never considered a tension or sustaining suture necessary, as a certain relaxation of the line of suture is obtained by the tampons of iodoform gauze which are placed in the lateral incisions. The operation is ended with the introduction of these tampons. It is to be remembered that with

Fig. 180.

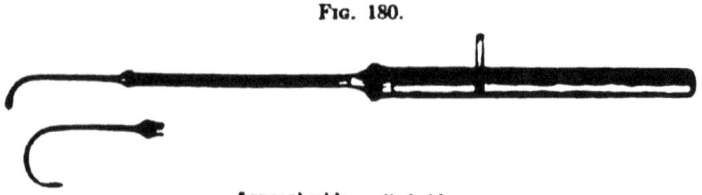

Langenbeck's needle-holder.

the introduction of the gauze between the bone and the flap the borders of the latter can roll upward, and it is from this that fistulæ arise later. Only the most posterior portion of the lateral incision can be firmly packed.

... involves only the soft palate and if a relaxation is nece ... incision is made on each side at the most posterior p ... process and the soft parts of the palate are detached ... palate. Small defects in the hard palate are operated o ... entirely similar to total clefts.

In ... double clefts of the jaw and palate, which are ope ... operation for harelip and the replacement of the pr ... maxilla, has been done previously, an opening remains a ... where normally the incisor canal (anterior palatine) is situ ... becomes slowly smaller. The further anteriorly it is po ... the palate cleft, the smaller is the opening which communi ... nose, which, in case it remains too large, can be closed ... freshening, together with lateral incisions and detachme ... of a small flap. In case it cannot be operated on, the cl ... behind the intermaxilla is attained by a dental appa ... palate. V. Eiselberg closed the opening by a flap of mu ... which he forms from the posterior side of the interma ... upward.

In the subsequent treatment rest of the line of suture is always ... the most important factor in the healing. Not onl ... condition of the patient, the absence of speaking and ... feeding with a long-nozzled cup or short rubber tube ... avoidance of superfluous testing of the strength of the sutu ... A pronounced chronic catarrh of the mucous membraue ... the temperature for several days after the operation can be ... tongue and palate then appear coated, small lymph-gl ... the angle of the jaw; these last are treated with moist w ... the individual stitch-holes become purulent, the su ... finally the entire suture may give way. In order to re ... from the nasopharynx during the first days after the o ... to check the inflammation of suture line, J. V ... douching the nose; the author has always been content ... inhalation of salt-water steam; slight inflammation ... the suture, while in severe infections accompanied with f ... possible in any way to remove from the suture-line the co ... of suppuration.

A week after the operation the lateral gauze packing and any l ... removed; the former is replaced again for a few days if ... need support. If this packing is removed, the palate fla ... attach themselves so quickly to the bone that the clef ... incisions diminish rapidly and close. Sometimes an ope ... into the nose remains at the site of the lateral incisio ... very narrow flaps and broad palate cleft with partial gang ... union of the flaps to the bone. If this does not close ... the aid of caustics, a closure must be subsequently attempted i ... and flap formation. In a large defect of this kind Ru ... employed a flap from the forehead, as the material fo ... was not sufficient on the palate.

Small openings in the line of suture are not infrequent. They arise most readily at the spot where the tension is the greatest, between the hard and soft palate, and where in movement of the soft palate a small dimple is formed. Very often such small spots are closed with the formation of granulation-tissue by means of slight cauterization. If a small defect remains, it is closed after a longer period of time by means of v. Langenbeck's method. If the entire line of suture gives way, it is well to wait not only for the complete healing of the cleft borders, but also for an improvement in the mucous membrane catarrh, which in most of such cases is the cause of the giving way of the suture.

The great advantage of v. Langenbeck's operation is the restoration of a hard and soft palate, which approaches the normal anatomical condition. This restoration, however, is not quite sufficient to make possible a pure normal speech.

The nasal speech continues in most of the cases. This distressing condition made the treatment of cleft palate by obturators popular for a time. The investigations of Passavant demonstrated the cause of this condition after suture of the palate to be above all things a velum which is too short or too rigid to be able to lie on the posterior pharyngeal wall as a flap which can completely close this off. After this was discovered a series of operations were invented for the relief of this main difficulty. They certainly improved the speech, but did not have any such brilliant results that they have become permanently adopted. Only Passavant's method may be mentioned, in which by means of his palate pharynx suture—i. e., suture of the uvula to the pharyngeal wall —he tries to bring about a closure between the nasal and buccal cavities, either by reflecting the soft palate posteriorly by means of a suture or by forming a prominence on the posterior pharyngeal wall. In addition there is Schönborn's staphyloplasty, which consists in suturing a flap of mucous membrane from the posterior wall of the pharynx into the defect of the soft palate. Küster's lengthening of the soft palate by means of a portion of the detached cleft border also belongs to this group, inasmuch as by this a better apposition of the velum to the pharyngeal wall is said to be obtained.

At the present time such operative procedures are abandoned and surgeons have learned to make the closure more perfect in other ways. It is plain that immediately after the operation and the healing, even under the most favorable circumstances, normal speech cannot be present. Many muscles which are necessary for the formation of the sounds act under altered conditions, and on this account must be exercised to become accustomed to the change. Not alone do the palate muscles come here into consideration, but also the tongue and the lips. The systematic exercise in speaking has been combined very advantageously with a mechanical treatment, massage of the soft palate and the pharyngeal wall (Gutzmann). The results which this author above all others has obtained with palate clefts operated on show that the nasal twang disappears from the speech as soon as the musculature of the soft palate functionates well, and that the length of this is very much

454

If the
a small le
of the alv
the hard
manner e
In con
on after
ing interr
spot whe
Later thi
to join th
with the
subseque
formation
of the de
or a thin
membran
with its b
In the
considere
general q
ing, a car
also an a
desirable.
present, t
high; the
appear at
compresse
loosen, ur
the secret
tion, and
employed
the less p
not harm
it is not p
quences o
A week
sutures ai
sutures sti
a couple o
the lateral
which lea
case of ve
or irregul.

lren begin to go to school and to come in contact with
it able to conceal their deformity, and the knowledge
e makes them shy, a circumstance which plays an
determining the time for operative treatment. The
another particular: it is permanent, while the ohtu-
f growth must be often controlled and changed.
ds are compared at the present time in regard to their
be reckoned of equal worth in view of the many cases
series of operative cases, as well as those treated with
res, nothing is left to be desired so far as the result
ut with both methods of treatment there are cases in
f attaining a pure speech is never completely gained.
to lack of intelligence and energy of the patient or
in the mucous membrane, especially atrophic condi-
igeal wall.
e two methods gives in many cases good results, since
operation is improved by appropriate mechanical
rmerly it was necessary, if it was desired to improve
ch after complete palate suture, to divide the soft
der to introduce the apparatus of Suersen, now it is
of Schlitsky's construction to leave untouched the
restored by operation. This obturator closes off the
a elastic balloon, which very readily adapts itself to
s in shape of the pharynx which occur during speech.
a is joined to a dental plate by an elastic spring or a
If the muscles of the pharynx and soft palate which
be closure of the pharynx are strengthened and exer-
obturator is gradually diminished in size, correspond-
' function attained, this obturator may in time become
t palate and pharynx finally bring about the closure
aus this obturator forms an important part in com-
menting the operative result.
ncerning the preparation of the obturators, the various
their application, may be obtained from dental publi-
ichlitsky, Grunent, Röse, Warnekros).
e question which has been discussed so much and for
isidered briefly: In what year of life may the opera-
e be best performed? The conditions here are some-
in operation for harelip, for here not only the closure
ion is to be considered, but also above all things the
nal activity of the soft palate. On this account, as
advised, it is best immediately after the healing of the
egin with systematic exercise of the palate muscles by
on in a language. This can be begun, according to
iences, in the fifth year of life at the earliest. At this
y circumstances and with strong children there is no
ie operation itself; according to Küster, absolutely no
after the third year. If in addition the fact, important

CHAPTER XI.

INJURIES OF THE SOFT PARTS.

Contusions and injuries of the face due to dull instruments are the result of fall, knock, or blow, and are also caused rather frequently during birth by the pressure of the forceps, especially over the prominences of the facial bones. Moderate contusions produce, besides slight abrasions, hemorrhage into the skin and soft parts; this remains circumscribed for a time in places where there is intimate connection of the skin with the underlying bone, such as over the malar bone, chin, and bridge of the nose; in other places the blood rapidly spreads and is soon absorbed with discoloration of the skin. A hæmatoma of the lids or cheeks may interfere with the venous return, so that the parts become œdematous, and the lids especially may thus present an alarming appearance. As a result of violence caused by blunt instruments, sharp edges of bone, such as the edge of the orbit or the free border of the incisor teeth, cut through the parts from within outward, so that many contusions have sharp margins like punctured or incised wounds. Severe contusions are complicated by fractures of the facial bones, or, when the force is directed obliquely, by lacerated wounds. These may be of great extent when a dull object, such as a cane, picket of a fence, etc., pierces the mouth or nose and tears open the cheek or nostril. Such lacerated wounds may also occur during birth. The finger introduced into the mouth to facilitate delivery of the after-coming head may tear open the lips and cheeks and even fracture the lower jaw; or lacerated wounds of the upper lid or bridge of the nose may follow the use of the forceps.

Comminutions of the soft parts and bones with separation of entire sections of the face follow the action of great violence. The severest injuries of this character are seen after explosions, in machine and elevator accidents, or result from being run over, dragged on the ground, or buried under earth, etc. The kick of a horse may also induce severe complicated injuries. Splintering of superficial bony structures and larger fractures with dislocations are present in the more extensive lacerated and contused wounds; often shreds of soft parts and skin are partially separated. Wounds caused by the bites of mad animals belong to this class and may leave large defects in the tissues.

The conditions necessary for healing are more favorable in the face than in other parts of the body, if one excepts the injuries of the most severe type, in which it is not surprising that part of the bruised tissues becomes gangrenous. Free circulation of blood and lymph gives abun-

dant nutrition to the skin of the face and enables the tissues to withst;
an infection better than is the case, for instance, in the skin of the
Hence it is usually the experience that wounds heal best of all in the f;
Nevertheless, one should not expect too much of these favorable coi
tions, and it should not be forgotten that bruised wounds, even tho
they involve the face, are predisposed to inflammation owing to
irregularities, pockets, and recesses of their edges.   Further than t
the tissues, lowered in vitality and infiltrated with blood, readily pei
bacterial invasion.   Although every contused wound should thus
regarded as liable to suppurate, it would be going too far to do a'
entirely with primary suture in the face. Moderately bruised and irr(
lar edges infiltrated with blood can be approximated, owing to the fa'
able state of nutrition of the facial skin described above, and the e
and very accurate suture of penetrating wounds of the lips, eyelids,
nostrils should even be regarded the rule. With the exception of tl
sites, the mistake must not, however, be made of applying the sut(
too closely, so that no intervening spaces are left, for suppuration in
depths and surroundings may then result from a slight infection and
be controlled only by opening widely the entire wound.   On the o(
hand, moderate infections and suppurations in the face may rap
subside without more than a narrow scar when the spaces between
sutures permit the inflammatory exudate or pus to escape freely into
dressing. With sutures sufficiently separated, one prevents the deve
ment of phlegmons and obtains smaller scars than when suppura'
demands a reopening of the wound.

   After shaving, the site of the wound is cleaned and disinfected for s(
distance. Coarse particles of dirt and blood-clots are then removed \
forceps and sponge. Much bruised edges and loosened shreds of ti;
are to be cut away with the scissors, and where very close approxima
is desired for cosmetic reasons the margins of the wound are to
smoothed as much as possible. Larger, much contused wounds \
flaps are best tamponed for one or two days with iodoform gauze
then sutured; or if primary suture is preferred, good drainage is ass(
at some site, if necessary, by counteropenings. Sterile gauze covers
wound or suture-line, and is held in place by loose turns of a band
If the soft parts are considerably torn and bruised in extensive, con
cated injuries, there is nothing to do but to await demarcation of
necrotic from the healthy tissues, and, with favorable local conditi
to repair the defect by means of a plastic operation.

   Injuries Caused by Sharp Instruments and Objects; Inci
and Punctured Wounds.—The smooth-edged wounds inflicted by s[
cutting instruments and weapons or by such objects as glass-splin
and broken fragments may be divided, according to their depth, i
superficial or deep; or according to their complications, into those \
injury to cartilage or bone and those with involvement of the oral
nasal cavities. In form they may be linear or with flaps, and of the la
may be distinguished those with partially or entirely separated flaps.
forcible cut may separate like a flap, not only the nose, with the except

ever, retract into the orbit and thus lead to ptosis. The muscle shou
be found, brought forward, and sutured to the lid at its line of divisi
(O. Weber).

TREATMENT.—Sharply incised wounds of the face are the best suit
of all accidental wounds for immediate exact suture. Although bacte:
are found in varying kind, number, and virulence in all wounds, especia
when treatment is begun late, their lodgement is prevented in large p
by the active bleeding and the smooth edges; and, after all, the exc
lently nourished soft parts of the face, as already stated, can readily de
with a moderate degree of infection without leading to suppuratic
Faulty technic, such as washing out the wound with a dirty rag a
water, as frequently practised by the laity, may, however, carry t
infection into the freshly injured tissues and result in severe inflamm
tion, phlegmon, or erysipelas.

The first condition necessary for healing by primary intention is abs
lute control of hemorrhage. The accumulation of blood beneath t
sutured wound assists the development of inflammation, for there
no better culture-medium for micro-organisms than a fresh blood-cle
Spurting vessels should be isolated from their surroundings and ligate
with catgut or secured with a deep suture. Bleeding areas are to I
grasped for a short time with hæmostatic forceps, and a more parench
matous hemorrhage is controlled by moderate compression exerted f
a short time. Particular care must be exercised in suturing the edg
of the natural openings of the face. In penetrating wounds of the I
or cheek the mucous membrane is also sutured, and catgut is the be
material to use. In larger wounds with flaps, for instance, in the regio
of the check or forehead, a small space is left between the sutur
leading to the pocket below the flap to permit the introduction of
small drainage-tube.

Completely severed flaps, consisting most frequently of the tip of tl
nose, but also of the auricle, lips, cheeks, or chin, have been known
heal under conditions most unfavorable for the wound. This observ
tion dates from a time when nothing was known of the cause of wout
infection and its proper management. As early as 1828, the Heidelbe
physician, Hoffacker, reported cases in which noses healed after havii
been cut off; in one case union was obtained when the tip had be
severed twenty-five minutes. This result was surpassed by Barthelém
in his case five hours had elapsed. Instances in which union is comple
and perfect may be more frequent at the present day; nevertheless tl
observation of all rules of aseptic wound treatment does not alwa
insure absolute success. Most often a partial union is seen; the edg
and the surface in part become necrotic and separate. The less tl
severed piece has been manipulated, the better are the chances for unio
A case like the one observed here, in which the injured man, a studer
of medicine, brought the tip of his nose well preserved in physiologic
salt solution, is, however, a unique one; the union here was very sati:
factory. Here also the most important condition is complete control e
hemorrhage, and compression with gauze moistened in physiological sal

solution does the best services. There should not be the slightest layer of fibrin or blood between the two surfaces (E. v. Bergmann), and the poor results after immediate suturing are solely to be attributed to imperfectly controlled hemorrhage. While the wound is compressed and its surroundings are sterilized, the severed tissue is placed in warm physiological salt solution, which also removes the superficial dirt; then we sew accurately with the finest silk, the sutures being placed close to the edge of the wound. If the septum is also separated, the mucous membrane should be united as far as $p_{os}s_{ible}$. Where the wound has penetrated the mucous membrane, a piece of iodoform gauze is placed loosely in the nostrils. The entire sutured tip is protected by means of a small piece of gauze, which is held in place without pressure by strips of plaster. Several cases treated by this method with good results have been observed in v. Bergmann's clinic. If necrosis or suppuration interferes with union, the various plastic operations are to be considered as soon as the wound granulates well. The prognosis is less favorable in the case of entirely separated auricles.

Wounds of the nose and of the face in general, if closely sutured after all hemorrhage has stopped, do not require protection with gauze and large dressings. V. Bergmann condemns all dressing in wounds of the face; he especially dislikes collodion applied to the wound, and lays the greatest stress upon rapid drying of the bloody transudate which exudes through the incision after the suture is complete and which protects the wound, as an adherent scab or crust, better than anything else. Wounds in which a few drops of blood escape after the sutures have been applied should be compressed for a short time with gauze.

Two phenomena are of importance in the after-treatment, namely, secondary hemorrhage and inflammation. Secondary hemorrhages are sometimes seen after slashes in the temporal region, where perhaps the temporal artery has been cut into at the angle of the wound and then caught with the skin suture without being isolated and doubly ligated. Large subcutaneous hæmatoma may follow and the suture must be opened, the blood removed, and the vessel ligated *lege artis.* Sometimes this imperfect ligation of the injured artery will show later in the development of a small aneurysm. Such aneurysms of the temporal and facial arteries following slashes and incised wounds have frequently been operated upon; they have also been observed after contusions and gunshot-wounds. Inflammation of the mildest grade, reddening of the surroundings, and stitch abscesses are not rare and rapidly disappear when the sutures at fault are removed in time. The wound should be opened at once and loosely packed with gauze to allow the inflammatory exudate or pus to be absorbed when a rapid rise of temperature, increasing œdema of the neighborhood, and progressive suppuration show the advent of a severe infection.

Punctured Wounds.—Punctured wounds are generally of a serious nature when they are inflicted by large instruments, pointed weapons, sharp sticks, etc. It must be considered a serious accident if the point of the instrument breaks off in the bone, in the temporal fossa behind the malar bone, the nasal, frontal, or maxillary sinuses or the orbit. If the end of the instrument has not been removed directly after the injury, the resulting inflammation and suppuration, the orbital phlegmon, or the empyema of the maxillary and frontal sinuses will soon demand its extraction. A large variety of foreign bodies have thus been removed from the nose, antrum, and orbits. In punctured wounds of the orbit the eyeball not rarely escapes, since, owing to its shape and mobility, it makes way for the penetrating objects, especially when these are not sharp. The results are much more serious if the instrument penetrates the skull through the orbits or through the nose by way of the cribriform plate. Cerebral symptoms may be absent at first, and it may not be until the symptoms of meningitis develop that the gravity of the injury, perhaps regarded as superficial and harmless, is evident.

When the instrument enters above the zygoma and runs downward and inward, dangerous and even fatal hemorrhage from the deeper parts may follow, owing to injury of the internal maxillary artery and its branches or to the deep temporal. In these cases ligation of the external carotid is the only method which controls the hemorrhage rapidly, since the region where these hidden vessels are injured can be exposed only with difficulty by resection of the zygoma and the coronoid process of the lower jaw. No time is to be lost in such severe hemorrhage.

TREATMENT of punctured wounds is carried out along general lines. The dangers of secondary infection make probing the depth and course of the wound undesirable. A suture is superfluous owing to the small size of the external wound and wound secretions readily accumulate in the deeper wounds if they were not left open. A sterile dressing protects the wound from external influences.

Gunshot Wounds of the Face.—Gunshot wounds of the face are complicated by injuries of the bones in the majority of cases. Trendelenburg's frequently cited case, in which the bullet from a rifle penetrated the face without injury to the bone, since it pierced both cheeks while the officer was shouting, is certainly an extreme rarity. Balls with much diminished velocity, small fragments from the bursting of shells, small shot, and the small projectiles of pistols or revolvers, can take a long subcutaneous course and penetrate the soft parts down to the bone without, however, injuring it. If the wound does not become inflamed, they remain beneath the skin or upon the surface of the bone without, as a rule, causing disturbance. In many cases it is difficult accurately to locate such projectiles, even with the aid of Röntgen rays, when they are hidden in the upper part of the nasal fossa, the orbits, the temporal fossa, or in still deeper tissues at the base of the skull. Injuries to the soft parts of the face are also caused during war by splinters of wood, etc., scattered by the bursting of shells or by fragments of metal torn from helmets.

In civil strife the most serious injuries of the soft parts are caused by shots fired with suicidal intent at close range into the mouth. They are generally accompanied by fractures of the jaw or other grave complications. Since the orifice of the weapon is often tightly grasped by the lips, powder burns or more serious disintegration of the soft parts of the mouth suggestive of explosion are common (Koehler). The skin-wounds

Fig. 181.

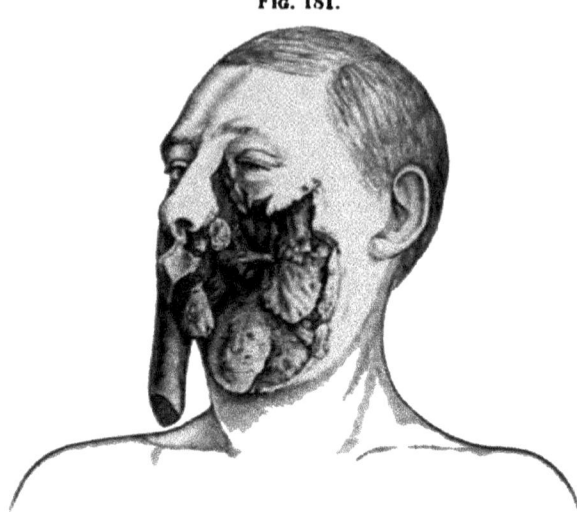

Recent wound of face from small shot at close range.

run radially about the mouth into lips and cheeks, and are characterized by their sharp, incised edges. If, in addition, the barrel of the weapon

Fig. 182

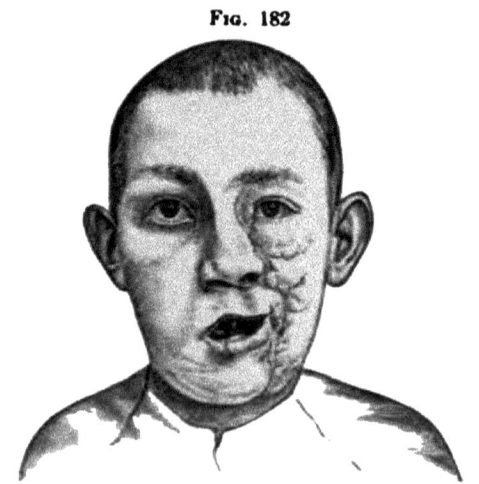

Same patient after healing of wound.

is filled with water, the extent of injury reaches its highest degree and the outcome, as a rule, is a fatal one, owing to severe damage to the base

of the skull or brain. The character of the inju1
mined by the variety and course of the projecti.
While the projectiles of small pocket pistols may
the hard palate or posterior pharyngeal wall, the b1
when taking an upward course, pierce the hard |
skull, reaching the anterior cerebral fossa, or,
medulla oblongata. The instinctive tilting back ‹
the missile a typical course through the hard pala᾽
(Trendelenburg).

Still more horrible mutilation is seen where sui᾽
through the mouth with the more recent military
of the mouth and cheeks are torn into shreds, the
base of the skull fragmented, and the brain conv
penetrating bullet.

Lacerations of the face of considerable exten᾽
fragments of shell or bomb. A large, irregular,
wound marks the defect, in the depths of which w
the mouth and nose. Death is caused by hem
pneumonia.

The accessory injuries are of great importan‹
course and treatment of gunshot wounds of the
complications as injury of the skull and brain ar‹
that with injuries of the mouth the chief dangers t‹
individual are interference with respiration and
larger vessels. Not only can large amounts of bl
from the lingual artery or the facial and its branch‹
or tongue has been wounded, but secondary h‹
vessels, extravasation of blood beneath the muco
matory swelling of the tongue extending to the la1
of the tongue after division of the anterior ling1
place the patient in imminent danger of asphyxi8

The life-saving value of immediate tracheotomy
ance of alarming symptoms with injury to mouth ‹
well-merited attention in the work of Lotzbeck.
ever, not only indicated in imminent suffocation
inflammation; it also prevents obstruction to brea
tory swelling at the entrance of the larynx and g1
ration of septic matter formed in the mouth. Th‹
found in difficulty in swallowing and breathing
mouth or tongue.

Injury to the bone is in great part responsib
hemorrhage occurring after gunshot-wounds of th‹
sels besides those originally injured may be affec᾽
splintering and dislocation. Simple packing and a
generally suffice for the superficial arteries and vei1
at the site of injury after the wound has been en
traversed by the bullet slit open is to be conside1
or temporal arteries. Hemorrhages coming from t

...ent **plastic operations. The lower lid particu-**
... I,.. traction **of the scar, so that the conjunctiva is**
.... known **as ectropion follows. The angle or**
..... grow **together and the entire palpebral fissure**
... scar, **especially after the destructive effects of**
... lid or **after ulcerations of the cornea. The**
... the nose **may undergo similar severe disfigurement.**
... the tip **or nostrils coalesce with the scar which**
...d the cheek, **especially when the scar is connected**
the nostrils **may become entirely closed. The angles**
... be pulled **upward and outward, the upper lip may**
... the nose **by scar-tissue, and the lower lip everted**

FIG. 184

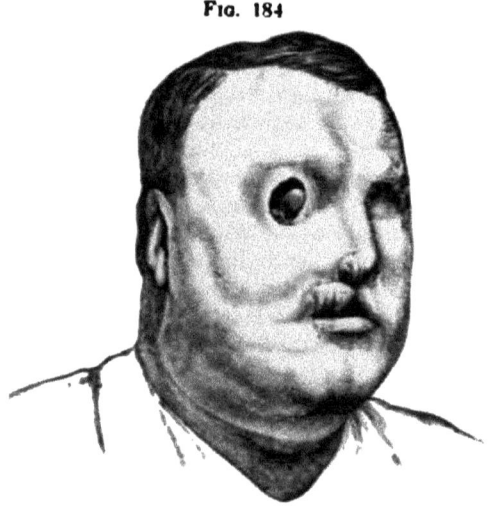

Extensive burn of face, healing after skin grafting.

strands to the chin and neck. Considerable disturbance of
thus follow, since in these cases the mouth can be closed
tely or not at all.

avoid firm, deforming masses of scar-tissue as far as pos-
he greatest importance to avoid a suppuration of the burn
atment. If pus is already present in deep wounds, denser
e expected and the growth of epithelium on the surface is
he grafting of large and broad pieces of skin by the method
i the best way quickly to cover the defect with epithelium
the formation of irregular, dense, cicatrical bands. But
: only when the granulations have a healthy appearance.
ould be made of the attempt to remove that peculiar tattoo-
e resulting from particles of unburnt powder lodged in
explosions, by means of Hebra's well-known remedy for

ĸn an attempt is
l ɷl-clots. The air
disappears in a few
k and chest, but also
ɷns were infiltrated.
malar bone, includ-
ʌ Since the point of
ɩeꙗe fractures show a
broken into a number
t as rare. The malar
. or the lower border
. dislocated fragments,
. ;rd. In the latter case
the two patients quoted
lly, the author has most
ɩɩꞓment of the bone. A
l ɩne from the rest of the
·· fractures do not exactly
ꞓ or less the proeesses of
lꙍnes. The zygoma fre-
mʌtic process of the upper
ɩ of fracture runs into the
n of the nerve by the dis-
lɷme is severed by fissures
ɩf the orbit and really con-
·ꞓ· malar hone thus becomes
n the direction of the force.
·he maxillary sinus is broken
mꞓ with the fractured zygo-
lɷcations take place posteriorly
ɩally into the orbits, and thus
sion so often complicate mul-

·hich are often accompanied by
ꞓ importance by their extension
ɩ l particularly to the base of the
ɩpon the malar hone. this, so to
·ortions of the facial skeleton, and
ʌnal, and alveolar border, as well
ꞓ roof of the orbit, as far even as
the fracture.
ɩsis of malar fracture is easy; it is
·· the presence and extent of injury
For evident reasons even Röntgen
rv results in all cases. Effusion of
skin shows the position; its extent
erity of the injury. Unless the effu-
malar bone can readily be palpated;

The only consequence of a non-complicated malar fracture which is approximately limited to the bone and not accompanied by much depression is a slight though often permanent deformity. If, however, the fracture extends through the roof of the orbit to the anterior cerebral fossa, the injury to the skull and cerebral tissues is of a most grave character. All such cases have ended fatally according to Gurlt's statistics. If subcutaneous, brain injury and intracranial hemorrhage form the chief danger; if wounds are present, purulent meningitis is to be feared, as in all other complicated fractures of the skull. The latter is most frequent in complicated fractures of the orbital walls, with or without simultaneous injury to the eyeball, since orbital phlegmons travel to the meninges through the cracks and defects in the bones, as well as along the ophthalmic vein. It is by this same route that furuncles of the lip may lead to fatal meningitis. Secondary hemorrhage may also cause a fatal termination, as in one case of Gurlt, in which the internal maxillary artery was probably eroded in the suppurating, gangrenous wound.

The presence or absence of wound infection, with its local and general consequences, determines the course of complicated fractures. The infection may enter through contused wounds or abrasions of the skin, as well as through the mucous membrane of the maxillary and oral cavities, which are often implicated. A meningitis, by extension through the venous channels, is the most serious outcome. If the patient escapes general sepsis or erysipelas, a prolonged suppuration, with separation of shreds of tissue and sequestra, follows the infection. Fistulæ may persist in the scar for a long time until all necrotic shreds and pieces of bone have been removed. All these local and general conditions of wound infection demand the greatest care in treatment to avoid a spread of the inflammation. As in all large lacerated and contused wounds, the healing is most rapid if all loose shreds and splinters are removed and the wound then treated openly with iodoform gauze, which should fill all pockets and recesses.

The complication of gunshot-wounds of the malar bone depend upon the direction and course of the projectile. The importance of injury to the large and deeply situated vessels in cases in which the projectile enters the vascular angle between the upper jaw and base of the skull has already been discussed. The vessels may still further be wounded by the fragmented zygoma and temporal process of the malar bone. Glancing shots may splinter the orbital margin, and the fragments may tear the eyeball. After comminuting the malar bone the projectile may penetrate the skull by way of the temporal fossa; it may reach the anterior cerebral fossa through the orbit or may travel from the orbit into the nose or other orbit. The course may be through the upper jaw or palate into the mouth, where the floor or the tongue may be wounded; and lastly, the temporomaxillary joint, the internal ear, and the facial nerve in its canal may be injured if the bullet takes an anteroposterior direction. Fragments of shell have been known to tear off the malar with of the nose and upper jaw and the entire cheek, etc.

given for the treatment of wounds with injury to the bone. If the injured site has once become inflamed, the infection spreads to the meninges by way of the veins of the nasal mucous membrane (ethmoid veins) or the orbit, which penetrates the skull, or through the agency of the injured and inflamed bone. The only method which prevents this course is immediate, free incision in the affected area, with exposure of the injured parts. The large wound, reaching, if necessary, to the brain or dura, should be cleared of all fragments and shreds and then tamponed carefully with iodoform gauze (E. v. Bergmann).

With extensive splintering the form of the nose may be permanently changed, even if the wound has remained aseptic. This so-called traumatic saddle-nose, with its more or less flattened bridge, requires plastic operations. Thickening through excessive callus is rarely to be feared, since, as in other fractures of the facial skeleton, it is very slight in amount at the nose. Stenosis or obliteration of the nasal duct is not so much due to callus formation as to the dislocations, especially of the frontal process of the superior maxilla. If the inflammation remains restricted to the site of injury, ostitis and necrosis may cause protracted suppuration with separation of a number of sequestra. The defect in the bony framework of the nose is thus considerably increased.

CHAPTER XII.

DISEASES OF THE FACE.

INFECTIOUS DISEASES OF THE SOFT PARTS AND BONES.

The Acute Inflammations Caused by Pyogenic Organisms.—T furuncle and the closely allied, though larger, carbuncle are found up the skin of the face. According to the experimental researches of Gar Bockhart, and Schimmelbusch upon the causation of furuncles, th are two conditions absolutely necessary for their development— accumulation of pyogenic staphylococci upon the skin and its mecha ical impregnation with them. But the skin of the face is favored a for other reasons. Not only must the special predisposition of the d batic, whose less resistant tissues easily permit development of furuncl be considered here, as elsewhere, but various changes in the skin, whi are known as eczema, impetigo, and sycosis, and which are merely d ferent forms of superficial staphylococcic infection (Unna), also play important part. The unclean skin of some individuals, whose face sho an abundance of large comedones and constantly develops new ac pustules, also favors furunculosis. With many patients it may be i sumed that the infection was transmitted to the face by means of a fing the seat of a felon or soiled with pus. According to the investigations Schimmelbusch on recent furuncles, the staphylococci travel along t shaft of a fine hair and become settled in its root and sebaceous gla Such small furuncles, in which the inflammation is frequently limited the immediate vicinity of the root and only a small pustule forms at t base of the hair, are especially frequent in the face. They disappe several days after the core has discharged. Their sites of preference i the vicinity of the mouth, nose, and forehead, and also the eyelids, so-called stye (hordeolum). Severe forms may develop from these har less lesions when they are subjected to mechanical irritation, as wh their crust is removed by scratching or their contents expressed. T inflammation then spreads, a very painful infiltration develops in the sl of the face, and it requires one to two weeks before a larger necrotic cc becomes loosened by suppuration. Generally others will follow throu new infection caused by the patient's fingers. The popular treatme with poultices favors distribution of the cocci in the vicinity, with dev opment of new furuncles. If the top of the pustule is cut off early ai the infected hair extracted, the furuncle usually remains small. Incisio best performed under local anæsthesia by freezing with ethyl chlorid hastens separation of the slough and hence the cure in the larger infi tration. Injections of cocaine or Schleich's solution should not be em ployed to produce anæsthesia, for, as in all acute inflammatory processes, there is danger of spreading the infection in the tissues. The incision is protected by gauze held in place by plaster or the turns of a bandage; the pus thus gets into the dressing and infection of the vicinity is prevented.

Furuncles of the median parts of the face, especially the upper lip, are well known and much feared, since they may be fatal in a few days. Often a harmless pustule appears as if it were healing, when considerable swelling of the lip indicates a local exacerbation, and high fever a general infection. In such cases the staphylococci have reached the lymphatics of the vicinity or the blood-stream, often owing to improper manipulation of the primary focus, such as removal of the scab by scratching, expression of the slough, piercing the furuncle with needles, etc. By examining blood taken from a vein of the arm during life, the author has proved that in these severe cases the entire body may be inundated by micro-organisms. Twice he has found *Staphylococcus pyogenes albus*, and frequently *Staphylococcus pyogenes aureus*. The infection spreads rapidly at the site. The dense infiltration of the primary focus, which has now turned into a carbuncle, involves the entire upper lip and rapidly spreads upward to the eye and inner canthus or downward into the submaxillary region. Indurated strands run along the course of the anterior facial vein and its first part, the angular vein, indicating that a purulent thrombophlebitis, soon leading to œdema of the lids, rapidly progresses from the inflamed area. Owing to anastomosis of the angular vein with the chief vein of the orbit, the superior ophthalmic vein, thrombosis of the cavernous sinus occurs, and this again is followed by meningitis if the general infection has not already killed the patient. The author has found suppurative sinus-thrombosis without meningitis at several autopsies. In other cases thrombosis of the jugular vein may be responsible for the most severe symptoms of embolic pyæmia, chemosis, and protrusion of the eyeballs, often bilateral, follow œdema of the lids, and are certain proof of the extension of the thrombophlebitis to the sinus.

In these most serious conditions all treatment is almost hopeless. As soon as a furuncle of the lip shows rapid enlargement with œdematous swelling of the cheek, particularly toward the eye, no time should be lost in making large incisions through the labial edge in its entire extent, and others, at right angles to these, through the infiltration of the upper lip and cheek. This is the only procedure which may save life. It is evident that in view of the great danger no regard should be paid to the possibility of subsequent scarring. Frequently the entire hard, infiltrated upper lip is riddled with small abscesses which reach to the mucous membrane, and may even break through this at different places and discharge very infectious pus into the mouth. Whether one believes in the efficiency of irrigating or sponging the wound with strong antiseptic solutions or not, the chief treatment must always consist in extensive incision. In v. Bergmann's clinic the wounds are kept open widely with iodoform gauze without the previous use of antiseptics, and several advanced cases could be reported cured by this method.

In another form of furuncle, which takes its origin as a rule from
fected sweat-glands (v. Wieniwarter), the inflammation extends to ₁
subcutaneous tissues, and the infiltration softens and forms the so-call
furunculous abscess. These small subcutaneous abscesses are oft
seen simultaneously on different parts of the body in poorly nourisl
nurslings, particularly about the nates and on the face about the chee
As a rule they open of themselves and then leave behind a dense indu
tion, which after some time again softens with the formation of p
These abscesses do not tend to progress acutely, and the inflammati
shows no signs of spreading. They heal most quickly after incisi
The frequency with which the author has found *Staphylococcus pyoger
albus* as cause of suppuration in these furunculous abscesses is strikii
Swelling of the lymph-nodes of the parotid region is almost alwa
present.

All forms of phlegmon occur in the face; they may be acute or chron
circumscribed, progressive, or necrotic. In severity they vary from t
slightest inflammatory infiltrate following infection of a skin-wound wi
any pyogenic organisms to the most extensive necrosis and suppurati
such as may be found in large, irregular wounds with torn tissues a
comminuted bone. These extreme cases may be associated with ga
grene if putrefactive germs reach the wound from the mouth. In gener
an accidental wound of the soft parts of the face is but rarely follow
by an intense inflammation. When infected, a transient inflammato
swelling, with slight purulent secretion, is generally all that is foun
Depth and irregularity of the wound and communication with the muco
membranes of the facial cavities predispose, however, to severe inflat
mation. A phlegmon in the region of the cheek can develop by tl
extension of a neighboring inflammation without any preceding injur
thus, after a suppurative parotitis a periostitis of the upper jaw or ₁
empyema of the antrum of Highmore. The origin may also be found i
the inflammatory processes of the lower jaw, such as the periostit
secondary to caries of the teeth or to the use of phosphorus. In tl
former the suppuration may in rare cases travel upward beneath tl
masseter to the temporal muscles (Gosselin's phlegmon profond tempor
sous-massétérin); in the latter diffuse suppuration may extend into tl
soft parts. If a phlegmon secondary to a periostitis, to inflammation
the deep lymph-nodes, or thrombophlebitis of the venous plexus betwei
the pterygoid muscles, extends from the pterygopalatine fossa and reach
the surface in the temporal fossa or beneath the zygoma, the clinic
picture often resembles actinomycosis or malignant neoplasm. Accon
ing to the investigations of Poncet and Albertin, phlegmons of the chee
may also originate from a small group of lymph-nodes which lie upc
the buccinator in front of the masseter, and which may be the seat ₁
acute suppuration after inflammatory processes of the nose, eyelids, an
the region of the cheek.

Acute phlegmons of the nose and upper lip are feared, as are furuncle
in these regions, for the inflammation may spread to the cavernous sinu
by way of the anterior facial and superior ophthalmic veins. Deer

phlegmons of the cheek take this dangerous route through the pterygoid plexus which communicates with the superior ophthalmic vein through the inferior ophthalmic.

If death has not occurred through meningitis or sepsis, the progressive inflammation of the orbital veins is often followed by phlegmon of the orbit. Like every suppuration of the retrobulbar tissue, these phlegmons are of importance in that they carry with them great danger of meningitis. Other causes besides extension of a thrombophlebitis are direct infection of the orbital tissues through injury, spreading of the inflammation from erysipelas of the lids, and inflammatory processes of the bone after suppuration in the neighboring cavities, notably the maxillary sinus. Any of the different pyogenic organisms may also set up an orbital phlegmon by way of the circulation in pyæmia, scarlet fever, and influenza. Besides fever and severe pains, there are œdema of the lids and conjunctiva and rapidly developing protrusion and rigidity of the eyeballs. Less severe but very protracted suppurations are often caused by foreign bodies which have remained behind in the orbits. The greatest danger of the acute phlegmons is extension to the interior of the skull, for meningitis, sinus-thrombosis, and brain abscess may follow. In addition to these most severe complications, disturbances of sight are of importance, since panophthalmitis or atrophy of the optic nerve can result. As soon as the first signs of orbital phlegmon develop, an incisiou should be made into either the upper or lower lid, depending upon the direction in which the eyeball is dislocated. Spontaneous rupture through the skin of the lids and the consequences enumerated are thus prevented. After incision and evacuation of pus sufficient drainage of the orbit should be assured. If the bone is affected or inaccessible foreign bodies are embedded in the depths of the orbital tissues, Krönlein's osteoplastic resection of the external wall of the orbit for orbital tumors is advised for the free exposure of the orbits.

In ineising facial abscesses one must particularly bear in mind the course of the facial nerve, so as to avoid subsequent disfigurement; as the deeper layers are penetrated, a direction parallel with the nerve should be maintained. One should also avoid dividing transversely the margins of the facial clefts, as, for instance, the lips.

After plastic operations a moderate degree of inflammation is sometimes seen, especially if the raw surface of the flap projects into the mouth or nose. Superficial necrosis of the raw surfaces, stitch abscesses, or a temporary hyperæmia in the region of the flap and its surroundings are usually the only signs, and these disappear rapidly after the suture is opened and the threads are removed.

Acute suppurative ostitis or **periostitis** has been observed as a spontaneous—*i. e.*, hæmatogenous—disease in only very few cases about the malar and nasal bones (Haaga, Fröhner).

Ostitis and necrosis occur much more frequently by the direct extension of infection from a wound of the skin or mucous membrane to the bone. It is generally in the suppuration readily developing after severe injuries, more particularly complicated fractures with extensive frag-

... communicating with the differe
... with necrosis of some of its injure
... suppuration complicating peri
... forms the starting point and
... In severe cases of phosphorus
... been affected besides the upper jaw
... reach the meninges by way of the
... complicated bone injuries. In m
... takes place from fistulæ which run
... large pieces of bone have separated as sequestra
... the bony framework.

... opening the abscesses, exposing the
... good drainage for the pus. By
... of the necrotic portions is hastene
... fistulæ requires exposure of the bo
... by means of spoon, bone-forceps, o
... may have its starting point in the
... membrane. The original lesion ma
... if the disease originated spontaneou
... in the epithelial covering may
... penetrate into the interstices and ly
...

... begins as a streptococcic angina or as an
... especially seen in the habitual forms
... reaches the face by way of the nose,
... Conversely, the mucous membran
... The mouth and pharynx in particul
... and even increase their virulence. In
... the adenoid tissue of the pharyngeal and palat
... the germs already exist in the ph
... more numerous when the latter is the
... and when the many crypts of the hyper
... a large bacterial flora (Stohr, L
... seen after operations on the face, b
... been banished entirely. As in
... the opening of the facial cavities, w
... membranes in the ulceration of
... Thus it may happen that aft
... involves the mucous membrane,
... fracture of the nasal bones with w
... operations in the interior of t
...

... most cases of facial erysipelas is a fa
... healthy individuals. Despite hi
... the duration does not exceed several da
... and there is no tendency to spread over larg
... which the inflammation spreads to the scalp
... mucous membrane, are frequent enough.

most serious local complication occurs when the infection extends into the skull by way of the lymphatics or the thrombosed nasal or orbital veins, with the possibilities of a fatal meningitis. Then, again, spreading of an erysipelas upon the mucous membranes may lead to œdema of the glottis or the so-called wandering pneumonias.

The phlegmonous form of erysipelas is not often encountered upon the face, and only rarely does a local suppuration, rather circumscribed in extent, accompany the inflammation of the skin. A more serious complication of this kind, however, is the appearance of an orbital phlegmon, on account of imminent danger of meningitis or destruction of the eyeball. Gangrene of the skin may be caused by the tension of the exudate interfering with the circulation. This occurs most readily in places with loose meshes of connective tissue. Other complications do not differ from those of erysipelas elsewhere; they are caused by general intoxication and by distribution of the germs through the circulation. Metastatic disease of the organs, pericarditis, pneumonia, etc., may arise. Besides the embolic form of pyæmia arising from the thrombosed subcutaneous veins, infection of the blood-stream is also possible, though this has been detected in only a few cases.

The multiple abscesses and subcutaneous foci of suppuration which occur in parts of the body not invaded by the erysipelas are also to be regarded as hæmatogenous inflammations, unless there is an obvious connection with the regional lymphatic nodes. (Compare the case of Landouzy with 69 and the one of A. Zeller and Arnold with 650 metastatic abscesses after facial erysipelas.)

Treatment.—As in erysipelas elsewhere, the therapeutics of facial erysipelas should above all insure a good state of nourishment and a forcible heart action. Many remedies and methods have been employed locally, no one of which has been much more successful than the other. Of the disinfecting ointments and fluids, the author will mention only the ichthyol and sublimate salve and the moist sublimate applications (1:2000) used by König; these stand in contrast to indifferent substances, such as lanoline and vaseline. The results in general are the same (Köster). Scarification is of advantage when there is marked œdema of the lids.

The use of antistreptococcic serum has not been encouraging; and control-experiments on animals have left serious doubt as to the efficacy of the serum.

In some cases, especially when the erysipelas has frequently recurred, peculiar changes in the face may remain behind. These are thickening of the skin about the nose, cheeks, lips, and lids, so that the patient's appearance suggests myxœdema. This pachydermatous condition, increasing fter every new erysipelatous inflammation, is caused, according to Friedreich, by an occlusion of the lymphatics leading to insufficient absorption and organization of the inflammatory exudate.

Attention has frequently been directed to the curative power of erysipelas in malignant neoplasms and in syphilitic and tuberculous lesions of the skin, especially since Busch reported a case in the year 1866 which

Softening leads to a breaking-down of the thinned and discolored skin, and large persistent ulcers with fungous granulations and undermined edges result. The process resembles the destruction of skin from within outward that is seen when tuberculous pus reaches the surface from the deeper parts.

Lupus occurs far more frequently in the face than in other parts of the body. According to v. Winiwarter, Raudnitz has estimated that of 100 cases of lupus, 76 involve the face, and of these again, 38 involve the nose. The female sex is more often affected than the male. The onset is usually between the tenth and fifteenth years, but often the disease begins in earliest childhood. In some cases the presence of the disease has been established in the parents; very often other signs of tuberculosis besides lupus exist (according to Sachs, in 85 per cent.; according to Bender, in 62.3 per cent.).

There are first disseminated nodules, varying in size from that of a pin-head to that of a pea, and showing as brownish-red spots which slowly increase in size and disappear but little on pressure. They are usually situated in the skin of the nose, particularly at the edge of the nostrils, or about the cheeks, chin, or forehead. During the very chronic course, exfoliation or ulceration of the foci takes place, and new nodules develop in the centre or at the periphery and increase the size of the lesion, while the parts first affected cicatrize. Thus, for instance, it may happen that lupus of the nose, in proceeding through its many detailed phases, may spread to the cheeks, forehead, and upper lip, and eventually involve the entire face.

Course.—The course varies with the depth of the affected cuticular layer and the degree of proliferation which the lupoid tissue undergoes. There are forms of lupus which show no tendency to ulcerate though they have persisted for years. A smooth scar covered by a thin layer of epidermis marks the site where the nodules have merely led to desquamation of the skin and have themselves undergone absorption, and the uniform, white, and shiny appearance of this scar is interrupted in places only by a few fresh eruptions. In the ulcerating forms, however, the infiltration soon reaches the subcutaneous connective tissue, and by slowly penetrating the depths spreads to the remaining soft parts, cartilage, periosteum, and even bone. In accordance with this, the resulting cicatricial tissue extends more deeply, becomes adherent to the surface of the bone, and causes disfiguring distortions. In part, the extent and depth of lupoid ulcers depend upon the co-operation of the usual pyogenic germs. Only too readily do these reach the open sores in the skin and settle beneath the dried secretion. Hence the old experience that the ulcers of lupus suddenly show a remarkable tendency to heal if they are kept clean, even if indifferent remedies are employed. If the diseased areas receive no treatment, the secretions of the ulcers dry to thick, hard crusts, beneath which bleeding readily occurs, especially at the nostrils and lips. The vicinity of the ulcers then shows considerable inflammatory swelling or œdema, which is especially apparent about the lips, lids, or nose. The frequency with which facial erysipelas occurs

(see below) is proof that streptococci may reach the lymphatics o
skin from the contaminated ulcers. Especially during the later st
of lupus, nodular swellings, seemingly diffuse hypertrophies of the
or soft, tumor-like thickenings varying in size from that of a chestn
that of an egg, may be seen within the affected areas. They are ca
by the presence of large masses or proliferations of lupoid granula
beneath a thin epithelial covering. Upon ulcers there may als
marked proliferations of granulation-tissue in the form of papillæ
jecting above the surface of the skin.

The surgeon, however, is more interested in the results of lu
namely, the disfigurements caused by the scar and the destruction
lowing deep infiltrations in the face, than in all the details of the n
fold process.

Since cicatrization goes hand-in-hand with the appearance of new
and the extension of the ulcerative process, the results of cicatricial
traction gradually become evident, especially about the lips and
The condition known as ectropion follows, since these parts bec
fixed to their surroundings and the eyes and mouth cannot be suffici
closed on account of shortening and immobility. Complete destru
of the soft parts is seen about the lips in severe cases when the mu
membrane of the lips, the soft and hard palate, and the gums are al
extensively diseased. Lupus of the lids may also extend to the conj
tiva and lead to blindness.

The nose is affected more frequently and severely than other p
The smaller scars pull the nostrils, with their defective edges, downv
or to the side. Simultaneous involvement of the mucous membrai
rarely absent and tends to implicate seriously the cartilage. The lu
infiltration and ulceration attack the framework of the nose from wi
and without, so that its entire cartilaginous portion breaks down. A
cicatrization the nose typical of lupus appears as if hewn off, sinc
the soft parts are destroyed down to the bony bridge. When lupu
the interior of the nose has perforated and destroyed the septum,
intact skin may sink in and the whole nose may appear as if it
formed by a plastic skin operation only. The bone is but rarely affe
to any extent. The edges of this pyriform aperture and of the b
framework only undergo necrosis and sequestration in severe c
The entire destruction of the nose goes on very gradually during
course of many years, but acute exacerbations occur with certain fo
especially where large tumor-like masses of lupoid tissue have for
and a sudden breaking-down of the deep and extensive infiltration t
place. Scarring is sometimes more pronounced after repeated cat
izations. For instance, narrowing of the month has been observei
that the tip of the little finger could hardly enter, and complete clo
of both nostrils may result when the lupoid proliferation and gran
tions upon the mucous membranes grow together and become cov
with skin.

Facial erysipelas following lupus deserves mention since it frequei
takes its origin from the ulcerations of skin or mucous membrane. 7

resulting inflammation of the skin assists the elimination and absorption of the lupoid tissues and thus shows a temporary curative influence.

It is clear that the ulcers may give rise to a phlegmon or to suppuration of the neighboring lymph-nodes of the neck as readily as to erysipelas. Hence the most pronounced glandular swellings are seen with the ulcerative forms.

Besides tuberculosis of the regional lymph-nodes and extension of the disease from the mucous membrane to the larynx, tuberculous disease of the organs, bones, and joints may develop. This may occur simultaneously with the onset of lupus or a long time after, and eventually the affection of the face may be of secondary importance when compared with the entire disease. In the absence of these complications the patients may reach an advanced age with good general condition if no'

FIG. 186.

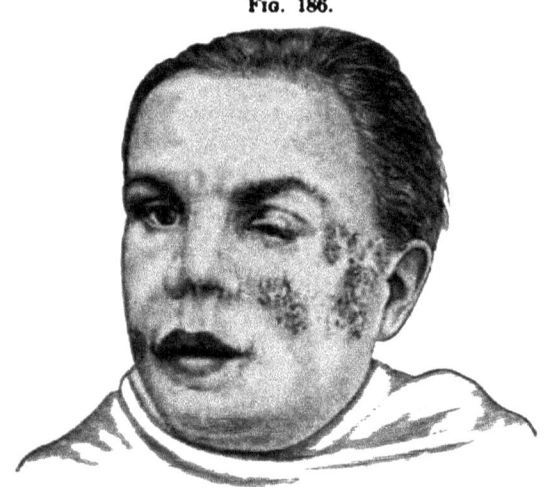

Cicatricial closure of nostrils.

extensive infiltrations or ulcerations form, and if the destruction of tissues is very slow owing to the exceedingly chronic course of the disease.

The development of carcinoma in the pathologically altered tissue forms a very serious turning point in the usual course of lupus. It may start from the scar as well as the recent ulcer. Of 83 cases of carcinoma of lupoid origin, 25 developed from the scar. It is particularly difficult to determine the first change within the lupoid ulcers. The carcinomatous tissue is, however, characterized by a different color, denser consistence, and more rapid growth, which cause it to project over the granulations.

Diagnosis.—If the diagnosis cannot be settled by the presence of distinct lupoid nodules at the periphery, it may be difficult to distinguish the ulcerations from those caused by carcinoma or syphilis. Besides the

peculiarities of both diseases, the entire previous course, elicited
personal history, is to be accurately studied.

Treatment.—The therapy of lupus and of the other forms
tuberculosis consists in the endeavor to remove the diseased t
radically as possible without causing too much disfigurement of
by cicatrization. Undoubtedly, excision of the skin down to the
taneous fatty tissue is the most thorough procedure and guards
local recurrence. But the treatment is only suitable for well-
scribed foci which do not extend to the margins of the orifices.
lesions of the cheek, forehead, or chin can be excised as spindle-

Fig. 187.

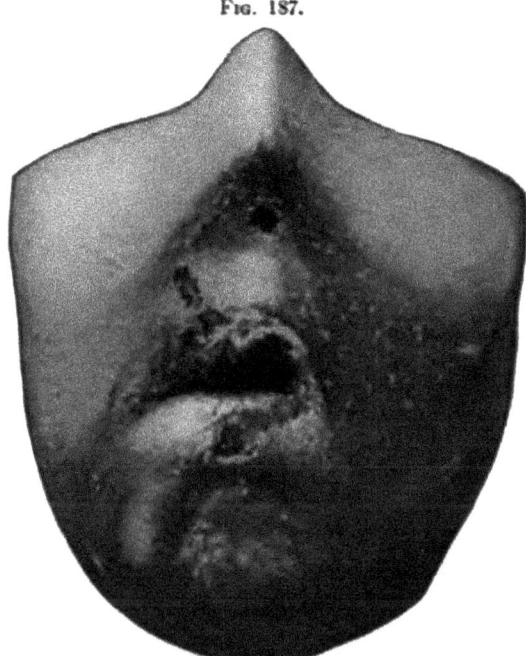

Atresia of mouth and nostrils following lupus. (Le Dentu.)

flaps and the edges of the wound then sutured. With larger d
is best to resort at once to skin-grafting according to Thiersch,
hemorrhage has been controlled. The larger and more unifc
grafts, the better the result obtained, for the scar is soft and even.
sionally, however, a pronounced keloid tendency exists $_{at}$ all the
operation, so that indurated strands recur after every excision an
plantation, as well as after other procedures. Good results are o
here only by using flaps from the neighborhood, with pedicles,
are usually employed after excisions involving the orifices. The
has also used repeatedly extensive flaps without pedicles (for in
for the entire cheek) to advantage, according to the directions of K

Lymphatics and Lymph-nodes of the Face.

Recurrences in the form of discrete nodules are rare after such radical methods.

In other cases in which the disease involves large portions of the face, the nose, cheeks, and lips at the same time, thorough removal of the diseased tissue can be accomplished by the sharp spoon, as first stated by v. Volkmann. If one scrapes with sufficient force, the soft infiltrated portions yield, and can thus be removed from all the pockets in the cicatricial tissue. After scraping, it is advisable to cauterize superficially with the Paquelin cautery, so that any foci left behind will be destroyed. The wound is then dressed with aseptic or iodoform gauze. If healthy granulations have sprung up in the region operated upon, especially with the aid of mercurial ointments, these should be removed with knife or spoon and resort had to Thiersch skin-grafting. The parts are thus rapidly covered with skin and distorting scars avoided as much as possible. Suspicious areas should be scraped repeatedly, so that the newly formed nodules are destroyed early. The method is also indicated if the mucous membrane of the nose is much diseased; the soft parts are widely slit open and exposed, and the interior then scraped and cauterized.

The results of these procedures are comparatively the most certain, although recurrences can never be absolutely prevented. Besides these methods, ignipuncture, as practised by Besnier with the pointed tip of the galvanocautery or the sharp point of the Paquelin cautery, is recommended for disseminated nodules. Hollander has substituted a hot-air apparatus for the Paquelin instrument to avoid extensive scarring. Although a smooth and soft scar results, the nodules often recur rapidly within it, since the method lacks penetration into the depths.

A number of remedies tend to favor separation of the diseased tissue by strongly irritating the skin. Among these are sublimate applications (1:1000) of Doutrelepont and the strong creosote-salicylic acid plaster of Unna. Another method of Unna consists in moistening small pieces of wood with liquor stibii chlorati and inserting them in the skin, where they remain forty-eight hours.

The most severe reaction takes place in the diseased region after the use of Koch's tuberculin.

Even though the investigations of v. Bergmann and Schimmelbusch have shown that the cells of the tubercle do not tend to undergo necrosis under the influence of tuberculin, and that even after a treatment continuing three months pieces of skin with tuberculous foci may still infect animals, the severe inflammation, which may be so intense as to cause gangrene, still aids in the separation of lupoid masses. The nodules and ulcers disappear and scarring sets in, as in lupus infected with erysipelas. The further use of tuberculin proves that the local reaction is the main factor in the breaking-down of the foci, for as soon as a tolerance is established and reaction no longer sets in, even the free and long-continued administration of Koch's remedy will not interrupt the rapid extension of the disease. The intense inflammation in the lupoid tissue which occurs after even a single dose of half a milligramme, may materially aid subsequent scraping with a sharp spoon in robust patients with

extensive lesions as yet free from internal tuberculosis; otherwise t
is little occasion to use this remedy.

Frequent trials have been conducted of late with the Röntgen
(Kümnaell). Their action, as well as that of the very slow light-thei
of Finsen, seems to depend chiefly upon an artificial inflammation in
cutis (Finsen, Lesser). For scars which remain hyperæmic, repeated r
tiple scarification with the finest sharp knife may be used (v. Volkma

The most difficult cases to treat are those in which the mucous m
branes are extensively diseased simultaneously with the face. W
in the nose radical measures, in the form of scraping and burning
the interior, may be resorted to, such procedure is obviously imposs
in the mouth. The cicatricial distortions and the defects which fo
lupus itself or its treatment frequently require plastic operations wi
may be of a very difficult nature.

Tuberculous Adenitis.—In the face the only important localitie
tuberculous lymph-nodes are the regions of the parotid and the ch
Palpable nodes with the characteristic formation of abscesses, ulcer
fistulæ are found most frequently in front of the ear. They occur toge
with the usual glands about the lower jaw and neck, which in lupus i
be considerably swollen. They originate from the superficial fa
lymph-nodes lying in and upon the parotid gland. Similar p
esses (abscesses, etc.) in the central region of the cheek are attribu
by Poncet and Albertin to

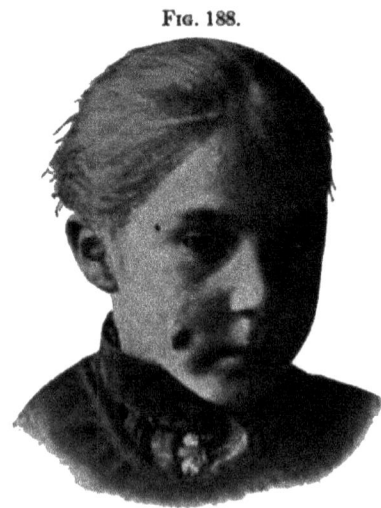

Fig. 188.

Tuberculous glands of the cheek in a child eight years old, swelling about 2 cm. from angle of the mouth.

largement of a group of lym
nodes, accurately described
the former. These so-called c
missural lymph-nodes lie in fi
of the masseter at about the n
dle of a line drawn between
angle of the mouth and the l
of the lobule of the ear. T
presence has been confirmed
Buchbinder and Küttner. (
188.)

**Tuberculosis of the fa
bones** is not rarely seen in c
dren, generally with tubercul
of the vault of the skull and
other bones and joints. '
margin of the orbit, especi
in its outer half, is most
quently affected, the upper qu
rant less often than the lov
A swelling below the lower
is the first prominent symp

which leads one to examine the abscess lying above the orbital mar
If this be opened and evacuated by means of an incision along
margin, the edge of the bone, usually pale and yellowish, is seen expo

at the bottom of a cavity lined with tuberculous membrane. Its more external portions are generally in a state of cheesy softening, and by means of a sharp spoon this softened portion can be easily scraped out down to the compact healthy bone.

The seat of the disease frequently corresponds to the junction of the malar bone with the upper jaw. After the tuberculous masses have been thoroughly removed by scraping, the entire wound is tamponed with iodoform gauze. Discharging fistulæ of long duration form in neglected cases after the abscess has ruptured spontaneously and sequestra of varying size have separated. In the meantime scar-tissue develops and the skin becomes united to the bone, so that disfiguring distortions of the outer palpebral angle and of the lower lid (ectropium) result. If the entire malar bone is sacrificed, either because it has been removed early by scraping away the diseased portions, or the bone has separated by itself as a sequestrum, disfiguring depression in the cheek remains behind. The tuberculous disease of the mucosa can extend to the bony framework of the nose, without, however, destroying the bone to any degree. According to F. Krause, primary tuberculosis of the bony structures of the nose is present in those cases in which cheesy sequestra are cast off.

Actinomycosis of the face starts most frequently from the mouth and then involves the region of the cheek, lower jaw, or malar bone and

FIG. 189.

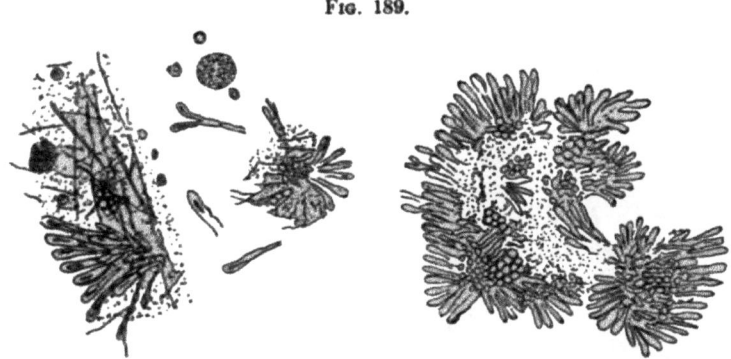

Actinomyces.

temple. Cases in which the lips and lids are affected are rare. Frequently the neck is affected with the face, and these localities are invaded far more often than the alimentary and respiratory tract or the skin on other parts of the body. This is proved by different statistics, notably those of Illich.

The possibility of an infection from outside has been shown by cases in which foreign bodies carrying the actinomyces have penetrated the skin. The clinical symptoms show, however, that the mouth is the most important starting place for the cases in which the infection is localized in the face. The fact that the disease appeared in the cheek

▓▓▓ ▓▓▓▓▓▓▓▓ in the vicinity of a carious tooth or after its extr ▓▓▓ ▓▓ ▓▓▓ ▓▓ ▓▓▓ frequent coincidence of the affection with ca: ▓▓▓▓▓, ▓▓▓▓ arouse suspicion that a close relationship existed betw▓ ▓▓▓ ▓▓▓▓▓▓▓. The fungus seems to resemble the leptothrix ▓ ▓▓▓▓ ▓▓▓▓▓▓ in that it finds favorable conditions for development ▓▓ ▓▓▓▓▓, and it may indeed be detected in the cavities of carious tee ▓▓ J. ▓▓▓▓ and Partsch have shown. Injury to the mucous membra ▓▓▓ ▓▓ ▓▓▓ occur from the friction of the sharp edges of a tooth or fr ▓▓▓ ▓▓▓▓▓▓▓ of a tooth, most likely favor entrance of the ray-fun▓ ▓▓▓ ▓▓▓ ▓▓▓▓▓. It seems that foreign bodies may also carry it fr ▓▓▓ ▓▓▓▓▓ membrane into the cheek, since infected barley-grains ▓ ▓▓▓▓ vegetable matter have been found in the actinomycotic foci. A ▓▓▓ ▓▓▓▓ of putting the husks or grains of cereals into the mo ▓▓ ▓▓▓▓▓ straw through the teeth is frequently admitted by patie▓ The portal for entry of lesions occupying the central region of the ch▓ ▓▓▓ be the vicinity of the parotid duct or the orifice itself (Schlange The beginning of the disease upon the mucous membrane is frequer ▓▓▓ noticed, since it manifests itself at first as small painless swellin which as a rule slowly increase in size. From the region primarily

fected the inflammatory infiltrat
invades all the soft parts slow
step by step, until by a direct
indirect route it reaches the sl
The peculiar inflammation cau:
by the ray-fungus is characteri:
by a strong preponderance of cellu
proliferation in contradistinction
the degenerative processes of ot
inflammation. It follows that
fungus, as it develops in small f
of flabby granulations, gives rise t
disproportionally large zone of ne▓
formed inflammatory tissue wit
the soft parts. The indurated gro▓
of connective tissue which result:
responsible for the term "boa
like" which has been applied m
properly to the entire infiltration
Esmarch). When a focus of gra▓
lation-tissue reaches the surface
ruptures with the discharge of
small amount of thin pus containing few actinomycotic granules. ▓ reactive proliferation of the tissues then brings the focus to the surfa where it is cast off like a foreign body (Schlange).

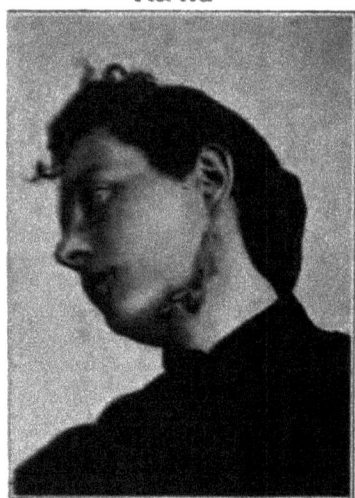

Fig. 190.

Actinomycosis of the submaxillary region.

The shortest route for this slowly progressive process lies through cheek in front of the masseter. A rather circumscribed infiltrati▓ which has developed within a few weeks, can be felt in the central lower parts of the cheek. By palpation from within and without thi▓

hard, dense, and nodular to the feel. If the por
at the upper or lower jaw, one frequently feels
tissue going to the starting point of the infectic
a carious tooth. Such strands are not infreq
places under the mucous membrane, and are
pletely absorbed inflammatory induration of the
the fungus has travelled. Thus they accurately si
fungus takes. As soon as the hard swelling a[
latter assumes a slightly reddish or more browr
occurs in different places with the formation of
break open spontaneously. A peculiar picture l
softened portions form rounded protrusions whi
side by side. About the cheek and neck they ha\
When the extent of infiltration is slight, there
abscess, such as is often found in the cheek.

Symptoms.—With all forms of facial actinom]
upper or lower jaw or the buccal mucous me
early symptom and is rarely absent, since the ii
soon spreads to the muscles of mastication and n
them. When the affection involves the cheek,
involved; while induration of the malar and ter
the pterygoid muscles as well as the temporal. '
a continuation of the process from the cheek, bu'
inner side of the ascending ramus of the lower ja'
of mastication are involved, the extension and c
explain the very obstinate course. If the patl
from the upper jaw, there are the additional dan[
from the pterygoid muscle to the base of the skull
latter. In neglected cases of actinomycosis of the
region extension to the temple may occur even
ths deeper softer parts; here the entire half of tl
of an indistinct, board-like swelling, which at fi
surface, but later shows softened foci, abscess
rarely the involvement is marked, the upper
affected.

Course.—In general the disease runs a c'
inflammation at the point of entrance is to b
organisms which can easily penetrate from l
developing with very severe symptoms in th
well as erysipelas or glandular abscesses ai
attributed to the same cause, since they do not (
mycosis. Foul-smelling abscesses may occur fr
with putrefactive germs. The combination and
infections can obscure entirely the characteristi
cosis. Inversely, the clinical symptoms sometim
invasion of inflamed tissue by the ray-fungus,
infiltrations appear in the vicinity of a dental fistu
after rupture of an acute periosteal abscess. Gr

the discharge. The co-operation of pyogenic germs may also manife
itself by the presence of fever, which in the pure affection is general
absent.

Diagnosis.—The symptoms and course are distinguished by certa
well-marked characteristics. The most important are the absence
fever and pain, the slow development of the advancing infiltration, i
hard consistence and not sharply circumscribed contours, and the te
dency of certain portions to soften and form abscesses. Despite all thes
clinical pictures may result whic
are hard to distinguish from oth
affections. When softening h
not occurred, a periostitis wi
thickening of the bone may
simulated, since the infiltratic
begins at the jaw and is close
connected with the bone.
mixed infection the characte
istics of actinomycosis may
entirely in the background.
large, extensive induration in t
region of the cheek, malar bor
or temple, may, in the absence
fistulæ and abscesses, suggest
malignant growth such as sa
coma or a gumma. As a ru
continued observation decid
these cases, since eventually t
characteristic softenings ta

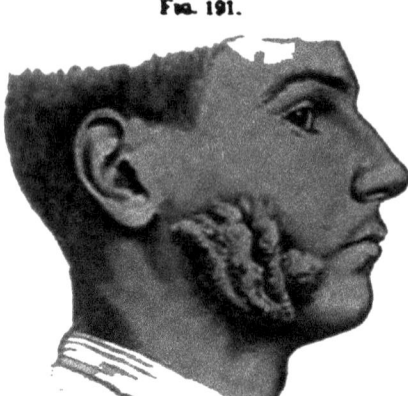

Fig. 191.

Actinomycosis of cheek originating in lower jaw.
(Illich.)

place and the granules can be detected in the pus. In the che
anterior to the masseter the process is frequently small and rather c
cumscribed, so that its disintegration results in a single small absc
whose base and surroundings show little or nothing at all of the cha
acteristic hard infiltration. One who is not familiar with this rather fi
quent form of actinomycosis may easily mistake it for an inflam
sebaceous cyst. Often examination of the buccal mucous membra
and detection of a strand leading to the jaw aid in the proper dia
nosis, even before the pus with its granules is detected on incision.
form described by Karl Koch as affecting the lower lip resembled cr
cinoma.

Despite the typical picture of actinomycosis, it may occasionally
difficult to detect a granule in the pus.

Prognosis.—The prognosis of actinomycosis is not so bad as w
formerly believed. As Schlange has shown, the affection shows a decid
tendency to heal spontaneously when it involves the face. The me
favorable forms are those of the cheek, including the processes exter
ing from the masseter and lower jaw. Inflammation ascending on t
inner side of the latter will even heal when an abscess forms and d
charges in the temporal region. The conditions are less favorable

extension takes place from the upper jaw to the bone of the skull or the anterior surface of the vertebral column. Otto, Illich, Partasch, and others report a number of permanent cures, particularly of affections of the face. In very extensive infiltrations the ray-fungus may penetrate the thrombosed veins within the inflamed tissue and thus be carried further by means of the circulation.

Treatment.—In view of the usual favorable course the treatment no longer consists in extirpation of the indurated areas. Resection of the jaw, formerly practised, has also been discarded, since it suffices to open the abscesses and scrape out the masses of granulation-tissue. Yet in large infiltrations a single operation may not achieve a cure; repeated incisions, as well as excision of fistulous tracts, may be necessary, since, owing to the peculiarities of the entire process, the separate, often small foci of granulation-tissue and pus may be enclosed in thick layers of inflamed and indurated tissue. Antiseptics have never been employed in v. Bergmann's clinic excepting the use of iodoform gauze for keeping open the Incision, just as it is used for other abscesses and phlegmons. The internal treatment with potassium iodide, so highly lauded by veterinary surgeons, is followed by excellent results in man, according to some authors, especially in the mild forms. In the above-mentioned clinic, however, healing was not more rapid or complete than after the simple procedures just described. In a recent examination of most of these patients to which Schlange and Otto refer, not a single recurrence was detected.

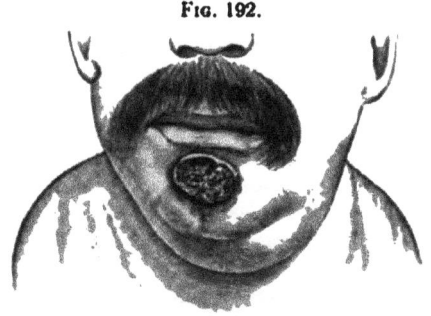

Fig. 192.

Chancre of the chin ten days after infection by a cut with a razor.

Syphilis of the Face.—Of all the different manifestations of syphilis, those which may give rise to mistake in diagnosis claim most interest.

The primary syphilitic lesion is seated comparatively often upon the lips, where it generally develops in connection with rhagades. It may also appear in other parts of the face, such as the cheek, nose, and chin, when as a rule special accidental factors are at play.

In v. Bergmann's clinic the author has seen the initial sclerosis develop three times upon the chin from the infection of a recent wound caused by a razor. When ten days old it formed a somewhat elevated ulcer the size of a twenty-five-cent piece, with hard and wall-like edges. At first sight it could easily be mistaken for a carcinoma, yet the rapid development of the ulcer, the greasy and smeary appearance of its surface, and the swelling of the lymph-nodes which soon follow, rendered the diagnosis easy. Finally, all doubt disappeared with the development of the general rash.

The later forms of syphilis may also simulate other diseases. The small ulcers are easily mistaken for the nodules and ulcerations of lupus wl they occur in large groups about the nose, forehead, upper lip, and che and in addition are accompanied by distorting scars or defects. They generally covered with crusts and follow papular and pustular syphilic and more particularly small gummatous infiltrations of the skin; resemblance is greatest with the last form. The base of these ulcer: excavated and covered with pus and their borders are steep; in cont distinction to this the ulcerations of lupus are shallow or more eleva and covered with granulations. During the slow course which char terizes lupus, the eruptions recur in large part in the cicatricial ar and extension into the surroundings is very gradual; the ulcerat syphillide, however, spreads rapidly along the periphery, while the cen heals. By the confluence of several ulcers their edges take on pecul shapes; since there is extension on one side and cicatrization on other, semilunar, kidney- or garland-shaped lesions result, the conce borders of which are always in a process of healing. To confirm diagnosis, one must, of course, look for other syphilitic processes up the mucous membranes of the mouth and pharynx, and for the eviden of earlier syphillides. The conditions are most uncertain in syph acquired by heredity or during childhood, for lupus is common in ea youth also. During the later stages the syphilitic saddle-nose is a w known sign differentiating lupus from syphilis. It is due to a gummate ostitis of the bony framework of the nose. Defects in its cartilagine portion may be a result of the destruction caused by lupus as well as the breaking-down of gummata.

Larger ulcerations which originate from gummatous syphilides of t skin or the subcutaneous connective tissue, and which are frequen seated in the face about the lips, angles of the mouth, nose, and fo head, may suggest carcinoma. The greatest difficulties are encounte in diagnosticating the condition when no other signs of syphilis are fou besides the gummatous ulcer, or when, as rarely happens, both disea: occur together, or the carcinoma develops later in a syphilitic ulcer. well-marked induration of the wall-like margin surrounding the e thelioma is generally present, and is the most important sign. It absent in the later syphilitic ulcers, where the sharply punched-out ed spread much more rapidly than in carcinoma. The base of an ulcerati gumma is covered with necrotic tissue which is still adherent to t deeper tissue, and which extends beneath the undermined edges. soon as it is cast off by suppuration granulations appear in its pla In contrast with this, the indurated and frequently elevated base of carcinoma is fissured and bleeds at the slightest touch or when attempt is made to remove the strongly adherent crusts. Frequen comedo-like masses of cells may be expressed from its depths. certain regions of the face, as under the eye and in the nasolabial fo traction on the skin will be noticed in cancer, so that folds are form which run radially to the tumor. In syphilis this occurs only wi cicatrization of gummatous ulcers which extend very deeply into t tissues (Lang). A syphiloma is generally not accompanied by swelli

10des, and these lack the hardness of the carcinomatous
1ermore, the other findings are important in enabling a
rphilitic ulcer to be made. The peculiar rounded, white,
scar which takes the place of the superficial gummatous
he skin after its disintegration, is often found next to the
e forehead and
the nose, or, if
arts of the body,
' preference, the
ce of the leg.
e tibial crest is
diagnostic value
1e mouth and
ld be examined
a of the disease.
:tion which fol-
1ata of acquired
reditary syphilis
ve in the face.
ot only does the
sult if the in-
1ose is diseased,
, of the skin of
destroy the tis-
The cartilage of
exposed at the
ummatous ulcer
wn, so that the
inous nose or
such as one ala

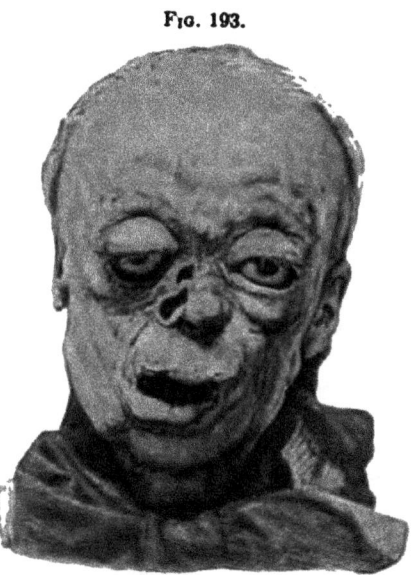

Fig. 193.

Results of syphilis of face, lids, lips, and cheek;
restored by skin-flaps without pedicles. Woman,
thirty years old, infected by wet-nurse.

inous septum, may be lost. Perforations of the bony
1r at the bridge of the nose. If destruction of the
1ce in earliest youth, an additional and usually very
1ity results from interference with growth. Extensive
stenosis of the oral and palpebral fissures may occur
and lids are diseased. Deep and extensive gummata
1se such pronounced ravages in the face as v. Bruns,
as pictured. Here small holes mark the site of mouth
1 open into the centre of an excavation covered with ray-
The everted eyelids complete the hideous sight, which
1rding to Trendelenburg, half-finished anatomical prepa-
head.
uated gummata do not break down and ulcerate early,
1 flat tumors the size of the fist. Owing to their rather
e and the slight bluish-red discoloration of the skin, they
malignant neoplasms; in the region of the cheek and
' at the lower jaw they may be mistaken for extensive
infiltrations if these lack the characteristic areas of

32

... so typical of this dis

... the face is rare when comp

... coming from the bones of

... and periostitis occasion

... At the latter site a

... or a mass of granula

... that accurate examina

... and that here the cours

... Finally, the effects of potas

... and newly formed tis

... one should not delay ger

... can be mater

... Superficial ulcers present a c

... in gray ointment is app

... infiltrations are s

... after the undermined skin

... scraped with a sharp spoon.

... pustules or anthrax carbun

... in individuals whose occupa

... with the cadavers or the hide

... The infection is probably brough

... contaminated finger. It is also poss

... the poison. W. Koch's statis

... involvement of the face as comp

... the body. The face without the foreh

... cases. The face and ha

... localization of anthrax, an

... the carbuncle, is most frequent.

... however, so rare, and both fo

... edema of the lips and lids acc

... anthrax is another very rare form

... by Weigert-Waldeyer. It appea

... pustules on the face of a man

... intestines.

... spot develops into a min

... forty-eight hours or several d

... filled with a serohemorrhagic f

... It is generally regarded as ha

... presses out its contents, or aids

... after ways. As soon as a dark c

... becomes more characteri

... common furuncle. Small amou

... places under the crust, arou

... swollen tissues rise like a w

... the periphery and into t

... and are converted in

a characteristic slough; thus the entire process may become very extensive and involve the entire half of the face. As a rule, however, the gangrenous portion is no larger than a quarter of a dollar; the œdematous swelling, however, extends far into the surrounding tissues. It is especially pronounced about the lids and lips, and frequently invades the neck when the pustules are on the cheek. In the inflamed and infiltrated zone surrounding the eschar and in the œdematous portions other small serohemorrhagic vesicles appear, which may also be converted into dark sloughs. If the common pyogenic germs participate in the process, the vesicles become filled with pus and purulent fluid exudes from under the crust. The lymphatic vessels and nodes are involved very early and swell into painful strands and nodes. According to K. Müller, pustulation is accompanied in one-fourth of the cases by fever which is often considerable. As a rule it disappears in a few days as soon as the swelling diminishes in the inflamed area. In the severest cases, in which the infection has become general, and diarrhœa, delirium, and somnolency characterize the disease, fever does, however, persist until death.

Course and Prognosis.—The course and result depend upon the development of general infection. This danger is imminent and to be feared in every case of anthrax. The germ of anthrax is properly regarded as one of the most dangerous blood parasites, since general infection with inflammation of the internal organs is fatal. Hence the efficiency of the various procedures which have been recommended for external anthrax are at present judged by their properties of either preventing or assisting the invasion of the general circulation by the bacilli. It is not surprising that in this disease simple cuts into the inflamed tissue have been followed by poor results. The lymph- and blood-channels are thus opened up for the microbes.

Treatment.—Notwithstanding the great danger of general infection, it is obvious that early destruction of the primary focus should prevent extension of the process. And, indeed, this has been accomplished. Many cases with favorable termination are reported by those authors who have excised the carbuncle of anthrax or cauterized it by means of heat or chemicals. But it is a question if these radical measures do not possess more disadvantages than advantages. If the germs are in a condition of diminished virulence, the opening up of bloodvessels by the incisions is probably followed by no ill consequence. Healing takes place after the carbuncle has been excised, as it would occur if this had not been done. If, however, the surgeon is dealing with very virulent germs, the slightest mechanical irritation to tissues laden with anthrax germs suffices to open the bloodvessels and thus bring about fatal general infection. This danger is present in all procedures which aim to destroy the primary focus, no matter whether extirpation, cauterization, the injection of antiseptic fluids, or, last but not least, extirpation of the swollen lymph-nodes, as practised by some, be resorted to. On the other hand, there is considerably less danger of general infection if external anthrax is treated by conservative measures. Here the tissues are left to combat the local infection without aid. The best

...the poison of tetanus may gain entrance the ... of the head is general and the infection ind... ...general picture the peculiarities of which ... The name "head tetanus" has been ap... ...since the portal of entry is an infected wound sit... ...by the twelve cranial nerves, and its chief symp... ...of the throat similar to those of hydrophobia or paraly... ...of the facial nerve, it has been called tetanus hydrophobi... ...facialis (Rose), or tetanus paralyticus (Klemm).

In the severe acute forms of head tetanus which develop a few ... after the injury, and which generally end fatally, spasm of the phar... and glottis, suggesting hydrophobia, soon sets in, owing to a very m...

increased irritability of the parts. There are tetanic twitchings of the muscles of the face and mastication, which are already in a state of tonic contraction, and paralyses of the cranial nerves, particularly the facial, appear. The muscular spasm may extend downward to the neck, trunk, and extremities (Brunner). Death occurs from suffocation in an attack of convulsions (by spasm of the glottis or diaphragm) or through cardiac paralysis.

Course.—The subacute and chronic cases run a course of from seven to twelve weeks and offer a much better prognosis. The different symptoms are not so severe; they develop more slowly and may be restricted to the cranial nerve region. Brunner distinguishes two groups of chronic cases. In the one the first symptom is a tonic contraction of the muscles supplied by the facial nerve at first on the side of the injury, or, if this be situated mesially, on both sides; this is soon followed by the so-called trismus, a spasm of the muscles of mastication, at first involving the injured side. In the other group paralyses, especially in the facial nerve region, accompany the spasms, and, like these, involve that half of the face which corresponds to the infection. Strangely enough, these paralyses never extend to the motor trigeminal region. When the wound has been situated about the eye, paralyses of the oculo-motor and trochlear have never been seen. The reason why the facial nerve is affected and why it is preferred over all the others by the infection is not quite clear. Fever does not generally accompany head tetanus.

Diagnosis.—The diagnosis may be particularly difficult in the chronic forms, especially when a wound can no longer be found and paralyses are absent, since trismus is present in all kinds of inflammatory infections of the face.

TUMORS OF THE FACE.

Lipoma.—Fatty tumors of the face are not frequent. According to Grosch's statistics, lipomata had their seat in the face in 13 of 685 cases, the frontal and temporal regions being excluded. This corresponds to 1.9 per cent., while Stoll's figures are somewhat higher, namely, 5.26 er cent.

p In part, these tumors take their origin from the subcutaneous fat, as in the rare growths seen about the lower jaw over the masseter or on the chin. The infrequent lipomata of the lids and the bridge of the nose are also seated directly under the skin. In the lips the tumor may orig-inate from the subcutaneous tissue, the muscular layer, or the structures about the glands, so that it may approach the mucous membrane or the skin. In contrast to the circumscribed subcutaneous fatty tumors of these regions diffuse growths sometimes occur in the subcutaneous tis-sues of the parotid region as offshoots of large fatty masses of the neck and back in cases of multiple symmetrical lipomata. The deep lipomata of the cheek are comparatively more frequent; they develop from its well-known fatty cushion, the corpus adiposum malæ, and may grow to a very considerable size (v. Bruns).

If these lipomata of the cheek grow toward the mucous membra their position is directly under this, and they project into the mo between the two rows of teeth. To understand the position of th growths, it is important to remember that the fatty cushion surrou the anterior edge of the masseter like a crescent, so that it stands in n tion with the skin as well as with the mucous membrane. This is sho by the horizontal sections of Fr. Merkel, which run through the ai of the mouth and the lobule of the ear.

Congenital lipomata are rare. Stoll has observed them in the che and eyelids; Weinlechner, in the latter position.

Anatomically these growths of the face are either simple lipomata v coarsely lobulated surface, or mixed forms, such as fibrolipomata i angiolipomata. They are not always well encapsulated. Small tum of the lips and cheeks can be readily shelled out of the tissues, but more extensive growths, especially those of fibrous or telangiect structure, may grow more diffusely into the surrounding tissue at cert places. The skin usually suffers no change, but it may be thinned, i a network of easily visible vessels may run through it where it cov large tumors or in the region of the lids and lips.

In many cases the disfigurement caused by even small tumors i sufficient indication for operation. Frequently, however, their remc is necessitated by annoying disturbances, as when they are seated in lids, lips, or under the buccal mucous membrane.

Diagnosis.—The diagnosis is not always easy, especially when lobulated structure of the surface, in general so characteristic, is pronounced. This is particularly the case in tumors of the cheek, wh can easily be mistaken for chronic abscesses or cysts, such as dermoic mucous cysts or cystic lymphangiomata. The history of a uniform, s development, the transparency of the cheek, and, in doubtful ca exploratory puncture make a diagnosis possible. Fatty tumors in parotid region have been mistaken for growths of the parotid gland.

Treatment.—The operation is very simple, especially if the grow lie directly under the mucous membrane; after this has been inci: the smaller tumors can easily be freed from their surroundings. In mucous membrane of the cheek the parotid duct must be guarded aga injury. Larger tumors of the cheek, in the parotid or facial region, more difficult to operate, and it may be best to excise the tumor in sn pieces, if necessary from different incisions, in order to protect the ne

Fibromata.—As elsewhere, fibroid growths of the face form a la group the members of which vary considerably in their external sh and histological structure. Very frequently they stand in relation to nervous structures of the cutis and subcutis, and not a few are acco panied by abnormal pigmentation of the skin.

The first stage of fibromatosis of the skin is found in the flat mented nævus. The surface of this may be smooth or the seat of abnormal growth of hair. The cutis here has a structure resembling i of the soft wart or soft fibroma of the skin (fibroma molluscum) in i a connective-tissue proliferation, starting from the finest nerve-filame

is present in all. Soldan has recently found nerve-fibres in the smallest foci of fibrous tissue and of cell-aggregations in the flat nævus and in the tissues of the soft wart, which latter has been classified by v. Recklinghausen among the lymphangiofibromata. The intimate relation between all these structures, the fibromata mollusca and other neurofibromata, thus finds an explanation, and the frequent transition of pigmented moles into massive nævi with plexiform neurofibromata seems clear. The pigmented nævus is a congenital anomaly of the skin, gen-

FIG. 194.

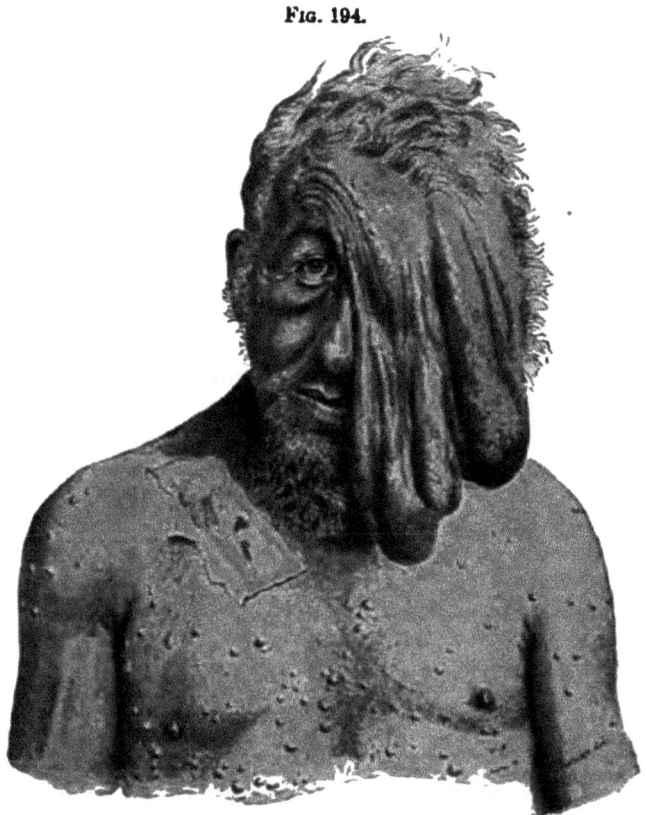

Fibroma molluscum. (Lanz.)

erally small and in rare cases only spreads over large portions of the face. Yet it may involve the entire half of the face, and its dark color and soft hairs may suggest the skin of different animals. In cases of multiple soft fibromata of the skin a number of pigmented spots or larger nævi covered with hair may be found disseminated over the entire body, and the patient frequently states that the site of the nodular and lobulated skin tumor has been occupied for a long time by a small mole. The soft wart is another similar manifestation of this generalized disease of the skin; by itself it forms a frequent and well-known lesion upon the ski of the face, where it may be pigmented and covered with hair, or smoot and like the normal skin. It is distinguished from the congenital wa: by its consistency, and from similar structures with cornified surface b absence of proliferation on the part of the epidermis. In some cases th wart is a congenital structure; in others it has appeared in youth. Bι rarely it exceeds a hazelnut in size; its connection with the skin is h means of a broad pedicle, and in shape it is rounded or more lobulate∢ According to Soldan's investigations, the soft warts pass over into th tumors known as fibromata mollusca, since in these also proliferatio of the connective tissue of the nerve-filaments is the most importaι feature, according to v. Recklinghausen.

· The soft fibroma begins as a very small neurofibroma in the papillaι body or in the subcutaneous tissue, and constitutes a superficial or dee nodule which is frequently covered by pigmented skin. In the face may be single or multiple, and in the latter case is often part of a tumₐ formation extending over the entire body. The first stages may be see at birth or during the period of development in the form of small sₒ protuberances of the skin. By a slow growth, larger, lobulated tumoₐ are formed about the nose, cheek, lips, and lids, and eventually enoₐ mous fantastical growths, such as are best pictured in the numerou illustrations of Esmarch and Kulenkampff, will result, together wit elephantiasis-like structures and skin-pigmentations. The more or les pedunculated fibroids of the skin which are occasionally seen in the faₐ of old people belong to this group.

In larger tumors hard tubercles can be palpated in the deeper parι provided subcutaneous nerves also participate in the process and whe a proliferation of their perineurium and endoneurium leads to the formₐ tion of large and small fibroids. Thus, each separate nerve-filameₐ will often take on the shape of a rosary. The interlacing nerve-plexusₑ of the subcutaneous tissue thus appear nodulated, and constitute th neurofibroma cirsoides of P. v. Bruns or the plexiform neuroma of Veₐ neuil and Virchow.

Frequently this structure is placed beneath a pigmented nævus, an more diffuse proliferations of the connective tissue of the cutis ma accompany it. According to P. v. Bruns, the most frequent site is th temple and the upper eyelid, and here shallow excavations and perforₐ ing defects in the underlying bone may give evidence of an early dispₒ tion to tumor-formation. The nose and cheek are less often affected. ₐ rare condition was noticed by the author in a child in whom the branchₑ of the facial nerve were converted into thick strands and beads in th deeper parts of a diffuse swelling occupying the cheek, and thus consι tuting the chief mass of the tumor. The case has been carefully describₑ by Soldan. By careful examination and palpation of soft fibroids of th skin, one may sometimes detect a similar plexiform structure in the cutι neous nerves which have undergone fibrous degeneration. A plexiforι neuroma on a small scale may thus be occasionally discovered even i smaller tumors or somewhat proliferated nævi. V. Recklinghausen hₐ drawn attention to this fact. In rare cases, plexiform neuromata have been found in the orbits (Berlin).

The rather indefinite term "elephantiasis" is frequently applied to the larger, more massive structures of this kind when the thickened skin forms long pads, folds, flaps, or bags, such as may hang over the face, neck, or chest in far advanced cases. Elephantiasis congenita nervorum or neuromatosa then corresponds to all tumors and thickenings of the skin which result from fibrous degeneration of the nerve-branchings.

All these forms, no matter whether they form large or small tumors, histologically stand in close relation with each other and with the same disease of the nerve-trunks, the so-called general neuromatosis. Hence the most manifold transitions and combinations are' seen clinically. Probably a congenital disposition must always be assumed, for the larger tumors generally develop from small skin-fibroids or beneath moles limited in size which were present at birth. Inheritance of the disease in its different forms has also been observed (Czerny, v. Esmarch, P. v. Bruns).

The disfiguring structures to which the name elephantiasis of the nose is given occur as lobulated protuberances of the nasal skin or as giant growths. According to their histogenesis, they belong in part to the fibromata mollusca or to the elephantiasis of the nerves in general. It may require a microscopical examination to decide definitely the nature of the growths here, as well as in similar lobulated tumors of the lids and lips, especially when a plexiform neuroma which might prove the nerve-involvement is concealed by the tumor or when everything that might suggest an extensive neurofibromatosis of the cutaneous nerve is absent. The elephantiasic structures developing from lymphangiomata, teleangiectasic, or inflammatory hypertrophies of the skin may have a similar appearance, and frequently there are transitional forms.

The growth of all these forms of neurofibromata is generally slow. The smaller structures rarely show an increase in size beyond the enlargement proportionate to the general development of the body. Even the lobulated tumors which develop from the small flat thickenings of the skin or nævi, which, as a rule, are present at birth, require years to assume a large size. Such enormous structures as Billroth, P. v. Bruns, and others have seen, and as v. Esmarch and Kulenkampff have pictured in their atlas, are rare in the face. Hence one has more opportunity to operate on the small soft wart, the fibroid involving the skin, and, above all, the pigmented nævus, and cosmetic reasons generally form the indication. Smaller tumors can be excised and the skin-edges sutured after they have been slightly loosened from the underlying structures and displaced; plastie operations may only be required about the nose. If, however, the defect has become so large that a suture would cause distortion about the eyes, mouth, or nostrils, the simplest way of assuring rapid and safe healing would be grafting by Thiersch's method. Elephantiasis, however, requires much more extensive operations, which may be very difficult in the face, for the fold of skin and the degenerated nerve-strands of the subcutaneous layer must not only be

removed, but large areas must be restored by means of plastic ope
tions. In extensive tumors hemorrhage prevents excision at one
ting. Billroth was obliged to perform twenty operations to obtair
good result in a case in which the entire upper half of the face was '
seat of long, pendulous folds, starting from the forehead and eyeli
The most serious problem in such large structures is always the plas
repair. Often it is impossible to use the neighboring skin on accor
of the size of the growth; or else slight lesions, such as soft fibro
or nævi, render it so brittle that hardly a single suture will hold. La
nævi of the face demand equally difficult surgical feats, often with uns
isfactory results, especially when they surround the palpebral fissures
involve the nose'and extend to the vermilion borders of the lips.

As a rule, removal at one sitting is a very extensive operation, parti
larly in children. Hence, one excises only small portions and cov
the defects by grafting. Cicatricial distortion about the orifices is to
avoided as much as possible, and here one succeeds best with pedun
lated skin-flaps from the vicinity. In many of the successful cas
however, the patient would have preferred the nævus to the appearar
which follows.

According to its histological structure, the *keloid* must also be clas
among fibroids. Although the form characteristic of the lobule of 1
ear does not invade the face, the so-called scar-keloid is very comm
after simple wounds, as well as after burns and ulcerative processes
the skin. The ugly, tumor-like scar following a wound is, as a ru
replaced by a permanent narrow cicatrix after excision and sutu
often, however, one encounters cases in which there is a striking t
dency to form thick strands, as, for instance, in lupus; and these 1
recur even after excision and grafting. The keloid developing upon 1
scar of syphilitic ulcers sometimes disappear with general antisyphil
treatment.

A rare fibrous neoplasm occurs at the bridge of the nose. It is rela:
to the sincipital encephalocele at its typical site. It is a flat or m
pedunculated tumor at the root of the nose, and may reach the size o
fist. Somewhat thinned skin covers the growth, which extends to '
downwardly displaced cartilaginous portion of the nose and to the li
By a careful histological examination such tumors sometimes se
related to fibromata or fibrosarcomata (Sklifowski); at other times tl
must be classed with other connective-tissue tumors.

V. Bergmann reports a number of such cases. Hildebrand descri
a large teleangiectatic glioma, seated upon an encephalocystocele. A
the author operated upon a broad flat tumor of the nasal bridge, wh
communicated beneath the raised left nasal bone with a meningor
which proved to be a lymphangiectatic fibroma (Grosser). In E
mann's congenital myoma at the root of the nose a connection with
cranial cavity is probable, although not proved (v. Bergmann).

Owing to their communication with the interior of the skull,
removal of these tumors carries with it great dangers of meningi
Infection may readily be transmitted by way of the nose in such case

The neuropathic papillary fibromata may occasionally form large and extensive tumors in the face. They are present in their first stages at birth or develop in earliest childhood. The lesion is also known as neuropathic papilloma (Gerhardt) and nævus unius lateris (v. Baerensprung), etc., and its pathological changes consist in a proliferation of the connective tissue of the cutis with marked hypertrophy of the papillæ. A certain relation with the nerves, possibly of a trophic nature, is suspected, since these tumors are unilateral and sharply limited in the median line, and often are grouped along the course of a cutaneous nerve. Perhaps they are also related to the fibroma molluscum (v. Winiwarter), yet a structure similar to the one found by Soldan in the soft wart and the pigmented nævus has not as yet been described. The peculiar unilateral distribution of these papilomatous growths gives evidence of a close relationship to herpes zoster. Spiegelberg records a typical case.

Lymphangioma.—Lymphangioma simplex or racemosum (Virchow), cavernosum and cystoides, with all their transition-forms, are rarely seen in the face. Generally they are present in their first stages at birth. As cavernous or mixed type, their favorite site is the region of the upper or lower lip (macrocheilia), or of the cheeks (macromelia). When diffuse, they are generally simple or cavernous, while the circumscribed tumors usually seen about the cheek are as a rule made up of one or more cysts.

Lymphangiomata enlarge very slowly though steadily. Sometimes they remain stationary for a time, to increase again in size by more rapid growth. Thus small tumors which involve a lip or only half of it, occasionally only one eyelid, stand in contrast to tumors in which the entire half of the face, including the lids, lips, temple, forehead, and side of the nose, is converted into a shapeless swelling. The consistency is either uniformly soft or rather firm, and compression often diminishes somewhat the size of the spongy tumor mass which has its seat in the cutis and subcutis or spreads through the entire thickness of the lips and cheek. The skin is intimately connected with it, and hence cannot be raised in folds. In appearance it does not differ from normal skin, and the bluish or reddish tinge characteristic of hæmangiomata is absent. Extensive growths with thickening of the skin and hyperplasia of the connective tissue have been termed lymphangiectatic elephantiasis in contrast to the telangiectatic and neuromatous forms. Even without much spreading, considerable swellings may form in rather circumscribed areas of the face, such as the lips; these may be three to five times broader and longer than normal; the upper lip may project forward as an immovable proboscis, and the lower lip may sink downward by its own weight so that the mouth remains open. In marked cases of macrocheilia the development of the upper and lower jaw may be interfered with. Such cases have been seen by Wegner and Trendelenburg. Congenital lymphangiomata may occur in the lids, but this locality is very infrequent. Esmarch and Kulenkampff cite only two instances, Beyer a third one. The neoplasms here appeared as elephantiasis-like thickenings of the upper eyelid, which overhung the eye as a large fold. In other cases

reported by Sachs the lymphangiomata of the lids and lid-edges w
only of slight extent. Extension of the growth from the cheeks to the l
is more frequent than their primary development in the latter situati
They may also spread still further into the orbits (Wiesner). Besi
the frequent combination of macrocheilia with macromelia, the con
tion of the tongue which is known as macroglossia may be present.
very peculiar case of bilateral macromelia is reported by Lannelong
   There are a number of pathological lesions of the skin which
generally classified among simple lymphangiomata. These are the c
ferent forms of pigmented nævi, the lenticular spots (lentigines), freck
(ephelides), and flesby warts (verrucæ carneæ). Ziegler states in
Text-book of General Pathology that rounded or cord-shaped areas
cells are found in all these structures within their connective-tis:
stroma. These must probably be looked upon as the enlarged a
proliferated cells of the lymphatics. Soldan has shown, as stated abo
that part of these structures belong to the neurofibromata.
   The cystic lymphangioma of the face is also congenital and most of
located in the cheek. It may, however, develop from the cavernous for
In the latter case, it generally spreads diffusely (E. Müller).
   Circumscribed tumors, on the other hand, belong more to the p
cystic types. In part the skin over these structures is non-adherent a
not otherwise changed; in part it is of bluish tinge, since the conte
of the cysts shine through. Both simple and compound lymphatic cy
may be found in the cheek, as in the somewhat more frequent hygro
cysticum congenitum of the neck (Ranke). An acute increase a
decrease in size belongs to the clinical picture of all lymphangioma
Inflammatory processes must be assumed in most cases as a cause
this condition. That inflammation really occurs can no longer
doubted after Tavel has found streptococci in the tissues. In lymph
giomata more than elsewhere the conditions are most favorable for
transport of germs from the mucous membrane of the mouth and l
into the tissues of the tumor. Other portals of entry are abrasions a
eczematous areas about the lips and cheeks or the lymphatic fistr
which sometimes develop when a varicose lymphatic of the skin ruptu
spontaneously. Depending upon the varying degrees of infection,
inflammation may disappear in a few days, or else the pus breaks throu
and discharges. The growth of the tumors is accelerated in success
stages by frequent inflammations, similar to the increase in size noti
in elephantiasis arabum after erysipelas. Occasionally inflammation
the lymphangiomatous tissue leads to occlusion of the lymphatics a
shrinkage of the connective tissue.
   Diagnosis.—The forms of lymphangiomata appearing as macrom
and macrocheilia hardly ever give rise to mistakes in diagnosis. T
unchanged condition of the skin distinguishes these growths absolut
from the closely allied angiomata. The discoloration of the skin ah
betrays the presence of bloodvessels in the latter, as in the two ease
Trendelenburg, in which the condition of macrocheilia depended up
diffuse angiomata.

The diagnosis is most difficult in circu
angiomata, which can easily be mistaken for c
cially when the skin is easily movable and c
tumor. Thus the general appearance of a
in which a walnut-sized lymphatic cyst exten(
lary fossa without being in relation with eitl
brane, corresponded very closely with an echi
v. Bergmann's clinic. In the parotid region
mind cystic tumors of the parotid gland, esp(
with an aggregation of cysts below and in fro
the skin over the tumor does not appear
Branchial cysts of this region may also reser
cysts when they extend to the cheek. If the
diagnosis, it can only be established by findii
or different forms of epithelium in the walls (
examination. Mucous cysts of the labial muc
guished by their seat, their rather rapid devel(
contents. On the other hand, the growths r
lipomata of the cheek, especially when small (
ated connective tissue and fat; with such c(
nature of the tumor may be undecided even
If a puncture is considered necessary to de
fluctuating tumor, it is better to perform this
the mucous membrane, since an infection m.
latter and there find conditions most favorabl
in the lymphangiomatous tissues.

Treatment.—The therapeutics of facial lym
the greatest difficulties, since only the few cir
extent are suited for complete extirpation. Ir
such extensive excisions as are practised at th
the body are impossible. One cannot operat
in those extensive cases of macromelia and l
abnormal tissue often reaches to the mucous n
injury to the branches of the facial nerve. If
tumor are left, these continue to grow. Sinc
children, all interference is rendered difficult
parts; and the fact that one cannot operate lo
radical removal of the tumor impossible. An
procedure recommended by Wölfler: to merel
apaees and then allow them to heal after pack
properly drawn attention to the dangers of an
which is almost unavoidable with this long-c
rapidly spreads in the intact portions of the
infection follows, a protracted discharge of lyr
children. Similar considerations hold good f(
sions in macrocheilia. Inflammation and sur
this procedure, which does improve the appea
it leaves tumor-tissue behind. Weinlechner a

satisfactory results after wedge-shaped excisions from the diseased
It follows that only procedures less difficult and dangerous, but a
less efficient, can be recommended for extensive lymphangiomata of
face of simple or cavernous type. Resort must be had to the parenc
matous injection of irritating fluids causing inflammation. Tincture
iodine (Trendelenburg) and solution of zinc chloride (Maas) have b
employed with success, especially in the cystic lymphangiomata.

In connection with lymphangiomata, there still remain those swelli
and tumefactions of the facial skin which depend upon chronic hyp
plasia secondary to chronic or frequently repeated irritation. Here th
generally is a connective-tissue proliferation with dilatation of the lym
and blood-channels in the skin and subcutaneous tissues. A thicken
of the skin, termed elephantiasis or pachydermia lymphangiecta
acquisita, has already been considered as a result of frequently recurr
erysipelas. The thickening of the skin, which involves the entire f
or only parts of it, is increased by every extension of the erysipe
The disease is only rarely seen in the face; it occurs more freque
about the extremities.

Fig. 195.   Fig. 196.

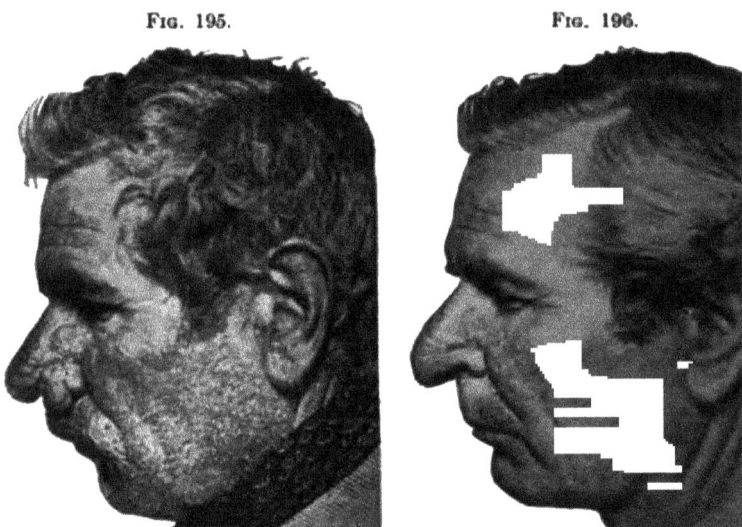

Rhinophyma before and after wedge-shaped excision.

The well-known scrofulous swelling which so frequently involves
upper lip of children is closely related to these growths of the skin.
condition is accompanied by abrasions and eczematous patches, w
set up a continuous or successive irritation and inflammation. As a
as the labial mucous membrane heals, the swelling slowly disappe
Similar thickenings are seen as a result of lupus affecting the lips.
The treatment of all these diffuse swellings requires removal of

cause; only extensive structures, such as occur about the lips and lids, demand operative interference.

The elephantiasis-like thickening of the nose developing after acne rosacea requires a distinct place. It is seen in elderly individuals, especially drinkers, and reaches its highest degree as rhinophyma. While in other parts of the face there are merely dark-red spots or soft nodules with widely dilated vessels, the nose is beset with dark-red tumor-like nodes and lobulated structures. Histologically these consist chiefly of a connective-tissue hypertrophy with dilatation of the bloodvessels and hypertrophy or cystic degeneration of the sebaceous glands. They are distinguished from other forms of elephantiasis in that they remain restricted to the nose. Part of the skin-follicles of the diseased area suppurate, while the excretory ducts of others appear like deep pores and give the dark-purplish soft tumors a spongy appearance. In addition to these changes, Brian encountered a chondroma of the nasal cartilage. A difference of opinion exists as to the primary cause of the lesion, whether this is the connective-tissue proliferation (v. Hebra), the degeneration of the sebaceous glands and inflammation of their surroundings (Lassar), the dilatation of the bloodvessels (Lesser), or the trophic disturbances following a primary angioneurosis (Kaposi, Dohi). Operative removal of the tumor-like masses has been accomplished with the knife or with the thermocautery on account of the profuse bleeding. An excellent result has been obtained by Dieffenbach in an advanced case by means of wedge-shaped excisions.

Hæmangioma.—It follows from the different statistics collected by Trendelenburg that the chief form of hæmangiomata, the simple and cavernous angiomata, have their site of preference in the face. Two-thirds of all angiomata are found here. It is a peculiar fact that about two-thirds of the cases occur in the female sex. According to their distribution among the different areas of the face, Virchow distinguishes auricular, labial, nasofrontal, palpebral, and buccal angiomata. According to Trendelenburg's collection of 170 cases, the tumors of the cheek and forehead exceed the others in frequency, then follow those of the lips, nose, aural region, and eyelids. In general, this corresponds with other statistics, for instance, those of Bittner. It is clear that all parts of the face can be affected. Virchow has attempted to explain their remarkable preference for certain regions by embryonal conditions, in so far as he assumed a certain relationship to the fetal clefts. Very slight irritations may suffice to bring about a more marked development of vessels in the margins and surface of these clefts, which in their normal state are very vascular. This may possibly show a nævus, or may remain latent for the time being, to become manifest later. Against this theory of fissural angiomata Trendelenburg has pointed out that angiomata occur in all parts of the face and are absent where clefts have formed.

The cutaneous form of the simple angioma is generally first noticed at birth or soon after. On account of its location the deep angioma, however, is frequently detected later, when the growth becomes more rapid and the skin is involved. The original spot resembles a flea-bite, with

and cicatrizations aid considerably. The hemorrhages occu
a simple angioma are not marked and can easily be controll
 Despite their slower growth, cavernous angiomata may appe
tumor-like structures, especially about the lips, lids, and che
proliferation of their peculiar spongy network they may also
beneath the mucous membrane of the lips, cheeks, and gums.
appearance of the growths may be traced to birth or to the fi
of life, but they may also develop later in life, and here the
said to be occasionally traumatic. As flat elevations of the
are spread diffusely over large areas, such as the cheek, temp

Fig. 197.

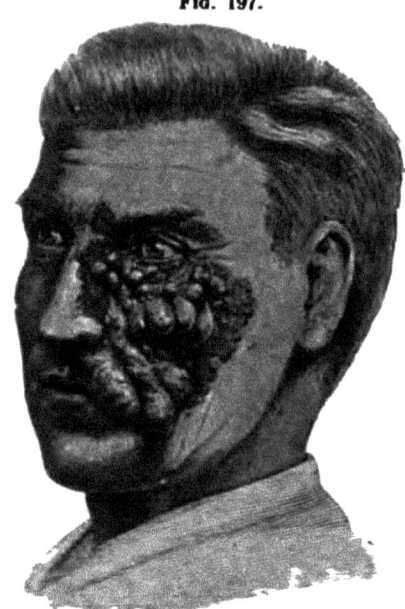

Lobulated hæmangioma.

maxillary region. Since the neoplasm develops in the sul
tissues, the skin is perfectly normal or else thinned out ii
places, with bluish discolorations. At other times the tumor
cumscribed, grape-like or lobulated, soft masses, over which t
epidermis is of bluish-black color. The cavernous growth rar
so much as in the case described by Bittner. Here the tumc
the entire half of the face and head of a thirteen-year-old gii
with the mucous membrane of the mouth, and its numerous
interstices stood in relation with the intracranial vessels.
 Symptoms.—Besides the bluish discoloration and the pain,
upon their intimate connection with the nerves, the chief si

swelling up. This is much more marked here than with the tu
subcutaneous angioma.

In rare cases the tumor of the lips and cheeks is made up of
convolution of varicose veins, which are in communication
blood with (angioma racemosum venosum). The cavernou
which develops as encapsulated or diffuse growths in the orbit
the eyeball and endangers it. One may suspect a cavernou
when there is diminution in size on pressing the eyeball back a
marked swelling on crying out or straining. The diagnosis is
certain when extension to the lids takes place and bluish tum
here. Elephantiasis-like structures have also been described a
lids and lips which are characterized by an abundance of dilate
vessels, and the structure of which suggests a cavernous growth (
tiasis cavernosa, teleangiectoides). Schüller saw a diffuse angi
in which the lids, lips, and cheek of the left side formed large p
folds.

Cavernous angiomata are subject to spontaneous changes.
grade development may occur by obliteration of the afferent v
by clotting within the network and shrinkage. Blood-cysts and
liths occasionally develop after this process. Considerable hen
may occur when the atrophic skin ruptures, but this can re
controlled by compression.

Diagnosis.—As a rule there is little difficulty in recognizing tl
ent types of hæmangiomata owing to their characteristic appea
certain forms which may occasionally be difficult to distingu
each other, such as the cavernous from the varicose or the simpl
ing from the plexiform angioma, be excluded. If the skin remain
an angiolipoma may be mistaken for a tumor of the parotid glan

Treatment.—The treatment of angiomata has been discussed
under neoplasms of the scalp; it is natural that in the face speci
must be paid to cosmetic results. Small superficial angiomat
require touching with fuming nitric acid, or needling with the fin
of the thermocautery. A superficial white and only slightly vis
follows. Excision, with subsequent suture or grafting, where d
of the lids or lips is apt to follow, must, however, be consid
larger angiomata. Since, however, the marks of the operatio
disappear entirely, many patients will prefer even a large flat str
mark to the scar. It stands to reason that the eyes must be p
as well as possible from the effects of heat or chemicals appl
surroundings. The removal of angiomata of the lids is diffic
their cartilage and edges must remain intact as far as possib
quently scarification with the finest knife is the most useful (F
Cautery with heat or chemicals is best for the tip of the nose, u
angiomata are large, when an excision followed by transplan
preferable.

Tumor-like growths consisting of simple subcutaneous or
angiomata should be excised as far as practicable. The o
should be performed rapidly on account of the active bleedin

wound and its surroundings are compressed and all bleeding points and vessels caught with hæmostatic forceps after the remaining tumor-tissue has been scraped out with a sharp spoon. Wedge-shaped excisions have repeatedly been resorted to about the lips. Encapsulated cavernous tumors of the orbit are easily extirpated, but the removal of the eyeball may be necessary where they have spread diffusely(Weinlechner). About the cheeks only the small cavernous growths are suitable for excision, and here the course of the facial nerve must be considered. In larger simple or cavernous angiomata resort is had to a combined method of treatment.

Tumor-like portions can be cut and scraped out, and the remaining parts obliterated gradually by the thermocautery or hy the injection of fluids (alcohol, silver nitrate, etc).

Occasionally good results have been obtained by ligating the afferent vessels (coronary or facial artery); at times improvement has followed ligation of the common carotid (V. v. Bruns). In the worst cases the latter procedure forms the last, as well as the most dangerous resort.

Plexiform Angioma.—Angioma arteriale racemosum is more frequent about the head in the region of the ear, forehead, or temple than in the face, but it may extend to the face from the other localities. When the tumor involves the cheek, its position corresponds to the course of the temporal artery and its branches, as in Lieblein's advanced cases; or else it follows the facial artery, with the trunk of which it descends into the submaxillary region. Rotgans saw a plexiform angioma develop within a few years in the lower lip after a dog-bite; in this locality the entire thickness of tissue may be converted into an interlacing mass of worm-like tumors. The characteristic symptoms, diagnosis, and treatment correspond with those of the same disease of the scalp.

Aneurysms.—Aneurysms of the face are rare. It can generally be ascertained that the dilatation is traumatic in nature; it develops either directly after the vessel is injured or slowly after contusions. Their size hardly ever exceeds that of a hazelnut if they remain circumscribed and do not form the first stages of a plexiform angioma by dilatation of a large portion of the vessel.

One can hardly mistake the small pulsating tumor which appears bluish through the skin and mucous membrane covering it, and which can be completely compressed, only to swell again when the afferent vessels are released.

Arteriovenous aneurysm developing after trauma is extremely rare. There are two cases mentioned in v. Brahmann's statistics.

Treatment.—The treatment of simple aneurysms consists in extirpation of the sac and ligation of the vessels.

Sarcoma.—Most sarcomata occurring in the face take their starting point from the bone or from the parotid glands. Retromaxillary tumors, tumors of the upper and lower jaw, the nose, and the parotid gland, are described in the respective chapters. The remaining sarcomata are growths of the skin, the fatty cushion of the cheek, and the orbit with its contents. Only the first-mentioned form a small group.

The congenital sarcomata of the face described and collected cially by Weinlechner, Kirmisson, and Zahn, are interesting, t rare. They occur as round-cell or spindle-cell myxosarcomata or sarcomata, and develop from the skin of the lids, lips, and nos fatty cushion of the cheek (Zahn), or the orbits (cited by Lannelo In a case of Ramdohr there were twenty-one analogous tumos tributed over the entire body besides the angiosarcoma of the chin. prognosis of these congenital sarcomata, as well as of those deve during childhood, is unfavorable on account of their rapid growt their tendency to form metastases over the body.

Sarcomata may develop from the skin of the face at any later of life. They then appear as papillary tumors consisting of so comatous warts, or else constitute small nodules in the deeper la the skin or in the subcutaneous tissues. From the latter, nodu lobulated tumors covered with delicate skin develop. Depending the kind of tumor-tissue, their clinical picture, aside from their growth, is an extremely varied one. Pigmented or melanosarc which are relatively most common, can be recognized with case. all, they are characterized by their light-brown, bluish-brown, or black discoloration. They take their origin from congenital ano of the pigment in the skin, and grow very rapidly to papillary t or to rounded structures with broad and pedunculated base. I vicinity new nodules soon develop from small black infiltrations skin. Since the tumor soon ulcerates superficially, with swelling nearest lymph-nodes, the clinical picture may closely resemble m carcinoma. This is, however, distinguished by the fissuring pecu carcinoma and by the crater-like excavation of the ulcer (v. Bergn

Among the remaining rare forms are myxosarcomata (Billroth). cases simulate lipoma of the cheek (Horteloup).

Treatment.—The treatment consists in radical removal as far a sible. In melanosarcoma especially the incision should be made i siderable distance from the growth, since the surrounding tissue freq contains small nodules which are hidden in the subcutaneous tiss are only exposed on incision. Since this variety so rapidly forms tases, one does not like to remove larger growths, and operation course, excluded as soon as there is reason to believe that metasta present in the internal organs. Skin defects remaining after excisi remedied by plastic operations.

The orbit forms one of the chief locations of sarcomata of th manifold type. Displacement and protrusion of the eyeball are th prominent symptoms of these tumors, which in part develop fro eyeball itself, as is frequently the case with melanosarcomata, i grow from the optic nerve and its membranes, the connective tissue orbit, the periosteum, the bone, or, lastly, the lachrymal gland. Oth comata grow into the orbits from the surrounding tissues (compare maxillary tumors, tumors of the nose and accessory sinuses and upper jaw). Although fluctuation and pulsation may be present in c forms of these tumors, one may sum up the diagnostic signs by s that a rapidly appearing tumor which can be felt through the intact skin at any region of the orbit, which forms a solid mass with nodular surface, and which is not fluctuating, pulsating, compressible, or of stony hardness, in a general way corresponds to sarcoma (Berlin). The consistence alone rarely permits one to determine the variety of sarcoma present.

An early and radical operation is indicated, since these orbital sarcomata may grow into the skull and extend to the dura and brain. It is rarely possible to remove the sarcomatous masses without injuring the eyeball with all its structures. Exposure of the orbit is necessary in doubtful cases to determine the character of the tumor and its relation to the eyeball. Temporary resection of the external orbital wall, according to Krönlein (Fig. 198), gives the necessary view of the interior of the orbit.

The skin-incision begins in the temporal region about 1 cm. above the supraorbital margin and runs downward along the external orbital margin in a curve, slightly convex anteriorly, to the level of the upper edge of the zygoma, where it turns backward to end over the middle of this process. After the periosteum has been incised at the external orbital margin it is raised, together with all the orbital structures, from the lateral orbital wall by means of an elevator, until the instrument can be introduced into the sphenomaxillary fissure. This indicates the point where the incisions in the bone should meet. The external angular process of the frontal bone is first chiselled through transversely somewhat above the distinctly palpable suture, between the frontal and malar bones, until the chisel enters the sphenomaxillary fissure; then follows division of the malar bone close to its base, near its articulation with the superior maxilla whereby the same fissure is again reached. The external orbital wall, now wedge-shaped and movable, is turned out together with the flap of skin, fasciæ, and muscles of the temple. If the periosteum of the orbit is sharply incised from behind forward and the edges opened up, the external rectus muscle will first come in view. By blunt dissection one may thus reach all retrobulbar structures as well as any tumor present.

Fig. 198.

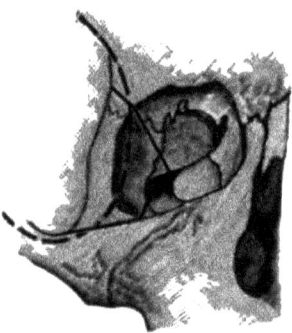

Opening the orbit. Krönlein's method.
- - - Line of skin incision.
—— Line of bone incision.

The indications for Krönlein's operation are all retrobulbar diseases with healthy eyeball. Cystic tumors (dermoids, blood or mucous cysts, echinococcus, and cysticerci), tumors of the optic nerve and its membranes, retrobulbar angiomata, lymphangiomata, osteomata, adenomata, and neuromata, are especially suitable, less so sarcomata and carcinomata. Retrobulbar injuries (foreign bodies, splinters of bone) and orbital phlegmons have been mentioned as forming other indications.

If the eyeball cannot be saved, Krönlein's operation may immediately be followed by removal of the orbital contents.

In order to perform an evacuatio orbitæ, it is only necessary to the palpebral fissure outward, so that the lids can be pulled far aps turned back over the margin of the orbit in an upward and dow direction. With a strong knife one then cuts through the conju down to the bony edge in its entire circumference. From this ii the periosteum is raised from the bone by means of an elevator up deeper parts of the orbit, so as to enable as far as possible a rem all the structures with the periosteum. The pedicle of this cone-s mass of tissues, which has now been loosened from its surroundi divided as deeply as possible with curved scissors. The entire ca at once tamponed firmly. If the tampon is removed in a short the spurting ophthalmic artery is seen distinctly, and can be graspe ligated by tying the thread with two anatomical forceps. If nec diseased portions of the bony wall can then be removed with sp chisel. If the tumor extends more deeply into the bone or even it skull, the results of the operation will be unsatisfactory, and it woul been better if it had not been undertaken. After all hemorrha been stopped, v. Bergmann at once covers over the empty orbit by of a plastic operation, as first recommended by Küster, otherwi deep cicatricial cavity pulling upon the lids leads to marked dis ment. The lids are employed in this operation after their edge the eyelashes and the remaining conjunctiva have been removec sewing both together a covering of skin results, which generally si It is gently pressed into the orbit with gauze, and will form its epic lining when it has firmly healed in place after two weeks. In or avoid an accumulation of blood behind the flap a small gap is left suture, which is kept open for the first few days by means of a s gauze. One proceeds differently, especially in carcinomata and sionally also in sarcomata, when the lids cannot be preserved. On cuts a flap with a pedicle from the forehead or temple and trans it into the orbit. The eyebrow should be avoided, as it must rem its place. The defect in the skin of the forehead is covered by gr Both procedures generally give such good cosmetic results th patients refuse the use of a bandage or of glasses to cover the region.

A part of those tumors which were classified by earlier authors different names (plexiform, alveolar sarcoma, angiosarcoma, cylind etc.) are now considered as belonging to the manifold group of theliomata. The angiosarcomata of Kolaczek belong to this class. have been observed in the subcutaneous tissues of the lower li cheek, and are characterized by slow growth, good encapsulatioi free mobility. Similar growths limited to the subcutis of the upp nose and cheek must be, according to the investigations of Nass R. Volkmann, looked upon as endotheliomata or mixed endot tumors resembling parotid tumors in structure. They form encapst rounded nodes covered with normal skin and of hard or soft and fl ating consistence. Besides these there are also diffuse new forms in the cutis; they are mushroom-shaped with smooth surface, or ulcers (v. Volkmann, König, Braun), or appear as slightly elevated, somewhat nodular structures. Ulcerating endotheliomata of the skin may closely resemble carcinomata owing to the extensive destruction reaching down to the bone. This has been observed by v. Volkmann in an ulcerated tumor involving almost the entire half of the face, and by Hinzberg with similar growths of the lids and nasal skin. Those clinical characteristics of endotheliomata which would enable one to distinguish them definitely from sarcomata and carcinoma are not as yet sufficiently defined. Emphasis is laid upon their slow growth, the rarity of recurrence in the encapsulated forms, their appearance at every age, and the non-involvement of the lymph-nodes. The latter is in contrast to the observation of Tanaka, who recently found that metastases may occur in the lymph-nodes. According to him, the enlarged lymph-nodes retain a soft fluctuating consistency and do not become adherent to the surrounding tissues.

Atheroma.—Atheromata are seen with considerable less frequency in the face than upon the hairy scalp. Their relative frequency has been referred to before. They usually occur about the cheek or in the neighborhood of the eye and lips, and, as far as origin, characteristics, and course are concerned, differ in no respect from those of the scalp. Such large structures as patients, who fear the operation, often have under the hair, are not, however, encountered in the face. About the lips, the skin covering the tumor may be so thin that its whitish contents shine through; by this the bluish cysts of the lips may be easily differentiated. Inflammation is comparatively frequent in these atheromata, and is generally caused by infection following attempts to press out the soft contents. They are easily recognized by their connection with the skin, mobility, and rounded shape; but when inflamed, it may often be difficult to distinguish them and the surrounding inflammatory infiltrate from an abscess of the skin. Mention of this has been made in discussing, for example, softened actinomycotic foci.

Atheromata which have become calcareous or carcinomatous may occur in the face. If the carcinomatous tissue has broken through the wall of the sebaceous cyst and the skin, the remains of the follicle carries the cancerous tissue upon it like a cup-shaped pedicle. As long as the follicle is still closed, as the author has seen it in one case, it is impossible to recognize its transition into carcinoma.

Atheromata are operated upon according to the rules which hold for sebaceous cysts of the scalp.

Dermoids.—As has been mentioned, dermoid cysts of the face have their most frequent seat in the upper and outer quadrant of the orbital margin and eyelid. Next in frequency are the inner canthus, the glabella, and the root of the nose. Other parts of the face are affected considerably less often.

Since the invagination of ectoderm in the course of the fetal clefts is recognized as cause of dermoids, it must seem very strange that they are so rare in the parts of the face mentioned and absent at the sites where clefts are most frequent, especially at the upper lip. V. Bramann explains this by the varying behavior of the amnion. V. Bergmann referred to this in discussing dermoids of the scalp.

The few cases observed, described by v. Bramann and Lannelor were noticed immediately after birth or in earliest childhood, and for small slowly growing cysts, usually seated upon the bridge of the 1 The rounded fluctuating tumor is generally immovable upon the fr work of the nose and is not adherent to the normal or thinned skin w covers it. According to v. Bramann's cases, the site is peculiar in the cartilaginous portion of the nose is involved, and that the upper of the cyst projects under the nasal bones, which it raises while the tilage is forced in. This repeated observation is explained by v. Bran by the development of the facial skeleton. As the nasal bones n their appearance in the second or third month, in order to cover ove structures they encounter the cartilaginous nose as remainder of primary cartilaginous cranium. In case the rudimentary dern extending far upward, is in the middle of this cartilaginous 1 the nasal bones must develop over it, just as a dermoid, de implanted at the root of the nose, comes to lie behind the frontal b and hence in the frontal sinus. The changes found in the l framework are regarded by v. Bramann as chiefly due to the pres exercised by the growing cyst, since deformity of any extent was seen in adults, and was absent when the tumor was small or had in existence for only a short time (in small children). The cases scribed consisted in part of intact cysts, in part of ruptured, compl or incompletely evacuated dermoids, from the opening of which a of hair protruded (dermoid fistula); or the cysts were in communic with a tract which was covered with epithelium, and which op externally after it had extended for some distance in the middle down to the tip of the nose.

Dermoids developed upon the edges of the primitive naso-or furrow are situated laterally to or directly above the nostrils. In ease of v. Bramann two strands of connective tissue were found run up and down from the main cyst in the course of the fetal tissue. 1 were firmly united to the periosteum and were covered with several s dermoid cysts.

Three cases described by Lannelongue, one observed by Verneuil, one by the author occupied the region of the intermaxillary or transv cleft of the cheek.

The histological structure, the contents, and the clinical peculiar of dermoids have been previously discussed by v. Bergmann.

Diagnosis.—The diagnosis is not difficult if a dermoid fistula is pre from which the hair protrudes or the characteristic pulp can be expres In adults the long existence of the cysts at the three typical sites l one to a correct diagnosis; in children, however, they may well be taken for abscesses. In suppurating dermoids the diagnosis is not e In the cheek the mobility of the skin over the dermoid excludes athero and cavernous lymphangiomata or hæmangiomata can be dis guished by the discoloration of the skin, their connection with it, a their indefinite outlines. The very rare carcinomatous degeneration of the cyst cannot be recognized if the follicle is closed (H. Wolffe).

Treatment.—The treatment involves removal of the entire follicle or fistulous tract. At the bridge of the nose the relation to the lower edge of the nasal bones, mentioned above, is to be considered.

Mucous Cysts, Echinococcus Cysts, Cysticerci.—Of the remaining cystic structures of the face, those of the lips which occur as retention-cysts of the mucous glands and have their seat chiefly in the mucous membrane of the lower lip, deserve attention. They form small rounded elevations of the thinned mucous membrane. Their growth is slow, but they may occasionally attain the size of a duck's egg. Their contents usually shine through the mucous membrane and give them a bluish appearance. Owing to this discoloration they may occasionally be mistaken for small carcinomata, or, if situated in the labial mucous membrane, for a small aneurysm. The treatment is simple. The external wall of the cyst is cut away with curved scissors; what remains behind is then destroyed with the thermocautery after the contents have been removed. Rarely, cysticerci of the lips have been observed (cited by V. v. Bruns and A. Broca).

Echinococcus cysts have been seen in the temporal region (Guttmann, Bertelé) and in the region of the cheek (V. v. Bruns, Bertelé, v. Bergmann, within the temporal and masseter muscles; they also have been repeatedly observed in the orbit (Preindlsberger). Cysticerci were found less often in the latter situation. An absolute diagnosis can only be made by a microscopical examination of the contents obtained from the cysts by puncture. While operating, care should be taken to extirpate the wall completely.

Cutaneous Horns.—Cutaneous horns (*cornua cutanea*) are considerably less frequent in the face than upon the hairy scalp or the frontal and temporal regions. They occur almost exclusively in advanced age, where one or more are seated upon the lids, lips, nose, or cheek. They first appear as small wart-like nodes which slowly develop into dark-brown horny structures, with spiral striping, 10 cm. or more in length. At the lower lip and lower lid ectropion results from the traction of these structures (Mitwalsky), and the weight of the horn may pull downward the upper eyelid (Herzog Karl Theodor). Several authors (Lebert and Spietschka) follow Malpighi in holding that the dermal papillæ play a part in the hyperplasia of the epidermis and the cornification, inasmuch as every hypertrophied papilla is in a certain sense continued into a column of epidermis (v. Winiwarter). Bätge, however, found the papillæ atrophic, and Mitwalsky considers them of no importance whatever. Occasionally a cutaneous horn develops from a papilloma or a sebaceous cyst (Home, Lebert, Franke). The base of the horn is sometimes ulcerated and may be the starting point of a carcinoma. The horn always grows again if it falls off spontaneously, or if it is cut off insufficiently or removed by tearing or ligation. A complete cure therefore can only be expected after radical removal with the knife, for which purpose an elliptical incision must be made around the base.

Adenomata of Sweat- and Sebaceous Glands.—Adenomat sweat- and sebaceous glands are chiefly interesting in that they may t the starting point of an epithelioma or may be mistaken for this when occur singly and ulcerate. An adenoma sudoriparum has been descr by Stilling from investigations at König's clinic. Its longest diam was 1 to 1.5 cm.; it projected about 5 to 6 mm. above the cutis and sisted of sharply circumscribed nodular, tumor-like elevations. T structures occur in the skin of the face of elderly individuals, near angles of the eye or jaw, where they slowly developed during many y The tumor has its seat in the cutis, and consists of the proliferated d and lobules of the glands, which show inflammatory infiltrations and formation. König draws attention to the resemblance which these flammatory adenomata of the sweat-glands, as he calls them, bet lupus. They frequently occur after an injury to the skin, and are tinguished by their persistence and their slight tendency to ulcera Microscopically they may be mistaken for teleangiectasiæ. If inf mation sets in after the cyst has ruptured, it may suppurate and b down and a persistent ulcer may follow. The malignant adenomat the sweat-glands described by some authors were probably, accor to v. Winiwarter, sarcomatous or carcinomatous growths after adenc Campanini has described adenocarcinomata of the sweat-glands in w the new tissue irritated the stricture of the glands.

Adenomata of the sebaceous glands (*adenomata sebacea*) occur in face as multiple growths usually situated about the nose and lids. Ba distinguished them from simple glandular hypertrophy. Several w or nodular growths of the lids, varying in size from a pea to the a walnut, are described by him as forming encapsulated tumor which the proliferated epithelium is contained in a fibrous stroma. 1 are frequently characterized by hyaline degeneration of the vessels connective tissue. Adenomata often have their origin in the cond of the skin known as seborrhœa; they may calcify or develop into cinoma.

Calcified Epithelioma.—The calcified epithelioma (Malherbe Chenantais) is regarded by Barlow as a calcified sebaceous adenoma. one case, however, Thorn could prove a continuation of the exte epithelium into the tumor mass of the calcified epithelioma. Accor to Van Noorden, this rare growth has been found several times abou eyebrows, forehead, cheek, the region of the parotid, and the lobu the ear.

Adenomata and epitheliomata should be removed with the knife cosmetic reasons if for nothing else. Besides, it must be rememb that the irritation following the frequent application of caustics to ul ating adenomata predisposes to carcinoma.

Epithelioma.—Epithelioma of the face plays a prominent part account of its frequency as compared with cancerous disease in o parts and tissues of the body. According to the statistics of Gurlt, cinoma of the external parts of the face constitutes one-seventh of cases of cancer; according to Heimann, about one-third.

Concerning distribution and frequency of carcinoma in the face, the different statistics (v. Bergmann, v. Winiwarter, Trendelenburg, Heimann) almost all agree. The chin is affected least of all; then come the upper lip, the eyelids, the cheeks, the nose, and, lastly, as the most frequent site, the lower lip. Of 499 cancers of the face, Trendelenburg finds that 241 involve the lower lip. It is remarkable that carcinoma of the lower lip affects the male sex almost exclusively; according to Heimann, of 509 cases, 473 were males and only 36 females. If the lower lip is excluded, about equal figures are obtained for both sexes, according to Heimann, and no marked difference is seen for any other part of the face, except that the upper lip is involved somewhat more often in females (Tricke).

The predisposition to carcinoma of the face increases in general up to an advanced age; the increase is especially rapid between the fortieth and sixtieth year (Trendelenburg). Epitheliomata have been observed in young individuals and children, but are extremely rare (v. Winiwarter). It is well known that inhabitants of the country are more frequently affected than those living in the city. Thiersch explains this by the more rapid withering of the skin of peasants owing to exposure to atmospheric influences. V. Volkmann lays stress upon uncleanliness of the skin as a marked predisposing factor.

Those changes in the skin which are of importance in the development of an epithelioma are present to a marked degree in the face. First of all, there are the congenital and acquired anomalies of the skin, benign epithelial growths such as warts, pigmented spots, papillomata, cutaneous horns, hypertrophies of the hair-follicles, the sweat- and sebaceous glands, adenomata of the latter two, atheromata, dermoids, etc. Then there are the skin diseases caused by chronic inflammatory irritation, such as frequently repeated erysipelas, chronic eczema, psoriasis, syphilitic and lupoid ulcers. These may all form the starting point for a carcinoma. It is well known that scars of different origin, whether after injury or ulceration of the skin, may occasionally form the foundation for a cancer. However, very few of the cases which are considered as directly the result of trauma are convincing. On the other hand, the importance of repeated traumatic irritation has been appreciated by Thiersch. An example of this is the lesion developing after shaving, which is seated especially at the junction of skin and mucous membrane of the lip.

Of the different skin diseases, congenital atrophy of the skin, termed by Kaposi xeroderma pigmentosum, and accompanied by peculiar alteration of pigment, has been found several times at the site of development in youthful subjects. At a more advanced age, two skin diseases often stand in relation to the development of carcinoma. It is often easy to trace the connection between the latter and the seborrhagic spots, the so-called seborrhœa senilis (v. Volkmann, Schuchardt, v. Bergmann). According to Schuchardt's investigations on old people, this lesion begins as a desquamative and cornifying process in the uppermost layers of the epidermis, especially in the hair-follicles, and is generally favored by

follicles induced by the
leads to a finely granula
ted epidermis. The
scale-like deposits of shie
they develop to wart-like
crusts, adhere rather fir
sened. Besides these fr
may also occur. The
lies and warts are remove
carcinomata, but th
intact spots, and they he
simple cleansing treatment.
elevated spots which occur
of the cheek and tongu
form an important etiol
upon increased prolife
As a rule there are several
the mucosal side of th
of the mouth and to the ju
The cancer may exist for thirty
and its surroundings b
of the proliferated
since it may be d
or the cauterization o
found in those who s
why the use of tobacco sta
of the lip, tongue, and m
irritation from the tobacco-
of the lower lip is said to d
particular spot. This, how
many cases the carcinoma dev
The spots characteristic of leuko
of a cancer of the lip;
carcinomata which follow each

and mucous membrane
carcinomata, it must not be for
upon absolutely normal skin.

that usually occurs on the
superficial ulcer which is
surroundings, very moderate
elevation of the edges. Cicatri
portions. These clinical signs
of epithelial cells, their tender
of the abundantly fo
the temple and forehea
the bridge of the nose, the no
the lids, and the skin of the c

The rather infrequent carcinoma of the upper lip generally belongs to this form. It is characteristic even of small ulcers that, owing to contraction, the skin forms radial folds. This is especially distinct about the lids (Fig. 199), where the growth is usually placed upon the mesial portion of the lower lid and the inner canthus.

At first the patient merely notices a crust, which always reappears if it is removed from the moist and easily bleeding spot upon the skin. Gradually he notices that the small ulcer is spreading beneath the crust. Then the edges become somewhat raised and indurated, the secretion increases in amount, and the crust shows fissures and is elevated in part by purulent matter. While the flat ulcer extends irregularly, complete cicatrization takes place here or there. The characteristics which distinguish this flat ulcer of carcinoma from the ulcer of syphilis and lupus have already been mentioned.

The further extension of a flat carcinoma may be so slow and interrupted by such long intervals that it may take years for a large portion of the face to be involved. As an example König mentions a woman ninety years old in whom an epithelioma of the lid required as much as twenty-five years to spread over one-half of the face. Where the extension is marked and the course long and undisturbed, the tumor does not, however, remain

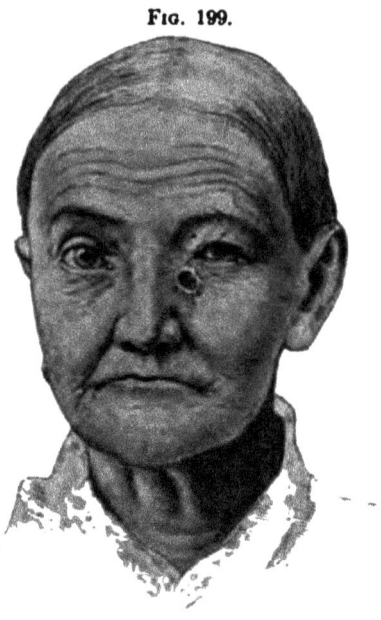

FIG. 199.

Epithelioma. (Von Bergmann's clinic.)

restricted to the face; it spreads into the deeper parts with much greater rapidity, destroys the lids and the nasal cartilage, and infiltrates the bone, so that the orbital wall, the frontal and the maxillary sinuses, and the framework of the malar bone and nose are destroyed. Eventually the greater part of the face is converted into a single deep ulcer. The destruction of the facial skeleton is very considerable.

The comparatively benign character of the flat carcinoma depends upon its slow growth at first and the rare involvement of the neighboring lymph-nodes. It is the ulcus rodens of the older authors and its clinical course, without microscopical examination would hardly justify its classification among carcinomata (Schimmelbusch). The property which it possesses to a high degree of contracting and cicatrizing may easily lead one astray. V. Bergmann has shown that these ulcers can be made to cicatrize by simple dressings or the application of ointments.

PLATE XI.

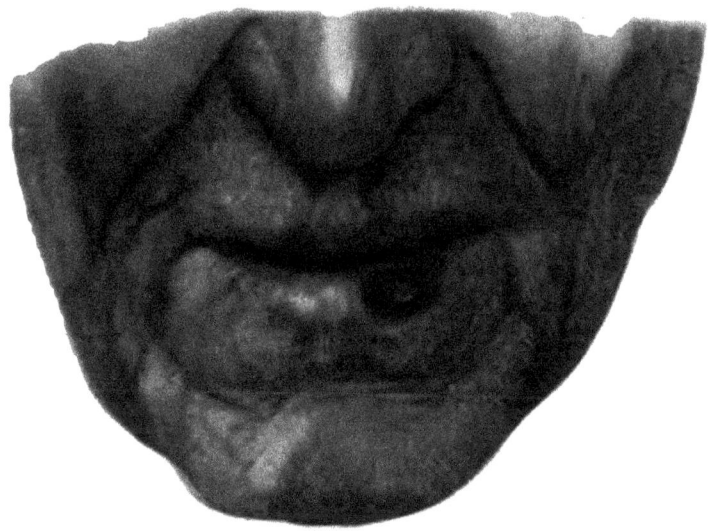

Epithelioma of the Lip. (Grünwald.)

more frequent. It appears at first as a small hard and superficial nodule, particularly at the junction of the mucous membrane of the lip with the skin, and more often between the middle of the lip and the angle of the mouth than in either of these places. Its surface breaks down soon and is converted into a fissured ulcer, or else papillomatous growths form which are covered with crusts or thick layers of cornified epithelium. In a short time there is a hard nodular tumor, the surface of which is the seat of cauliflower growths or irregular, crater-like ulcers with easily bleeding dirty and fissured bases. Owing to the growth of the tumor the edge of the ulcer forms a steep indurated wall which is somewhat inverted on the side of the mucous membrane; it is surrounded by the

Fig. 202.

Fig. 203.

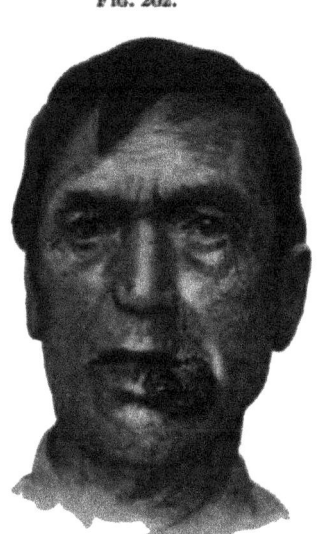
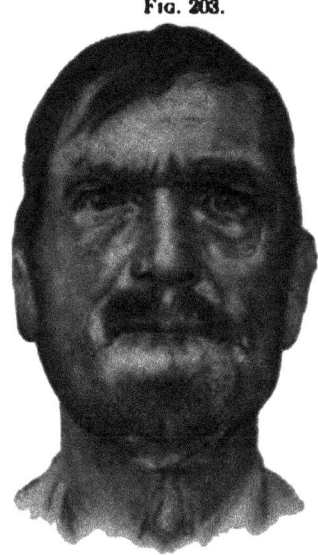

Epithelioma of lower lip.

Same after removal and plastic operation in a man aged seventy.

sharp edge of the mucons membrane. The regional lymph-nodes of the submental and submaxillary region soon show their participation in the disease by becoming larger and hardened, and the nodular growth extends further from the lip to the lower jaw. Finally the entire lower lip and angle of the mouth, with a large part of the skin of the chin and mucous membrane of the lower jaw, are converted into a dense putrid mass of cancerous tissue from which a hard infiltration extends to the floor of the mouth, the cheek, and the upper lip, and continues almost without interruption into the much swollen lymph-nodes.

The very malignant melanocarcinoma is found very rarely in the face. It may develop from pigmented moles or warts, and must be classified among the deeply reaching forms of epithelioma. Like the more fre-

... ... forming the fla[
... ... region. Frequ
... ... scale, it the sub

... ... are to be fou
... ... extent an
... ... of large ca
... ... in spite of
... ... success. High
... ... these were exam
... after a few years or
... ... of the current
... ... expedition
... ... well as in th
... in large tumors of
... ... companie
... ... recurrence
... ... very extensive
... ... the skin and th
... ... healing and for th
... ... and gene
... ... of an opera
... ... patience is
... ... upon th
... ... characterization
... ... alteration. F
... acetate or hydrog
... ... alteration of
... ... which exi
... after sets in after he

CHAPTER XIII.

PLASTIC OPERATIONS.

RHINOPLASTY.

THE history of rhinoplasty is the history of plastic surgery. The old Indian and Italian methods were devised to cover defects of the nose probably because mutilations of the face were so common in those days. Since then plastic operations have been improved and altered constantly. Formerly only reparation of the cartilaginous part of the nose was attempted. Dieffenbach was the first to operate where the nose was completely absent (Zeis). To him belongs the credit of having placed rhinoplasty on a scientific basis. Many procedures are only of historical interest, while certain features of others are embodied in common and useful methods of the present day.

The different plastic operations upon the nose are the operation for saddle-nose and complete and incomplete rhinoplasty.

Operation for Saddle-nose.—The cartilaginous nose, consisting of the tip, the alæ, and the septum, is preserved but pulled upward, while the entire bridge of the nose is deeply depressed. This well-known lesion occurs in varying degrees, and most frequently follows syphilitic processes of the interior of the nose which may destroy the entire bony framework with the bony septum, all the turbinated bones, and the floor of the nasal cavity. The traumatic saddle-nose is caused by depressed fractures of the bridge of the nose or by suppuration and necrosis after complicated injuries of the frame of the nose. Very rarely it is due to an acute or a tuberculous ostitis of the nasal bone.

The operation for saddle-nose has a twofold task in view, for, besides restoring the bridge, the cartilaginous nose, which has been pulled upward by the cicatricial contraction of the interior, must be loosened and brought to its normal position.

According to König, the steps of the operation are as follows: A transverse incision at the deepest portion of the depression renders the soft parts of the nose movable so that they can be pulled down to where normally the tip of the nose would be. The resulting defect, which reaches into the nasal cavities, is covered by means of a flap from the forehead. This flap is a prolongation of the nasal bridge with its base at the root of the nose; it is cut out of the forehead so that it is from 6 to 7 cm. long and only 1 cm. or less broad. (Fig. 206, a.) After the skin and periosteum have been incised, the cortical portion of the bone is chiselled through along the cut in the periosteum. The flap of skin and bone thus demarcated is now separated from the diploë from above

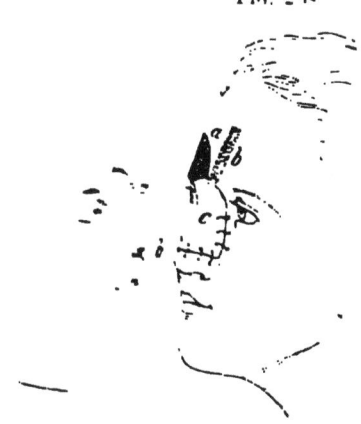

530

for this.
plastic
surgeon.
region
In o;
much i
tion of
of the
growth
remain
four to
patient
and of
ever, i
nodes
lip wh
adhere
certain
the rea
portion
conditi
play a
allevia
Beside
it is fr
somew
renewe
ide di
helps
the re
from

Fig. 2's

n-flap from forehead.

place by catgut sutures. Ts

ead sutured in place over the

ad once been introduce
ens and improvements
eration for saddle-nose, in

e osmetic result after Kö
ts the flap of bone ha
does not become too br
sured to the soft parts of
a curved transverse incis
sures. The flap is at first
and cicatrize. In the meanti

the skin will grow over the plate of bone for some distance from the edges, and can later be employed in lining the interior. When cicatrization has taken place, the bridge-like flap from the forehead is drawn somewhat to the side and the skin of the depressed nasal bridge, which lies underneath it, is incised in its length. A transverse incision to each side is placed at the upper and lower ends of this longitudinal incision, so that two door-shaped, quadrangular flaps are formed after the skin has been loosened freely. As soon as the new bridge of the nose—that is, the cicatrized side of the frontal flap—has been freshened by dissecting off the skin which has grown around the edges and folding it backward, the quadrangular flaps from the side of the nose can be placed over the bony plate and be almost completely brought together. They receive a support and their internal lining of skin from the flaps of skin dissected off the plate of bone.

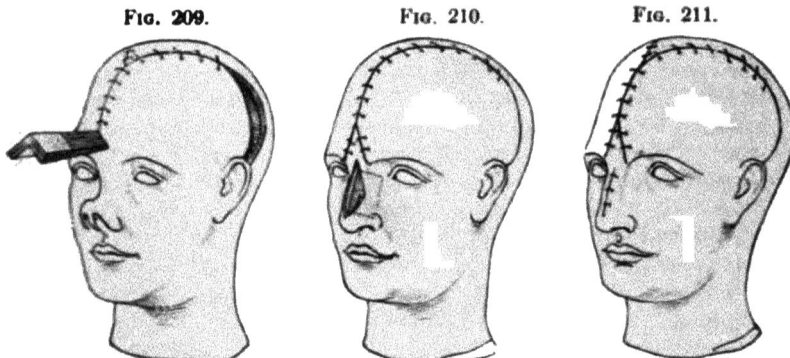

Fig. 209. Fig. 210. Fig. 211.

Fig. 209.—Defect caused by frontal flap replaced by large cured flap from scalp.
Fig. 210.—Flap transplanted into nasal defect.
Fig. 211.—Result of the plastic operation.

Helferich has modified König's method in a similar way. By means of a curved incision reaching up to the nasal root he separated the skin of the nose in the form of a flap and at the same time loosened the soft parts of the nose. The frontal flap with its plate of bone was transplanted into the defect under the dissected skin and its pedicle divided as soon as the flap had healed in place. Those parts of the frontal flap which were still exposed were covered by skin from the nasal root, which was drawn over by means of lateral flaps.

In using the flap of skin and bone according to Schimmelbusch, the newly formed bony nasal bridge rests like a roof upon the edges of the pyriform aperture. The frontal flap is cut so that one end is very broad (6 to 9 cm.). (Figs. 209 and 211.) It contains a plate of bone wider than it is long, while its more narrow pedicle consists of skin only. The large defect upon the forehead can be covered by transplantation; according to Schimmelbusch, it is, however, more advisable to bring about a linear scar by the displacement of large curved flaps cut out of the scalp. The

downward by means of a flat chisel. After this the f
its pedicle, inverted, and transplanted into the defect.
will thus form the external and the skin the internal s
The lower part of the inverted flap is sutured to the
so that the skin-edge of the latter is on top. The a
taken from the forehead in the usual manner, is sut
surface of the first flap and forms the external skin of
bridge of the nose.

At the place where the flap which forms the bri
small bridge of skin remains, which König closes
by cutting around the openings on each side and
after longitudinally placed elliptical pieces of skin
By this the form of the root of the nose is improved

FIG. 206.   FIG. 207.

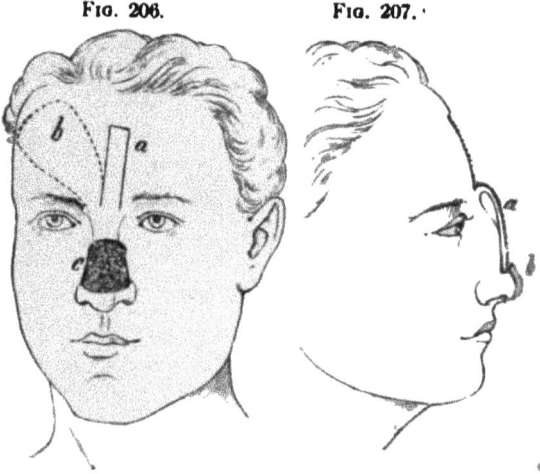

FIG. 206.—a. Bridge of nose flap (skin and bone). b. Sk
formed by transverse incision.
FIG. 207.—a. Bridge of nose flap turned down. b. Held in p
at b remains free for union with forehead flap.
FIG. 208.—a, b. Defects in forehead. c. Skin-flap from forehe
of the nose.

After the use of flaps of skin and bone ha
this method of König, a number of alteratio
suggested. In part they apply to the operati
to the restoration of the entire nose.

A considerable improvement upon the co
operation is recommended by Israel. He
0.75 cm. wide, so that the bridge of the nose
The flap is then turned downward and sec
nose, which have been freed by means of
The wound of the forehead is closed by sut
uncovered, and is allowed to granulate and

flap of skin ⬛⬛⬛ shrunken mass of skin, often
is covered wi⬛ ⬛⬛ take the place of the nose.
adhesive pla⬛ ⬛⬛ flap, whether from the cheek
meantime ⬛⬛ ⬛⬛ in general a French, an India
and the ⬛⬛⬛ ⬛⬛.
time to be⬛⬛ ⬛⬛ developed especially by Serr
edges of the ⬛ ⬛⬛ part of which must still be in pl
knife. The ⬛ ⬛⬛ shaped flaps taken from the c
its middle, ⬛⬛ ⬛⬛ to the defect from their bridge si
surface to ⬛⬛ ⬛⬛ root to the region of the nas
defect. The ⬛⬛ ⬛⬛ flaps provide for the alæ na
and freeing ⬛⬛ ⬛⬛ the flaps are brought together t
nections of ⬛⬛
sected off ⬛⬛

Fig. 213.

placed in ⬛⬛
of the pyr⬛
covers only
the pedicl⬛
an inner l⬛
so that it ll⬛
quent ⬛⬛
formed fr⬛
  Excellent
method, ⬛⬛
each indiv⬛
method of
sive oper⬛
scar resul⬛
of the im⬛
give a m⬛
would be ⬛
the eyebr⬛
  Attemp⬛
was found⬛
support to
manner w⬛

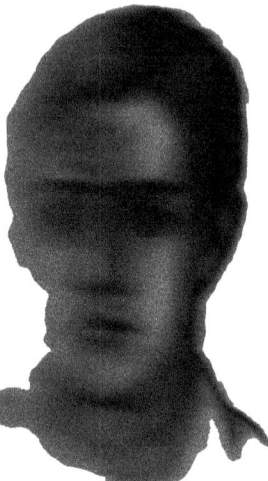
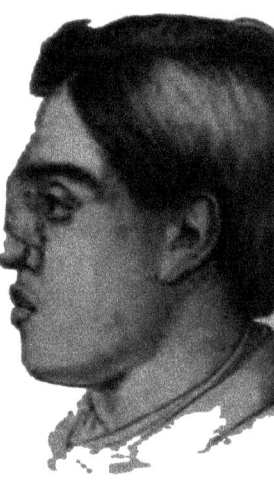

⬛⬛ nose" due to syphilis nearly two and a hal
⬛⬛ operation. (König.)

of the ⬛⬛ ⬛⬛ has developed as the site of the su
a longit⬛ ⬛⬛ lateral traction which Nélaton tri
underm⬛ ⬛⬛ periosteum with the flap, so that the sca
decalcifi⬛ ⬛⬛ For the same reason Hüter left a n⬛
it is im⬛ ⬛⬛ edge of the defect and the flap which
mitted, su⬛ ⬛⬛ support to the latter after its displace⬛
the scar⬛ ⬛⬛ nose will soon fall together unless a
mentioned ⬛⬛ septum is present, since it lacks support a⬛
that the ⬛ ⬛⬛ The method is mentioned here only be⬛
separation ⬛⬛ sonally to cover with skin a flap of skin
a part of ⬛ ⬛⬛ some other place.
and this ⬛⬛ ⬛⬛ only those retain a practical value at
⬛⬛ principle of which consists in the form⬛

of a flap of skin and bone. Here, even more so than in operations for saddle-nose, the chief condition necessary for a satisfactory and permanent result is the construction of a strong and firmly placed support.

Several procedures show how the skin- and bone-flap of König may be used. König himself has applied his method of operating upon saddle-nose to total defects of the nose. As in the former condition, the frontal flap is turned over and allowed to heal in the defect after freshening the edges; after several weeks the raw surface is covered over by a flap from the soft parts of the forehead.

The method of Rotter and Schimmelbusch differs chiefly in that the transplanted bone is supposed to form an osseous frame firmly seated upon the pyriform aperture. According to Rotter, a skin- and bone-flap 3.5 cm. broad is cut out of the forehead. It is then inverted at its base

Fig. 214.   Fig. 215

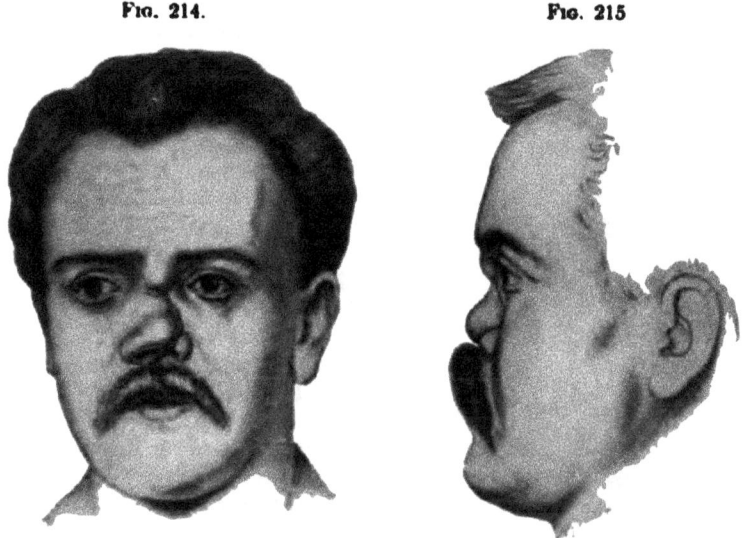

Deformity of the nose due to injury.

over the nasal root and upon the total defect, so that its skin surface lies internally. After several weeks the plate of bone is firmly incorporated in the flap with the formation of abundant granulations, so that it can be divided lengthwise with a pointed saw into three strips. The middle one is intended for the new bridge of the nose, while the lateral ones are separated from their underlying support so far that they only remain in connection below at the future tip of the nose. By turning them downward they will become the supports of a tripod-like bony nasal framework. By bringing the skin from the margins of the defect in approximation with the flap, the former is employed as much as possible for an external covering. The skin at the pyriform aperture will thus line

... the edges of the flap. The remain...
... by flaps of epidermis.
... gives a much firmer support from Sch...
... it is formed of bony walls in its entire ex...
and since it is sought to proc...
bony union with the pyriform a...
ture. The frontal flap is cu...
for saddle-nose (Fig. 217); in...
it should be too large rather t...
too small. The base meas...
from 2 to 3 cm. between the...
brows, and the upper end fro...
to 9 cm. close to the hair-line.
thin plate of bone is remo...
from the frontal bone with a...
broad chisel in the entire exten...
the flap. If the bone splinters,...
must above all try to keep the f...
ments connected with the per...
... and for this purpose latt...
shaped sutures are placed...
the bony side of the flap.
latter is then wrapped in iodof...
gauze and the plastic closure of...
large defect upon the forehead...
dertaken at once, as in sad...
nose. (Figs. 218 and 219.)
In the meantime all hemorrh...
from the flap has ceased and...
fragments are found in the b...
plate, one can then cover this...

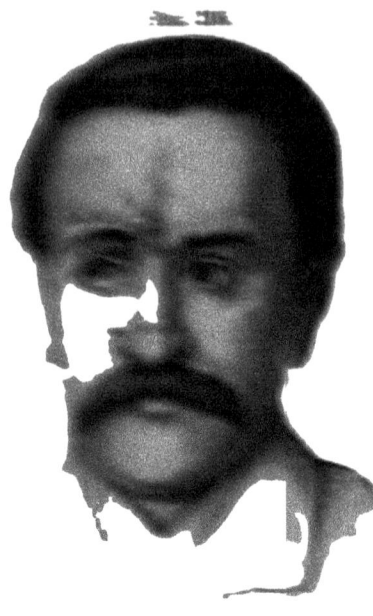

... these, if not all, will grow.
... in several places, one does...
... to await the formation of granulations
... weeks, when the necrotic porti...

... with skin it is transplanted into
... The plate of bone is sawed through in the mid...
... and then placed upright like a roof, but so that
... In the mean time the pedicle has a...
... so that it must be separated in order to...
... the bony edge of the pyrif...
... and the nasal flap, the sides of which have...
... upon it. If possible, it is fixed...
... through the bone, while the skin-edge of the flap
... of the cheek. If parts of the alæ nasi have remain...
... with the skin-edge of the flap.
... sure of the roof-like shape of the bony plate a...

start a wire may be pulled transversely through the nose at the depressions above the normal nostrils. This is then tied in a knot at both sides over rubber tubes. The imprints subsequently produced circumscribe the alæ nasi, the appearance of which will be almost normal.

If one intends to construct a septum, this can be taken from the skin-edge of the pyriform aperture after it has been freshened, in the form of two thin flaps of skin. (Fig. 218.) Their pedicle retains its connections with the normal insertion of the cutaneous septum, and they are joined to each other as well as to the tip of the nose. In three weeks

Fig. 217.   Fig. 218.   Fig. 219.

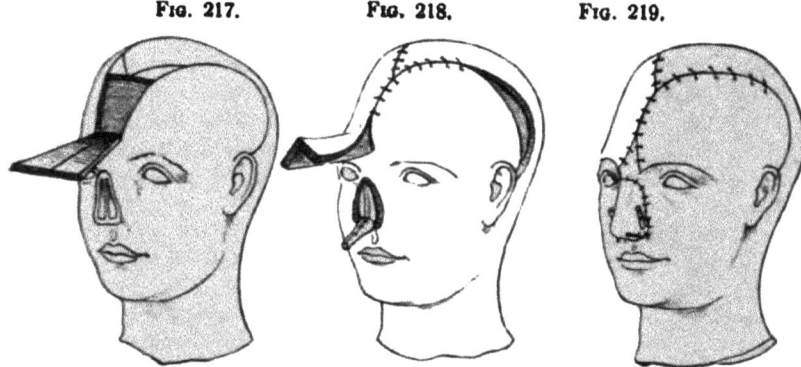

Fig. 217.—Bone flap from forehead turned down.
Fig. 218.—Defect in forehead closed by transplanted curved scalp-flap.
Fig. 219.—Result of plastic operation.

the pedicle of the frontal flap is cut through and replaced. After the shape of the newly formed nose has been improved, if necessary, it is completely sewed into the defect. (Fig. 219.)

This method has been frequently employed for total defects in v. Bergmann's clinic and has been followed by excellent results. When the fleshy nose is absent or depressed, a tip which will permanently retain its prominence can be constructed in the same way, although it will never possess the delicate structure of the natural tip.

Volkmann and König especially advise against the construction of a septum, so that the free passage of air through the nose is not impeded. If the nostril has a tendency to contract, König lets the patient wear a small tube of celluloid. This attracts as little attention as the absence of the septum if the tip of the nose is well arched below. V. Bergmann introduced two small silver tubes connected by means of a spring; they preserve excellently the form and shape of the nostrils even when their septum is present. After several weeks the patient need only wear this apparatus at night.

V. Hacker does not use König's frontal flap to build up the complete bony nose, but only for the bridge and septum. According to his method, the flap contains only a narrow plate of bone, the end of which is broken and turned over, so that the site of fracture will form the tip of the nose

the nostrils, that of the nasal root the edges of the fl
raw surfaces are covered by flaps of epidermis.

The newly formed nose receives a much firmer si
melbusch's operation, since it is formed of bony wall
and since it i:
bony union wit
ture. The fr
for saddle-nos
it should be t
too small.
from 2 to 3 c
brows, and th
to 9 cm. close
thin plate of
from the fron
broad chisel ii
the flap. If tl
must above all
ments connec
teum, and for
shaped sutur
the bony side
latter is then
gauze and the
large defect u
dertaken at
nose. (Figs.
in the meanti
from the flap

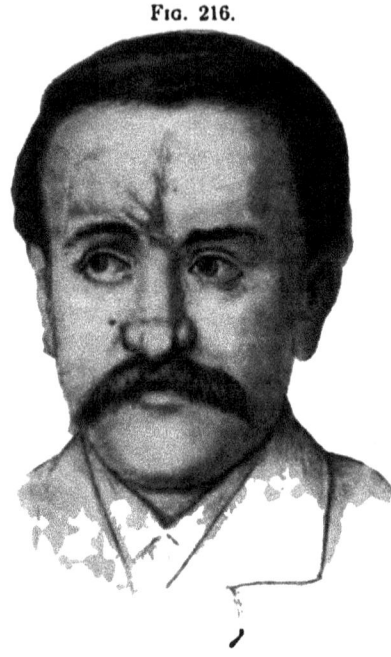

FIG. 216.

The same after plastic operation one year later.
(König.)

fragments ar
plate, one can
strips of epidermis. The greater part of these, if n
however, the plate of bone is fractured in several
according to Schimmelbusch, to await the formatio
to graft only after from four to eight weeks, when
have come off.

After the raw surface is covered with skin it is
defect upon the nose. The plate of bone is sawed
as in saddle-nose, and then placed upright like a
skin forms the external surface. In the mean tim
in part healed in place, so that it must be sepa
the flap over. By freshening the defect the bon
aperture is exposed, and the nasal flap, the sid
been freshened, is placed accurately upon it. If
further by sutures through the bone, while the
united with the skin of the cheek. If parts of the
they are raised and sutured with the skin-edge
In order to make sure of the roof-like shape

is turned do
direction. W
egin over the l
right side of t
unnecessary; it
si. The resultin
rt; the remainin
ck.

flap is constructed
rectangular flap is
lose above the edge
isions run obliquely
athus of the diseased
ar area is left, over
latter from the car-
The new margins
s at once covered with

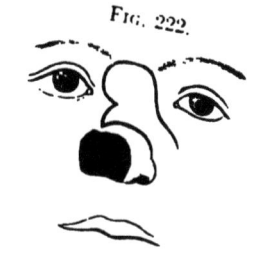

Fig. 222.

ap of nose are absent

the skin of the cheek at
ort-Malgaigne. Since its
rts which replace it should
the inner side of a Langen-
d inverted into the nose.
lateral portion of the nose.
small flap from the cheek
d turn it into the defect
Fig. 223.) For the shape of
imilar flap (v. Hacker). Its

ing to the scars of lupus, for
pedunculated flap from the
Weber. It is turned upon its
am. After several weeks the
nasi hemmed.
as well as the lateral portion.

the skin of the bridge and the root of the nose can be used by means of a flap formed according to W. Busch. (Fig. 222.) The pedicle lies close to the lateral portion of the healthy side. An inner lining with an inverted flap from the cheek is desirable in such a case.

The deformity caused by a small defect at the edge of the nostril or by the cicatricial distortion of this in an upward direction can be corrected very simply by dissecting off the skin from an angular or curved incision. The edge is then moved into its normal position, and is retained in its new place by suturing the V-shaped wound in the form of an inverted A (Fig. 224), or, with a curved incision, a flap of cutis, without pedicle, is placed into the defect. (Fig. 225.) The successful attempt of Fritz König to cover the defect of the lateral nasal parts by a corresponding piece from the auricle is worthy of imitation.

FIG. 223.   FIG. 224.   FIG. 225.

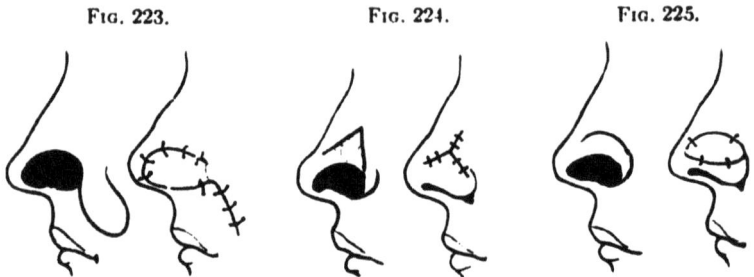

The missing tip of the nose can be best replaced by a skin-flap without pedicle, if the defect is only superficial. The flap heals well as soon as it is placed upon a broad freshened surface. If this is impossible, when the cartilages of the nose are also gone, pedunculated skin-flaps from the forehead, the bridge of the nose, or the cheek may be employed. For cosmetic reasons a flap from the region of the nasolabial fold is to be preferred above the others, since the resulting scar corresponds exactly to the fold. An inner lining is necessary only with larger defects of the nasal cartilages. Helferich here forms two flaps from the cheek and inverts one of these. If it is improbable that a flap without pedicle would heal in place, and if there is an objection to even the slightest scar in the face, one is forced to employ the Italian method (Kuster). By allowing the raw surfaces of the flap to heal together an inner lining can be provided for. If the cutaneous septum must be restored with the tip, it is advisable to cut the flap with or without pedicle so freely that a process may be used as septum after it has healed.

In a larger defect of the tip and the entire cartilaginous septum Payr took a long flap on each side from the region of the nasolabial furrow, the pedicle of which was placed close to the nose. They were rolled up with their raw surface outward, so that in forming the septum both of their ends came into contact with the surface of the wound. After dividing the pedicles the tip was constructed by uniting the flaps with the freshened remainder of the lateral portion of the nose.

Narrow strips taken from the nose (Dieffenbach, Hüter) or from the upper lip (Dieffenbach, Wutzer, v. Langenbeck) are to be used to replace the missing cutaneous septum. The former method is, however, recommended only in too large artificial noses. The flap is cut in the middle line from the tip of the nose in order at the same time to improve the form of the latter. It is then inverted so that its end can be sutured into a corresponding place of the nostril. The raw surface which is turned outward is at once covered with a strip of epidermis. The fact that the raw surface may thus be rapidly covered with skin makes the use of older methods unnecessary. An example is the one of Dieffenbach, who gave the septum an external covering by cutting a flap from the region of the philtrum, inclusive of the mucous membrane, and then turning it upward. The base of Wutzer's flap was situated at the labial mucous membrane; the flap was raised upward and allowed to heal in place with elevated lip. Its pedicle was severed later.

If a flap from the upper lip is used by rotation, the fact that the pedicle does not lie in the centre will always be a drawback. Its lateral position will necessitate subsequent modifications. If the tip of the nose is

FIG. 226.   FIG. 227

Lance-shaped flap for repair of septum when tip is shrunken and nostril stenosed.

shrunken and at the same time the nostril is stenosed, one can construct the end of the small flap lancet-shaped, according to Nicoladoni. (Figs. 226 and 227.)

CHEILOPLASTY.

The object of plastic operations upon the lips is to replace defects or to correct anomalies of shape. The absence of a lip, in part or entirely, may be due to severe injuries of all kinds—noma, spontaneous gangrene in typhoid, and most often to neoplasms or their operative removal. Among the latter, carcinoma of the lower lip plays the most important part. Tuberculous and syphilitic ulcers, as well as burns, may alter the form, and their cicatrization may bring about a marked distortion of the edges. The upper lip is everted toward the nose and the lower toward the chin. In other cases the same lesions may lead to an abnormal stenosis of the mouth.

The fact that defects of the lip are so manifold, and that their configuration depends, of course, upon the seat and extent of the disease in question, has given rise to so large a number of operations that they can hardly be recorded. In 1859 v. Bruns collected about fifty such operations from the accounts of the various authors. Of this long list, only those operations have practical value which satisfy the requirements of a newly formed lip. The result should not be an immovable mass of skin covering the lower jaw and firmly adherent to it, with a contracted and cicatrized internal surface and an inverted free edge, but a lip which approaches as nearly as possible the normal. Its edge and also part of its inner side should be covered with mucous membrane, so that it does not grow to the gums. It should, at the same time, afford protection to the teeth and prevent the saliva from flowing out. The repair of a lip should not affect the shape of the mouth, nor should the newly formed lip or the plastic repair itself be particularly prominent or disfiguring from a cosmetic point of view. Methods the only object of which is repair of the defect are only justified when the neighborhood of the mouth is unsuited for the removal of a flap covered with mucous membrane.

For the complete or incomplete repair of the lower lip, such as is most frequently necessary after operations for carcinoma, the choice of the procedure depends in part upon the extent of the disease, in part upon the shape of the resulting defect. The latter can, however, be formed so as to correspond with the intended plastic operation. Lining the newly formed lip with mucous membrane is the most important feature.

Smaller operations on the lips, such as wedge-shaped incisions, can very well be performed under local anæsthesia. In all, the coronary artery is compressed in the left angle of the mouth by the assistant's fingers, in the right by the operator himself. After incision the vessel is at once caught and ligated.

While for small superficial neoplasms of the margin of the lip a transverse elliptical excision with subsequent suture is sufficient, larger tumors extending to the skin are best excised in the form of a wedge, so that the gap may easily be drawn together by the sutures. The width of the lesion determines how far the point of the wedge extends into the skin of the chin. Since the lip is very dilatable, half of the lower lip may be removed by means of a wedge-shaped excision without appreciably narrowing the mouth; in people more advanced in years, this limit may be exceeded, as König does, to avoid more extensive operations.

In order to avoid marked stenosis of the mouth, Serre carried a horizontal incision through the entire thickness of the cheek from the angles of the mouth on each side. The buccal flaps so formed were loosened somewhat from the lower jaw. After suturing the wedge-shaped defect the missing part of the lip was replaced by sewing together the buccal mucous membrane with the edge of the skin. The procedure is simple, but a disproportion of the parts readily results, the upper lip projecting over the tense lower lip, owing to the traction on the skin of the cheek. An improvement can then only be reached by excising two triangles above the horizontal incisions and suturing these according to Burow.

On the other hand, tension is avoided even when the lip is completely absent, by resorting to Dieffenbach's lateral displacement of two flaps from the neighborhood of the lesion. In the course of years this operation has undergone many alterations. According to Dieffenbach's directions, the flaps should be from 3.5 cm. to 4 em. broad; Adelmann constructs them larger by dividing the cheek up to the masseter and then prolonging the incisions up to the ear through the skin only; in this way the posterior portions of the flaps at once cover the two large holes in the cheek, which otherwise discharge saliva for a long time until they heal by granulation. The incisions forming the flaps of Jäsche and Ried have a downward curve, so that the secondary defects may be closed at once.

Dieffenbach's method may be employed for complete as well as partial absence of the lower lip. In the latter case flaps are cut out on one side only. (Figs. 228 to 230.) According to v. Bergmann, in whose clinic large and complete defects after removal of cancers of the lip are often restored after Dieffenbach's method, the operation is as follows:

The excised area has the shape of a triangle or heart with its apex pointing toward the chin and its base occupying the site of the missing vermilion border. While the soft parts of the cheek are held taut, the incision is carried from the site of the former angle of the mouth through the cheek in a direction toward the external auditory meatus,

Fio. 228.   Fio. 229.   Fio. 230.

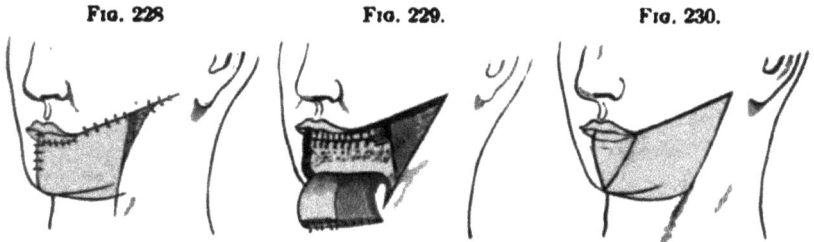

Cheiloplasty.   Dieffenbach's method.

across the masseter up to about a finger breadth anterior to the auricle. At first only the skin is incised, then layer after layer is divided between the edge of the defect and the masseter up to the connective-tissue stroma of the oral mucous membrane. In the outer part of the wound the masseteric fascia must be kept intact, so as to avoid injury to the parotid gland. After all hemorrhage has been stopped (vena facial. ant.), the mucous membrane is divided with one cut of the scissors close to the upper margin of the gaping skin-incision up to the edge of the masseter, and then along this perpendicularly downward to where the mucous membrane turns over at the lower jaw. In this way the mucous membrane remains in connection with the anterior Part of the flap. Then another incision is run downward to the submaxillary region and parallel with the edge of the defect. It begins at the lateral end of the incision through the cheek, in front of the ear. Here also the masseteric fascia must be spared. Separation of the flap from the fascia and the lower jaw, after transverse division of the reflected fold of the oral mucous membrane, must be carried so far that the lower margin of the lower jaw is reached and crossed by one to two finger breadths. Further

bluntly with sponges of gau
the trunk of the facial arte
In this way the submaxilla
lymph-nodes must here be d
being taken not to injure the fac
upon the other side the su
extirpation of glands. The t
cover the entire defect a
middle line. As soon as these ed
edges of the flaps are lined with
inner surface. Then the two recta
the mesial edges of which are a
margin of the lip and its inner coati
the mouth the outer edge of each squ
with the border of the upper lip, whe
sutured into the wound of the che
on each side is drawn together
most extreme angle of the incisi
left open in order to av

show the formation of flaps a
partial defect at the lips. Here the ec
must, of course, be closely appro

since the facial artery has been p
with by too tight bandages, so tl
formed margin. It is therefore b
with a simple funda maxillæ.
out in the described fashion, co
all requirements. The resulti
prominent, since they only form narr
off so far, even large losses
can be covered. The method may e
conjunction with resection of the mid
severe cases in which carcinoma l

entire lower lip, but does not exte
cannot be formed according to Dieff
from the chin. In such cases
more simple way by other methods
defect is cut out and two qu
from the entire thickness of the che
of the mouth and reach up to
downward at their base next to the def
The secondary defects can be brou
lip is formed of the mucous membrane
In carcinoma the region of the lymp
incisions.

It is impossible to save a narrow strip of mucous membrane after all
• the diseased tissue has been removed between the defect and the fold;
where the mucous membrane is reflected on to the lower jaw, this strip
may serve to line a flap displaced from the region of the chin. The lesion
is circumscribed by carrying the first incision from one of the angles of
the mouth obliquely to the other side in a slightly downward direction
until it meets the second incision running from the other border of the ·
neoplasm or from the other angle of the mouth perpendicularly downward. The second incision then describes a wide curve over the sub-

Fig. 231.	Fig. 232.

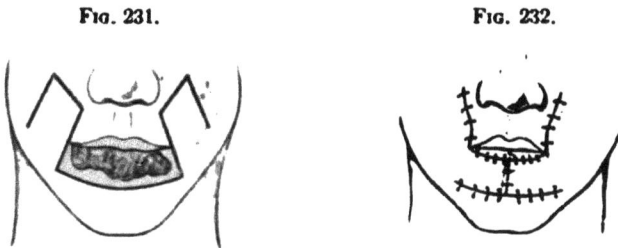

Restoration of under lip. (V. Bruns.)

mental region and is prolonged into the submaxillary region of the
opposite side. After the mucous membrane has been transversely divided
at its point of reflection (Fig. 234, the dotted line), the entire circumscribed flap can be dissected off with exposure of the region of the submental and submaxillary lymph-nodes. No secondary defect results if,
after forming the labial margin, the flap is displaced upward and fixed.
(Fig. 234.)

Aside from the method of lining, this method resembles somewhat the
cheiloplasty of Berg. It can be employed with good cosmetic result in
complete as well as incomplete defects, provided there is sufficient mucous

Fig. 233.	Fig. 234.

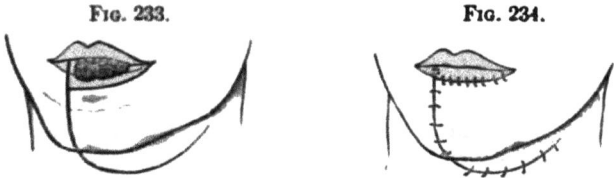

membrane upon the internal surface. Owing to the formation of a single
flap the appearance is better than if one takes two flaps from the skin of
the chin (Blasius), by running curved incisions from the middle of the
defect to both sides.

The upper lip is used in various ways to replace the defect of the lower
lip in order to form a lining from its vermilion border or to improve as
much as possible the functional result by a simultaneous displacement
of muscular fibres. However, the normal shape of the mouth is often
lost, in so far as it will become distorted or like a proboscis.

Dieffenbach dissected off two pointed flaps from the upper lip
means of two small oblique incisions running from the angles of t
mouth toward the septum, so that he could line with these a skin-fl
formed from the cheek. V. Langenbeck dissected off the margin of wl
remained of the lower lip and of the entire upper lip on both sides, wh
necessary, so that only a narrow bridge of tissue remained at the pl
trum. By this method of displacing the lip-edges one can well prov
for the missing vermilion border of the lip in all cases in which one
obliged to replace the lower lip by means of flaps without mucous me
brane lining. (Fig. 237.) V. Bruns not only freed the labial margin, I
also the lateral portions of the entire upper lip in the form of two flt
by running two curved incisions around the angles of the month fr
the lower corner of the partial quadrangular defect. The small round
outline of the month which results after such displacements of the up|
lip has been again converted into a cleft by Dieffenbach and Maass
means of lateral incision in which the mucous membrane is sewed ext
nally to the skin.

Fig. 235.   Fig. 236.   Fig. 237.

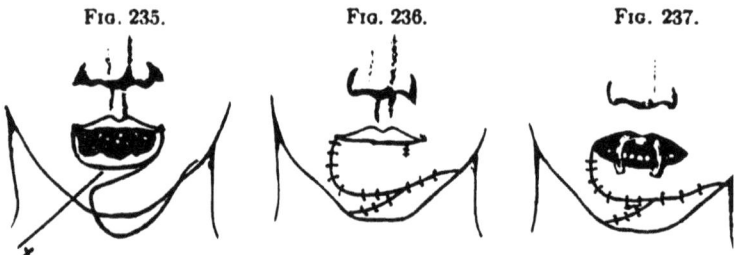

Cheiloplasty.   V. Langenbeck's method.   Fig. 237 restoration of vermilion border.
                   X Spur.

In partial defects of the lower lip a triangular flap is formed out
the entire thickness of the upper lip in Estlander's operation. Its a|
reaches upward to beyond the nasolabial furrow; its base, lying up
the margin of the lip, extends with one of its corners into the angle
the month, while the other possesses a small bridge of tissue in the vicin
of the philtrum in which the coronary artery runs. The flap is turr
downward and sewed into the wedge-shaped defect; the second:
wound of the upper lip and cheek is closed by sutures. By this p
cedure the loss of substance in the lower lip is replaced by normal a
functionating labial tissue, but the mouth is unsightly, shortened up
the side operated upon. The latter disadvantage is overcome by t
somewhat more difficult procedure of Schultén. Here the upper lip
turned upward and a bridge-shaped flap of mucous membrane a
muscle containing the coronary artery is formed. It is from 1 to 1.5 c
broad and has a pedicle at each angle of the month. This bridge
mucous membrane is inverted and turned downward and accurat:
sutured upon the lower lip, which is constructed of a flap of skin.

By means of v. Langenbeck's displacement of the labial margin or Schultén's procedure one can supply skin-flaps containing no mucous membrane, such as those from the region of the skin or neck, with a margin of mucous membrane, and thus prevent shrinkage or crumpling in of their margin. In this way methods which would otherwise be unsatisfactory on account of the absence of mucous membrane are rendered serviceable.

Above all, v. Langenbeck's method of cheiloplasty may be combined with a method which constructs a labial margin. Fig. 235 shows that a small tongue-shaped area of skin (X) remains between the oval defect and the loosened skin after the flap has been circumscribed. This so-called spur is used by v. Langenbeck as support for the flap when it is displaced upward. This spur has been freed by v. Volkmann (Ranke) so that the secondary defect could be better closed. If a pad forms at the upper edge of the flap, this can be excised. (Fig. 236.) (Krönlein.) According to Krönlein, this procedure has been used in v. Langenbeck's clinic in total and partial defects; in the latter it was altered so that by increased rotation of the flap its narrow end and not its upper margin formed the edge of the lip.

If the skin of the chin is also gone, similar pedunculated flaps may be cut from the skin of the neck. The latter is, however, less suitable to replace defects and readily becomes gangrenous in old individuals. A flap taken from the skin of the chin with a double pedicle, like a bridge, possesses better nourishment. A large curved incision is run from one submaxillary region to the other parallel to the curved edge below the chin. The bridge of tissue thus defined is separated from the underlying tissues and is displaced upward. This procedure is fashioned after Morgan's operation (1829), and was preferred by Regnier in Wölfler's clinic on account of its simplicity. By lining the upper edge with labial mucous membrane the drawing in of the former is avoided.

The less common defects of the upper lip can be covered by methods similar to those used for congenital clefts by drawing forward the soft parts of the lips and checks which are separated from the jaw, provided they are merely narrow and wedge-shaped. If the vermilion border of the lip is drawn into the edge of the cicatrized defects, it must be loosened as in operations for harelip. For cosmetic reasons, one cannot draw together wedge-shaped defects to such an extent as in the lower lip, for the slightest tension causes the upper lip to fall behind the latter, or, if the defect is not in the centre, the philtrum will be pulled toward the side.

If dealing with larger partial or with complete loss of substance, the lateral portions of the upper lip and the adjacent portions of the cheek will form a good substitute covered with mucous membrane. In order to draw forward and displace them in incomplete defects, Dieffenbach's wave-like incision around the nostrils, if necessary, with a slight prolongation in an outward direction, is suitable. With complete absence, however, both cheeks must be used to form flaps. They may lie horizontally with their pedicles on the outside, but the resulting tension in a transverse direction of the newly formed lip does not give good results.

━━ and removed from the e
━━ their base directed up

━━ that for the lower lip.
━━ of the mouth, while t
━━ to the nostrils. As s
━━ in the middle line, t
━━ the outer limits of the qu
━━ the newly formed lip, wl
━━ Sédillot placed the pec
━━ the narrow end below.
━━ inward and upward; t
━━ mucous membrane as is ne
━━ suture.
━━ to the lower lip are sev
━━ them and the ugly scars al
━━ suited for a plastic operat
━━ forehead, as in plastic v
━━ from the skin of the r

Fig. 240.

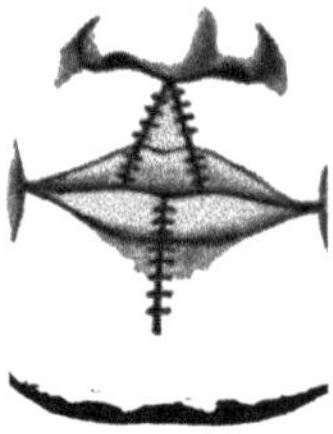

maxillary region. The inner
once with skin-grafts as far a
to the defect only after they
diminish considerably in size v
is little to be feared. The l
or neck is covered chiefly by
drawing together its edges o
lip has healed in place, it is l
asplanting the labial margin al
culated flaps of mucous memb
the bridge of tissue at the ar

d lip—that is, an internal as
y only to prevent shrinkage v
stored at the same time.
es behind the lower lip, as oc
from the cheek, Estlander's op

tion can be employed to correct the disproportion between both lips in the following manner, according to Abbe. (Figs. 238 to 240.)

A triangular flap is taken exactly from the middle of the lower lip and is turned 180 degrees upward upon its pedicle, which is formed of labial mucous membrane, at one corner of the base of the flap. It can then be sutured into the upper lip after this has been split along its middle. In the author's cases he has cut the pedicle as early as the fifth day. If the labial margin is accurately united all around after this procedure, the upper lip will be considerably larger at the expense of the lower lip. This procedure was introduced by Abbe, and after him by Neuber, as a secondary operation in harelip; its results are excellent if the wedge is not too narrow.

A flap consisting only of the vermilion border of the lower lip may, of course, be transplanted into the upper lip in the same way.

The defect of both lips is always combined more or less with loss of substance in the check. This is replaced by the various methods of meloplasty.

STOMATOPLASTY. ·

Aside from congenital anomalies of form, it is indicated to improve the shape of the lips by plastic operation in cicatricial distortion and stenosis of the oral orifice.

Ectropion of the lip should be operated upon, according to Dieffenbach, as is the same condition of the lower lid. A V-shaped incision marks off a triangular flap, which is dissected off down to its base at the labial margin and displaced upward with it. The lip is retained in its new place by suturing the wound in the form of a Y. This method can be used in complete as well as incomplete ectropion of both lips, provided the skin has not changed into a dense mass of scar-tissue. If this is the case, the scars are to be excised as completely as possible with preservation of the labial margin; they should be replaced by pedunculated or bridge-shaped flaps from the chin or upper margin of the neck. In ectropion of the upper lip it may be necessary to reconstruct the alæ nasi or the septum at the same time. If the skin of the neck is the seat of extensive scars, as after severe burns, it is best to transplant skin-flaps without pedicles upon the defect after dissecting off the vermilion border and excising the cicatricial masses.

In a stenosed oral cleft lateral incisions permanently widen the opening only when it is possible to unite accurately the edges and the newly formed angle of the mouth with mucous membrane, as was first accomplished by Dieffenbach. He cut a narrow strip out of the skin in the direction of the month which he desired to form, and freed the outer side of the mucous membrane by dissecting off scar-tissue, fat, and muscle before he severed it by means of an incision ending several millimetres in front of the outer angle of the mouth. The mucous membrane was then sewed externally.

A recurrence of the stenosis may very well take place from the angles

of the mouth, and one can take care of these angles still better by shap
ing a small triangular flap at the end of the incision (Velpeau) whil
severing the mucous membrane. This is sutured toward the outsid
into the angle of the skin-wound. According to Roser, one can cut ou
a similar flap of skin, which is then turned toward the inside and unite
with the mucous membrane.

For Dieffenbach's operation, the mucous membrane should not hav
become entirely changed into scar-tissue.

If the stenosed mouth still possesses a well-preserved labial edge, th
can be dissected off on both sides of the mouth without being divide(
according to v. Langenbeck and v. Szymanowski. Then one forms th
angles of the mouth from the cheeks and displaces the labial mucou
membrane on both sides into the resulting defect and secures it ther
V. Langenbeck has also employed this method in cases of macrostom
After separating the labial mucous membrane the wounds in the chee
are here closed up to the normal site of the oral angles before the labi
edge is again sutured in place.

MELOPLASTY.

The plastic repair of the cheeks is frequently done in association wit
stomatoplasty or cheiloplasty and is indicated in defects of the cheek o
cicatricial ankylosis of the jaw. In the last-mentioned condition the fre
mobility of the lower jaw is restored by removing and replacing th
cicatricial tissue; hence the chief precaution in every plastic operatio
upon the cheek is the avoidance of shrinkage in the flap, so that th
jaw will not be ankylosed. In carcinoma of the buccal mucous mem
brane, as well as in cicatricial ankylosis of the jaw, the loss of tissu
either involves only the mucous membrane or the entire thickness
the cheek after all the diseased tissue has been removed.

If a complete defect of the cheek were to be closed so that the ra
surface of the transplanted flap lines the oral cavity, the shrinkage
the newly formed cheek would soon form an impediment to the fre
mobility of the jaw. Hence, Thiersch covered the raw side of the fla
with skin-grafts before he transplanted it (Plessing). This simple pr(
cedure is sufficient for small defects of the cheek; for larger ones, how
ever, other operations are preferred, since a shrinkage of the flap s
covered is not entirely exclud . In these the defect in the mucou
membrane itself is replaced hyed skin-flap according to the method
Gussenbauer (1877). By permanently curing a cicatricial stenosis of th
jaw by this method a way was shown to prevent a similar condition
a result of plastic repair of the cheek.

Gussenbauer cuts a trapezoidal flap out of the cheek on each sid(
the pedicle of which is placed in front of the lobule of the ear. Afte
dividing the entire cheek with the scar-tissue from the angle of the mout
to the masseter, he turned the free edge of the flap around the edge
the muscle into the mouth and sutured it to the mucous membran

placed behind it. In the second stage of the operation, after four weeks, the pedicle was severed, the flap inverted in its entire extent into the mouth and secured at the jaw. A second similar flap of the skin of the cheek was later placed upon the raw surface of the first flap.

The principle of Gussenbauer, the restoration of the mucous membrane of the cheek by means of a plastic operation, has been employed in a number of methods which in part simplify the operation, in part improve the cosmetic result by avoiding scars running through the cheek.

First of all, the mucous membrane itself from the neighborhood of the defect can be used in suitable cases. By cutting a flap to cover the defect in the mucous membrane, Bayer removed a pedunculated flap of mucous membrane from the hard palate; while in a case of carcinoma of the mucous membrane of the cheek, Oberst first split the entire cheek from the angle of the mouth to the edge of the masseter, then removed the neoplasm and dissected a flap with its pedicle above from the upper lip and one with its pedicle below from the lower lip. Both flaps of mucous membrane were turned backward and brought together so that they bridged over the middle of the defect. The outer wound of the cheek was then again closed by sutures.

However, sufficient mucous membrane is not present in all cases for such flaps. In cases in which there are defects in the mucous membrane only, the simplest way of replacing what is missing by skin-flaps is by means of Gersuny's method, since it renders all subsequent operations unnecessary.

If one divides the lower lip and the skin of the chin in the middle, or, as Gersuny preferred, close to the angle of the mouth, perpendicularly downward to the margin of the lower jaw, and then carries the incision along this up to a finger breadth anterior to the angle of the jaw, one has excised a flap from the cheek which will give a sufficient survey of the oral cavity if it is dissected off the lower jaw and turned outward. Masses of scar-tissue or neoplasm can then be sufficiently removed from the inner side of the cheek. To replace the resulting defect of the mucous membrane, a flap is formed out of the skin of the neck corresponding in size to the loss of substance. According to Gersuny's procedure, the flap is peculiar in that the incision which outlines it reaches into the wound at the margin of the jaw, so that no pedicle of skin can be formed; for, as soon as the flap is dissected off up to the margin of the jaw, the periosteum is here divided and somewhat loosened, so that there will be a movable pedicle consisting of periosteum and subcutaneous tissue. The flap, now severed in its entire circumference, is turned over into the mouth and closely sutured everywhere with mucous membrane. The edges of the flap from the cheek placed over it are secured at the lower jaw and at the lip, and the defect of the neck, which is very favorably placed for the extirpation of lymph-nodes, is closed by sutures, or, if necessary, by skin-grafting.

The method of forming flaps according to Gersuny has been successfully employed in its different modifications in defects of the cheek

(v. Hacker, v. Eiselberg). The latter recommended that not the ski
from the margin of the jaw, but from a beardless portion of the chee
be employed in men.

Although the method of Gersuny possesses the great advantage (
completing the entire plastic operation in one sitting, yet other methoc
in which the flap is allowed to heal in place with a broad bridge of tissu
to nourish it are preferred on account of greater safety. The peduncu
lated flaps can be taken from the hairless portions of the neck, if or
wishes to avoid scars in the face. To remove cicatricial or disease
mucous membrane, and in order to suture accurately into place the flaj
it is necessary to get a good view of the inner side of the cheek; henc
the author prefers turning open the cheek as in Gersuny's operation, (
dividing it transversely (Gussenbauer, Oberst) to the slit-shaped opei
ing, which Rotter placed at the anterior edge of the masseter, or whic
Bardenheuer recommended as running from one ala nasi to the mala
bone, in order to introduce a flap from the arm or forehead, respectivel:

FIG. 241.　　　FIG. 242.　　　FIG. 243.

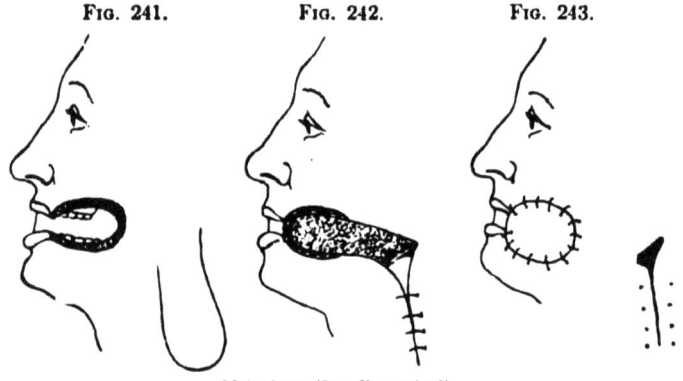

Meloplasty (Israel's method).

If the skin of the cheek is also gone—in other words, if a comple
defect is present—a plastic operation must supply a substitute wit
internal and external covering of skin. This can be accomplished i
various ways. The simplest procedure consists in forming a flap froi
the immediate vicinity, then suturing it into place with the skin on th
inside and covering the raw outer surface with skin-grafts. Kraske, wh
performed meloplasty in this way, circumcised the flap completely ar
with Gersuny allowed it to retain its connection with the subcutaneou
tissue only (Ritschl).

In order that the outer part may be covered with skin, Hahn ar
Israel have allowed flaps with very long pedicles to heal into the defe
with the skin surface on the inside. The long pedicle is then divide
then placed and fixed over the raw surface of the healed end of the flaj

While Hahn constructs a large flap from the skin of the chest wit
its base at the clavicle and its end at the nipple, Israel circumscribes

long flap from the angle of the jaw to the clavicle, which he turns over at its superiorly placed pedicle so that the free end can be sutured to the mucous membrane at the upper and lower margin of the defect. The epidermis thus comes to lie on the inner and the raw surface on the outer side. The large wound of the lateral cervical and the supraclavicular regions can be brought together in greater part by sutures. After from two to three weeks the pedicle is divided, the granulations are scraped off with a sharp spoon, and the end of the pedicle is turned over, so that it lies with its raw surface upon the freshened side of the flap already healed in place. It can then be sutured to the denuded upper and lower margin of the defect of the neck. This is followed by the third stage, the construction of the angles of the mouth, if the loss of substance also involves the lateral portions of the lips. The vermilion border of the lips is dissected off for a distance from the upper and lower lip, and is then used to line the wound, which is to be cut out of the newly formed cheek in the form of a wedge to correspond to the angle of the mouth. Finally the slit which runs into the mouth at the posterior edge, where the flap is turned, must be closed. For this purpose the double flap is here denuded and its inner part sutured to denuded mucous membrane, its outer to the skin.

Czerny brought about a reduplication of the flap in a more simple manner. In a defect of the cheek and the outer third of the lip resulting from an operation for carcinoma, he cut out a flap from the cheek and neck by beginning behind the loss of substance. Its pedicle was placed at the zygoma, its free end at the middle of the sternomastoid. The flap consisted of skin and platysma, and was so long that its end could be turned over and hence at once reduplicated. By turning it laterally this double portion was placed into the defect. It was here accurately secured to the edges of the skin and mucous membrane, so that the defect in the mucous membrane as well as in the cheek was replaced in one operation. The wound of the neck was closed by suture after the lymph-nodes had been extirpated. After the flaps had healed, it was only necessary to construct the angle of the mouth, as in Israel's method, and to excise a redundant portion of skin where the pedicle of the flap was turned.

A fourth method, the formation of two flaps as practised by Bardenheuer and Schimmelbusch, must still be mentioned. Since the operation constitutes a much greater interference than other methods, it can only be recommended for very extensive defects of the cheek complicated by complete or incomplete loss of the lips. The first flap, which should not be hairy, is taken from the lower part of the neck or the forehead. It is inverted and secured in the defect, where it replaces the mucous membrane, by being turned at its pedicle, which is situated at the margin of the lower jaw in the former and above the zygoma or nasal root in the latter case. Over this one at once suture the second flap which is taken from the same regions—that is, the forehead or the neck. It acts as a substitute for the outer skin and is sutured to the skin-edges of the wound.

Grafting the secondary defects, gradually dividing and replacing both perfidious, completely sewing the inner and outer flaps into the cheek, and finally constructing the angles of the mouth with mucous membrane lining are further stages of this prolonged method.

In conclusion, several points must be mentioned which are to be taken into consideration in every meloplasty. The first refers to the condition of the transplanted skin within the mouth. The expectation that the skin would become like mucous membrane, and above all would lose its growth of hair, has not been realized, despite the atrophy of the epidermal structures which Ritschl has detected. Long hairs may grow out of the mouth after years; Thiersch recognized evidences of this growth after twenty-one years. Hence, one should replace mucous membrane only by skin which is hairless.

Furthermore, the parotid duct must be considered. If one approaches it while operating upon a carcinoma of the cheek or excising scar-tissue, one should look for the divided end, so that it can be secured to the raw edge of the mucous membrane with a few sutures. The branches of the facial nerve should be protected from injury as much as possible while the defect and the flap which is to cover it are being shaped.

BLEPHAROPLASTY.

The eyelids may be absent in whole or in part owing to injuries of all kinds, syphilitic or tuberculous ulcers, gangrene following erysipelas or anthrax, or after the removal of neoplasms, and it may be necessary to restore them after all these conditions by a plastic operation. The superficial loss of substance which is seen after a cicatricial ectropion is corrected requires the same treatment, if a recurrence is to be avoided.

In order to insure the success of a blepharoplasty, it is of the greatest importance to determine whether the outer layer of skin alone is destroyed or, with it, the edge of the lid and the conjunctiva. No matter how good the result of a plastic operation in the former case, the simple skin-flaps will be entirely inadequate where there is complete absence of the lids. Since the flap lacks an inner lining, it shrinks and becomes adherent to the eyeball which it covers only imperfectly. Its edge becomes inverted and irritates the conjunctiva on account of the scar-tissue and fine hairs. The sensitive condition of the conjunctiva of the bulb renders it difficult to find a suitable material for lining the under surface of the flap. A large number of experiments in this direction give evidence of how much trouble has been taken to find a proper substitute for the missing conjunctiva, for besides using the skin, mucous membrane, and conjunctiva of animals, attempts have been made to heal into place small flaps of mucous membrane from the lips, vagina, and rectum and pieces of human prepuce.

Owing to the varying position and size of the defect at the upper or lower lid or the inner or outer canthus, the varieties of plastic operations are many. In general, however, four groups can be distinguished.

The first group includes the construction of flaps according to the Indian method, as was first suggested by Fricke in 1829, and modified by v. Ammon, Blasius, and v. Langenbeck. The main feature of this method is the construction of a pedunculated flap of sufficient size, the pedicle of which lies directly adjacent to the defect and the free part of which is taken from the temple for the upper lid and from the cheek for the lower. The form of the flap is regulated by the shape of the defect; thus, when it was necessary to construct a new palpebral angle, Hasner cut it out with two processes at the end. In v. Langenbeck's method (Figs. 244 to 246) the pedicle can be rotated without tension by turning

FIG. 244.   FIG. 245.   FIG. 246.

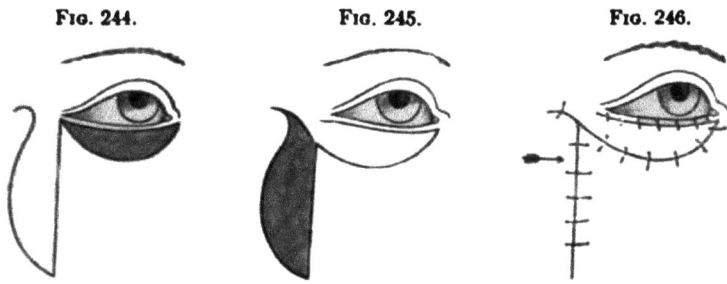

over the blind end of the incision; the secondary defect is brought together by sutures. The upper edge of the flap is sutured to the retained edge of the lid or else to the palpebral conjunctiva which still remains. A flap taken from the side of the nose with its base above (Blasius) can be used, especially for defects at the inner canthus. If, owing to scars, one places the pedicle of the flap at some distance from the defect by constructing a frontal flap with its base at the nasal root or at the temple, it follows that the pedicle must be cut through and replaced after the flap has healed in place.

FIG. 247.   FIG. 248.

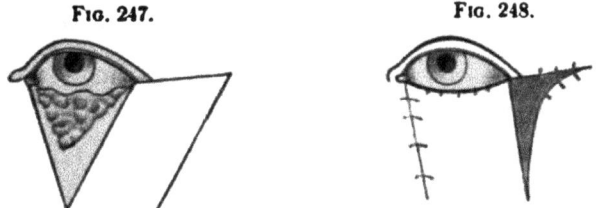

The method of laterally displacing a flap from the immediate vicinity was used in the construction of lids for the first time by Dieffenbach in 1834. It necessitates an approximately triangular defect, like the similar method of cheiloplasty, and is suitable for complete and partial losses of substance of both lids, especially, however, of the lower one. (Figs. 247 and 248.)

If it is desired to construct a new lower lid where this is entirely absent, an incision somewhat longer than the base of the defect is carried horizontally outward from the outer canthus. From the outer end of this incision a second one is carried downward, parallel to the outer margin of the defect. A rhomboidal flap is thus outlined which is dissected off and placed upon the defect. According to Szymanowski, the first incision is not horizontal, but runs somewhat obliquely in an upward direction; this will permit the closing of the secondary denuded surface almost completely by sutures starting from the outer angle of the wound. In v. Arlt's modification the flap is cut out about 1 cm. broader than the base of the defect. After lining the edge with conjunctiva or lid margin, as the case may be, the outer part of the upper border of the flap can be brought together with the skin external to the palpebral angle, so that the flap is given a better hold. In partial defects of the lid at the inner portion of the eye Dieffenbach's plastic operation can also be performed, unless, with flaps shaped as above (Figs. 247 and 248), one wishes to retain the healthy part of the lid or preserve it as a small triangular spur (Hillroth). The method of Celsus has also received a trial. In imitation of this, Knapp has rendered two lateral flaps movable by means of horizontal incisions from the rectangular defect. The defect was covered by pulling them over. This method has the advantage of avoiding the downward pull of the scar.

The transplantation of skin-flaps without pedicles is a fourth method at the surgeon's disposal. It was introduced for the repair of lids by Wolfe especially, but the directions of Krause are at present followed. It can be employed to advantage in all skin defects of the lid, especially in cicatricial ectropion (Silex). Here the V-shaped incision of Dieffenbach followed by the Y-shaped suture is appropriate only in the slight distortions; in more marked ectropion the edge of the lid must be loosened and rendered movable by means of an incision down to the conjunctiva running parallel with the margin of the lid at a distance of 1.5 mm. from it. The larger strands of scar-tissue are excised and the entire defect is then covered by a piece of cutis cut of corresponding shape. This method is to be preferred to the grafting of strips of epidermis on account of the dangers of subsequent shrinkage.

If, in addition to the skin, the margin of the lid and the conjunctiva must also be repaired, the flap can be lined on its inner side in a simple and safe way by the methods of Uhthoff and Jordan.

In a defect of the lower lid secondary to carcinoma the first author marked off a rectangular flap in the delicate skin of the upper lid. This he dissected off up to its base at the ciliary edge and then turned it downward like an apron. By securing the lower edge of the flap to the conjunctiva of the bulb the missing conjunctiva of the lower lid was replaced. A frontal flap with its pedicle at the nasal root supplied the outer covering. The secondary defect of the upper lid and forehead was covered with strips of epidermis. By the seventh day the turned-down flap was divided directly beneath the margin of the upper lid and thus the palpebral fissure was again restored.

Like Czerny in his meloplasty, Jordan constructs a comparatively large frontal flap. After the subcutaneous tissue has been removed, its ends are turned over and it is transplanted in this way into the defect. If the latter is situated in the outer half of the lid, the pedicle is placed in the temporal region; in defects at the inner half, at the root of the nose. In partial defects of both lids the tissues at the palpebral angle are restored by folding upward and downward from an incision at the end of the flap before suturing the latter in place.

The more tedious grafting of small strips of mucous membrane has been attempted frequently since Wölfler tried it. According to Uhthoff, de Vincentiis, after dissecting off the pedunculated skin-flap, succeeded in grafting mucous membrane of the most varying origin upon its raw surface. The flap was transplanted only after these had become adherent.

As long as only partial defects are restored, the lids continue to functionate sufficiently. If, however, the entire lid is gone, the plastic repair only imperfectly protects the eyeball even under the most favorable conditions, since the lid lacks mobility. Its disadvantages are especially apparent in the upper lid. Owing to this fact, one is frequently justified in removing the contents of the orbit in cases in which there is carcinoma of the lids.

Attempts have been made by Rapier to replace the completely destroyed lid by functionating tissue. He transplanted a bridge-shaped flap consisting of skin and muscle from the forehead to take the place of the upper lid, and a similar one from the upper lid for the lower.

Küster's plastic lining of the orbit, the contents of which have been removed, has been described.

THE NEURALGIAS OF THE HEAD.

By Prof. Dr. FEDOR KRAUSE.

CHAPTER XIV.

TRIGEMINAL NEURALGIA.

Etiology.—A neuropathic, hereditary taint, exhausting diseases with their resulting anæmia and cachexia, arteriosclerosis, and premature senility, play a rôle in the etiology of facial pain; but men and women in the best of health are affected equally by the disease. The neuralgia may be brought on directly by many infectious diseases; of these, intermittent fever must be mentioned first. This shows itself not rarely in the form of a supraorbital neuralgia, thus forming a masked malaria. Of the acute infectious diseases, influenza is most often followed by a typical neuralgia, which generally affects the supraorbital, less often the infraorbital nerve. Facial neuralgia has also been observed after typhoid and smallpox.

Certain poisons have a like effect, especially when they have acted for a long time. Among these are mercury, lead, alcohol, and nicotine. The neuralgias which accompany diabetes mellitus and gout can, in a similar way, be traced to a defective composition of the blood and tissue-juices. The third branch is generally affected in diabetes, and occasionally the disease here is bilateral.

Of the chronic infectious diseases, syphilis deserves mention. In the first place, the swellings of the periosteum bear a relation to the affection. The nerves lie so closely in the bony canals that besides the nerve there is room only for the nerve-sheaths, the accompanying vessels, and finally the thin periosteal layer. It follows that the slightest swelling disturbs the relations. In this respect the smaller canals are of most importance, such as those for the dental nerves, and the canals in the malar bone, etc. In the second place, the nerve or its sheath may be attacked by the specific inflammation itself. It may be impossible to diagnosticate anything else but a neuralgia from the symptoms at the beginning of the disease and occasionally throughout the course. It is thus clear why the question, if a true neuralgia can follow syphilis, has not been answered. Syphilitic inflammations of the meninges must also be mentioned here.

Other etiological factors are rheumatism, colds, and digestive disturbances, especially chronic constipation. Lastly anæmia, disease of

the female sexual organs, and mental excitement must be mentione
Many patients regard a previous injury to the corresponding bones
the face or skull responsible for the appearance of their neuralgia.

CENTRAL OR PERIPHERAL SEAT OF THE NEURALGIA.—It is of tl
greatest importance to know if the cause of the neuralgia is seate
peripherally or centrally. It is to be looked for in the periphery
changes which are known to cause facial pain are found here. Amor
these are scars, foreign bodies, and new formations. The surgeon ma
also decide upon a peripheral seat if the neuralgia has developed aft
a severe cold or after injury to certain parts of the face, and is main
restricted to these parts. One must always remember here that tl
nerve-change (Möbius' neuralgic changes), once started, progress
toward the centre.

According to the law of excentric phenomena, the cause is to be looke
for higher up in proportion to the number of subdivisions of a brane
that are really diseased. The area of irradiation should not be include
In those rare cases in which all three branches are affected from tl
first in their entire distribution, one can therefore conclude with son
probability that the etiological factor lies within the skull. It may ha
its seat near the anterior aspect of the ganglion where the branches st
lie close together, in the ganglion itself, more centrally in the trigemin
root, in the course of the sensory fibres up to the nuclei of the nerv
and even beyond these. A periostitis of the middle cerebral foss
spreading also to the three branches, would have the same effect.

Generally, however, the neuralgia is restricted to only one or sever
branches, and here the conclusion that the cause is peripherally seate
is by no means justified. Even where tumors or aneurysms of the intern
carotid compress the trigeminus in its intracranial course, only sever
branches may be the seat of neuralgic symptoms. The harmful pressu
is resisted longest by the motor root, but even the sensory fibres are I
no means affected uniformly, for occasionally anæsthesia instead
neuralgia develops in the trigeminal area in such cases.

If a patient suffering from facial pain gives evidences at the same tin
of cerebral disease, the neuralgia is referred to a centric cause; ofte
enough this assumption is proved to be without foundation, for thei
need be no connection between the cerebral disease and the neuralgi
In other cases the cause of the disease lies within the skull, though a
cerebral symptoms have been absent, even where this condition ha
lasted for years.

From these few statements it can be seen how difficult it frequently
to determine the cause, and that sometimes it may be impossible to dir
cover it. A. Wagner says: "We can most properly assume that a nei
ralgia is of cerebral origin if several branches only, and not the enti
peripheral distribution, are the seat of neuralgia, and if with this n
peripheral cause can be ascertained, and if the presence of other sym
toms of cerebral disease is afforded in cranial nerves, the origin of whic
is not restricted to a small space, but is convergent from different par
of the brain."

This is not the place to discuss the pathological changes. Those who wish to study them, and especially the microscopical lesions in the Gasserian ganglion, are referred to the author's monograph, *Die Neuralgie des Trigeminus*, Leipzig, 1896.

Symptoms and Course.—PAINS, PAINFUL POINTS, AND DISTRIBUTION. —Those pains are termed as neuralgias which occur in attacks (paroxysms) of more or less marked severity, and which are restricted, at least in the beginning of the disease, to the course of some particular nerve or nerve-branch. Of all the peripheral nerves, the branches of the trigeminus, next to the sciatic, are the most frequent seats of neuralgia. It is difficult to say whether this is due to physiological peculiarities of the fifth pair, which has the most manifold and important functions, or whether anatomical conditions must be held responsible. The course of the branches through long bony canals, their abundant subdivisions spreading over large areas, and the superficial position of many branches which exposes them to all kinds of injuries, may be determining factors.

Occasionally the pains are initiated by a sort of aura (itching, feeling of tension, unrest of the facial muscles, etc.). Generally, however, they come on suddenly, like a flash of lightning from a clear sky. They vary considerably in their severity, and there are all transitions from a slight burning to a feeling as if the face were cut by red-hot knives. In other cases the pains are described as pricking, tearing, boring, lancinating, and in the subsequent course reach an unendurable degree of severity, so that the patients are driven to suicide. The attacks come on without cause or are incited by trivial movements (touching the skin, draught of cold air, slight motions, talking, chewing, swallowing, etc., also psychical excitation). They at first last minutes or seconds, later often much longer; they may be repeated up to many dozen times during the day. Finally, in the very severe cases, the intervals are of considerably less duration than the attacks, so that really one can no longer speak of paroxysms. The night, too, is often not free from pain. Sometimes there is a periodical return of pains, as in the spring, for example.

As the disease continues the skin generally becomes more sensitive to touch. There are, however, many exceptions. Occasionally a continuous sensation of painful tension will remain in the affected area.

Certain points in the course of the diseased nerve may be particularly sensitive to pressure (painful points); from them the attacks may be induced. But even in severe neuralgias the painful points may be absent; occasionally strong pressure lessens the severity of the pain during an attack.

In general the painful points are situated at places where the nerves pass from bony canals or bony furrows into the soft parts, where they can be pressed against firm underlying tissue. They also have their seat where the branches of the nerve pass from the more deeply placed soft parts into the skin or mucous membrane, in order to subdivide there; and finally where the ends of two branches communicate with each other.

In neuralgia of the first branch of the trigeminus such points are the supraorbital point at the supraorbital incisure, the palpebral point in

the upper eyelid, the nasal point upon the bony lateral wall of the no
in neuralgia of the second branch the infraorbital point at the inf
orbital foramen, a point in the upper lip lateral to and beneath the i
nasi, a point at the anterior part of the temple, and the point of
cheek at the malar bone; lastly, in inframaxillary neuralgia, the po
of the chin at the mental foramen, the temporomaxillary point in
region where the nerve enters the canal in the lower jaw, and a po
directly in front of the tragus.

A painful spot in the region of the parietal eminence or a little hig
up may belong to the region of the first as well as the third branch
is often particularly sensitive (parietal point). Since, however,
nervus occipitalis major and even the minor occasionally send branc
as far as this area, accurate examination and observation are necess
to determine to which district the spot belongs in each case.

The author draws particular attention therefore to the fact tha
number of the described painful points may lie in the area of more tl
one trigeminal branch. The anatomical peculiarities of the branc
readily explain this. Generally, though not invariably, the brar
which is diseased can be determined by carefully searching for ɛ
other painful points and by accurately observing the attacks and stu
ing the history of the case. Occasionally one must remove the ad
cent subdivisions of two branches, for instance, the infraorbital ɛ
the inferior dental nerves where the pains are seated just at the an
of the month.

Every sensory twig of the trigeminus may be neuralgic. Often
attacks will be restricted to one particular terminal filament dur
the entire course of the disease. Thus the supraorbital nerve of
first, the infraorbital of the second, and the mental of the third brat
may be affected. Accordingly one speaks of the neuralgia as sup
orbital, infraorbital neuralgia, etc. At first the pain frequently con
from a rather sharply circumscribed area, but it rarely remains limi
to such a point during the entire disease. The pains are very soon l
along the entire course of the diseased branch and even radiate
neighboring areas.

Generally the surgeon is here dealing only with symptoms of "irrad
tion" or shooting of the pain into the territory of neighboring nerv
These may affect extensive areas; thus they may reach into the tempo
region (auriculotemporal nerve) when the inferior dental is diseas
In severe cases these irradiated pains are no less severe than the origi
ones, and where the disease has lasted for a longer period the patie
are no longer able to locate accurately the area primarily affected. T
pains are described as vague; they uniformly involve one-half of l
head and face and even radiate to the nape of the neck and the ne
itself. During the examination one may occasionally get the impressi
that the case is not one of trigeminal neuralgia; above all, it is impossil
to decide in which of the three branches the neuralgia has its seat. T
author has experienced this in several patients on whom a number
peripheral nerve-resections had already been done and from whom t

Gasserian ganglion had to be removed. The entire hyperæsthetic skin. of the diseased side was hardly less sensitive to pressure than the typical painful points.

DETERMINING THE DISEASED NERVE-BRANCHES.—It is the surgeon's duty to determine the primarily affected nerve or nerves in every case. The following points may give a clue: In the beginning of the disease the pain is restricted to a smaller area; irradiation occurs only later. The different attacks begin in the primarily diseased area even in the later stages, but the radiated pains are superadded after a shorter or longer interval, indeed in many cases in but a few moments. Furthermore, the latter are not constant; they do not appear after some attacks or they change their course, and in general they are not quite so severe as the pains in the primarily diseased nerve-area.

FIG. 249.

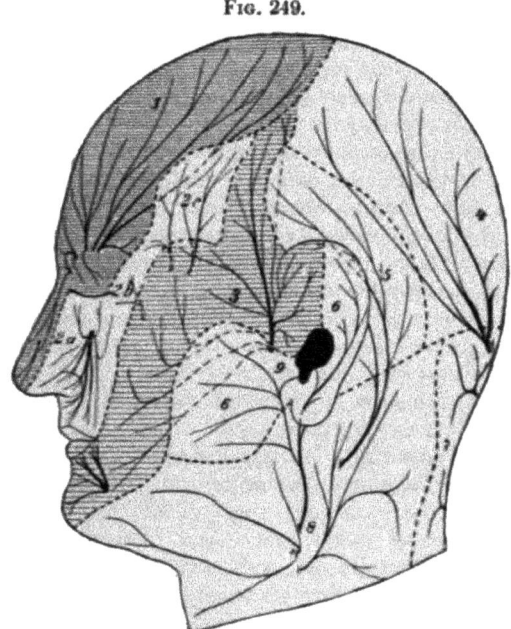

Schematic drawing of the sensory nerves of the head according to F. Frohse (from F. Krause, *Die Neuralgie des Trigeminus*, etc., Leipsig, 1896). Area of the first (1) and third (3) trigeminal branch shaded transversely; area of the auricular branch of vagus black. 1. First trigeminal branch. 2. Second trigeminal branch: (a) infraorbital nerve, (b) malar branch of the second division, (c) temporal branch of the second division. 3. Auriculotemporal nerve. 4. Occipitalis major nerve. 5. Occipitalis minor nerve. 6. Auricularis magnus nerve. 7. Posterior (dorsal) cervical nerve. 8. Lateral (ventral) cervical nerves. 9. Auricular branch of the vagus.

The sensations which continue in the intervals between the attacks are generally seated in the primarily diseased area. If strong pressure is exerted upon certain regions by the patient to moderate the pain, these generally indicate the area first affected and not the area of irradiation.

An injection of morphine occasionally prevents the radiating pa
without checking the attack itself; consequently it may be used
purposes of diagnosis. But in very severe affections all these char
teristics are of no value. Only an accurate investigation of the ori
of the disease helps, and, as in all cases of facial pain, the histor)
the case is of the greatest value.

As soon as the extent of the primarily affected painful area is cl‹
it is usually not difficult to ascertain the diseased nerve-branch with
aid of anatomy. When one becomes conscious that a sensory nerve
been irritated one always refers this sensation to the peripheral dis
bution of the nerve no matter in which part of their course the ner
filaments have been stimulated; this law of excentric phenomena m
be taken into consideration here. Furthermore, it must be remembe
that with present anatomical knowledge the areas which the differ
branches innervate are by no means so definitely and regularly de‹
mined as one has been accustomed to believe. The investigations
F. Frohse have shown that very variable conditions prevail, not only
far as the subdivisions of one and the same chief branch are concern
but also even in the relations the three chief branches bear to each otl
One must also take cognizance of the investigations of Zander, accord
to whom some areas are supplied by several nerves. Despite the di
culties which these anatomical conditions present, they neverthel
coincide with the fact, known to everyone who has had experience, t'
the areas of the different nerves affected are accurately defined.

It is exceptional to see the branches of both trigeminal nerves involv
this occurs in some constitutional diseases, such as diabetes, influen
or after certain intoxications (mercury, lead). It is also exceptional
see the neuralgia pass from one side to the other. All the cases in wh
the neuralgia is caused by a central disease and hence only form.
symptom, are, of course, excluded here.

CONCOMITANT SYMPTOMS.—During the attack symptoms of irritat
on the part of the secretory, vasomotor, and trophic branches of
trigeminus appear, such as reddening of the conjunctiva; increa:
secretion of tears, nasal mucus, and saliva; reddening and swelling
the skin of the face, perspiration, and increased perception of warm
Herpes, generally affecting the forehead, must also be classed am‹
the trophic disturbances. The facial nerve may also be affected: fib
lary contractions and twitchings are noted, much more rarely tonic c
tractions. In some cases the motor part of the trigeminal nerve
irritated (contraction of the muscles of mastication); in others,
muscles of the tongue.

Together with the facial pain there may be neuralgic affections in otl
parts of the body, such as intercostal neuralgia and sciatica. T
occipital pains which are observed in severe trigeminal neuralgias sho‹
not be regarded offhand as occipital neuralgia; they frequently depe
upon irradiation.

In severe attacks the entire body may participate: the patients tremt
the action of the heart is excited, and the irritability in general is

creased. Nausea, and even vomiting, sets in. Occasionally one notes retardation of the pulse.

RESULT AND RECURRENCES.—Where a trigeminal neuralgia is cured without operation, it generally does not terminate suddenly. As a rule there are exacerbations and remissions, finally a gradual cessation of the pains. Even after successful operations the neuralgic pains do not always disappear at once; they may recur during the first days with diminishing severity and of shorter duration, until they finally vanish entirely. The author has found this peculiarity only in peripheral nerve operations; in his 36 cases of extirpation of the Gasserian ganglion, the neuralgic pains had completely left the patients when they recovered from the anæsthesia.

Trigeminal neuralgia has a marked tendency to recur, and relapses occur especially after any one of the peripheral nerve resections, no matter which method is employed. As a rule they generally affect the nerve-area originally involved, but occasionally their seat is in other twigs of the same branch or even in another branch of the trigeminus. The pain of recurrences is sometimes slight, fortunately rendering further operations unnecessary. In other instances, however, they reach the intensity of the former attacks; in severe cases they cause terrible torture and radiate to new areas.

Diagnosis.—One should not be guided by any one symptom alone, but should take all the signs of the disease into consideration when making a diagnosis. Above all, the beginning of the disease must be accurately determined, since the symptoms are much more distinct here than during its later course. In addition, the surgeon must assure himself in every case that the neuralgia is not caused by disease of the facial sinuses or the teeth, tumors in the peripheral course of the nerves, or in the cranial cavity in the neighborhood of the trigeminus. Here the neuralgia would merely be a symptom of a disease. In the same way neuralgia can be caused or simulated by aneurysms in the course of the arteries of the head, especially the internal carotid near the Gasserian ganglion, or by syphilitic inflammations of the bone and the periosteum. Diseases of the central nervous system, such as multiple sclerosis, may also give rise to typical facial pains; they occur among the first symptoms at a time when the diagnosis of this causative disease cannot yet be made. Symptoms, clearly defining the nature of the condition, only develop in the further course.

The author can merely refer here to the neuralgia of hysteria, headache, and migraine. Occasionally these conditions make the diagnosis difficult. Each of the three trigeminal branches sends a twig to the dura mater, to supply it with sensory fibres. It does not seem impossible that these twigs may also be the seat of neuralgia, and many forms of headache would then be included in this disease.

Prognosis.—In itself trigeminal neuralgia does not endanger life, and it always seems remarkable that even those who are affected with a severe form of the disease look comparatively well and possess considerable strength. But a severe cachexia not rarely develops if the patients do

... ... These unfortunate patients whose attacks com
... ... sleep, suffer much more than the other
... ... attack has not been observed as far as th
... ... where organic disease of the brain was presen
... ... of pure and simple neuralgia. It is true tha
... ... the organism renders the patients less resistan
... ... Yet many suffering from severe facial pai
... ...

... ... in general upon the cause of the neuralgia
... ... a cure may be achieved in many cases wit
... ... When the neuralgia is not of long duration
... ... young and well nourished, the prognosis
... ... A cure is less probable after the disease ha
... ... attacks are frequent and severe and the patien
... ...

... ... in many respects if operative procedures ar
... ... Often one still meets with the opinion tha
... ... only after all other methods have failed
... ... strongly opposed. Not infrequently patient
... ... have been freely dosed with morphine, even b
... ... after all other internal remedies had failed, instea
... ... surgeon. Morphinism is almost as harmful a
... ... besides, the good effects of morphine are onl
... ...

... ... treatment is begun one should try to ascertai
... ... trigeminal neuralgia. As soon as this has bee
... ... should be first directed against it. To accom
... ... of the history of the case will not suffice, but on
... ... examine all those organs from which the disease mu
... ... include the teeth, the ears, the eyes, and the faci
... ... teeth appear healthy externally exostoses ma
... ... and thus cause the facial pain. The neuralg
... ... alveolar process without the teeth ceas
... ... of the frontal sinus sets up a supra
... ... application of the nasal douche (lukewar
... ... 3 per cent. boric acid solution) will cure i
... ... the mucous membrane of the nose and catarr
... ... proper treatment.

... ... after a tooth has been pulled, or if foreig
... ... present in the course of the nerves, they mu
... ... saw a severe neuralgia heal after
... ... removed from the mucous membrane

... ... the use of quinine and eucalyptol, of arseni
... ... preparations of iron, potassium iodide, and me
... ... purgation, and baths, as well as change
... ... But even after the cause has been found an
... ... neuralgia unfortunately continues in many case

The use of morphine is best avoided entirely in chronic facial pain. The danger of becoming accustomed to the use of this drug is especially great in so protracted a disease. A few quiet hours for these pitiable patients should not be regarded as an excuse. In really severe cases of neuralgia the drug gives relief for a short time only, and soon even large doses fail. Then morphinism follows as a permanent drawback. Where internal treatment has proved inefficient the surgeon possesses a number of operations which may help the patient. In the most unfavorable cases the last and most radical one, the removal of the Gasserian ganglion, is still to be preferred to the habitual use of morphine. Cocaine is still more dangerous. The anodyne antipyretics, antipyrin, phenacetin, apolysin, etc., are to a certain degree substitutes for morphine, and are efficient in some cases. Occasionally pyramidon (0.15 to 0.5 gram) and asperine (1 gram) act very well.

Of the numerous other remedies which have been recommended, mention will be made only of 1 per cent. solution of osmic acid for subcutaneous injection ($\frac{1}{10}$ to 1 syringeful); strychnine (0.005 to 0.025 gram per dose); aconitine nitrate (Merck) (0.05 to 25 grams given in drops eight times daily; increase the number of drops carefully); methylene blue (0.01 to 0.08 gram subcutaneously, or internally up to 0.1 to 1 gram daily). The value of electrotherapy is judged by E. Mendel in the author's monograph, mentioned above, as follows: "The constant or faradic current is to be recommended for the treatment of the real, atypical trigeminal neuralgia to diminish the pains or even bring about a transient improvement. But only in the most exceptional cases is it followed by a cure or a remission of several months."

PERIPHERAL OPERATIONS.—*Indications.*—When a rational general treatment, but not one that has been continued for a long time without a definite plan, has proved inefficient, operative interference must be taken into consideration. The author must emphasize here that this is not to be looked upon as a last resort, as unfortunately still happens so often. It is without question that owing to this view many neuralgias which could be cured by small operations at their onset are aggravated by their long duration. The neuralgia-changes which are at first situated in the peripheral parts of the nerves progress centrally, and eventually no extracranial operation is of permanent value. One can expect a cure more readily from an extracranial operation if the cause of the neuralgia can be found in the peripheral distribution. But one is justified in performing a peripheral operation even when the seat of the disease cannot be ascertained; for experience has shown that even in cases in which a permanent cure does not set in after this method, the pains at least disappear for a longer or shorter period. Theoretical discussions are out of place here, as elsewhere; the best proof · is afforded by the large number of patients who repeatedly present themselves for operation. Every busy surgeon has had such experiences, and W. W. Keen reports the case of a dentist who had fourteen operations for trigeminal neuralgia performed on himself within thirteen years. Besides this, the late recurrences after operations have frequently been much milder than the

not take enough food. Those unfortunate patients, ... their condition, on during the night and prevent sleep, suffer much ... ation. Death during the neuralgic attack has not been ... removed. The author is aware, except where organic disease of ... difficult one; but these were not cases of pure and simple neu ... tology. A thor the enfeebled condition of the organism renders th ... ody of the his to intercurrent diseases. Yet many suffering ... are absolutely reach advanced age.

The prognosis depends in general upon the ... up to where all If this can be removed, a cure may be ac ... division is not proper care and treatment. When the neural ... and where the patients are young and well ... need not be con generally more favorable. A cure is less pro ... lace. The excision taken root, where the attacks are frequent ... omy) is more likely exhausted and decrepit. ... in 1 cm. But even

The prognosis is better in many respec ... vented. included in the treatment. Often one sti ... of the peripheral sub an operation is to be considered only after ... e or the regeneration This opinion must be strongly opposed ... return of the disease, come for treatment who have been freel ... an. Hence the prin skilled neurologists, after all other into ... in a centric direction of being referred to a surgeon. Morp ... hes which run through the original disease, and, besides, the ... these. temporary in severe cases. ... ward the centre and

Treatment.—Before treatment is l ... tion as introduced by the cause in every case of trigeminal n ... free from its surround determined, treatment should be fir ... onstructed forceps with plish his purpose a study of the histor ... this forceps is concave must accurately examine all those ... are ribbed transversely take its origin. These include the t ... or uses a forceps the arms sinuses. Even where the teeth app ... result, since some of the be present about the roots and tho ... do not follow the traction. caused by sclerosis of the alveol ... forceps must be avoided so after this is resected. If catarrh ... After the nerve has been orbital neuralgia, the regular app ... about their axis. Thiersch 0.7 per cent. salt solution, 3 p ... but a still slower rotation Chronic inflammations of the m ... pheral portion, including its of the middle ear require prop ... he central portion, one can

If splinters of bone remain ... u, provided it runs in the bodies, scars, or tumors are p ... bony canal; it tears off clos be removed. Thus Bretsch ... the case may be. It must b splinter of porcelain had bee ... pherally, only those nerve the cheek. ... forceps follow its slow pull

Causal therapy include ... pulled upon and usually d antipyrin, salicylic acid, p cury. Treatment by swe ... a nerve can be removed. I climate, may be indicat ... especially of the muscles o removed, the trigeminal ... after the operation, since th

TRIGEMINAL NEURALGIA. 571

[...] portions of the anastomosing filaments of the facial nerve may also [...] removed. These pareses generally, however, disappear in a short [...]

[...] advantages of this method are evident; insignificant wounds [...] to expose and extract very large pieces of a nerve. On the other [...] the author regards it as a great disadvantage that of all the operations which will be described there only remains the extirpation of the Gasserian ganglion in case a recurrence sets in. For if Thiersch's method is carried out properly, the nerve in question is removed up to the skull and even into it, as the author's investigations on cadavers have shown. As an example, the third branch pictured in Fig. 250 may be mentioned; a grayish-red mass was attached to the white nerve above and a microscopical examination showed that there were ganglion-cells present; in other words, a small portion of the Gasserian ganglion came out with the nerve. If, however, the nerve has been cut off centrally, one can free the patients for months and years from their pains in case of a recurrence, and even now heal them completely by a repeated resection somewhat further toward the centre. Several cases of this kind have been observed.

But no matter which method is given preference, it is always advisable to extract the peripheral branches as thoroughly as possible.

Success and Prognosis of the Peripheral Operations. Peripheral Operations. — All the peripheral nerve operations resemble each other in that the neuralgic pains do not always disappear immediately. Frequently the attacks come on as before during the first days after the operation, but they soon diminish in frequency and severity and finally disappear

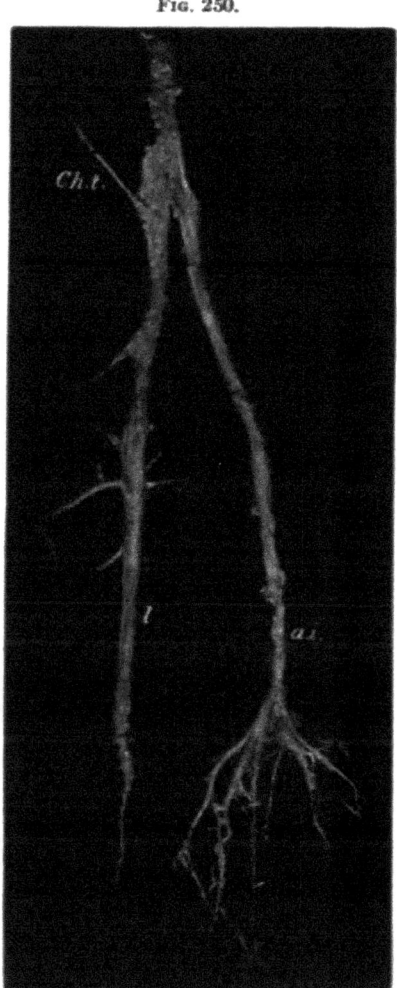

FIG. 250.

Inframaxillary nerve, extracted according to Thiersch, from a man aged forty-three years. *Ch.t.*, chorda tympani; *l*, lingual nerve; *a.l.*, inferior dental nerve. Five-sixths natural size.

altogether. Evidently the cause of this lies in the laceration to which the nerve is exposed in every interference, and, above all, in its division. One must draw the attention of the patients to this fact before the operation, so that they may not worry unnecessarily afterward.

Concerning the prognosis of peripheral nerve operations, most of them, including those done after Thiersch's method, must be regarded as insignificant procedures. The wounds heal in a few days and leave slight scars. The resulting anæsthesia annoys the patients very little; besides, the anæsthetic area becomes much smaller in the course of time. The fact that the author has seen a very severe keratitis develop in one case after extraction of the supraorbital nerve, deserves special attention; as in healing it left behind a spot on the cornea.

On the other hand, all extracranial operations which must be conducted at the base of the skull are to be regarded as severe measures.

FIG 251

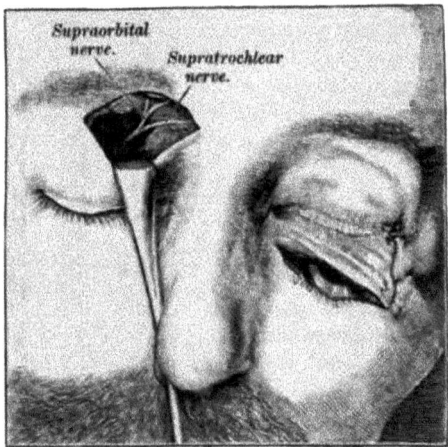

Exposure of the supraorbital and supratrochlear nerve at the right eye. Incision to expose the infraorbital nerve at the left eye. Two-thirds natural size.

Though life is endangered only exceptionally, considerable scars often remain behind and occasionally severe disturbances in the motions of the lower jaw.

Of the large number of methods, the author will mention the most practical; yet it is absolutely necessary to be able to select from several of the difficult operations at the base of the skull, since previous operations with their scars may render the one or the other impossible. It is also necessary to be familiar with the technic of these operations at all times.

In some, fortunately infrequent, cases the neuralgic pains continue with undiminished severity after the peripheral operation. The author has observed only one case of this kind.

First Trigeminal Branch, Ophthalmic Nerve.—After shaving off the eyebrow, a curved incision, 3.5 cm. long (see Fig. 251), is made along the upper edge of the orbit, so that the supraorbital incisure, which generally can be plainly felt through the skin, approximately occupies its middle. After the periosteum is bluntly raised from the orbital roof the supraorbital and frontal nerves will be exposed or will shine through the uppermost layers of the periosteum. If the periosteum and with it the entire contents of the orbit are carefully held downward by means of a broad hook, the nerves can be easily loosened from their surroundings. One should avoid tearing the periosteum, since the orbital fat will protrude and interfere with the free view. The branches of the ophthalmic nerve are not always developed in the same way.

FIG. 252.

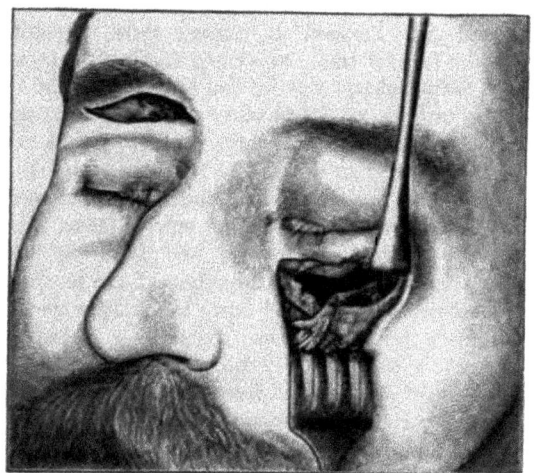

Exposure of the infraorbital nerve at the left eye. Incision to expose the supraorbital nerve at the right eye. Three-fourths natural size.

The supraorbital incisure is exposed by dividing the connective tissue which covers it or chiselling away the bridge of bone if it is present. Finally search is made for the trunk of the supraorbital nerve in the back parts of the orbit before it has given off the supratrochlear nerve. It is possible to reach the point where the lachrymal nerve leaves the ophthalmic by penetrating very far back into the cavity of the orbit, but it is impossible to reach the origin of the nasal nerve.

If it is intended to operate in the region of the latter nerve, one of its end-filaments, the ethmoid nerve, is exposed where it enters the skull through the anterior ethmoidal foramen at the inner and upper aspect of the orbit. By lifting off the periosteum the ethmoidal nerve becomes tense and thus visible about 2 cm. behind the mesial end of the supraorbital margin. If it is wished to reach the nasal nerve itself, a feat which is possible on the cadaver but very difficult in life, one ascend carefully along the ethmoidal nerve with blunt instruments until th origin of the infratrochlear nerve is reached. Directly above the poir of division the trunk common to both these branches is isolated.

In milder cases of neuralgia one may also use the method sug gested by Thiersch for exposing the ethmoidal nerve. He looks for at the pyriform aperture, where it reaches the surface between the nasa bone and the nasal cartilage. It must be remembered that in this wa only a branch of the ethmoidal, the lateral, is reached.

Second Branch of the Trigeminus. Superior Maxillary Nerve. Resec tion of the Infraorbital Nerve.—The incision begins 0.5 cm. beneath th mesial end of the infraorbital margin and runs somewhat obliquel downward and outward to the posteroinferior border of the malar bon The beginning and the end lie in about the same vertical line as the corre sponding points of the supraorbital incision. The length of the incisio is 4 cm. At first the incision is carried only through skin an fasciæ down to the levator labii superioris (musculus quadratus lab superioris), care being taken to avoid the branches of the facial nerv The fibres of the muscle run downward and cross the incision. Th upper branches of the infraorbital nerve (palpebral and nasal) appea in the incision, since they run upward to the upper edge of the woun They are to be spared. Search is then made for the infra-orbital for men; it lies in the uppermost part of the canine fossa, as a rule 1 cn beneath the bony infraorbital margin and generally somewhat c the inner side of its centre. Over it the origin of the levator labii sup rioris and the periosteum are divided down to the bone transversely, ar the periosteum then reflected downward with a raspatory until th infraorbital plexus is completely exposed. The latter is dissecte free from the infraorbital artery, freed bluntly for a distance fro. the surrounding fatty tissue, and grasped with a clamp. Now the perio teum of the orbital margin and of the floor of the orbit is reflected as fa as possible into the latter. If the entire contents of the orbit are car fully raised with a broad hook, the nerve can almost always be see shining through the thin upper wall of the canal as a white streak a soon as the hemorrhage, which is always slight, has ceased. Furthe backward it is often seen lying free in the sulcus. The canal runs rather straight course from behind forward; its bony walls are thin, excep in its most anterior portion, where for the distance of about 0.5 cm. th upper wall is formed by the broad infraorbital margin. Here a wedg shaped piece of bone is removed with a small chisel; further backwai the protecting layer of bone can generally be broken off with anatomic forceps. In this way all the structures filling the infraorbital canal ar laid bare up to the sphenomaxillary fissure, and are then bluntly lifte out of the bony furrow. They consist of the infraorbital nerve, arter and veins; the artery accompanying the nerve lies on its inner and und side.

Resection of the Temporomalar or Orbital Nerve (Nervus Zygomaticus —Disease of this nerve alone seems to be rare; the author has been abl to remove it in the following way: An incision 2 to 3 cm. long, starting from the outer canthus, is carried downward along the outer margin of the orbit through skin and orbicularis palpebrarum to the bone. The periosteum of the lower, lateral orbital wall is then lifted up sufficiently far back to expose the trunk of the nerve at its entrance into the zygomatico-orbital canal. If the nerve has already divided into its two branches (temporal and malar) in the orbit, instead of as usual in the zygomatico-orbital canal, both branches are found under the periosteum. These or the trunk are carefully freed into the depths of the orbit, after which the nerve can be extracted with the forceps or else a sufficiently long piece removed from it.

Third Branch of the Trigeminus, Inferior Maxillary Nerve. Resection of the Inferior Dental Nerve.—An incision 3 cm. long is made midway between the anterior and posterior borders of the ascending ramus of the lower jaw. It is carried layer after layer through skin, fascia, mas-

Fig. 253.

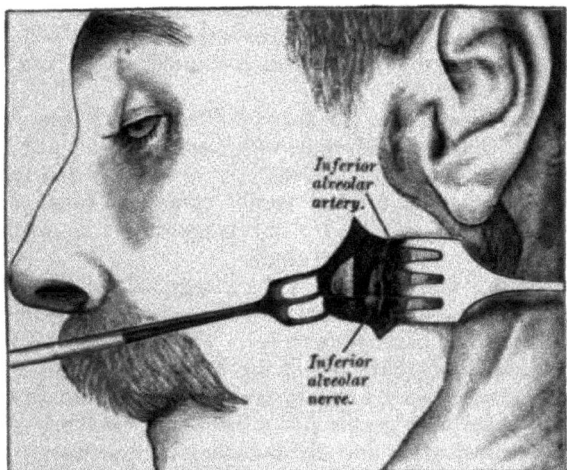

Relation of the inferior dental artery to the inferior dental nerve in the canal in the lower jaw, chiselled open for operation. Three-quarters natural size.

seter, and periosteum down to the bone in a longitudinal direction. The surgeon should avoid injuring the fibres of the facial nerve and Steno's duct; the latter occasionally appears beneath the masseteric fascia, and should, if necessary, be displaced upward. The periosteum is raised and retracted, thus exposing a sufficiently large piece of bone.

In order to open the canal in the lower jaw with the aid of a small chisel, up to its inner (upper) opening, the surgeon must remember that it is placed about 3 cm. above the angle of the jaw and is almost equidistant (easily 1.5 cm.) from the anterior and posterior borders of the raruns of the lower jaw. Anteriorly this opening is somewhat covered by a projecting platelet of bone, the lingula. Within the bone the canal

itself runs somewhat nearer to the mesial than to the lateral surface
the jaw. Accordingly the surgeon chisels away the outer bony lam
from the middle of the ramus in a right-angled area until the cana
exposed. He then proceeds upward in the same way to its internal op
ing. Above, the artery lies on the posterior; further below, on the me
side of the nerve. The vessel is bluntly dissected off and then the ne
is resected or extracted. In this way the mylohyoid nerve, which c
rarely contains sensory fibres, is also removed.

Resection of the Lingual Nerve.—After this nerve has entered the t
of the tongue between the ramus of the lower jaw and the palatoglo
arch, it lies directly under the mucous membrane in the region of
three last molar teeth. This corresponds to where the mucous membr
is reflected from the lateral margin of the tongue to the floor of the mot
The nerve can occasionally be seen shining through the mucous m
brane. The mouth is opened widely, the tongue pulled to the heal
side and somewhat upward with a ligature. The mucous membran
then incised for a short distance at the corresponding place anterior
the last molar tooth. The incision should be from before backward
not too close to the tongue. The nerve is then exposed, and can be
sected out or extracted. The wound is sutured. Such simple wou
of the tongue heal readily.

Simultaneous Resection of the Inferior Dental and Lingual Nerve
The operation must be performed with hanging head, and prefers
with obliquely reclining chest, so that the structures lying on the in
surface of the ramus of the jaw readily come into view. Light fr
above, or at least high up from the side, is necessary; an electrical he
mirror may also be used with advantage.

The incision divides the skin at the margin of the lower jaw to
extent corresponding to the insertion of the masseter (Sonnenburg),
facial branches being carefully avoided. The lower part of the par
gland is exposed and pulled out of the recess behind the angle of
jaw and then lifted upward firmly toward the ear by means of a retract
which at the same time grasps and protects the branches of the fa
nerve. The periosteum is now divided along the free margin of the j
and bluntly dissected off the mesial surface of the ascending ramus u
the projecting lingula can be distinctly felt. The internal pteryg
muscle will be raised from the bone at the same time; if its tendin
insertion makes blunt dissection difficult, the tendinous fibres are divi
with scissors. The inferior dental nerve entering the inner open
of the inferior dental canal can be seen when the slight hemorrhag
checked, the angle of the jaw pulled forward firmly with a hook, and
loosened periosteum displaced mesially, with the soft parts lying und
neath it, with a Lagenbeck retractor. The opening is somewhat cove
from in front by the lingula. The author forces his way into the dep
along the nerve to the base of the skull until the point where the ling
nerve is given off from the common trunk is reached. By bluntly pu
ing back the external pterygoid muscle, the common trunk of the ling
and inferior dental nerve can be isolated still higher, and can then

resected or grasped with a Thiersch forceps and extracted. Where the operation is rendered difficult by excessive development of the jaw, Thiersch recommends sawing the bone on its inner surface along a line extending 2 to 2.5 cm. above and below the angle. The bone is then broken with a blunt forceps and turned outward. After the operation is completed the piece is placed in its original position.

Resection of the Auriculotemporal Nerve.—The terminal branch of this nerve (nervus temporalis superficialis), which occasionally breaks up into two branches, can be reached by a small operation where it leaves the upper pole of the parotid and turns upward to the temple in conjunction with the superficial temporal artery in the loose subcutaneous tissue in front of the auricle. This terminal branch is exposed by a longitudinal incision which begins directly in front of the tragus and close under the root of the zygoma and then runs upward about 2.5 cm. By dividing only skin and fascia the superficial temporal nerve with its accompanying vessels comes to view; the nerve lies behind the artery, toward the ear. The branches of the auriculotemporal nerve going to the external auditory canal and to the skin of the auricle are not affected by this operation.

EXTRACRANIAL OPERATIONS AT THE BASE OF THE SKULL.—If severe recurrences develop after resection of the peripheral branches of the trigeminus, so that another operation is indicated, then the second and third chief branches can be exposed and removed at the base of the skull immediately after their exit from the foramen rotundum and the foramen ovale. The same operations are indicated in those rare cases in which the neuralgic nerves cannot be reached in any other way on account of their deep position. Examples are the palatine branches of the superior maxillary nerve. Finally, the operations are indicated when from the onset the disease affects the entire area of one of these two chief branches.

Second Branch.—In order to reach the second branch at its exit from the foramen rotundum at the base of the skull, one must do an osteoplastic resection of the malar bone and then enter the sphenomaxillary fossa.

Lücke originated the first suitable method. It will be described as modified by Lossen and Braun. The incision forms a right angle and begins 1 cm. above the outer canthus and 2 to 3 mm. from the external orbital margin. It runs somewhat obliquely forward and downward to the neighborhood of the third upper molar, where the malar process of the upper jaw can be felt as a projecting angle. The incision at once divides the periosteum. down to the malar bone; the periosteum is reflected from its mesial side and the bone divided in the direction of the incision with the pointed, chain, or wire saw. The second part of the right angle runs from the upper end of the first incision backward to the zygomatic process of the temporal bone and divides the temporal fascia. The zygomatic arch behind is stripped of its periosteum in front of the articular tubercle and is cut through. The flap, consisting of skin, zygomatic arch, and masseter, is now turned downward at its base and held here with a hook with four prongs.

The author does not recommend the incisions just described, branches of the facial nerve are injured. Besides, it is better to fi divide the zygomatic arch with cutting bone-forceps at its thin porti anterior to the articular tubercle, and then to saw or chisel throu the body of the malar bone in front. If one proceeds in reverse ord the thin and tough root of the zygomatic arch is easily splinter and the temporomaxillary articulation may thus be opened up. T anterior cut with the saw should separate the entire zygomatic ar from the body of the malar bone; hence it should be carried obliqu from behind and above, downward, and forward, and should end front of the tuberosity at the junction of the malar bone with the up jaw. This procedure makes the narrow field of operation more roon (See Fig. 255.)

The path to the sphenomaxillary fossa is now free; if necessary, t anterior fibres of the temporal muscle going to the coronoid process m be divided. In penetrating into the deeper parts one should keep to t front, along the posterior surface of the upper jaw. Here the fat, c taining within it a venous plexus, which is of some importance, is push backward and held with a broad, blunt hook; this will also protect t internal maxillary artery from injury. If the fat disturbs the view ir the depth, it can be carefully removed with dissecting forceps. The s geon now pushes his way toward the sphenomaxillary fissure, who position can easily be determined by means of a probe.

At the narrowest portion of the funnel-shaped wound, whose dep is about 6 cm., the superior axillary nerve finally appears as it lea the foramen rotundum. It passes from behind and mesially, forwa and outward, and at the same time somewhat from above downwai through the sphenomaxillary fossa, to the infraorbital canal. It c be caught here with a small sharp hook, bluntly dissected from the inf orbital artery (from the internal maxillary), which runs upward fr without, behind and below, and finally pulled forward. If the nerve now grasped tightly in Thiersch's forceps and slowly and steadily pull it can be dissected free with the elevator for another considerable d tance, and can then cut off behind the forceps, close to the foram rotundum. The peripheral portion is extracted according to the meth of Thiersch.

Gussenbauer and v. Friedländer have exposed the second branch to the base of the skull by a temporary resection of the entire malar bo instead of the zygomatic arch. For this purpose the connections of t malar bone with the frontal, sphenoid, and temporal bone and with t upper jaw must be severed. The method is more radical than that Lücke, but gives a good view. The facial nerve is endangered more Gussenbauer's incision than by Friedländer's; hence the latter will described.

The skin-incision begins at the outer end of the eyebrow, descen along the posterior border of the frontal process of the malar bone, a then proceeds along the upper margin of the zygomatic arch in a wi curve, concavity upward, up to the anterior end of the zygomatic proc of the temporal bone. The temporal fascia is divided in the same direction and extent, then the zygomatic arch is cut through behind. The fibres of the temporal muscle are now separated from the posterior surface of the malar bone, and the posterior surface of its frontal process is thus cleared. In order to expose this process also from the inner side the skin-wound is pulled forward, the tarso-orbital fascia is split, and finally the periosteum of the orbit is reflected with an elevator as far as the inferior orbital fissure. The connection of the malar bone with the frontal bone and the large wing of the sphenoid is now severed with a chisel, and after loosening its connection with the upper jaw it is turned downward. The temporal muscle is pulled backward and the fatty tissue removed, and the sphenomaxillary fossa thus rendered accessible. By raising up the orbital contents the superior maxillary nerve and its branches come to view from the foramen rotundum to the infraorbital canal, since by breaking off the malar bone the lateral wall of the infraorbital canal will also follow. The antrum of Highmore will not be opened, according to Friedländer. The nerve can be separated without trouble from the artery which accompanies it and can be resected sufficiently. Finally the malar bone is replaced.

It is said that exposure of the third branch at the foramen ovale according to Krönlein's method is rendered easier by the above operation on account of the free access to the base of the skull. The author has employed similar incisions for a long time in doing Krönlein's temporal method; yet he has always found the temporary resection of the zygoma according to the method of Lücke, in connection with the resection of the mandibular coronoid process, perfectly satisfactory to reach both the second and third branches at the base of the skull. Hence the osteoplastic resection of the entire malar bone seems unnecessary. Besides, experiments on the cadaver prove that by turning the malar bone downward the antrum of Highmore may readily be opened, since it occasionally extends into the body of this bone. An accident of this kind would involve considerable risk, because it interferes with asepsis.

Third Branch.—The retrobuccal method of Krönlein serves to expose the third trigeminal branch at the base of the skull. In those cases of neuralgia in which the pains affect all subdivisions of the third branch, and in which an accurate localization is not possible, this method enables the surgeon to expose the peripheral course of the lingual, inferior dental, buccinator, and auriculotemporal nerves from a single wound, and to follow them to the base of the skull. As the case may demand, one can, from the same wound, simply remove one of the nerves mentioned or else resect the trunk at the foramen ovale.

The head of the patient is placed upon the side so that the affected half faces the surgeon and is well illuminated. The incision divides the skin of the cheek in the direction of a straight line drawn from the angle of the mouth to the lobule of the ear. It begins about 1 cm. from the angle of the mouth and ends behind about 1 cm. in front of the lobule of the ear. The subcutaneous fat is divided in exactly the same direction and extent, while the buccinator muscle and the buccal mucous membrane

remain uninjured. The fibres of the facial nerve are avoided by tl
incisions, approximately parallel with the nerve. The masseter is no
divided in the same direction from before backward, but only whe
the muscle is not covered by the parotid (about two-thirds of the breadtl
The gland and Stenson's duct, which runs above the incision, should n
be injured.

Search is now made for the base of the coronoid process and it is free
from the adherent muscles (masseter laterally, internal pterygoid mesiall;
by several lever-like motions with an elevator. With a strong bon
forceps the projecting bone is cut as far down as possible and oblique
forward and downward from the semilunar incisure (compare tempor
method). If it is now drawn upward in connection with the ten
poral muscle with a sharp retractor, the nerve district will be so f;
accessible that the surgeon can proceed to isolate the nerves with blu
instruments (forceps, director, fine elevator, blunt strabismus-hook
For this purpose the fatty cushion of the cheek (corpus adiposum mal;
Boule graisseuse of Bichat), situated at the anterior edge of the massete
is freed bluntly and removed. In the same way the deeper layer of f;
which surrounds the nerves and vessels on the lateral side of the intern
pterygoid as far as the external pterygoid is removed. Here one mu
carefully look for the buccinator nerve. which crosses this fatty cushic
as a rather thin nerve-twig to run downward and forward. Furth
above it lies upon the muscle-fibres of the buccinator, just where tl
coronoid process has been divided. It can be followed up centrally
the external pterygoid muscle. When it is desired to resect the bucc
nator nerve alone. it follows from the above that it is not necessary
incise the masseter or resect the coronoid process. The skin-incision he
need only begin at the anterior edge of the masseter (Zuckerkandl).

The surgeon must now determine the direction and course of the in
ferior dental nerve and the lingual nerve, by palpating for the lingu
on the inner side of the ramus with the index finger. It is generally ea;
first to isolate the lingual nerve and then the inferior dental, which
placed behind it upon the internal pterygoid, and to follow the
upward to the lower margin of the external pterygoid muscle. By caref
blunt dissection with a director the chorda tympani will also appear,
well as the internal maxillary artery as it crosses the two large nerv
(inferior dental and lingual nerves).

In order to trace the nerves still more centrally to the foramen ova
or to find the auriculotemporal nerve, which has not yet come to vie
it is necessary to pull the external pterygoid muscle firmly upward, pre
erably with a Langenbeck retractor. If necessary, the fibres which ru
over the nerves from in front backward must first be torn through I
means of a director or an elevator. (In the temporal method this musc
is pulled downward, since it is desired to reach the foramen ovale from
its upper margin.)

If the internal maxillary artery is in the way, it is caught further dow
ward and backward—i. e., centrally—and ligated. One then finds tl
auriculotemporal nerve behind the lingual and inferior dental nerve

as it surrounds the middle meningeal artery with its loop. The separate subdivisions of the third trigeminal branch from the periphery may thus be followed up to the base of the skull and a large portion of each resected. If one prefers nerve extraction according to Thiersch, the opportunity to do this on the nerves which in part are freely exposed has presented itself before.

When the operation is finished, the divided masseter is brought together by a few catgut sutures and the coronoid process sutured in place, if one does not prefer to remove it entirely. The skin-wound is closed, except for a drain which is introduced into the posterior angle.

The method is simple and does little damage, and hence is free from danger. The wound heals quickly and the resulting scar is not conspicuous. Yet trismus may develop after this operation, and one should bear this in mind during the after-treatment.

In the extrabuccal method of Mikulicz, with temporary resection of the lower jaw, the incision runs from the mastoid process at the anterior edge of the sternomastoid, downward to the level of the hyoid bone and then turns upward and forward in a curve to the margin of the lower jaw, which is reached at the anterior border of the masseter   Here the incision reaches to the bone; the periosteum is completely reflected, particularly from that portion of the body of the lower jaw behind the wisdom tooth. The oral cavity should, however, not be opened. The jaw is now divided obliquely with a chain or wire saw at the anterior insertion of the masseter, and the internal pterygoid muscle is sparated from the bone at its insertion with scissors. The ramus of the lower jaw can be brought upward and outward in an almost horizontal direction and the body of the lower jaw well pulled forward with a bone-hook. A funnel-shaped space results between the ramus of the lower jaw, the internal pterygoid muscle, and the parotid gland, whose apex is directed toward the foramen ovale. Upon the loosened internal pterygoid are here found the divided inferior dental nerves, mesial to it the lingual nerve. By ascending along these two nerves are reached first the muscular branches, and lastly the auriculotemporal nerve. Finally the divided bone is sutured.

Second and Third Branch Together.—A round skin-flap is outlined in the region of the temple and cheek. Its base corresponds to the upper margin of the zygoma; anteriorly it reaches to within a finger's breadth from the outer orbital margin, and behind close to the tragus. Its summit lies in a line drawn from the nostril to the lobule of the ear. The flap is dissected off the masseteric fascia, the zygoma and the lowermost portion of the temporal fascia, and care should be taken to protect the branches of the facial nerve, Stenson's duct, and the temporal artery.

Now the temporal fascia is separated transversely from the upper margin of the zygoma. The periosteum is cut through in front and behind to correspond to the two vertical incisions, and is pushed back a little with an elevator; then the zygoma is cut through in front and behind, as in Lücke's method. While the skin remains turned upward, the flap, consisting of the masseteric fascia, the zygoma, and the masseter,

is turned downward so that the temporal muscle with its insertion at
coronoid process of the mandible is now freely exposed. By several incisions it is freed from the muscles attached to it (externally
masseter, internally the internal pterygoid), and then chiselled off
its base or cut off with a bone-scissors and extirpated. Now the in
temporal fossa is free and with it the external pterygoid muscle.
internal maxillary artery runs upon it or occasionally between its
heads of origin; it is ligated in two places and divided.

FIG. 254.

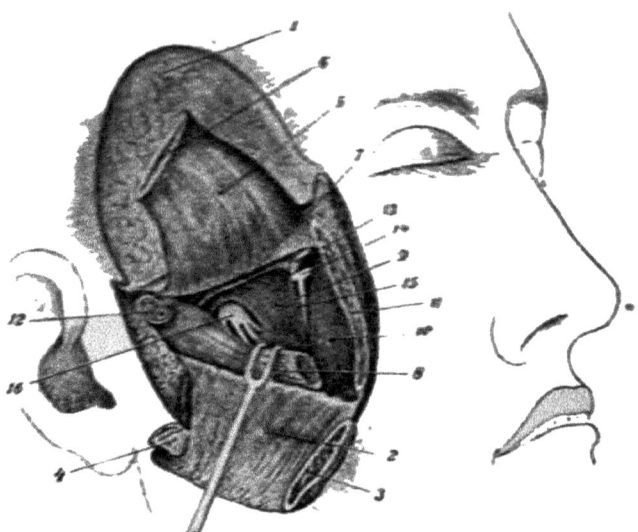

Exposure of the second and third branch of the trigeminal nerve close to the foramen
ovale and foramen ovale (Krönlein's temporal method): 1, turned-up skin-flap; 2, turned-
flap of zygoma and masseter; 3, anterior sawed surface of the zygoma; 4, posterior sawed
face of the zygoma; 5, turned-up flap of coronoid process and temporal muscle; 6, cut surfa
the coronoid process; 7, infratemporal crest; 8, external pterygoid muscle; 9, pterygoid pro
10, maxillary tuberosity; 11, sawed surface upon the upper jaw; 12, sawed surface upon the
mastic process of the temporal bone; 13, spinous tubercle; 14, superior maxillary nerve
palatine nerve; 16, inferior maxillary nerve at the foramen ovale.

In order to get at the foramen ovale and the third branch of
trigeminal the surgeon must bluntly dissect off, with an elevator,
upper head of the external pterygoid muscle from its origin at the in
temporal crest and the lower surface of the great wing of the sphen
While it is being held downward, the surgeon should work his
down toward the middle line, from the upper margin of the mu
and close to the base of the skull. The pterygoid process sho
serve as a landmark; the foramen ovale is directly behind its b
The large nerve-trunk issuing from it is freed with blunt instrume

The Eustachian tube lies directly internal to the foramen ovale; aside from the danger to the organ of hearing, asepsis is impaired if it is opened. As soon as the third branch has been freed far enough toward the middle line to be grasped, the surgeon should go no further toward the centre. After freeing the external pterygoid muscle, the second branch is found by penetrating into the sphenomaxillary fossa toward the sphenomaxillary fissure. The surgeon must work his way into the deeper parts with blunt instruments and in an anterior direction. The steps are exactly the same as have been described in Lücke's operation.

FIG. 255.

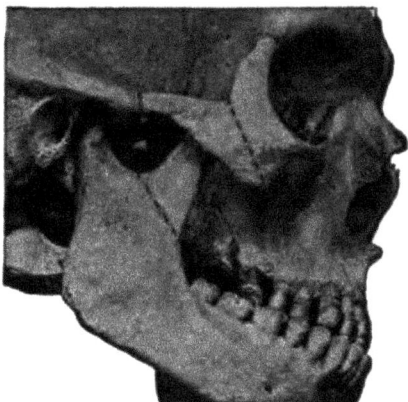

Sites of the bone incisions for the temporal method of Krönlein. One-twelfth natural size.

By the above methods the sphenopalatine ganglion may be removed with the second and the otic ganglion with the third branch.

After the operation is finished the zygomatic arch is secured in place by periosteal sutures of catgut and the skin-flap sutured over it. Where hemorrhage has been entirely controlled it is well to place a drain into the deeper parts of the wound toward the sphenomaxillary fissure. The process of healing is generally uninterrupted, so that the patients can be discharged after eight or ten days.

As soon as cicatricial contraction sets in, however, the mobility of the lower jaw is impeded in many cases. This may reach a very high degree; and will require careful treatment with Heister's mouth-gag.

The narrow entrance into the depths of the sphenomaxillary fossa may be encroached upon still more by an excessive development of the maxillary tuberosity. In two such cases the author has pushed a small blunt hook, bent to a right angle, directly inward from the distinctly palpable infratemporal spine (the spinous tubercle of the infratemporal crest) to the median border of the infraorbital fissure. The entire contents of the latter, consisting of fat, infraorbital artery, and superior maxillary nerve, were pulled forward; the nerve was then readily isolated and resected. Another method has also proved successful in the author's

hands in several cases. As the palatine nerves pass downward from th
sphenopalatine ganglion, their position is more superficial directly befo
they enter the pterygopalatine canal, where they lie between the po
terior surface of the upper jaw and the pterygoid process, than high
up toward the ganglion. They can be found more readily here; and
one follows them upward by carefully putting them on a stretch with
small hook, one has no difficulty in reaching the sphenopalatine ganglic
and the second branch of the trigeminus.

If the different methods for exposing the second and third branch
at the base of the skull are compared, it is seen that as long as they ai
accompanied by an osteoplastic resection of the zygoma there is dang
of cutting through branches of the facial nerve. Such division should b
avoided wherever possible. Injuring the nerves which supply the sphin
ter of the eye is not always without consequences, for the author
observations, as well as those of other surgeons which have come to h
knowledge, have convinced him that their reunion is not always certaii
The symmetry of the face suffers when the lids remain half open, an
besides there are the disturbances following irritation of the conjunctiv
and increased secretion of tears. If extirpation of the Gasserian gai
glion is contemplated when a recurrence takes place, then even a sligl
paralysis of the lower lid greatly endangers the eye. The author perfectl
agrees with Kocher, who makes it a rule to avoid branches of the faci
nerve wherever possible. In exposing the second branch at the base
the skull, the author therefore in part employs the incision recon
mended for the third.

The author finds that the following incision suffices if the tissu
possess their normal elasticity and no scars of previous operations ai
present in the temporal region; it has the advantage of dividing only th
branches of the facial nerve running to th

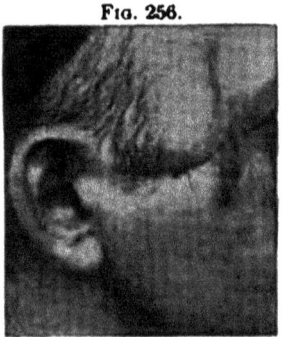

Fig. 256.

Incisions to remove the second
and third branch at the base of the
skull. Photograph sixteen days
after the operation.

frontal muscle. The skin-incision begins
finger's breadth below and external to th
end of the eyebrow, and descends along th
posterior margin of the frontal process
the malar bone. It then describes a wid
curve with its concavity above and passe
backward and downward to the lower mai
gin of the zygomatic arch. This it follow
to the anterior aspect of the articular tube
cle. Here the incision ascends a little an
passes obliquely backward, to end directl
above the zygomatic arch, in front of th
ear. The temporal fascia is divided in it
entire extent along the upper margin of th
zygoma, after corresponding displacemei
of the skin. The zygoma is now chiselle
or cut through with the cutting bone-forceps directly in front
the articular tubercle. While the skin and subcutaneous tissue ai
strongly retracted so that the facial branches running over the bod

of the malar bone are protected, a Gigli wire saw is run through underneath the anterior insertion of the zygoma with the aid of a curved,
eyed probe. This part is then sawed through in the very oblique
direction shown in Fig. 255. If the parts possess normal mobility,
the zygoma, now severed from its connections, and the masseter with
the skin covering it, can be pulled down so far with a strong four-pronged
hook that the vertical incisions of Krönlein are unnecessary. The one
or the other of them can still be added in its required length if the case
demands it. Otherwise the author follows Krönlein's direction; the
author's other modifications have been referred to under the last section.

INTRACRANIAL OPERATION, REMOVAL OF THE GASSERIAN GANGLION
ACCORDING TO KRAUSE.[1]—*Preparations.*—The external auditory canal
is cleaned mechanically, and wiped with a 3 per cent. solution of boric
acid and sterile gauze inserted. The eye is washed out before the operation only with boric acid solution so as not to irritate it. The author
does not believe in suturing the lids as recommended and practised by
others, since the cornea cannot thus be examined. Healthy eyes in
general do not become inflamed after the Gasserian ganglion is removed.
The danger, however, is greater if suppurative disease of the lachrymal
sac is present. The author has here seen keratitis with hypopyon develop
in two cases. One healed with a hardly visible spot upon the cornea
after applications of atropine and chlorine water. In a second case,
however, paralytic lagophthalmos had remained behind after a Lücke
operation performed elsewhere; the corneal suppuration progressed,
probably on account of the insufficient closure of the lids and the drying
up of the part which followed, and the eye was finally destroyed. Other
surgeons have seen cases of corneal ulcer after the operation.

These observations show that particular attention must be given to
those cases in which earlier peripheral operations have interfered with
closure of the lids on account of facial paralysis. In these cases the
eyes always remain open to some degree, and though the cornea is
rolled upward underneath the upper lid when awake, this occurs imperfectly or not at all when the patient sleeps. In two cases of this kind
the author has seen a defect develop upon the corneal epithelium in the
form of a long, transverse streak which corresponded exactly to the edge
of the upper lid when the lids were closed. Pressure was caused by a
moist dressing applied to the eyes. Although regularly changed in the
morning and evening, the weight of the bandage was sufficient to bring
about this lesion of the cornea, which suffered loss of innervation. The
ulcer corresponded exactly to the sharp inner margin of the lid.

Since this observation the author no longer uses a bandage to protect
the cornea, for it always exerts some pressure. He now uses a large
unground watch-glass, such as is employed in suppurative inflammations
to protect the healthy eye. A round hole, half the size of the watch-
glass, is cut in the centre of a large square piece of zinc oxide plaster,

---

[1] The operation was devised and performed by Dr. Frank Hartley, of New York, several
months before Dr. Krause performed his first operation, and is known in America as the
Hartley-Krause operation.

and by means of this the watch-glass is secured all around the orbital margin. The inner surface of the glass will soon be covered by moisture and this moist chamber is the best protection for the cornea. In it small defects of the epithelium readily heal, if necessary with the aid of atro pine. The author changes this plaster dressing every twenty-four hours he then carefully pours boric acid solution into the eye, but never wipe the eye. The protecting glass is used as long as any tendency to irrita tion and inflammation remains.

The patient is almost in a sitting posture; the head rests upon the occiput and an assistant holds it forward in a straight direction, or, i necessary, turns it a little toward the diseased side. In this position the blood and the exuding cerebrospinal fluid, which would otherwise collec at the bottom of the funnel-shaped wound, will flow out and thus the view will not be so readily obstructed. A second assistant holds the brain retractor firmly.

In extirpating the Gasserian ganglion the field of operation should be kept absolutely dry, as in all operations in aseptic regions. The autho uses sterile gauze exclusively as sponges.

The operation consists of three stages.

First Stage. Opening the Cranial Cavity.—According to Wagner'. method the author constructed a flap, with base below, in the region of

FIG. 257.

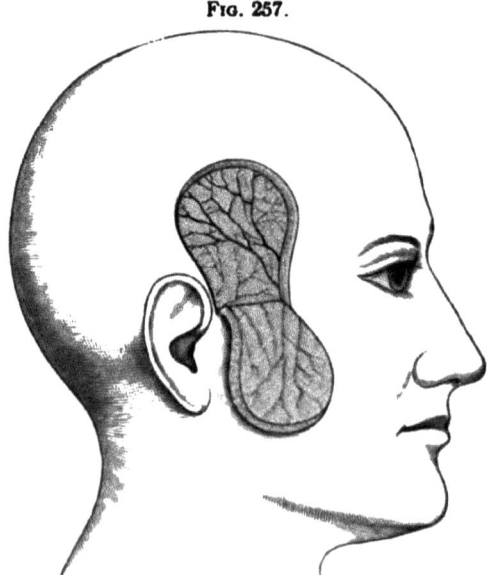

Bone flap turned down and dura exposed.

the temporal muscle. It includes the skin, fascia, muscle, periosteum and bone. The incision begins directly in front of the tragus and over the zygoma, which need not be injured in any way. It turns upware and backward with a convex curve, then describes a semicircle, and again descends to the malar bone with another convex curve. The base of the uterus-shaped flap should measure 3.5 cm., its height 6 cm., while its greatest width above should be 5 cm. The entire operation is performed extradurally.

The incision penetrates all the layers down to the bone. All hemorrhage is carefully checked. The periosteum is then pushed aside a little, and the skull opened along the entire line of the incision. The author usually starts this with the aid of Doyen's perforators. With these he bores one opening down to the dura in front and behind, along the upper margin of the flap; from these he cuts out the entire bony flap with Dahlgren forceps. A lever is then inserted and the flap broken downward so that the dura is freely exposed. (See Fig. 257.) The fracture-line in the skull runs about 1 cm. above the zygoma; the crest of bone which remains here and which interferes with the view is removed with gouge-forceps down to the base of the skull—that is, to the infratemporal crest. This precaution should not be forgotten, for the base of the skull must be freely exposed. The flap hangs mainly on the skin, temporal muscle, and periosteum; it is turned down so that its skin side rests upon the skin of the cheek. It is grasped in its entire thickness by means of a toothed forceps, surrounded by a sterile bandage, and in the almost sitting posture of the patient, simply allowed to hang down. The dura mater is then exposed to where it turns in below.

While the author has never performed the temporary resection of the zygomatic arch, this has recently been recommended by Lexer, together with removal of the base of the skull into the foramen ovale. At the same time he places the temporal flap lower and sacrifices the bone.

Second Stage. Ligation of the Middle Meningeal Artery.—By carefully raising the dura from the upper surface of the base of the skull, the finger and a dull raspatory penetrate into the middle cerebral fossa between the bony base and the dura mater. The foramen spinosum is first reached with the trunk of the middle meningeal artery, which here enters the dura. In order to ligate this the brain, surrounded by the dura, is now carefully elevated by an assistant with the aid of a right-angled retractor 2.75 to 3 cm. broad. The elevation should be no further than is absolutely necessary to get a clear view. Immediately after opening the skull the dura appears very tense, but by this time it will be relaxed considerably, so that the surgeon has sufficient room to obtain a clear view and to operate. By raising the dura the middle meningeal artery, surrounded by its two accompanying veins, comes to view as a distinct strand running upward to the dura from the foramen spinosum. The bundle of vessels is isolated on all sides if the dura is raised from the base of the skull with an elevator internal to the artery, so that the second and third branches become visible. Without difficulty the surgeon can then pass a thread of catgut or silk around the vessels with a flexible eyed sound, and thus ligate them. On account of the depth of the wound this is best done with two anatomical forceps.

and by means
margin. The
and this mois
defects of the
pine. The an
he then carefu
the eye. The
tion and infl

The patient
occiput and as
necessary, to
blood and the
at the bottom
view will no
brain retrac

In extirp
kept absolut
uses sterile ga

The oper
First Sta
method the

the temp
and bon
the zyg

pressure. The small sponges on holders (Péan's artery-forceps with some dry gauze), which are used to wipe the blood from the wound cavity, may lift the dura from the bone in many places if somewhat more pressure is exerted. Sometimes the operation must be interrupted for a few minutes to check the hemorrhage. The author then loosely packs the wound beneath the retractor by inserting sterile gauze down to its deepest portion. By allowing it to be compressed firmly against the base of the skull, the hemorrhage from the bone is checked completely; the hemorrhage from the dural veins soon stops, as the brain, surrounded by its dural sac, falls more into its natural position. If exceptionally this should not be the case, the author then removes the brain-retractor and introduces more gauze.

Fig. 259

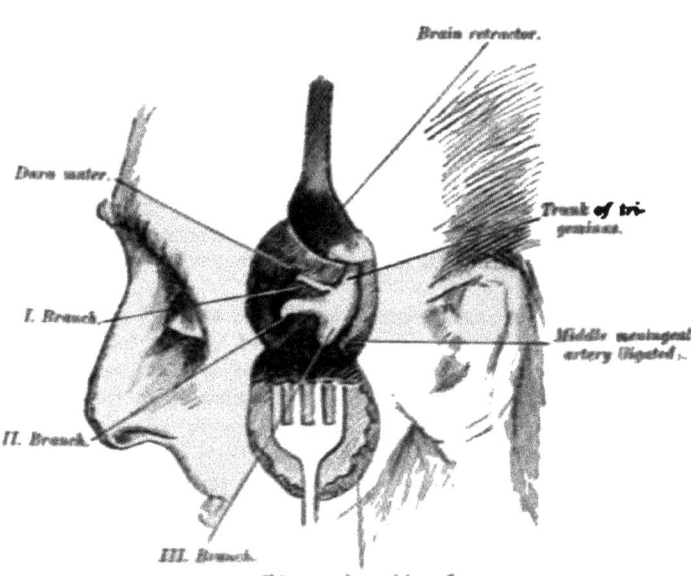

Field of operation to remove the Gasserian ganglion according to Krause. The brain had to be pulled up more with the retractor as the cadaver than is necessary during the operation, so that the deeper parts received enough illumination to be photographed. One-half natural size.

V. Bergmann recommends sitting the patient up, so that the venous hemorrhage ceases and the brain is able to fall back. The author always has the patients take an almost sitting posture from the first. One can often observe that a slight change in the position of the retractor or its slight displacement forward or backward is sufficient to check the hemorrhage from the dural veins. The brain-retractor (see Fig. 259 is 5 cm. long; its anterior 5 cm. are modelled so as to form a number of furrows. For exceptionally broad skulls, it may be desirable to prolong the so-

tractor by 1 to 2 cm. It should elevate the brain with its dura very slightl
but should not push it toward the middle line.

If the brain-retractor is well placed, the third branch is freed with a
elevator and then the more mesially placed second branch in its enti
extent from the Gasserian ganglion to the foramen ovale and the for
men rotundum; to this end, the dura is lifted off the nerves and then th
latter raised from the underlying bone. This same procedure is no
applied to the Gasserian ganglion itself; it succeeds perfectly if sever
thin but particularly firm strands of connective tissue are cut throng
here and there with the tip of a scissors. In general, however, it is suffi
cient to push back the parts bluntly with small sponges on holder
Occasionally there may be a small tear in the dura, and cerebrospina
fluid may flow out; this, however, is of no account in an aseptic operatio

This stage of the operation may be simplified by grasping the thir
branch with a Péan forceps and rendering it taut, so that the ganglic
is brought forward somewhat; for this reason the branches should I
cut through last of all, since by them the ganglion is anchored, so t
speak, in its place. At all events, the author has in every case succeede
in dissecting free the ganglion to its inner edge, and so far backwar
against the upper margin of the petrous bone that the trigeminal trun
just became visible. The ganglion appears like a network of fibres an
is grayish-red, the trigeminal trunk is almost white and its fibres ru
longitudinally. When finally the ganglion is loosened from the bon
underneath it, the second and third branches as well as the ganglion ai
completely free.

The author has purposely exposed the first trigeminal branch only i
its immediate junction with the ganglion and has not followed up i
further course, since it runs forward in the wall of the cavernous sinu
Besides this, the abducent and trochlear nerves lie in its immedia
vicinity, and more mesially the oculomotor nerve; all injury to the:
nerves must be avoided.

Should the cavernous sinus be wounded, the resulting alarming hen
orrhage can be checked by pressing a small sponge or a holder again:
the site, as described above. As soon as the brain falls into its norm
position the hemorrhage stops without further effort; otherwise a sma
strip of gauze must be pressed against the bleeding site. It should I
left in place and its end carried out of the wound. The pressure withi
the sinus is very slight.

Before proceeding further, the surgeon should grasp the expose
Gasserian ganglion transversely with a longitudinally ribbed force
at its posterior portion where it passes over into the trigeminal trun
This is directly in front of the upper border of the petrous bone, an
directly underneath the superior petrosal sinus. Great care should t
exercised that none of the structure lying mesially, not even the smalle:
fold of dura mater, is caught in the tip of the forceps.

The surgeon must now cut through the second and third branche
with a sharp tenotome or a small curved scissors close to the intracrania
opening of the foramen rotundum and the foramen ovale. The forcep

which has grasped the Gasserian ganglion can now be slowly rotated around its axis. The entire ganglion will always follow, and with it a larger or smaller piece of the centrally—*i. e.*, posteriorly—placed trigeminal trunk. The first branch generally tears off close to the ganglion, but since only peripheral portions of it remain, it is as good as gone.

Fio. 260.

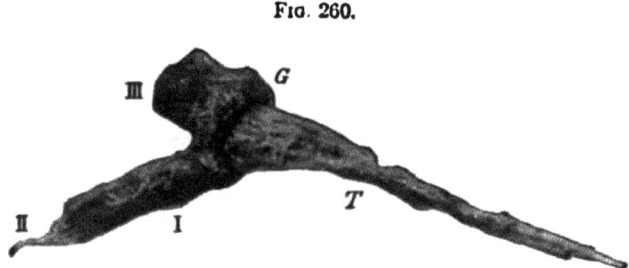

Extirpated Gasserian ganglion (man, fifty-eight years of age) in natural size. *I* Site where first branch is torn off. *II.* and *III.* Second and third branch. *G.* Gasserian ganglion. *T.* Trunk of the trigeminus (sensory and motor root).

In conclusion the author presses the peripheral stumps of the second and third branch as deeply as possible into the foramen rotundum and the foramen ovale with an elevator. Once more the under surface of the cavum Meckelii should be inspected, which is now deprived of all

Fio. 261.

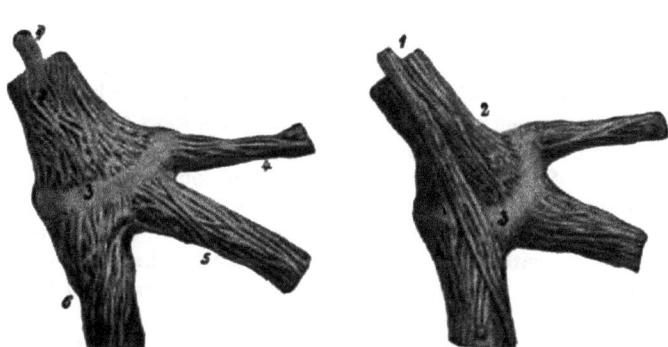

Gasserian ganglion, with its roots, enlarged: (*a*) external view; (*b*) internal view. 1. Small motor root. 2. Large sensory root. 3. Semilunar ganglion, over which the motor root passes to get to the third branch. 4. First branch. 5. Second branch. 6. Third branch. (After Rüdinger.)

its contents and is exposed in its entire extent, to the upper margin of the petrous bone. Beyond this the foramen ovale and the intracranial orifice of the foramen rotundum are seen to be empty. The bone is exposed everywhere, but in some cases there is no bone behind the foramen ovale but a grayish-red mass distinctly outlined from its bony surround ings. It is dense fibrous or fibrocartilaginous tissue which occasionall forms the upper and lateral wall of the carotid canal, directly anteric to where the internal carotid enters the skull. Together with a thi layer of periosteum it forms the only structures between the lower sui face of the Gasserian ganglion and the large artery. The author assure himself of these relations in three operations. Hence one should neve use sharp instruments in dissecting the Gasserian ganglion from th bone, and the elevator should not have too sharp a point. Furthermon the carotid artery lies very close to the inner margin of the ganglio and the trunk of the trigeminus after it has passed out of its cana but the distance is sufficiently far to guard it from injury with ordinar precaution. Besides, it is surrounded by the cavernous sinus. If on should penetrate too far to the inside and beyond the mesial border o the trunk and the ganglion, the sinus would be torn first and would war the operator by a very disturbing hemorrhage.

The author has never injured the internal carotid in any of his opera tions; but if this misfortune should occur, one must check the hemorrhag by tightly packing the carotid canal with gauze. Owing to the larg size of the vessel and the high blood-pressure, the tampon must be lef in place at least five days, and it would therefore be advisable to use or 10 per cent. sterilized iodoform gauze.

Duration and Difficulty of the Operation.—The duration of the opera tion depends chiefly upon the severity of the hemorrhage and the tim required to check it. Where there is severe bleeding the surgeon i obliged to work slowly and to interrupt the operation again and agai by a temporary packing, so that he may accomplish all the necessar manipulation at the bottom of the wound by sight. But even if th operation takes long, the author prefers to finish it in one sitting, an resorts to the operation in two stages only in the extremest cases. Fo he does not consider it without risk to expose patients, who have been e> hansted by protracted severe pains, twice within a short time to the dar gers of a narcosis and an operative procedure. Besides, the aseptic cours is endangered if the deep wound remains open long, even if the flap i secured over the iodoform tampon with a few sutures. In general, th operation in one sitting, where the bone was preserved, required one an one-half hours; with slight hemorrhage the author has frequently re quired only twenty to twenty-five minutes after the bone had been cu out of the skull.

The technical difficulties of the operation seem to the author no greate than those of Krönlein's temporal method.

Care of the Wound and After-treatment.—As soon as the operation i finished and the brain has fallen back into its normal place the hemor rhage stops of its own accord or can be checked by temporary compres sion. Hence the author has never found it necessary to pack the entir wound with iodoform gauze, as is done by others. One must remembe that the operation is considered as done in one stage. Should, howevei a serious hemorrhage continue, then resort must be had to careful tam ponade. The flap is accurately fitted into place and the bone secured with periosteal sutures of catgut. A medium-sized drainage-tube passes through the entire depth of the wound, between the dura and the base of the skull. It is placed into the posterior angle of the wound after a small piece of bone has been cut out of the skull with the gouge-forceps to give it room. It will give exit to any blood or to cerebrospinal fluid if the dura has been injured. This drainage-tube is better than a strip of iodoform gauze, since the latter becomes adherent to the skin, and dries up so that it leads to retention of blood. The tube remains in place from three to four days.

The amount of cerebrospinal fluid which flows out during the following days, when the dura is injured, is generally slight, but it may be so excessive that the dressing must be changed daily. In such cases the author uses 10 per cent. sterilized iodoform gauze for the more superficial layers of the dressing so as to provide for an antiseptic protection; otherwise he uses only sterile mull. The discharge of cerebrospinal fluid soon becomes less and finally ceases. The wound generally heals in a short time. The majority of the author's patients get up in seven to twelve days after the operation, and are discharged in from eighteen to twenty days.

In two cases the author has seen the usual course of healing interrupted; in both there was necrosis of the bony flap. In the first case (the author's second case) the operation was performed in two sittings, and the wound had been tamponed for four days, the second case was done in one sitting and was complicated by a severe hemorrhage, which prolonged the operation to three hours. Other surgeons have made the same observation. If the bone is unintentionally stripped of its periosteum to a larger extent, it should be removed altogether, so that the patients may not be subjected to this danger of necrosis of the bone and to a second operation—the removal of the bony plate.

Dangers and Results.—The two chief dangers of the operation are the hemorrhage and the pressure to which the brain must be exposed. The latter is exerted by the retractor which raises up the brain; but the general cerebral pressure is also increased by the displacement of the cerebrospinal fluid. The author has discussed above how both dangers should be met. Up to the end of 1899 the author collected 128 cases which were operated according to the method described. Of these, 20 died, which gives a mortality of 15.6 per cent. Sepsis, affections of the brain, and shock are given most frequently as cause of death. Concerning the age at which the intracranial resection was done, there is a wide range; though the majority of patients were in middle life, the extremes are twenty years (Capanotto) and seventy-nine years (Tiffany).

The author's experience (beginning of 1902) is limited to 36 operations. Of these, 3 cases died as an immediate result of the operation.

As far as the final results are concerned, the author has never seen a recurrence in any of his cases in which the ganglion was removed for typical trigeminal neuralgia, though nine years have elapsed since his first extirpation. In one of his patients severe pains developed later upon the side which was not operated; in two others slight pains appeared here. All patients operated on are happy that they are freed from their terrible tortures with but slight subjective disturbances.

These disturbances sometimes include a slight difficulty in opening the mouth, due probably to cicatrization within the temporal muscle. This can be remedied, if necessary, by dividing the tendon of the tem-

Fig. 262.

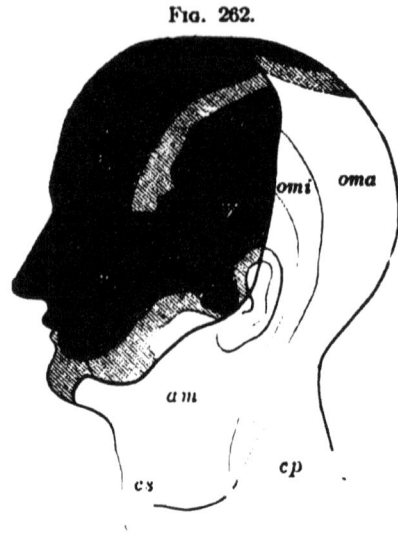

Scheme showing effects of total extirpation of Gasserian ganglion forty-seven days after operation. Sensation of heat spoken of as slightly warm; sensation of cold absent. V_1 V_2 V_3. First, second and third branches of fifth nerve. *oma.* Occipitalis major. *omi.* Occipitalis minor. *am.* Auricularis magnus. *cs.* Suboutaneus colli. (Freidrich.)

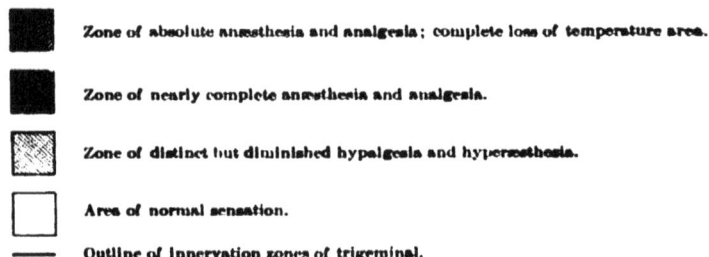

Zone of absolute anæsthesia and analgesia; complete loss of temperature area.

Zone of nearly complete anæsthesia and analgesia.

Zone of distinct but diminished hypalgesia and hyperæsthesia.

Area of normal sensation.

——— Outline of innervation zones of trigeminal.

poral muscle or by removing the coronoid process of the mandible, for the temporal muscle is paralyzed.

Of course, patients all have symptoms directly due to the absence of the Gasserian ganglion. These are, however, considerably less marked than one would expect. It must especially be emphasized that the paralyzed muscles, especially the masseter, temporal and internal

Fig. 263.

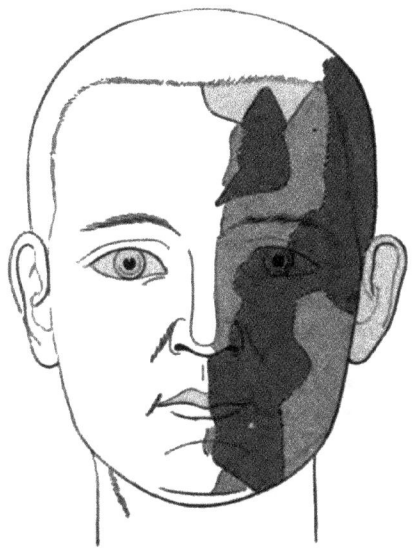

■ Zone of absolute anæsthesia and analgesia   Sixty-three days later than in Fig. 262.

Fig. 264.

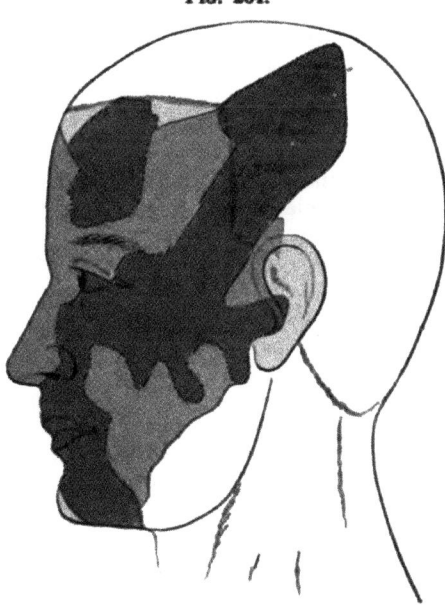

■ Zone of hypalgesia and hyperæsthesia.   Sixty-three days later than in Fig. 262.

pterygoid, are so thoroughly compensated by the same muscles of the healthy side that no deviation can be noticed on closing the jaw. Naturally the power of chewing on the operated side is diminished, but this is not noticeable, since the unilateral anæsthesia of the oral mucous membrane makes the patients chew on the side with normal sensation.

The general condition which has suffered to a considerable degree, owing to the long-continued pain, improves rapidly. Nervousness and insomnia disappear; the patients are no longer dependent upon the help of others and can again resume their work. In one case the author has seen insanity disappear after the operation. It had lasted for several years, as had the neuralgia which caused it.

Indications.—In every case in which the intracranial method is in question on account of the severity of the pain, the ganglion and the trigeminal trunk should be extirpated. Surgeons should never restrict themselves to the intracranial resection of the different branches, since recurrences may follow here as readily as after the peripheral resection, and the danger is no less than after the radical method. The operation may be attempted even where the patients are much exhausted; the author has operated on several cases of this kind with success.

In general an extirpation of the ganglion should only be considered after less serious operations have failed. Should, however, further experience teach that removal of the Gasserian ganglion cures permanently the most severe cases of trigeminal neuralgia, it is probable that the stage will be reached when the operation will be undertaken in these cases from the very beginning, especially since it is to be hoped that with further advances in technic the risk may be still less than the author has experienced. It would be cruel to suggest a peripheral nerve resection if on account of the severity and course of the disease we can at best expect only a temporary alleviation of the pain.

Under very favorable conditions the cause of the neuralgia may be found to lie in changes in the Gasserian ganglion or the trigeminal trunk; here, of course, the intracranial method must be suggested from the first.

While discussing diagnosis, the neuralgias in the course of the recurrent branches which supply the dura mater with sensory fibres were mentioned. The recurrent nerve of the third branch alone takes its origin within the foramen ovale or directly beneath the foramen. Its first part could be extirpated by any one of the extracranial methods for finding the third branch at the base of the skull. It is possible even to succeed here in removing a small part of the ganglion from below.

The recurrent twigs of the first and second branches, however, take their origin from within the skull, and hence can only be reached by the intracranial method. But the three recurrent nerves are not always implicated in the exceptionally severe, unilateral, and deep headaches, such as the author has observed in severe trigeminal neuralgia, for occasionally the meningeal branch of the nasal nerve is at fault. It innervates the dura mater in the anterior cerebral fossa and in the frontal region, and can be exposed in the orbit.

CHAPTER XV.

NEURALGIA OF THE OCCIPITAL NERVES.

CASES of trigeminal neuralgia in which several branches or subdivisions are affected simultaneously are not rare. This peculiarity is present to a still higher degree in severe cases of occipital neuralgia (also termed cervico-occipital neuralgia). Very frequently it is thus difficult or impossible to localize accurately the primary diseased nerve-area. The nerves which are especially involved are the occipitalis major and minor and inner branch of the posterior division of the third cervical (the third occipital nerve), as well as the auricularis magnus; the subcutaneous colli and the supraclaviculares are affected less often. (See Fig. 262, *am, cs, omi, oma.*)

The neuralgic area (Fig. 265) generally comprises the area of distribution of the four nerves mentioned. It therefore includes one side of the occiput, the lateral portion of the skull up to and including the auricle, the region of the lower jaw, especially in its posterior part corresponding to the temporomaxillary articulation, and finally the upper portion of the neck up to the level of the hyoid bone.

The nature of the pain and its cause are in the main the same as with trigeminal neuralgia. Every motion of the head, especially stooping, will excite an attack; there is hypersensitiveness to noise, touch, and light. In the same way psychical excitation may lead to an attack.

Symptoms.—The pain is as intense as that of severe trigeminal neuralgias, and the phenomenon of irradiation is also present. The pain involves the entire front and back of the neck; it radiates to the clavicle and shoulder and along the lower jaw to the chin, and the temporomaxillary joint may become painful. Occasionally the attacks are accompanied by muscular twitchings and spasms which rotate the head, turn it rigidly toward the side, or pull it backward. Sometimes the facial muscles are also involved. At the height of the attack there may even be vertigo, nausea, and vomiting. Vasomotor symptoms, such as reddening of the ear and the nape of the neck, and lachrymation in the corresponding eye have been observed.

The painful points are situated where the nerves become superficial and where they can be reached with the finger. That of the occipitalis major is situated where it penetrates the tendon of the trapezius and comes to lie underneath the skin; this is half-way between the tip of the mastoid process and second cervical vertebra or from 2 to 3 cm. external to the external occipital protuberance. The painful point of the occipitalis minor is situated more laterally at the lower part of the posterior margin of the mastoid process, occasionally somewhat above the following; that of the auricularis magnus is found at the posterior margin of the sternomastoid, at about its middle, at the level of the hyoid bone or somewhat lower.

Diagnosis.—In diagnosticating occipital neuralgia the surgeon must above all exclude caries of the upper cervical vertebræ. Severe neuralgias which not rarely are bilateral develop owing to direct irritation of the nerve-roots. Similar symptoms may be caused by arthritis deformans

FIG. 265.

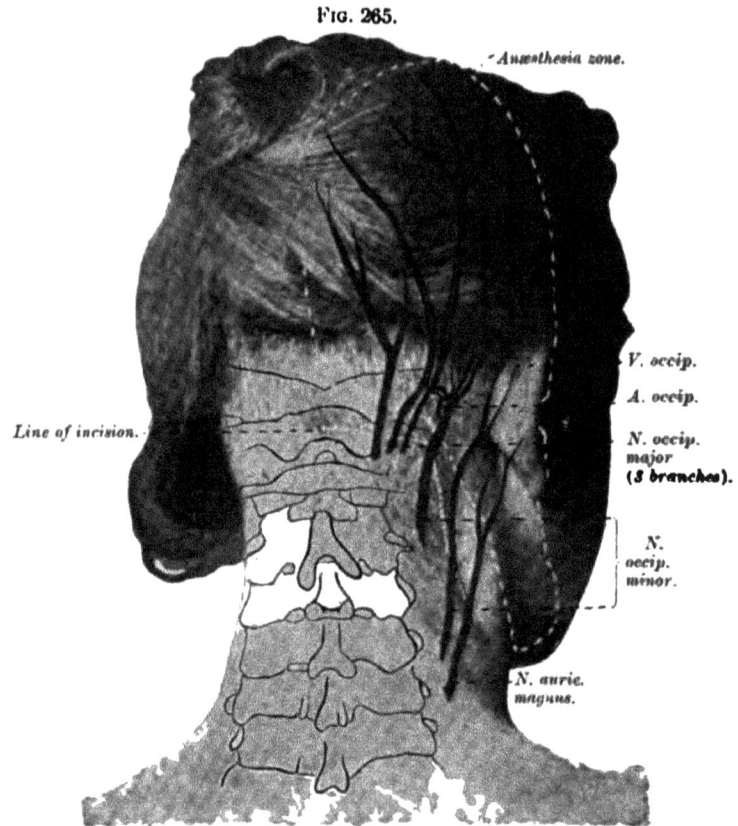

- Anæsthesia zone.

V. occip.

A. occip.

Line of incision.

N. occip.
major
(3 branches).

N.
occip.
minor.

N. auric.
magnus.

Patient, thirty-three years of age, photographed sixteen days after the operation. The fresh scar was not plainly visible, hence has been filled in. The contours of the bone and the nerves in their superficial course have been added according to Fig. 13 of Merkel's Handbuch der Topographischen Anatomie, Braunschweig, 1885-1890, and the occipital artery and nerve are merely indicated at the site where they reach the surface. The anæsthetic zone, nine days after the operation, is included in the dotted white lines.

of the upper cervical articulations. Furthermore, disease of the ear must be thought of; of these, severe persisting pains are caused especially by sclerosis of the cortical portion of the mastoid process.

The differential diagnosis also includes the occipital pains occurring with neurasthenia and hysteria. They may also assume a neuralgic character, with muscle pain. There may be tenderness or moderate pressure over a larger or smaller district of the soft parts of the occiput, but these areas do not correspond to the typical neuralgic spots which are seated in the course of the nerve. The muscular pains are felt very frequently at the insertions and over the body of the occipitalis muscle, and then have their seat along the superior semicircular line of the occipital bone. In such cases there may possibly be an exudate into the muscle or its tendinous insertion; occasionally small nodules may be felt. But it must not be forgotten that painful tubercles may also occur along the cervical nerves.

As contrasted with bony lesions, it is of importance to remember in the diagnosis of neuralgia that even where this has persisted for years no changes occur apart from trophic disturbances, reddening, thickening, and swelling of the skin and hyperæsthesia.

Concerning etiology and prognosis, everything that was said under trigeminal neuralgia holds good here; concerning general treatment, reference should be made to the section on trigeminal neuralgia.

There are good reasons why it is difficult and even impossible to locate accurately the primarily diseased nerve-area in severe occipital neuralgia, for here the anatomical relations vary within very wide limits. This point is of great importance for the surgeon; concerning it the reader may consult the author's article in Bruns' *Beiträge zur klinischen Chirurgie.*

Operative Treatment.—The operative procedure must follow a course which takes all possibilities into consideration. Besides this, the nerves should be removed as far as possible toward the centre, since typical or atypical branches are given off here which also supply the painful area with nerve-twigs.

With these precautions the author proceeds to operate as follows: The patient lies flat upon the healthy side; the head is held by an assistant so that it can be brought into the required position at any time. The incision through the thick skin (see Fig. 265) begins at the occiput near the median line and 3 cm. below the external occipital protuberance. With only a slight deviation downward it is carried toward the tip of the mastoid process, but stops short 2 cm. from this. It then runs obliquely down and forward about 7 cm. to the posterior edge of the sternomastoid and ends a little below the level of the hyoid bone. With the exception of a small portion, the entire incision runs within the limits of the hairy scalp, so that but little can be seen of the scar when the wound has healed.

Exposure of the Nervus Occipitales Major and Tertius.— The skin-incision was purposely laid out beneath the place where the occipitalis major nerve pierces the back muscles to gain the surface. The subcutaneous fat here appears as indurated tissue in which the different structures, especially the fine nerve-branches, cannot be readily distinguished; they would be cut through at once unless great care were exercised if the incision were placed directly over them. Besides this, the most superficial muscle of this region, the trapezius, is not covered by a distinct fascia, but merges almost directly into the subcutaneous tissue.

By the above incision the peripheral distribution of the nerve is not injured; it is discovered by carefully dissecting upward the skin of the upper wound-edge from the underlying structures to the extent of from 1 to 2 cm. As soon as the beginning of the terminal distribution is found, no matter whether this consists of one or more branches, the surgeon can follow it or them down into the deeper structures and toward the centre. In general the surgeon proceeds with anatomical forceps and scissors, and the knife is only occasionally necessary to divide tense or obstructing muscle-fibres or tendon-fibres.

The place where the occipitalis major passes through the muscles and tendons to the skin is along a horizontal line drawn 2 cm. below the external occipital protuberance (Luschka). Its distance from the median line varies; it may be only from 1 to 2 cm. (Schwalbe) or as much as from 3 to 4 cm. (Henle). In general the occipital artery reaches the surface under the skin more externally about half-way between the external occipital protuberance and the posterior aspect of the mastoid process in a line which connects the protuberance with the base of the mastoid process.

Just as the occipital artery and nerve enter the dense subcutaneous tissue in different places, so do their respective courses differ in the deeper tissues. Following the nerve from the periphery toward the centre, it penetrates the outer part of the tendon of the trapezius. This muscle is very delicate in its uppermost portion; if it is very poorly developed here, the nerve enters the deeper parts along its lateral edge. Accordingly the insertion of the trapezius must be divided or merely displaced toward the centre. Exceptionally the occipitalis major penetrates the sternocleidomastoid in its posterior portion, where this muscle has a particularly broad insertion at the superior nuchal line.

Below the trapezius lies the splenius capitis, a strong muscle whose fibres run from below and within, upward and outward. The occipitalis major nerve runs into the depths along its mesial border; and in rare cases it penetrates this muscle. It then pierces the thick semispinalis capitis, whose fibres are almost parallel with the spine. If the nerve is divided in its more superficial course, it generally consists of only one trunk in this region. The fibres of the splenius and the semispinalis must be divided transversely as far as necessary, so that a better view is obtained as the surgeon penetrates still further into the deeper parts.

Before the deepest layer of back muscles is reached, it is noticed that a number of muscular branches are given off from the nerve. An ascending branch goes to the splenius capitis, longissimus capitis, and occasionally also to the obliquus capitis, superior and inferior; sometimes it also gives origin to a cutaneous nerve which runs up to the occiput from the mesial edge of the splenius. A descending branch goes to the semispinalis capitis and anastomoses with the posterior branch of the third cervical nerve.

Besides the inconstant cutaneous nerve just mentioned, there is another constant one which comes from the posterior branch of the third cervical nerve and which ascends in a straight line along the inner side of the occipitalis major nerve to the lower part of the occiput (third occipital nerve, nervus occipitalis tertius). One must be aware of the presence of this nerve, so that it is not taken from the occipitalis major. In its superficial course it may anastomose with the latter or join it altogether. Depending on the position of the occipitalis major, the distance between both is from 1 to 2 cm.

Measuring from the periphery to the centre, the third occipital nerve penetrates the tendon of the trapezius about 4 cm. below the external occipital protuberance. It then pierces the semispinalis and reaches the deeper parts. If the trapezius is displaced toward the middle and divided, the semispinalis transversely, as stated above, the surgeon will here encounter the nerve even where it could not be seen distinctly at the periphery on account of its small size. Here also may sometimes be found an anastomosis between it and the occipitalis major.

Fig. 266

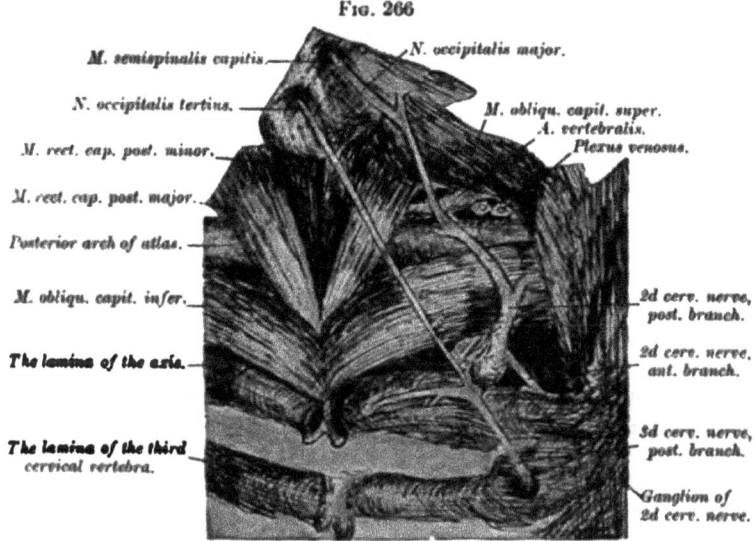

Prepared specimen of about natural size looked at from behind. The semispinalis capitis has been transversely divided at the nape of the neck; its upper part has been turned upward. The occipitalis major and tertius nerves pass into it. The occipitalis major is here pushed a little to the right side, so that it hardly touches the rectus capitis posticus major muscle. The right obliquus capitis inferior muscle is raised somewhat, so that the ganglion of the second cervical nerve becomes visible. The posterior branch of the first cervical nerve (suboccipital nerve) appears above the posterior arch of the atlas and beneath the vertebral artery, just where our illustration has placed the occipitalis major nerve. Since it gives off no cutaneous nerve, according to Henle it is unimportant for us, and is not shown.

Returning now to the latter it is found that after this nerve has pierced the semispinalis capitis it rests upon the deepest layer of the back muscles, upon the posterior surface of the rectus posticus major, and then upon the same surface of the obliquus capitis inferior. It crosses both muscles in the direction of their fibres; for the rectus runs from the spinous process of the axis to the median portion of the inferior semicircular line of the occipital bone, and the obliquus from the same spinous process to the transverse process of the atlas. The nerve now runs in a lateral direction, and finally reaches the depths by curving around the lower edge of the obliquus. In this part of its course the nerve constitutes the entire posterior branch of the second cervical nerve. Here it also unites with the anterior branch to form the trunk of the second cervical nerve. The ganglion of this nerve lies from 3 to 5 mm. external to the ligamentum obturatorium atlantoepistrophicum. The author has never extirpated this ganglion on the living body, but has restricted himself to dividing the trunk. Numerous investigations on the cadaver, however, have convinced him that this extirpation is technically possible, and can be done without injuring the spinal column. It would be of the same significance as removal of the Gasserian ganglion in trigeminal neuralgia.

The third occipital nerve runs along the inner side of the occipitalis major, also crosses the rectus capitis posticus major and the obliquus capitis inferior along their inner portion, and then unites here with the muscular branches to form the posterior branch of the third cervical nerve. To the extent of about 2 cm. more it runs across the arch of the axis in a downward and outward direction to the intervertebral foramen between the second and third cervical vertebræ. Even in this most deeply placed portion of its course there may be an anastomosis between the major and the third occipital nerve.

While the posterior trunk is the smaller with all other spinal nerves the reverse is the case with the first and second; the posterior branch is the larger with the latter especially.

Another peculiarity of the second cervical nerve is of great importance. In all other spinal nerves the trunk divides within the intervertebral foramen, so that it is already split into an anterior and a posterior branch as it issues from the lateral foramina of the vertebræ. In all, the spindle-shaped ganglion of the posterior root lies directly above the undivided trunk; it possesses a furrow along its anterior surface for the anterior root. Thus the spinal ganglia lie within the intervertebral foramina and at the same time outside of the dura mater. The trunk of the second cervical nerve, however, lies external to the spine; its ganglion is accessible from the incision without removing bone since there is no intervertebral foramen between the atlas and the axis, but in its place an intervertebral cleft more than 1 cm. wide. The ganglion is placed in its lateral corner, lateral to the origin of the posterior arch of the atlas.

Thiersch's method is not to be employed for the cervical nerves, since it drags upon the nerves for quite a distance toward the centre before they tear off. The posterior branches are frequently united among each other by loop-shaped anastomoses; between the anterior branches they are always present. If it is considered that the phrenic nerve takes its fibres entirely or in greater part from the fourth cervical nerve, yet often receives fibres from the third cervical nerve as well, it must be agreed that for this reason alone caution is necessary. But besides this the spinal cord is in close proximity and withal a part particularly essential to life. Hence the nerves should be cut through as near to the centre as the above dissection will permit. If the author's directions are accurately followed, all anastomoses with neighboring nerves will be severed. The subdivisions peripheral to the line of division can then be slowly extracted.

Hemorrhage in the superficial layers is not marked. In its normal course the occipital artery does not appear in the incision, but runs above it; if necessary, it can easily be ligated. The vertebral artery is found in the deep parts of the wound from 1 to 1.5 cm. lateral to the trunk of the second cervical nerve; it ascends almost vertically up to the axis, in the foramina of the transverse processes of the cervical vertebræ. It then forms a large curve with its convexity to the outer side, since it must bend outward to reach the transverse process of the atlas lying more than 1 cm. externally, and then again inward to reach the foramen in the occipital bone. In this way the artery is not covered by muscles above the atlas (see Fig. 266), but only enclosed in a layer of fat; it runs transversely directly above the bone. If its course is regular, the artery is so far from the field of operation that it does not come to view. Exceptionally it does not enter the foramen in the transverse process of the axis, but loops around the process with a curve convex posteriorly (the artery would here be close to the field of operation, since directly external to the trunk of the second cervical nerve), and then enters the foramen in the transverse process of the atlas in the regular way.

The well-developed plexus venosus cervicalis posterior of Breschet lies in immediate proximity to the vertebral artery. It drains the deep muscles of the nape of the neck and also communicates with the occipital vein.

Since the occipitalis major and tertius may be surrounded by parts of the plexus in their deep course, one should proceed carefully and if possible with blunt instruments. In such depths venous hemorrhages are more troublesome than arterial ones; they can only be controlled by compression. The deep and narrow wound should be held apart firmly by retractors such as are used for the hip-joint; the pressure exerted by the retractors at the same time checks the hemorrhage, if this is not too excessive.

EXPOSURE OF THE NERVUS OCCIPITALIS MINOR AND THE AURICULARIS MAGNUS.—The author's incision exposes the two nerves where they appear at the posterior edge of the sternomastoid at about the level of the hyoid bone. From this point they continue their course upward in an almost vertical direction. (See Fig. 265.) One should be careful not to injure the nerves in dividing the subcutaneous colli muscle and the fascia lying underneath it. It must also be remembered that the sternomastoid is covered only by very thin fascia. Both nerves may have branched beneath this muscle or they divide into two or more subdivisions in their further course.

The occipitalis minor either lies very close to the auricularis or is placed higher, up to 4 or even 5 cm. above the auricularis behind the

sternomastoid, and may penetrate the posterior margin of the latt
Generally the nerve ascends close to the margin, more rarely parallel
it; it then passes over the splenius capitis up to the occiput.   Occasic
ally the occipitalis minor appears high up beneath the superior nucl
line and under the posterior edge of the sternomastoid, or it penetra:
in addition the anterior edge of the trapezius shortly before its inserti

Fig. 267

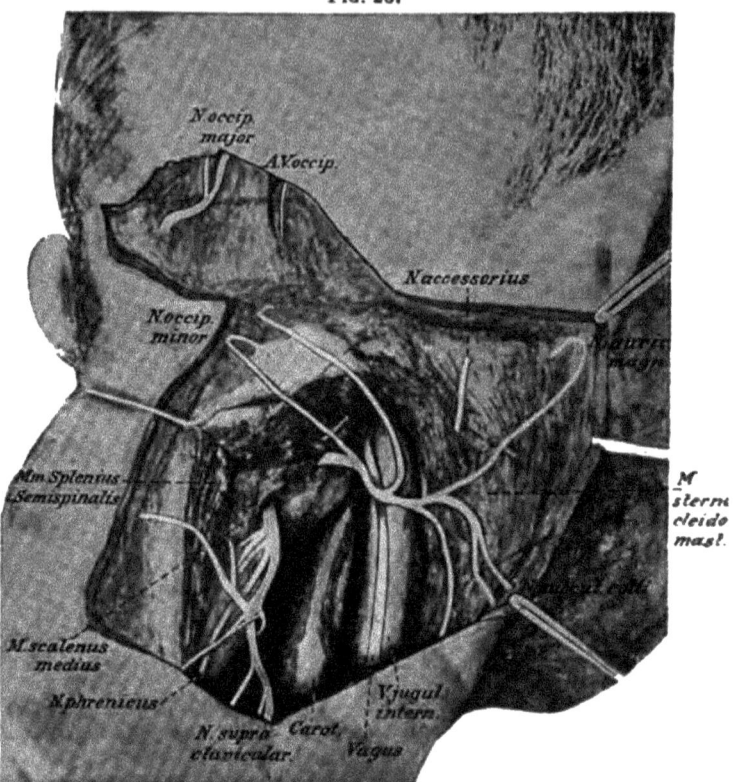

The anterior branches of the third and fourth cervical nerves in their relation to the surround
ings. Photograph of an anatomical preparation. The contours of the carotid, the internal jug
lar vein, and the superficial nerves have been filled in to render them more distinct. The vag
is rendered visible by being placed upon the jugular vein and the muscles of the nape of the ne
are pushed backward. The occipitalis minor issues from the third cervical nerve in the form
two branches. The spinal accessory is divided; its central end is turned upward over the stern
cleidomastoid.

at the superior nuchal line. Still further, the occipitalis minor may l
so small that it does not reach the occiput. If the nerve cannot be four
on account of its aberrant course or its small size, search should be ma(
for the auricularis magnus first and follow this into the depths.

The auricularis magnus may be double; directly underneath it tl subcutaneous colli inferior runs almost horizontally forward as a flat band; somewhat more deeply the supraclavicular nerves appear from under the sternomastoid and run down to the clavicle. The last-mentioned nerves are not dissected free in the above operation unless they should also be involved in the neuralgia.

The relation of the occipitalis minor and auricularis magnus to each other, as far as size is concerned, varies considerably. Generally the latter is the largest nerve of the cervical plexus, but there are many exceptions. Usually one nerve is more prominent if its neighbors are less developed.

As the occipitalis minor and the auricularis magnus are traced more toward the centre (see Fig. 267), the sternomastoid must be displaced forward and the splenius capitis with the other muscles of the nape of the neck backward. The posterior external branch (muscular branch) of the spinal accessory nerve is dissected free and lifted forward with the sternomastoid. This nerve is peculiar more on account of its course than its size; when in doubt the surgeon will find that the shoulder twitches when it is irritated. The nerve frequently anastomoses with the cervical plexus; above all, the occipitalis may communicate with it by one or even two twigs. The nerve-trunks pass out of the lateral portion of the upper cervical spine.

A bundle of structures rests on the transverse processes of the vertebræ. Besides lymph-nodes and lymph-strands it consists of the internal jugular vein, the vagus nerve, and the ansa hyperglossi, and is surrounded by connective tissue, which is as a rule free from fat. These structures rest not only on the transverse process, but also on the muscles taking their origin from them (musculus longus atlantis and longus capitis or rectus capitis anticus major, the scalenus medins and levator scapulæ). The descending ramus of the hypoglossal nerve lies upon the anterior aspect of the carotid and forms the ansa hypoglossi with a branch of the third cervical nerve at the level of the larynx. This branch lies close to the jugular vein and generally runs obliquely downward along its outer side.

The vertebral artery may show an important abnormality in its course; it may lie entirely or partly in front of the transverse processes without entering their foramina; in such cases the vessel is placed behind the common carotid.

The vascular cord, composed of so many different structures, can be bluntly lifted forward from the lateral portion of the spine as a whole, without dissecting free its integral parts. The lower portion of the cervical plexus is always covered by the internal jugular vein.

The anterior branches of the four upper cervical nerves, together with their anastomoses, form the cervical plexus. As they leave the spinal column they lie in a furrow on the upper surface of every transverse process. They are then placed between the anterior and posterior intertransversales, and more lateral to these between the musculus scalenus medins posteriorly and musculus longus capitis or rectus capitis anticus major anteriorly. The nerves are only accessible to the knife after they have pierced the intertransversales. They should be divided as closely as possible to the spinal column so that any anastomoti branches which may continue the neuralgia are excluded.

By dividing the nerves in the depths, the author encountered an active venous hemorrhage in one case. It ceased after tamponade. Other wise the bleeding was not worth mentioning.

No disturbances are evident after the motor branches have been divided. The muscles are numerous and are supplied by so man branches of the cervical nerves that a permanent disturbance is no produced.

If the occipital neuralgia is restricted to a very marked degree to onl one of the nerves discussed, the surgeon may resect only this. Th course of the incision need not be modified to any extent, but it shoul be limited so that the nerve to be removed approximately occupies th centre.

ANOMALIES, INJURIES, AND DISEASES OF THE SALIVARY GLANDS.

By Prof. KÜTTNER.

CHAPTER XVI.

ANOMALIES OF THE SALIVARY GLANDS.

APART from the cystic structures resulting from a congenital atresia of the excretory ducts, the anomalies of structure occurring about the salivary glands are of more anatomical than surgical interest. Only a few cases of absence and abnormal position of the different salivary glands have been reported. In a well-developed male Gruber observed a congenital absence of both submaxillary glands; Turner also records a case in which these glands were not in the digastric triangle on either side, but instead were on the dorsal surface of the mylohyoid, adjacent to the sublingual gland. Another of Gruber's cases proves that under some circumstances such transpositions may be of importance to the surgeon. The parotid gland was missing at its normal site; instead there was a very voluminous gland at the posterior border of the buccal region which corresponded in position to the accessory parotid. On account of its size it suggested a real tumor. A similar case has been described by Cruveilhier.

The author must also record an abnormal orifice of Wharton's duct, eleven lines behind the sublingual caruncle, observed by Bochdalek; and a case of congenital salivary fistula reported by Gherini. In a young girl two openings as fine as a hair were found a few centimetres above the sternum on the inner side of the sternomastoid muscles. Saliva exuded from these, especially on chewing, and by injecting a colored fluid into the fistulæ this appeared at the sublingual caruncle. Another case of congenital salivary fistula, observed by Roser, is cited by König.

CHAPTER XVII.

OF injuries to the salivary glands only those of the parotid are of importance. The submaxillary and sublingual glands and their excretory ducts are hardly exposed to trauma on account of the protection which their position affords; if they are injured from the mouth, no unpleasant consequences follow, since the resulting salivary fistula communicates with the oral cavity.

INJURIES OF THE PAROTID.

In severe trauma of the parotid region by blow, stabbing, or gunshot wound, the injury to the important nerves and vessels situated here is generally of such importance that the involvement of the gland is easily disregarded. In general it is of slight consequence. In operating the gland is frequently wounded, and one observes that it heals readily. The anatomical relations rather than the direct inspection of the wound make it evident that the parotid has been injured. The very vascular tissue generally bleeds freely, so that the granular gland-substance is recognized only with difficulty, and the blood generally masks the flow of saliva, which is not abundant. Generally the injury to the gland becomes evident after a few days, when the wound has not united completely or when a subcutaneous accumulation of saliva breaks through the suture line and discharges externally. Phenomena of this kind are not of great importance, for the outflow of saliva need not interfere with the primary union of the rest of the wound, and the fistula closes sooner or later, even when the wound is lacerated and primary union improbable. Obstinate protracted fistulæ of the salivary gland are unusual signals of these injuries.

Treatment.—Complete primary union is the best way of preventing a result of this kind. To bring this about, the wound should be sutured as accurately as possible, and the deep parts included in the suture, so as to avoid the formation of cavities and pockets. If the edges of the wound are irregular and torn, sufficient tissue must be removed to permit of a primary union. As soon as this is done, pressure is exerted by means of a bandage, and talking and chewing are interdicted for from five to seven days, so as to restrict the movements of the lower jaw and the secretion of saliva. Only fluid diet in small amounts should be given.

(608)

during this time. If, despite this, saliva accumulates beneath the suture-line, dressings which exert pressure, if continued for some time, generally suffice to make it gradually disappear.

INJURIES OF THE PAROTID DUCT.

Injuries to the excretory duct of the parotid are more important, though less freqnent, than those of the gland itself. The surgeon is usually dealing with wounds inflicted by swords or broadswords, less often with lesions after operations, gunshot-wounds, or other injuries. According to the observations of Desault and Malgaigne, subcutaneous ruptures of the duct may also occur from the effects of blunt force. Since the direction of Steno's duct corresponds to a line drawn from the base of the lobule of the ear to the vermilion border of the upper lip (Merkel), one must look for an implication of the salivary duct in all deeper injuries which cross this line. It also follows that the duct is more frequently involved if the wound is vertical than if it is horizontal and more or less parallel with it. Complete divisions are the rule, on account of its small diameter.

Diagnosis.—The diagnosis of an injury to the duct is not difficult if the wound gapes widely. After carefully checking the hemorrhage the saliva is seen to exude from the central end of the duct on directing the patient to chew or by placing an irritating substance upon the mucous membrane of his mouth. In very recent injuries the divided ends may even project freely into the wound for a short distance, and thus be clearly exposed to view; they soon, however, retract. To insure the diagnosis one may also sonnd the duct from the month[1] and then try to make the sound appear in the wound of the cheek.

Prognosis.—Formerly it was generally believed that primary union of the divided duct did not occur, and that a salivary fistula always developed. This is not so, and König properly emphasizes the fact that many ducts divided in a sharply incised wound have healed by primary union before anyone thought of its injury. If a primary union does not occur, the severed ends retract. The peripheral portion is now without function; occasionally it remains patent; more frequently it undergoes cicatrization. One can become convinced of its closure by introducing a sound from the month after the injury has healed. The central portion of the duct which still remains in connection with the gland is kept patent by the flow of saliva. This runs outward or inward; in the latter direction, of course, only when the injury is a penetrating one. If a non-penetrating wound has been sutured and the ends of the duct do not unite primarily, there will be a complete external salivary duct fistula when the dressing is changed, or else a tense fluctuating accumulation

[1] In attempting to sound the parotid duct from the mouth, it is desirable to correct its curves. This can be accomplished by raising the cheek from the teeth and drawing it forward. This motion is necessary anyway to render the orifice accessible.

of saliva will appear under the suture-line from which a fistula wil
develop when the suture is removed.

Treatment.—From the foregoing, the treatment of an injury of Steno';
duct would be as follows: A clean, non-penetrating wound with dividec
salivary duct must be united primarily with great care. Both ends arc
accurately approximated by sutures of catgut which do not enter the
lumen. The after-treatment should restrict the secretion of saliva and
the movements of the lower jaw in the manner already described. If
notwithstanding an accumulation of saliva under the suture-line occurs
one should first empty the contents through a fine opening and then try
to prevent the saliva from breaking through to the exterior by means of
dressings exerting pressure; a permanent result does not often, however
follow this procedure. Formerly a sound or bristle, or something similar
was inserted into the two ends of the divided duct and sutures placec
over it. Such methods are, however, no more justified than the estab
lishment of immediate communication with the mouth; since primary
union of the divided duct is possible, it would be wrong to dispense with
it from the start. The surgeon is only justified in making a communication with the month when the degree of laceration or contusion renders
primary union improbable. In such cases the surgeon may use one of
the methods employed in dealing with fistulæ of the duct.

In a penetrating wound of the cheek, the outer wound is sutured and
the mucous membrane left ununited. The saliva finds its way to the
mouth alone; an internal fistula of the salivary duct develops which wil
functionate as well as a normal orifice of the duct. Special methods to
keep the wound in the mucous membrane open can be dispensed with.

CHAPTER XVIII.

DISEASES OF THE SALIVARY GLANDS.

SALIVARY FISTULÆ.

A SALIVARY fistula is an abnormal communication through which the saliva reaches the surface. According to the part involved, salivary gland and salivary duct fistulæ may be recognized; in the former only the smaller ducts are involved, but in the latter the chief duct. A fistula is termed external if it opens upon the skin of the exterior, internal if it communicates with the mouth at an abnormal site.[1]

It is evident that only the external fistula can have surgical interest, and, since this occurs only in connection with the parotid, the term salivary gland fistula practically corresponds with that of parotid fistula, and the term salivary duct fistula with that of fistula of Steno's duct.

Although a salivary fistula is not dangerous, it is very troublesome, and may become unendurable when the communication of the chief duct with the skin of the exterior allows the entire secretion of one parotid to be discharged upon the surface. Such patients are obliged constantly to wipe off the saliva as it runs down; they are unfit for social intercourse and the constant wetting of the skin leads to obstinate eczema. Nutrition also suffers, since the food is not sufficiently mixed with saliva, and since the excessive, often hardly controllable secretion from the fistula during meals does away with all desire for eating.

As has been stated, trauma is the most important etiological factor. Besides this, salivary fistulæ may follow as a result of abscess formation or ulceration starting from the salivary glands or extending to these (carcinoma, lues, tuberculosis, noma). The existence of congenital salivary fistulæ has been mentioned.

Salivary Gland Fistulæ.—*Parotid Fistula.*—Fistulæ follow rather frequently after operative or other injury of the gland-substance of the parotid; but it is rare that a fistula of this kind does not close by itself in the course of weeks or, at the most, months. If a parotid fistula is particularly obstinate and shows no tendency to heal, the surgeon is probably dealing with a fistula of the glandular portion of the duct— that is, with a duct fistula, and not a gland fistula.

Symptoms.—The fistulæ occur about all parts of the parotid gland and generally communicate with the surface by means of a very short fine tract. Exceptionally the orifice does not lie within the normal limits

---

[1] Angléras has observed a communication of Steno's duct with the maxillary sinus. The duct had been injured during an operation. The profuse excretion of saliva through the nose ceased after the fistula was cauterized.

of the parotid. Then an accessory parotid is involved or the gland is abnormally large, or finally there is a long, fistulous tract, as after the rupture of an abscess.

The surgeon will generally find in the slightly altered skin a single very fine opening lying in the middle of a small mass of granulation-tissue. Slight or moderate amounts of saliva as clear as water exude from it; during the act of eating the discharge is more abundant. With a parotid fistula the secretion is naturally much less than with a fistula of Steno's duct, since the secretion of only part of the gland flows out; if the secretion is excessive, one should always think of a duct fistula. The gland fistulæ generally cause no other symptoms apart from this discharge of saliva, though sometimes occlusion of the outer opening may lead to inflammation of the parotid, and inversely inflammatory swellings may occasionally cause closure of the fistulous orifice.

Treatment.—If a salivary gland fistula shows no tendency to heal, it should be aided with the different therapeutic measures. Generally one succeeds by cauterizing the fistula energetically with a silver nitrate pencil from time to time, say, every four or five days. A bandage should then be applied which does not exert too firm pressure. This local treatment must be assisted by measures which restrict the secretion of saliva, hence the patients should be kept on fluid, non-irritating diet, and should as much as possible avoid moving the jaws. Burning out the fistula with the galvanocautery is still better than cauterizing with silver nitrate. The cautery should be introduced cold as far as possible into the tract and then brought to a glow. If this does not cure it, the edges of the fistula should be freshened and this followed by suture, or resort is had to a plastic operation. The latter is indicated especially if the fistula did not result from an injury, but from ulcerative process. In very obstinate cases a partial extirpation of the parotid must be done, avoiding carefully the facial nerve.

Salivary Duct Fistulæ.—*Fistulæ of the Parotid Duct.*—Salivary duct fistulæ are of much greater practical importance than salivary gland fistulæ, since they cause considerably more inconvenience, and since they heal much less often without operative aid. A fistula of Steno's duct is to be regarded as permanent and incapable of healing sponta- neously (1) if mucous membrane and skin have grown together to form a lip-shaped fistula; (2) if the peripheral portion of the duct lying toward the mouth is occluded; and (3) if larger defects of the duct are present.

Symptoms.—The appearance of a salivary duct fistula resembles that of a salivary gland fistula. The outer orifice is generally very narrow and passable only for the finest sounds; the communication between the opening on the skin and the one in the duct is usually short. One is not always successful in introducing a sound far into the salivary duct from the fistula; in suitable cases, however, one can enter both the peripheral and the central portion of the duct if the mouth end is open and not too much shrunken. The skin around the fistula is generally unchanged. Rarely the skin is undermined and forms a kind of pocket in which the saliva collects before it reaches the surface. In such cases the opening in the tract is deeper than the orifice upon the skin, and there was an undermining of the soft parts before the external fistula formed. In exceptional cases there may be more than one opening; the saliva may even run out of numerous holes as out of a watering-pot.

The seat of the fistula is important from a therapeutic point of view. Corresponding to the three subdivisions of the duct, buccal, masseteric, and glandular fistulæ are recognized; the buccal are the most frequent and the most easily treated.

That it is easy to see why the secretion from a fistula of Steno's duct is much more excessive than from a gland fistula has been stated. If the peripheral portion is not occluded, part of the saliva can still find its way into the mouth, and in such cases the fistula does not secrete so profusely as if the oral end were closed. How much saliva may flow out of the fistula in the latter case, especially during meals, is evident from the observation of Duphénix, who collected 70 grams in a quarter of an hour, and from a patient of Jobert who voided several cupfuls in twenty-four hours. Such large amounts naturally signify considerable loss of fluid for the body.

Diagnosis.—The diagnosis of salivary fistula is easy and lymphatic fistulæ alone may give rise to error. But the error is soon made evident by the increased secretion of salivary fluid during meals and by the examination of the voided fluid.

It may be more difficult to distinguish a salivary duct fistula from a salivary gland fistula. In the first place, the seat is characteristic. A fistula anterior to the margin of the masseter would hardly belong to the gland itself, although it is possible that an accessory parotid may be involved or that exceptionally a salivary gland fistula may communicate with the parotid by means of a long tract. Besides the seat, there are the following differential points: In many fistulæ of Steno's duct a sound can be passed into the tract for quite a distance; in real parotid fistulæ this is impossible. The secretion of a duct fistula is much greater than that of a gland fistula; in accordance with this the discharge of saliva from the normal opening in the mouth is entirely absent in the duct fistula or is much less than with the gland fistula. These symptoms are especially of importance for fistulæ situated in the neighborhood of the parotid itself, since here the seat is of no value in differential diagnosis. A fistula should be pronounced incurable if the impermeability of its peripheral portion is evident by sounding (if necessary, with two instruments introduced from the mouth and from the fistula) if the injection of colored fluids into the oral opening of the duct has failed, and if the absence of all discharge of fluid from the latter is established, or if it has a lip-shaped external opening. It is thus seen how important for the therapeutical management it is to take all these facts into consideration.

Treatment.—Here a distinction must be made between those salivary duct fistulæ which, in the above sense, are still capable of a spontaneous cure and those concerning which so favorable an outcome is no longer to be expected.

TREATMENT OF FISTULÆ OF THE PAROTID DUCT TENDING TO HEA
SPONTANEOUSLY.—In duct fistulæ which have not yet become permanen
spontaneous cure can be assisted by proper precautions, as in salivar
gland fistulæ. Besides limiting as much as possible the secretion o
saliva, resort must be had to cauterization with the silver nitrate penci
and with heat; both can be combined with moderate compression.

If a still curable duct fistula will not close by these methods, especiall
by cauterizing, resort must be had to one of the procedures enumeratei
under the treatment of permanent duct fistulæ. At any rate, it is advis
able to wait several months to make sure that the spontaneous cure o
the cure induced by simple methods is really impossible.

TREATMENT OF PERMANENT FISTULÆ OF THE PAROTID DUCT.—Pei
manent salivary duct fistulæ have always given the surgeon trouble; thi
is clear from the report of Delarue, according to which no less tha
twenty-six operations had been reported as early as 1895. Recently
still others have been added to these. In accordance with the object c
this text-book, only the most important and the really practical method
will be described.

A duct fistula may be cured (a) by restoring the outflow of saliv
through the normal route by way of the peripheral end of the duct, (b
by converting the external salivary fistula into an internal one, or (c
by bringing about complete cessation of salivary secretion with oblitera
tion of the corresponding gland.

*Restoring the Normal Flow of Saliva by Way of the Peripheral End c
the Duct.*—Nicoladoni has recently shown that under certain circum
stances it may be possible to restore the discharge of saliva into th
mouth, even in permanent fistulæ of any part of the duct. In a masse
teric fistula he succeeded in exposing the duct, excising the scar, am
then closing the defect in the duct by means of a fine catgut suture. ι
plastic operation by means of a flap from the skin of the cheek was the
done, so that the skin suture would not lie directly over the duct suture
He also succeeded in this way with a glandular fistula of the duct. Th
descending part of the main duct was severed by the blow of a fencing
sword; the part lying nearest to the mouth was occluded. The end c
the peripheral part of the duct lying toward the fistula was found b
sounding from the mouth, and was then sutured to the correspondin
end of the central part of the duct. Although at first the fistula reopened
it healed permanently after frequent sounding from the mouth with th
finest catgut.

Nicoladoni has rendered this method applicable in an ingenious wa]
even for those particularly unfavorable cases in which large defects ar
present at the end of the masseteric or the beginning of the glandula
portion. He believes that the condition can be improved only by a kin
of prolongation of the buccal portion of the duct, and proceeds as follow:
After exposing the masseteric portion of the duct he dissects free th
buccinator around the place where Steno's duct is inserted. A curve
incision, passing anterior to the normal orifice of the duct, is then carrie
through the buccal mucous membrane; a well-nourished tongue-shape

flap, consisting of mucous membrane and muscle, with its base at the anterior edge of the masseter, is thus shaped. By turning this flap around the edge of the masseter the orifice of the duct can be displaced more than 1.5 cm. backward; hence the peripheral end of the duct can be approximated by as much to the central end and united with this. The wound in the cheek is sutured. The peripheral portion of the duct must be in a suitable condition before this method can be carried out. Yet a similar plastic operation can be done even when a direct union of both ends of the duct is no longer possible.

Converting an External Fistula into an Internal One.—On account of its simplicity this is the method of choice for all permanent fistulæ of the buccal portion of the duct. In certain modifications it is also, however, suitable when more posterior portions of the duct are involved. The French distinguish between a "procédé de la ponction unique" and a "procédé de la double ponction," and most of the exceedingly numerous methods can indeed be classed under these headings. To these must be added v. Langenbeck's method of direct implantation of the central end of the duct into the mucous membrane of the mouth, which has also been modified repeatedly, and, finally, the construction of a new duct by a plastic operation upon the oral mucous membrane.

1. *Simple and Double Puncture of the Mucous Membrane of the Cheek at the Site of the Fistula (Ponction Unique, Double Ponction).*—In the "ponction unique" the cheek is penetrated at the site of the fistula by means of a trocar (Desault) or a thermocautery (de Roy), so that the saliva can flow into the mouth. Since, however, the new tract has a tendency to close, it must be kept open artificially by introducing a foreign body. It is best to use a drainage-tube, according to Richelot and Kaufmann.

Kaufmann's drainage of the cheek is carried out as follows: The canal is formed by means of a trocar 4 mm. thick. A rubber tube from 3 to 4 mm. thick is drawn through the canal into the month, so that one end projects into the month, while the other is cut off somewhat obliquely and placed so that the saliva can flow directly into the tube. One can also simply permit the tube to project outward upon the cheek. The tube remains in place eight days and is then shortened on both sides close to the level of the skin and the mucous membrane. In eight or ten days more it is removed entirely. The saliva will now flow through the new canal into the mouth and the external fistula will close by itself or after cauterization or direct suture. Kaufmann's method is simple and rational, and suited for buccal as well as masseteric fistulæ. With a buccal fistula it is simply necessary to puncture the cheek at the abnormal orifice of the duct in a straight direction, or with a slight deviation toward the front; with a masseteric fistula, however, one must be careful not to push the cannula through the masseter, for a foreign body in the muscle is not borne well, since it causes severe pains with trismus; besides, the long tract will readily close again if it runs between muscle-fibres. Hence in a masseteric fistula the trocar must first be pushed from the opening of the fistula subcutaneously to the anterior edge of the masseter before the oral mucous membrane is perforated.

Following the simple comes the double puncture of the mucous membrane of the cheek (procédé de la double ponction). Deguise was the first one who operated in this way; his simple method is still in use. With two elliptical incisions the fistula is first excised for half the thickness of the cheek; the floor of the wound is then punctured twice, so that both openings are 0.5 cm. distant from each other upon the oral mucous membrane. A wire of lead or a strong piece of silk is carried through both isted together or tied inside the mouth. (Fig. 268.)   If a silk thread is used, it is best to pass a straight needle through

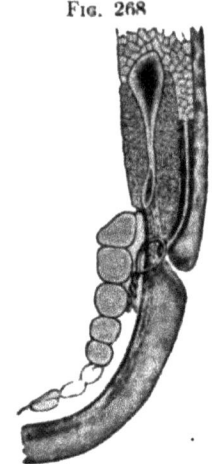

Fig. 268

each end, pierce the mucous membrane of the mouth with these in two places, and then to tie the ligature tightly within the mouth. The outer wound is allowed to take care of itself or else is sutured. It is clear that this method differs from the above only in that the canal is kept open in a different way—by a necrosis of the bridge of tissue surrounded by the wire or thread.

1. *Direct Implantation of the Central End of the Duct into the Mucous Membrane of the Mouth.*—This method was originated by v. Langenbeck, and consists in dissecting out the central end of the duct and implanting it into the opening in the oral mucous membrane after the cheek has been pierced. In this form the method is applicable only if sufficient of the duct is present, as in fistulæ of the buccal portion; but even here difficulties may arise, if the fistula is placed in the posterior portions of this part, near the anterior edge of the masseter.

Operation for salivary duct fistula according to Deguise. (Duplay-Reclus.)

In one case Nicoladoni was obliged to cut out a large piece from the anterior edge of the muscle, for otherwise it would have been impossible to bring the loosened end of the duct up to the oral mucous membrane. Nicoladoni was aware at the same time of the close proximity of the ascending ramus of the lower jaw, which may sometimes render the operation impossible.

3. *Formation of a New Duct from the Oral Mucous Membrane by Means of a Plastic Operation.*—The credit of having introduced this operation belongs to Nicoladoni and Braun. Reference has been made to a plastic operation of Nicoladoni which resulted in a posterior displacement of the orifice of the duct and its peripheral portion.

The following methods are indicated for those difficult cases in which the peripheral portion of the duct is much shrunken or embedded in scar-tissue, so that it can no longer be employed, and in which the duct ends upon the masseter or at the transition from the masseteric to the glandular portion. If the mucous membrane of the mouth is movable in the normal way and there are no cicatricial changes, Braun's method may be followed: The soft tissues of the cheek are divided transversely in the direction of the duct and the mucous membrane of the cheek is laid bare for some distance from without. On account of the ease with which it can be displaced, this mucous membrane can now be pulled out to quite an extent without being divided. The projecting fold of mucous membrane is now cut in the direction of the skin-incision, and thus two flaps of mucous membrane are formed which can be pushed far behind the anterior edge of the masseter toward the parotid by means of two sutures running through their edges. If the two sutures are now secured next to the stump of the parotid duct on both sides, upon the outer surface of the masseter, the stump can easily be placed between the flaps and even fixed to them directly. Finally that part of the wound in the mucous membrane which was formerly in front, but now is on the outer side, is sewed separately, and the remaining wound in the soft parts is closed. The final result of this method is a funnel of mucous membrane which, when viewed from the inner side of the cheek, deepens behind and externally and takes up the central end of the duct.

If the mucous membrane of the cheek is not displaceable in the normal way, it is advisable to cut out of it a tongue-shaped flap with its base behind, according to Nicoladoni. This flap is turned back into a deep excavation cut out of the anterior edge of the masseter and brought together by means of fine sutures, so as to form a tube into which the central end of the duct is led.

Artificial Checking of the Salivary Secretion and Obliteration of the Gland.—Obliteration of the gland from which the diseased duct springs has been recommended as a last resort. Louis, Dupuytren, and others have attempted to accomplish this by such inappropriate methods as compression of the gland or of the part of the duct lying between fistula and gland. The suggestion of Viborg seems more rational. Based upon the results of animal experiments, he recommends ligation of the central end of the duct. This has recently been done by Bramann in 3 cases, and in 2 of these the flow of saliva was checked. Nevertheless he advises against tying the duct, for the results are doubtful and there always is more or less reaction with pains, fever, and marked swelling which may extend from the parotid region to the neck. Even alarming symptoms, such as intense inflammation, suppuration, perforation of saliva or pus into the external auditory canal, etc., have been observed. Hence ligation of the duct is not to be advised.

If a salivary duct fistula cannot be closed in any other way than by excluding that part of the parotid from which it springs, as would be the case when the fistula lies deeply at the bottom of the recess formed by the gland, it would be more proper and more in accordance with modern principles to resort to the knife. After the facial nerve has been dissected out carefully, the part of the parotid at fault, in the case mentioned the tail of the organ, should be removed.

If it is considered after this review which method is most suitable for the cure of permanent fistulæ in the different parts of the duct, it is found that the method of Deguise or drainage of the cheek of Kaufmann is to be recommended for buccal fistulæ in which direct union is not

Kaufmann's method may
operation may be done
cannot be accomplished
masseteric fistulæ are also
glandular portion of the duct.
involved, direct union should
direct the saliva into the mouth;
of the parotid with careful

CALCULI.

in the excretory ducts as well
In general, a foreign body passes
and then finds its way toward
in the case of a projectile, that it
even heal in place here. Foreign
submaxillary duct, which seems
of its position, of its orifice, and
such as fish-bones, bristles, hairs,
duct on account of its more
position. Naturally, the foreign
elongated form, with pointed ends,
tract. Besides the above-men-
splinters of wood, the seeds of

by the entrance of a foreign body
alarming; on the other hand,
be absent altogether, and more
gradually when the foreign body
More commonly an intense
the body gains entrance. This is
stasis with painful swelling of the
disappear after a time, but soon
removed. If it remains impacted
complex of the "coliques salivaires,"
generally develops. These will be
stones.
changes occur. The excretory
inflammation by the purulent dis-
orifice, the dilatation and thick-
enlargement of the gland. After the
develops which is, however, inter-
paroxysms induced by stasis of the
at last forced out of the duct during
or obstinate salivary fistulæ may
until the object is passed through the

orifice of the duct or the fistula or until it is removed by operation. Then the symptoms generally disappear all at once, the fistula closes, and the chronic inflammatory changes gradually recede. If a salivary stone has formed around the foreign body, the symptoms are similar to those described, since the salivary stone also acts as a foreign body.

Diagnosis.—The diagnosis is easy only if the presence of the object can be determined by inspection or examination with sounds. If this is impossible, then the sudden appearance of very severe disturbances accompanied by symptoms of salivary stasis speaks very much in favor of a foreign body. The diagnosis, however, is hardly possible when the object cannot be felt with the sound, and when its entrance has caused slight symptoms or none at all and a chronic inflammation of the duct and gland only develops gradually. The intermittent appearance of a salivary tumor with salivary colics is not characteristic of a foreign body it proves only that there is some impediment to the discharge of saliva, no matter whether this consists of a foreign body, a stone, or an inflammatory swelling of the duct.

The examination with Röntgen rays is only of value if the surgeon is dealing with very opaque bodies, especially metallic ones, such as pieces of shot, as in a case of Rochs.

Prognosis.—Prognosis and treatment are about the same as with salivary stones. By itself a foreign body in the salivary organs is not dangerous; at most a progressive suppuration following it may become threatcuing. It is always, however, followed by marked disturbances with considerable reaction upon the general well-being and nutrition.

Treatment.—The treatment consists in removing the foreign body as soon as possible. The extraction is, of course, simple when the object projects from the salivary duct. If more deeply situated, it may be possible to press it out of the orifice of the duct; generally, however, an incision is necessary to bring the sharp and often encrusted body to light. In other cases the indication to operate is on account of abscesses or fistulæ, and the foreign body is found, expectedly or unexpectedly, during the course of the operation. If a submaxillary salivary gland containing a foreign body is much changed by inflammatory processes, it may be advisable to extirpate it entirely or in part; concerning the parotid, this is not indicated on account of the danger of injuring other structures.

Salivary Stones.—The disease leading to the formation of salivary stones (sialolithiasis) is a rare affection which affects the salivary glands less often than their excretory ducts. Salivary stones are usually found in the submaxillary duct; they occur considerably less often in the submaxillary gland; then follow the parotid with Steno's duct, and, lastly, the sublingual gland with its excretory ducts.

According to the statistics of Czygan, Buchwald, and Wenzel, 61.4 per cent. of all salivary stones belong to Wharton's duct and the submaxillary gland, 20.4 per cent. to the parotid and duct, and 18.2 per cent. to the sublingual and their excretory ducts.

Salivary stones occur decidedly more often among men than women. The middle years of life are especially predisposed. Children may also be affected, though but rarely. Bundel has even seen a congenital case. The size and number of the stones vary considerably and stand in a certain relation to each other; the more numerous the concretions, the smaller they generally are. Stones occurring in the glands are generally more voluminous than those found in the ducts. In the large majority of cases there is but one stone which does not exceed the size of a pea or bean and weighs from 5 to 30 grams at the most; but very small ones, the size of a grain of millet or sand, and on the other hand very large ones, have been observed. Three exceptionally large concretions of Wharton's duct, observed in v. Bruns' clinic, are reproduced in Fig. 269.

Fig. 269.

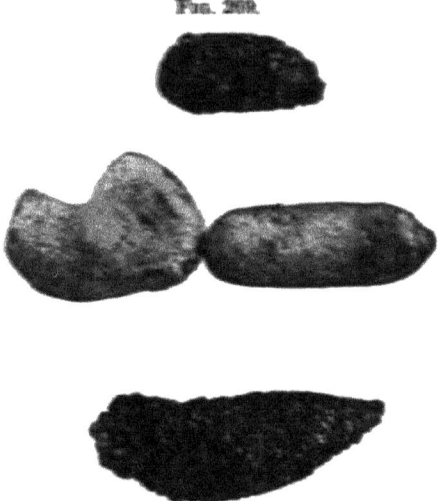

Salivary stones observed in von Bruns' clinic.

Stones of the excretory ducts are generally elongated and cylindrical, not unlike the pits of dates or olives; more rarely they are club-shaped. Rounded or very irregular structures generally belong to the glands. The surface is rough and irregular, but perfectly smooth concretions also occur. Stones of the excretory ducts not rarely show longitudinal furrows; they run along the outer surface in a straight or spiral (Després) manner and are due to the saliva as it pushes the stone forward. If several stones lie close together, they are generally flattened. The consistency varies within wide limits; some stones can be crushed between the fingers; others are so hard that they cannot be scratched with the nail. The color is grayish-white or yellowish; other colors are less frequent.

Every salivary stone consists of organic and inorganic material. If the lime-salts are dissolved out by means of acids, the residue consists chiefly of bacteria and salivary bodies. The most important of the inorganic substances is phosphate of lime, then comes carbonate of lime. Strangely enough, potassium sulphocyanide could not be detected.

The origin of salivary stones has only recently been cleared up. In a number of cases the entrance of foreign bodies into the salivary glands or their excretory ducts is to be regarded as the cause of the stone-formation, as has been pointed out. Perhaps small particles of tartar also play a rôle as foreign bodies. For the great majority of salivary stones, however, an infectious origin must be assumed, as for the formation of concretions elsewhere. The biological activity of bacteria is to be held responsible for sialolithiasis, according to the researches of Klebs and Galippe. The masses of bacteria which are found in the interior of the stone and which form its skeleton are not accidental, as was formerly believed, but give rise to the stone, according to the authors mentioned. The bacteria of the mouth find an opportunity to settle when, owing to moderate inflammatory processes, there is a rough spot or a defect upon the mucous membrane or even an inflammatory structure with retardation of the flow of saliva.

The anatomical changes which a stone can bring about in the course of the salivary passages may be considerable. If situated in the excretory duct, it causes a dilatation at the place where it is located, and, since it is a foreign body, it sets up a severe inflammation of the duct with ulceration and suppurative catarrh. Abscesses may develop which rupture into the mouth or upon the outside, so that the stone is either passed or else a salivary fistula forms. Instead of circumscribed abscesses, progressive phlegmons may develop after perforation of the duct; this is especially the case along the floor of the mouth with stones of Wharton's duct. According to Mikulicz and Kümmel, these processes are always located in the posterior part of the floor of the month next to the base of the tongue and easily spread to this and to the pillars of the fauces. With stones situated in the ducts the inflammatory changes also assume considerable proportions in the salivary glands, especially when the stone is large and the lumen of the excretory duct occluded. The resulting stasis of saliva favors the spreading of the inflammation to the remaining portions of the duct and to the gland; the latter will be swollen, firm, and adherent to its surroundings, and may simulate a malignant tumor. Microscopical examination shows a chronic interstitial inflammation with infiltration of round cells, hypertrophy of connective tissue, and more or less marked atrophy of the glandular parenchyma.

If the stone or more frequently the stones are situated in the gland itself, the latter will be much inflamed and infiltrated and sometimes permeated by miliary abscesses; the concretions are either embedded in dense, inflammatory indurations or they lie in the interior of an abscess which may communicate with the excretory duct.

Symptoms and Course.—The clinical picture of sialolithiasis varies considerably. The beginning of the stone-formation generally causes but few symptoms unless the surgeon is dealing with a foreign body, and it may happen that stones have existed for years and have attained a considerable size when the first symptoms come on. It is, however, exceptional that a stone suddenly makes its appearance in the mouth, as during a meal, without having manifested its presence before. In general, the disturbances are more serious with stones situated in the ducts than with those located in the glands. They are particularly marked at their most common site, the duct of Wharton, and exceptionally slight if the stone is placed in one of the smaller sublingual ducts and the other ducts are free. Here the chief cause of the disturbances, the salivary stasis, does not take place.

The most characteristic symptom of sialolithiasis, the intermittent appearance of a salivary tumor, is due to salivary stasis. Owing to the severe pains which accompany these attacks, the French have applied the name "coliques salivaires" to them. While generally there is only a dense, more or less tender tumor over the site of the stone, which interferes with talking and chewing to a moderate degree, and occasionally gives rise to radiating pains, the symptom-complex of a "colique salivaire" is entirely different. Very severe pain comes on suddenly during a meal, sometimes also by the mere sight of food. With stones in Wharton's duct, the pain is referred especially to the tongue and the floor of the mouth. At the same time a very distinct swelling forms which involves the entire gland and the portion of the duct lying behind the stone. Pain and swelling increase more and more until there is a profuse discharge of saliva or perhaps pus from the orifice of the excretory duct. The symptoms then gradually recede, but it may require hours before the previous condition is resumed. These disagreeable crises are explained by the fact that the more abundant discharge of saliva during a meal causes a stagnation behind the stone, so that the saliva cannot escape until the duct is dilated sufficiently to allow the saliva to find an exit beside it. In severe cases the attacks develop with almost every meal, and it is clear that the nutrition and general well-being may suffer to a very high degree.

Another, not constant, symptom, the pyorrhœa salivalis, is caused by a catarrh of the mucous membrane of the duct. The discharge which exudes from the swollen, reddened, and occasionally widely gaping orifice of the excretory duct in question is only rarely profuse; frequently only a few drops of pus are voided during the day. Other inflammatory symptoms, such as stomatitis and salivation, are virtually never absent, especially during the salivary colics.

It has been mentioned that the salivary glands are frequently enlarged and inflamed. This swelling develops either slowly and insidiously or more acutely with severe symptoms of inflammation. Severe phlegmonous processes and abscesses in the floor of the mouth give their own symptoms.

Diagnosis.—The diagnosis of salivary stone is easy only when the concretion can readily be felt with the finger or the sound; if more or less of it is exposed after the tissues which cover it are destroyed, a mistake is, of course, impossible. It is otherwise, however, if the signs are less prominent. If the characteristic attacks are present, a salivary stone always suggests itself, though the surgeon must not forget that other conditions (inflammations of the excretory ducts, foreign bodies) may also be followed by the periodic development of a salivary tumor. A close examination of the excretory duct will then decide. This is first conducted bimanually from the floor of the month and outside, and then with a sound. If one cannot feel the stone with the sound on account of its deep position or the marked swelling of the mucous membrane of the duct, one may pass a needle into the suspicious site; an exploratory puncture has frequently led to the right diagnosis. While sounding one must take care not to come in contact with the teeth, since this may simulate striking a stone. The reports of Alsberg and Gerota show that the Röntgen rays give valuable assistance in diagnosis.

If the inflammatory symptoms are in the foreground, the condition may be mistaken for an alveolar periostitis, especially when marked tenderness and perhaps trismus render examination difficult. With an acute inflammation of the gland itself, caused by stones, it may occasionally be very difficult to exclude a simple inflammation of the salivary gland or even of a lymph-node. Severe phlegmons of the floor of the mouth or abscesses secondary to a perforation of Wharton's duct may be mistaken for an angina phlegmonosa, an angina Ludovici, or, again, for an alveolar periostitis.

If the swelling of the salivary gland develops insidiously and without marked inflammatory symptoms, a malignant or an "inflammatory tumor" may be thought of, especially since swelling of the lymph-nodes and adhesions with the surrounding structures are rarely absent. Tuberculous lymphomata, gummata, and even bone tumors have been diagnosticated by mistake.

Prognosis.—Marean has pronounced sialolithiasis "une affection généralement plus incommode que dangereuse," and this applies to most of the cases. Yet it should not be looked upon as an innocent disease, for the disturbances are sometimes so considerable that they take all pleasure out of life. Above all, the system may suffer considerably from the constant recurrence of salivary colics by interfering with eating. If suppuration or perforation leads to an external salivary fistula, this will also be a very troublesome condition. The secondary phlegmons of the floor of the month are directly dangerous, for general sepsis or suffocation may follow; fortunately these complications are rare.

Treatment.—The stones should be removed from the month if at all possible. The exceptions to this rule are (1) if an external fistula leads to the concretion, (2) if this lies in an external abscess, and (3) when the parotid or submaxillary gland itself is the seat of the stone. Removal by way of the mouth may be very simple, if the stone is freely exposed or lies directly behind the orifice of the excretory duct; it will suffice to divide the tissues lying over it somewhat more extensively or to slit open the duct and grasp it with plain or dressing-forceps. Stones lying directly behind the orifice may occasionally be pressed out.

The removal may be difficult if the stone is located in the deeper parts of the excretory duct or if it is in the substance of the sublingual gland. It is best first to brush the mucous membrane with cocaine; after incising the mucous membrane the hemorrhage may be considerable and may obscure the field. If the stone is removed, the wound requires no further attention, and the after-treatment merely demands that the mouth be kept clean and be frequently rinsed with antiseptic gargles. Should the wounded duct remain open, a salivary fistula opening into the month forms, which is without significance. The relief experienced after the stone is extracted is very great and generally no recurrence follows; if it does, a fragment has been left behind or some small stones have been overlooked, hence' one must be sure to remove all concretions during the operation. If the stones are situated in the sublingual gland, this may be extirpated entirely if necessary.

Stones in the tissues of the parotid or submaxillary gland cannot be removed from the month; they must be exposed from without. This is not always easy, especially when numerous stones are embedded in dense masses of connective tissue and are firmly fixed. In case of the submaxillary gland, recurrences may best be avoided in such cases by removing the entire, often very adherent organ. Total extirpation of the parotid is, of course, not indicated; in its place the surgeon must carefully extract all stones and resect those portions of the gland which have undergone particularly severe changes. The facial nerve must be carefully protected.

INFLAMMATION OF THE SALIVARY GLAND.

According to the most recent investigations, it seems probable that all non-specific inflammations of the salivary gland start from the oral cavity, and, by ascending, involve either the chief excretory duct or the corresponding gland. This mode of infection was never disputed for inflammations of the excretory ducts and for certain forms of glandular disease, as in parotitis developing after mercurial stomatitis; for epidemic parotitis the evidence seemed less convincing, while for the so-called metastatic salivary gland inflammations, infection from the mouth was denied as being altogether improbable, since it was thought that the gland became infected by way of the circulation.

Although the cause of epidemic parotitis is not yet known, or at least the investigations on this point have not been verified, it can hardly be doubted that the process takes its start from the mouth. This mode of infection is rendered probable especially by the fact that a more or less intense stomatitis is never absent in the prodromal stage; from two to ten days before the parotid begins to swell (Soltmann).

The conditions are less clear with reference to the secondary inflammations of the salivary glands. Even at present these are frequently termed metastatic in view of the fact that their origin by way of the blood was generally accepted. Orth and Hanan especially have shown, by exact microscopical investigation, that even in septic patients metastatic sialoadenitis is caused by micro-organisms which reach the salivary ducts from the glands; hence this form of salivary inflammation has nothing to do with the metastatic distribution of a virus primarily located elsewhere.

For most, if not all, salivary gland inflammations, an infection from the mouth can be considered as settled. As an argument in favor of infection by way of the blood, it may be stated that foreign bodies are at times excreted by the parotid gland, and that quite recently typhoid bacilli and pneumococci, besides the usual pyogenic organisms, have repeatedly been found in the parotitis secondary to typhoid and pneumonia (Janowski, Duplay, Fishl). As far as the pneumococci at least are concerned, even these findings do not, however, militate against an infection of the mouth.

The inflammatory change may remain restricted to the chief excretory duct, or it may spread to the corresponding gland.

Inflammation of the Chief Excretory Ducts (Sialodochitis).— Besides the sialodochitis which has already been discussed in connection with foreign bodies and salivary stones, there is an independent inflammation of the chief excretory ducts, which, however, is rather rare. It involves the parotid duct more frequently than the duct of Wharton. The inflammation may affect more or less of the duct; it takes its origin from the mouth, but the evidence is not always so palpable as in a case of Walther, in which carious teeth at the level of the orifice of Steno's duct kept up the inflammation. Injuries are repeatedly mentioned as the primary incitor of the process.

Symptoms.—On examination the orifice of the duct will be found swollen, reddened, and somewhat gaping. If pressure is exerted upon the course of the duct, a droplet of pus or a fibrinopurulent clot will appear, to be followed by clear saliva (sialodochitis fibrinosa). The course of the disease is always chronic, but variations are present in as far as typical attacks of salivary retention dominate in some of the cases, while in others gradual and painless thickening and dilatation of the inflamed duct develop.

The attacks, if they occur, are exactly like those which have been discussed under foreign bodies and stones. An acute retention of saliva generally takes place while eating, a salivary tumor forms, the gland swells with a feeling of great tension, and the skin covering becomes hot and red. The flow of saliva is here not impeded by a foreign body, but the duct is occluded by a plug of pus and clots of fibrin. If the pressure of the pent-up saliva is sufficiently great, the plug is extruded from the duct; a large quantity of clear saliva discharges and the salivary tumor then becomes smaller. These paroxysms do not occur as often with sialodochitis as in the presence of foreign bodies or stones, and there may be intervals of weeks or months between the different attacks. But they generally last longer, and cases are known in which the swelling persisted eight days.

Gradually a permanent dilatation of the diseased duct with thickening of its walls develops so that the duct may sometimes be felt through the cheek as an elongated tumor. The corresponding gland may also show chronic inflammatory changes when the disease has lasted long, but these are only of secondary importance to the affection of the duct.

It is an interesting fact that air can collect in the dilated duct, esp
cially where the masseteric joins the glandular portion and in the begin
ning of the latter (Walther). By pressing upon the duct one can fe
distinct crepitation, and frothy fluid can be seen to discharge into th
mouth. The dilatation of the duct and the gaping of its orifice perm
the air to enter, especially if it is under high pressure. Hence suc
accumulations of air are especially found among glass-blowers (Tillau:
Regnault), and the primary disease also seems to stand in relation wit
their occupation. Sometimes the phenomenon is very marked; one ca
see how the air enters the duct on distending the cheek and how th
tumor again collapses on ceasing to blow.

Diagnosis.—The diagnosis of sialodochitis is not very difficult; i
typical attacks of salivary retention occur, the presence of a foreign bod
or of salivary stones must be excluded.

Treatment.—Since inflammation of the salivary ducts is a very obsti
nate disease, the treatment is not very satisfactory. Only in those case
in which a definite cause can be discovered can a rapid cure be achieve
by removing this, as by the extraction of carious teeth. For other case
sounding of the salivary duct is especially recommended; it can gen
erally be done easily and it gives relief, especially during the attack o
salivary retention, since the occluding plug is loosened and follows th
sound. According to the author's experience, dry warmth is also pleas
ant during the acute swelling. It is probable that the disease itself i
favorably influenced by carefully keeping the month clean and by inject
ing dilute antiseptic solutions into the diseased duct from an Anel syring
(Walther); with more marked dilatation of the duct, and particularl
when there is an accumulation of air, a systematic moderate compressio
is of decided advantage. In severe cases more energetic methods ma
be considered; thus, the injection of tincture of iodine into the disease
duct has been recommended. An operation consisting in splitting th
duct from the mouth is to be preferred. This splitting is indicated i
there are many painful attacks of salivary retention in succession; whicl
seriously affect the general well-being and the ability to work, and whicl
do not disappear after a less radical treatment.

Acute Inflammations of the Salivary Glands (Sialoadenitis Acuta)
—The inflammations of the salivary glands, especially those with acut
course, are by far more frequent and important than those which remair
restricted to the excretory ducts. The acute inflammations are divide
into primary and secondary. The parotid is most often the seat of th
disease, far less frequently one of the other large salivary glands.

Acute Primary Inflammations of the Salivary Glands.—Among thes
must be classified epidemic parotitis, known generally under the nam
mumps (Ziegenpeter, Bauernwetzel of the German, oreillons of th
French). Since this infectious disease possesses more medical than sur
gical interest, and only its complications really belong here, the descrip
tion will be brief.

The disease is probably contagious. It occurs in epidemics and
endemics (barracks, schools), and chiefly attacks children and young

individuals. After a period of incubation lasting about fourteen days, and a short prodromal stage which is always accompanied by stomatitis, the disease begins with a unilateral and general left-sided swelling of the parotid. The tumor is covered by tense, œdematous skin; it increases during the next few days with moderate fever and may become very extensive so as to reach to the clavicle. Regularly in a few days the other parotid begins to swell, though generally not to such an extent as the first one. The face then assumes a peculiarly idiotic expression which has given rise to the popular German names. Besides the parotid, the submaxillary and sublingual glands are sometimes affected on one or both sides, and it may even happen that the parotid remains free altogether, and that only the submaxillary gland, with or without the sublingual gland, is diseased.

The course is nearly always favorable. After about seven days the fever falls by crisis, the swelling recedes and has disappeared entirely in from two to four weeks at the most. In rare cases the tumor does not become smaller, but an abscess develops, and this is especially frequent in some epidemics. The suppuration may sometimes run a very severe course; it can simulate an angina Ludovici or can even develop into extensive, noma-like gangrene (Demme). Induration sometimes remain behind in the gland after the acute symptoms have subsided.

A special therapy is hardly indicated in the mild cases; keeping the mouth clean, cold or ice applications to the parotid gland, some fat for the skin to relieve the tension, rest in bed, and fluid diet are all that is necessary. When resolution is tardy, Strümpell recommends the application of iodoform collodion (1:15) or tincture of iodine with a brush. Abscesses are to be incised early.

The most important complication is the *inflammation of the testes.* No definite explanation for this occurrence has as yet been given. The inflammation generally develops several days after the beginning of the parotitis with renewed fever, but occasionally it may precede the affection of the salivary glands. It occurs almost exclusively in sexually mature individuals and generally affects only the testes, while the epididymis and seminal cord remain free. A very tender swelling forms of one, more rarely of both testicles, which, however, recedes in a short time with proper treatment, In other cases there is suppuration, and this complication does not seem to be so very rare. Remarkably often testicular atrophy develops after the orchitis of mumps; according to Kocher's calculation, in about one-third of the cases. The atrophy is either total or partial, and if both testicles are affected impotency may follow. Sorel has drawn attention to the fact that the atrophy is the more likely the longer the testicular swelling lasts. The treatment of metastatic orchitis consists in elevating the parts and carefully applying cold; if an abscess forms, it is to be incised at once, not only to remove the symptoms, but also to save as much as possible of the testicular tissue.

Of other complications oöphoritis must be mentioned, perhaps analogous to orchitis; mastitis, vulvovaginitis, prostatitis cystitis, and nephritis, endocarditis and pericarditis, affections of the eye (in all forms, from conjunctivitis to optic neuritis) and of the ear (otitis media, genera after the perforation of an abscess, unilateral and bilateral deafness a result of labyrinthine disease). Even without ear affections, seve cerebral symptoms are occasionally seen.

Besides the epidemic form, there are few *acute primary inflammatio of the salivary glands.* A sialoadenitis occurring in nurslings durii the first weeks and months of life is mentioned by Hennig, Mikulic and Kümmel; strangely, it affects only the submaxillary and sublingu gland and never the parotid.[1] Though the glands swell rapidly, wit fever, and abundant pus is discharged from their excretory ducts, th nutrition of the children need not suffer considerably. Only rarely doe the pus merely discharge through the excretory duct; generally mor extensive abscess-formation sets in.

In general the prognosis is favorable in otherwise healthy children, bu in weakly nurslings the suppuration and the difficulty of feeding owin; to the painful tumor may bring dangers with them.

The treatment consists in careful attention to the mouth with exten sive incision and drainage at the proper time.

Acute Secondary Inflammations of the Salivary Glands.—Secondar; sialoadenitis is of much greater surgical interest than primary, sinc it does not possess the benign character of the latter, but generall; leads to suppuration which often is of very progressive nature. Thes secondary inflammations may develop as a result of local or genera disease. Local affections are foreign bodies and stones, where th original inflammation of the duct has spread to the gland, infectiou: processes of the surroundings (suppuration of lymph-nodes, etc.), am the different forms of stomatitis, especially the mercurial, in which however, a direct participation of the salivary glands is not exclude (salivation while taking mercury). Very extensive and dangerous sup purations of the parotid may also develop after trauma (as the wouns inflicted by the blow of a broadsword).

A parotitis may accompany every severe disease, but particularly ofter it complicates the febrile infectious diseases, above all typhus, scarle fever, pneumonia, variola, cholera, plague, pyæmia, and sepsis. It is most frequent with typhus; rarely it is observed with severe non-infec tions disease, such as carcinoma. The parotitis developing after opera tions also belongs here and is of particular interest to the surgeon. Formerly it was believed that it only came on after ovariotomies, but it is now known that it may appear after other not necessarily severe interference, though most frequently after laparotomies.

In all of the last-mentioned secondary inflammations, the surgeon is probably also dealing with infections from the mouth. But other con ditions favoring the immigration and settling of bacteria also exist—a weakening of the general constitution and a diminution or cessation of the salivary secretion. The latter has been regularly observed in fever,

---

[1] Hennig thinks that these inflammations have some connection with puerperal diseases of the mother. This is probably not so for all cases.

and, according to Pawlow's animal experiments, also with operations on the abdominal cavity. Furthermore, the salivary and sexual organs are probably connected with each other by nerve-tracts, which would tend to explain parotitis after ovariotomy (Bumm, Eisenhardt). In fever and after operations the mouth is dry, so that the bacteria which wander in find conditions favorable.

This is also the place to mention that inflammatory changes in the salivary glands besides the functional disturbances of salivary secretions have also been observed in severe nervous diseases. Thus, Klippel found diffuse catarrhal inflammation in the large excretory ducts and degenerative processes in the gland-cells, in a patient suffering with tabes and salivation. A settling of bacteria at a predisposed site must also be assumed here.

Symptoms.—In discussing the clinical picture the author will limit himself to describing the acute sialoadenitis following infectious diseases and operations, since that dependent upon local causes, especially foreign bodies and stones, has already been discussed in detail.

Almost always the parotid gland alone is involved. The other salivary glands are affected considerably less often, and then either alone or in conjunction with the parotid. The beginning of the disease is about the same as with the epidemic form, but it is frequently obscured by the severe general disease. The time when the salivary glands become affected varies; with infectious diseases it may be soon after their onset, in other cases when the febrile stage approaches its termination. The sialoadenitis developing after operations, especially ovariotomies, generally. appears in from five to seven days, sometimes, however, as early as the third and in other cases as late as the eleventh or twelfth day.

If the gland affected is the parotid, a swelling develops in its region, with considerable constitutional disturbance and pains radiating to the head and face. The swelling generally manifests itself first in those parts which are not enclosed in tense fascia—that is, below the angle of the jaw at the neck. But soon the swelling is distinct in the other parts of the parotid; it reaches from the lower temporal regions to the neck and from the middle of the cheek to the mastoid process, and is most prominent in the region of the lobule of the ear, which is considerably elevated. The appearance is very characteristic on account of the broadening of the face, especially if the affection is bilateral. The disturbances increase with the swelling, the radiating pains become very intense, moving the jaws is hardly possible, and swallowing and breathing may occasionally be difficult. The skin covering the tumor becomes red, adherent, and œdematous, the superficial veins dilate, the entire face is somewhat swollen on account of the compression of larger venous trunks; not rarely the condition represents a progressive phlegmon from the very first. The facial nerve is generally not involved, but hearing may be very much reduced, especially in the bilateral affection, on account of the pressure of the swollen gland upon the auditory canal.

All symptoms increase up to the third or fourth day and then recede, or, much oftener, suppuration occurs. The presence of pus cannot always

be determined with safety by palpation, for the parotid is covered b
dense, unyielding fascia where it is accessible to touch. It may t
happen that the pus ruptures into the external auditory canal bef
distinct fluctuation can be detected at the cheek. Hence one can
depend upon this symptom, but must expect the process to termin
in suppuration if there is no recession by the fourth day, but inst
an additional, sometimes very rapid increase of the swelling with ris
temperature and aggravation of the general condition. In cases
spontaneous resolution the process runs its course in from one to t
weeks without other consequences except, perhaps, a permanent indu
tion of the gland, which has no significance. When suppuration occ
the course is, of course, more protracted, especially when suppurat
takes place in different sites or involves the entire parotid. Necro
of larger portions of the gland is then the rule, but it leads only exc
tionally to the formation of a salivary fistula.

Rather frequently the disease assumes a serious character and dea
are not rare. This unfortunate termination may have different caus
occasionally the process runs its course as a putrid phlegmon leading
extensive gangrene and general septic infection; in other cases the exi
comes on as a result of a spreading of the suppuration into the ret
vesical or antevisceral space or to the cranial cavity.

Since the posterior portion of the parotid in the region of the styl
process communicates with loose meshes of connective tissue which a
exceedingly well suited for the extension of a suppurative process,
follows that abscesses may burrow behind the pharynx and œsophag
into the mediastinum, and that perforations into the air-passages m
take place. The suppuration extends to the interior of the skull by w
of the vessels and nerves, and frequently by softened venous thron
(König). Thrombosis of the jugular veins and of the sinus has be
observed several times (Smith, Bloxam), also severe arterial and venc
hemorrhages and destruction of the facial nerve (Nélaton, Gillett
Rupture into the external auditory meatus is, as already mention
rather frequent, and may be followed by purulent otitis media and
its complications.

The same affection of the submaxillary gland is not nearly as comm
as that of the parotid; it resembles it closely, and also tends to spre
to the sublingual. The inflammation is generally less ominous, but
may also lead to very dangerous, deep phlegmons of the neck, runni
the course of an angina Ludovici.

Diagnosis.—The diagnosis of secondary salivary gland inflammatic
is not difficult. There will hardly be any doubt as to the nature of t
affection if a swelling of the parotid region develops with fever duri
a severe infectious disease or after an operation. The beginning of t
disease may indeed escape observation, and one may at first seek
the cause of fever in other places than about the salivary glands af
operations which otherwise may run a perfectly aseptic course. If t
submaxillary gland alone is diseased, the diagnosis may be more diffic
since the isolated involvement of the gland is very rare and enlargeme

of the submaxillary gland does not cause such characteristic symptoms as a swelling of the parotid. Here the condition may easily be mistaken for suppuration in the lymph-nodes, affections of the jaw, and deep phlegmons of the neck of other origin.

Prognosis.—The prognosis of secondary sialoadenitis is serious, since it affects individuals whose powers of resistance are diminished by the general febrile disease or by the operation. Besides this form of inflammation has little tendency to recede spontaneously; it has a decidedly malignant character and can give rise to the most serious complications. The older physicians were of the opinion that the development of a parotitis during an infectious disease might be a favorable sign; this idea is not now held and the appearance of this affection should be regarded as a very unwelcome and serious occurrence.

Treatment.—The treatment first of all consists in prophylaxis. The mouth of a patient seriously ill or recently operated upon should be regularly and thoroughly cleansed. It should be wiped out frequently with a piece of gauze dipped in water containing tincture of myrrh; this will be agreeable since it alleviates the thirst. As soon as the inflammation of the salivary glands has developed, expectant treatment should not be continued too long. During the first days an energetic application of cold is recommended, and particularly in the inflammations after operations one or two coats of iodine (König). If the process then shows no tendency to recede and the fever, swelling, and the various disturbances increase, one should not hesitate to resort to the knife, even if fluctuation is not certain in the accessible portions. Especially in those cases which run their course from the very beginning as progressive phlegmon or which are accompanied by gangrene, one should not postpone the incision too long. This is probably efficient by relieving the tension of the unyielding fascia and thus preventing as far as possible the dangerous extension of the process.

About the parotid the operation is best performed by dividing only the superficial layers and the parotid fascia with the knife and then continuing bluntly. The incisions are to be made so that they interfere as little as possible with the facial nerve and the larger vessels. Generally one encounters diffuse suppuration and necrosis, occasionally even gangrene, as soon as the fascia is divided, so that several incisions will be necessary. Loose necrotic shreds are removed and the deep incisions are carefully drained and tamponed. If the submaxillary gland is affected, the operation is simpler; the surgeon simply makes an incision into the submaxillary region, parallel with the margin of the jaw, and then pushes his way bluntly into the depths. Complications are guarded against and serious results forestalled if secondary inflammation of the salivary glands is treated according to these rules and if at the same time resort is had to proper measures to support the patient's strength.

Chronic Inflammations, Inflammatory Tumors.—The non-specific chronic inflammations, developing without definite cause (foreign body, stone, sialodochitis), are among the least known of the various diseases

be determined with safe
dense, unyielding fascia
happen that the pus ru
distinct fluctuation can
depend upon this symp
in suppuration if there
an additional, sometime
temperature and aggrav
spontaneous resolution
weeks without other con.
tion of the gland, which
the course is, of course,
takes place in different
of larger portions of the
tionally to the formation
   Rather frequently the
are not rare. This unfo
occasionally the process
extensive **gangrene and**
comes on as a result of
vesical or antevisceral sp
   Since the posterior po
process communicates w
exceedingly well suited
follows that abscesses m
into the mediastinum, a
take place. The suppur
of the vessels and nerv
(König). Thrombosis c
observed several times (.
hemorrhages and destr
Rupture into the exterr
rather frequent, and ma
its complications.
   The same affection of
as that of the parotid; i
to the sublingual. The
may also lead to very da
the course of an angina l
   Diagnosis.—The diagn
is not difficult. There w
affection if a swelling of
a severe infections disea:
disease may indeed escu
the cause of fever in otl
operations which otherw
submaxillary gland alone
since the isolated involve

and develop slowly on both sides without particular symptoms. They are observed after chronic lead-, copper-, mercury-, iodine-, and opium-poisoning, and are of no surgical interest. Perhaps the swellings of the salivary glands noticed in uræmia belong to the same class.

ACTINOMYCOSIS OF THE SALIVARY GLANDS.

Actinomycosis generally affects the salivary glands secondarily from foci in the soft parts and bones in the neighborhood; thus the author has operated upon a case in which a small focus in the lower jaw had spread to the entire parotid. Besides this secondary form, there also seems to be primary actinomycosis of the salivary glands, in which the fungus travels to the gland by way of the excretory duct. In advanced cases of parotid or submaxillary actinomycosis it is only rarely possible to determine where the process started; one may assume a primary involvement if the characteristic granules are discharged through the excretory ducts during an early stage.

A suppuration of the submaxillary gland, probably caused by *Leptothrix buccalis*, has been observed by König.

TUBERCULOSIS OF THE SALIVARY GLANDS.

The salivary glands belong to those organs which for a long time were considered immune to tuberculosis. Cases of tuberculosis, of the parotid especially, have been published only in recent years. With the exception of the doubtful cases of Tripier and Kiesow, there are up to the present 10 undoubted observations. Of these, 1 involved the submaxillary (Aievoli) and 9 the parotid (v. Stubenrauch, de Paoli (2), Leguen, Bockhorn, Parent, Küttner, Lecène, Mintz). A tuberculous affection of the sublingual gland has not yet been described.

Tuberculosis may affect the salivary glands in different ways. Most often extensive portions of the gland are involved diffusely. The tissue will then be grayish-white and brittle, as in a malignant tumor; or it is permeated by small or large caseous foci or abscesses, around which the gland-tissue is œdematous and brittle, occasionally indurated, owing to fibrous tissue. A more circumscribed tuberculosis is less frequent; this will have the appearance of a tumor, a cold abscess, or, as in v. Stubenrauch's case, a salivary cyst.

Tuberculosis of the salivary glands is generally a purely local disease. The cases observed were in non-tuberculous individuals from thirteen to sixty-one years old and without hereditary taint. The case observed by Mintz was an exception; the patient here was a child three years old with bad heredity. The majority were of more advanced age. The onset of the disease is very insidious; generally the swelling of the salivary glands is noticed only by accident and disregarded on account of the slow growth. The tumor grew rapidly in Mintz's case

_____ _____ developed aft

_____ _____ visible.

_____ _____ an enlargeme

_____ _____ fluctuating tum

_____ _____ of softer consistenc

_____ be reddened, tens

_____ diminish the size of t

_____ communication betwe

_____ duct, which explains t

_____ patient. Swelling of t

_____ tenderness has be

_____ in two cases. In thr

_____ of neuralgia, whi

_____ exacerbated with

_____ affected gland. Besid

_____ of de Paoli's case

_____ affection and the absen

_____ cannot be made with safet

_____ usually absent. In mo

_____ mixed tumor, or saliva

_____ character of the disca

_____ tion. In most cases it w

_____ decide between a parot

_____ developing in the interior

_____ swering the gland are mu

_____ resemblance to actinomycos

_____ favorable. Later examin

_____ fluence has always cured t

_____ in other respects, as o

_____ nature of the condition. On

_____ year after the operation t

_____ The facial paralysis fr

_____ treatment was not influenc

_____ operative paralysis and saliva

_____ culosis of the salivary glands

_____ is diseased, the entire gla

_____ tuberculosis total extirpation

_____ injuries and the serious ch

_____ appears in the form of a c

_____ the diseased portion. Whe

_____ they should be removed

_____ should be spared and t

_____ can generally be done witho

_____ are as a rule very brittle a

_____ soon. If one is not sure of t

diagnosis and has reason to suspect a sarcoma or a gumma, first excise a portion and let the result of the microscopical examination decide upon the further course.

SYPHILIS OF THE SALIVARY GLANDS.

Syphilis of the salivary glands is somewhat more frequent than tuberculosis, nevertheless the glands belong to those organs which only exceptionally are the seat of a syphilitic affection.

About 20 cases of syphilis of the salivary glands are found in literature, of which the large majority concern the parotid. The submaxillary and sublingual glands have been found diseased much more rarely; in one case a luetic affection of Blandin-Nuhn's gland was observed (Neumann). All cases of syphilis of the submaxillary, sublingual, and Blandin-Nuhn's gland belong to the late stage; the parotid, however, has also been found involved in the early stage. A case of hereditary syphilis of the parotid (Mandowsky-Schüller) is not generally regarded as unquestionable. Occasionally several salivary glands are affected at the same time.

It seems that a gummatous as well as an interstitial fibrous form of syphilis involves the salivary glands, as in the other organs, but the formation of gummata seems to predominate. On account of the infrequeney and curability of the disease, anatomical and histological examinations could be made only in a very few cases, but the changes which Mandowsky found in the parotid, and Lancereaux in the submaxillary, give evidence of the occurrence of both forms of syphilis.

Symptoms and Course.—It has been stated that the salivary glands have been found diseased in both the early and late stage of syphilis. Only Neumann has observed the disease in recent syphilitics, and in all of his 5 cases the parotid was involved. All of his patients were weak and anæmic individuals, in the first year of the disease, with macular and papular eruptions. In all there were more or less severe disturbances, profuse salivation, trismus, and difficulty in chewing and swallowing. The diseased salivary gland could be felt in front of the ear as a firm tumor, with irregularly nodular surface; the pre-auricular lymph-nodes were enlarged and could be well marked off from the parotid; and the skin covering the gland was reddened and œdematous to a greater or less extent. This form of parotitis usually ended in resolution and absorption.

The symptom-complex is different in the more common affection of the salivary glands in the later stages of lues. The onset of the disease is slow and without symptoms, and the patients only become aware of a glandular swelling after a distinct tumor is visible. The development of this generally requires two to three months. The tumor may reach the size of an apple, it is not very movable upon the deeper parts and the skin is also frequently adherent. Softening and rupture are not rare; large parts of the gland may then be destroyed through ulceration, and salivary fistulæ may remain behind (Lang). Often the disturbanc are only slight; in other cases the patients are much troubled by mark« salivation, difficulty in speaking, chewing, and swallowing, and gre tenderness over the tumor. Cases of lues with involvement of the sal vary glands have generally, though not always, belonged to the seve types.

Diagnosis.—The chief clinical interest rests on the diagnosis, for wh holds true for syphilis in general and for syphilitic disease of the moui in particular, also applies to prognosis and therapy here. It is of tl utmost importance to recognize this disease, since a gumma of the paroti may easily be mistaken for a malignant tumor and the patient thus sul jected to an operation endangering life. The diagnosis is facilitated t the fact that almost always other symptoms of syphilis can be discovered if these are absent it may be difficult or even impossible to recogniz the true nature of the disease.

The luetic parotitis of the early stages bears a certain resemblance t the common acute parotitis, but the inflammatory changes, the fun(tional disturbances, and the general symptoms of the acute infectio are so much more pronounced with the latter that a mistake can b easily avoided, especially if other early syphilitic manifestations ai present at the same time. The differential diagnosis between gumm and tumor may be much more difficult. This refers less to the slov movable benign tumors than to the malignant growths, and it is ju: here where the correct diagnosis is of such paramount importance. 1 other symptoms of syphilis do not aid, it is hardly advisable to insur the diagnosis by a course of antiluetic treatment, since the proper tim for the operation may thus be missed. In such cases a piece should b excised for examination. The diagnosis between syphilis, simple chroui inflammations, and tuberculosis may also be very difficult, but is of le: practical importance.

Especially in the case of the parotid gland, it may be difficult to decid whether one is dealing with a gummatous affection of the gland itself c of a lymph-node, for a gummatous lymph-node in the interior of th parotid gland will in general give the same symptoms as a gumma of th parotid itself. But it is of more theoretical than practical interest t distinguish between the two.

SYMMETRICAL DISEASE OF THE LACHRYMAL AND SALIVAR' GLANDS (MIKULICZ'S DISEASES).

Mikulicz has called attention to this peculiar condition as being i typical, well-marked disease. It is characterized by prominent sym metrical swellings of the lachrymal and salivary glands.

The clinical course is as follows: The patients are generally indi viduals in the twenties or thirties, who are otherwise healthy; mor rarely they are younger or older. A uniform swelling of all the organ of the head belonging to the type of the salivary glands appears ver slowly in the course of months. The glands involved are both parotids, with their accessory organs, the submaxillary, sublingual, and lachrymal glands. (Fig. 270.)

Besides this, v. Mikulicz, Tietze, and Kümmel saw enlargement of the palatine glands, Kümmel swelling of Blandin-Nuhn's gland, and Osler hypertrophy of the labial and buccal glands. Not all these glands need be affected in every instance, but in order that a case be considered one of Mikulicz's disease it is necessary that several large glands of the head, of the type of the salivary gland, be diseased. The affection need not be equally severe on both sides.

The swelling gradually increases in size and may reach varying degrees in the course of years. Thus the parotid glands have attained the size

FIG 270.

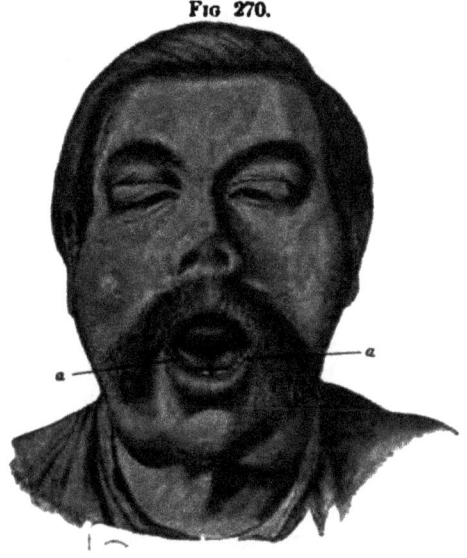

Symmetrical affection of the lachrymal and salivary glands. *a.* The enlarged sublingual gland. (After Mikulicz.)

of a goose-egg to that of a fist, and other glands have been found increased to twice their size. In all cases the entire gland is swollen uniformly and the outlines of the tumor correspond to the enlarged contours of the gland. The disease never spreads beyond the gland capsule, hence the tumor remains movable under the skin and mucous membrane and upon the deeper parts. The consistence is generally rather firm, less often soft, but not fluctuating; the surface is smooth or distinctly lobulated. Inflammatory symptoms do not occur. In some cases there was a general swelling of the lymph-nodes of a moderate degree (Hirsch), Osler, and in one instance a palpable enlargement of the spleen was present (Osler). Blood-examination was always negative.

Symptoms.—The disturbances are generally not severe. The tumo are not tender, they only cause disfigurement and, owing to their siz occasionally difficulty in speaking and chewing. Serious general di turbances have not been observed. The mucous membranes may gi rise to very troublesome symptoms; above all, a very disagreeable dr ness of the mouth and conjunctivæ was repeatedly complained of, whi is probably to be ascribed to imperfect function of the diseased gland Falling out of the teeth has also been observed.

Course.—The course of the disease varies. In some cases the tumo remain stationary after they have slowly attained a considerable siz In other cases the tumors recede after intercurrent febrile disease or a a result of treatment.

Prognosis.—The prognosis is therefore favorable as far as life is coi cerned; the deaths which were observed had nothing to do with Mik licz's disease. No cases passed into a pernicious form. Concerning cur the prognosis does not seem to be so absolutely favorable, for in son cases the use of drugs was without effect or renewed swelling followe after a temporary improvement. Surgical interference, which is no however, indicated in all cases (parotid), guards against recurrence.

Diagnosis.—The diagnosis is easy and mistakes are avoided by tl symmetrical involvement, the uniform enlargement of the affected gland the absence of inflammatory symptoms, and the absolute restriction the process to the diseased organ. Outwardly there is a certain resen blance to malignant lymphomata, which may be increased by the fa that the spleen may be enlarged, and that a general though slight swel ing of the lymph-nodes may be present. Kümmel speaks of trans tional forms between Mikulicz's disease and this malignant process.

This corresponds with the explanation which v. Mikulicz, Tietze, an Kümmel give to this disease. Since microscopically the most prominei feature is a diffuse, very marked infiltration of round cells, these autho believe that there is a new formation of lymphadenoid tissue, which spread around the acini as centres and which leads to destruction of tl specific gland-tissue. Tietze regards the process as similar to the hype plastic changes so frequently observed in the lymphatic ring of tl pharynx; he terms the disease "adenoid proliferation of the lachryma and salivary glands," while Kümmel suggests the name "achroöcytosis.

The process is interpreted differently by Hirsch as a result of h microscopical examinations. He found the same extensive and unifori collection of round cells, but besides that an independent degeneratio of epithelial cells and a transition of the round-cell infiltration into coi nective tissue. Since in his case only stony-hard, shrunken rudimen of the glands were left, he considers the chief lesion to be a "cirrhosis the lachrymal and salivary glands."

The etiology of this peculiar disease is as little settled as its patholog Most authors speak of a chronic infectious process in which the inci ing agent passes from the mucous membrane to the excretory ducts an finally reaches the glands. No relation to syphilis or tuberculosis coul be discovered.

Treatment.—Arsenic and potassium iodide have repeatedly had good therapeutical effects. If medicines fail, extirpation of the diseased glands is indicated, provided marked disfigurement or functional disturbances make it necessary. If an operation is decided upon, the glands in question should be removed completely, since recurrences have been observed after partial excisions. For this reason surgical interference is not recommended in case of the parotid, whose enlargement causes the most marked disfigurement, for its total extirpation is not without dangers and the disfigurement will be greater than before.

CYSTS OF THE SALIVARY GLANDS.

The salivary glands not rarely show retention of secretion; it has already been stated that this occurs as "tumor salivalis" with inflammations of the chief excretory ducts or their surroundings, with cicatricial stenosis, foreign bodies, stones, and exceptionally with tumors compressing the excretory duct. Generally the saliva again finds exit and the retention is transient, or it occurs periodically; if, however, the closure is permanent, true cystic dilatations form. According to the seat of the obstruction, these involve either the excretory duct or the gland, so that cysts of the salivary ducts and cysts of the salivary glands must be distinguished.

Cysts of the Salivary Ducts.—Cystic dilatation of the excretory duct occurs with all the large salivary glands, especially with the parotid and submaxillary. Such cysts have also been repeatedly observed in case of Blandin-Nuhn's gland (Stoltz, Dubois, Foderl).

If the cases of salivary retention, which do not belong in this chapter, are excluded, it is found that cysts of the salivary ducts depend either upon a permanent, acquired, and generally cicatricial occlusion, or else upon a congenital imperforation of the chief duct. In some rare cases, which have not been thoroughly explained, this mechanical factor cannot, however, be discovered. A "deficient power of propulsion on the part of the walls of the salivary ducts owing to inflammatory changes" or a "primary hypertrophy of the walls with widening of the lumen" has been suggested in these cases. Sonnenburg even noticed a congenital cystic dilatation of Wharton's duct without evident obstruction.

If the parotid duct or Wharton's duct is cystically dilated, examination reveals an elongated, cylindrical or spindle-shaped tumor, whose long axis lies in the direction of the diseased duct. The dilatation, evident externally, corresponds either to the entire length of the duct or to only part of it; frequently the corresponding salivary gland itself is also enlarged, for the retention of secretion and the dilatation must naturally be transmitted to the entire system of excretory ducts if the chief duct is occluded. The tumors are generally thin-walled and covered with normal skin or mucous membrane; they are sharply circumscribed and not tender. On account of the yielding floor of the mouth, fluctuation can be elicited less readily with cysts of Wharton's duct than with those of Steno's duct. The cysts contain saliva, which, as in a ranula, undergoes considerable chemical changes in the course of time. In a case observed by Latour-Marliac the inner surface of the wall of a very large salivary cyst of the cheek was incrusted with lime.

Sultan found a peculiar condition in a child three and one-half months old. Here there was a bilateral congenital occlusion of the submaxillary duct which gave rise to two cysts in the region of the sublingual gland the size of a plum-pit. Each of these cysts gave off an anterior cylindrical process, whose end projected 1 cm. into the mouth and which crossed with the opposite one in front of the lingula of the tongue. The most interesting feature of this case was the free projection of the ends of the tumor underneath the oral mucous membrane; probably the accumulation of secretion in the excretory ducts permitted these to be raised from the floor of the mouth and to assume an erect position, and the freely movable mucous membrane of the mouth readily adjusted itself to this change of form.

The excretory ducts can only be sounded in those rare cases in which there is no mechanical obstruction, or at least an incomplete one. If pressure is exerted upon the cyst in such cases, saliva will flow out of the orifice of the excretory duct; if, however, the latter is closed, sounding will fail, and if any irritating substance, such as a drop of vinegar, be placed on the mucous membrane of the month, it is easily seen, especially upon the sublingual caruncles, that saliva flows only from the healthy side.

If the cyst is due to dilatation of an excretory duct of Blandin-Nuhn's gland,[1] a transparent, more or less mesially placed, thin-walled cyst is found about the tip of the tongue or directly underneath it. The appearance may be that of a malformed tip of the tongue; in young children the cyst often projects between the lips.

It would be fair to assume that salivary cysts caused by an occlusion of the chief duct show an unlimited growth. But this is not so, and clinical experience teaches that such cysts do not reach an excessive size. After some time they remain stationary, and may even become smaller spontaneously where the permanent occlusion of the duct has led to atrophy of the corresponding gland. In other cases there will be a spontaneous rupture, with or without the aid of an infection, and a salivary fistula will form. If perforation takes place into the month, this is akin to a spontaneous cure; if, however, a cyst of the parotid duct breaks through the skin, a troublesome external salivary duct-fistula results. This will also be the case if one carelessly punctures or incises such cysts from the outside. Congenital cysts of Wharton's duct or of the excretory duct of Blandin-Nuhn's gland interfere considerably with the nutrition of the nursling, since they make the act of sucking difficult; hence their operative removal should not be postponed.

Treatment.—The treatment must supply a new permanent opening of the dilated portion of the excretory duct into the mouth. The simplest

---

[1] Concerning cysts of the sublingual gland, see under "Ranula."

way to do this is to follow the principle of Deguise's operation for salivary duct-fistulæ (see above). As near as possible to the natural orifice, a needle with silk thread is passed from the mouth through mucous membrane and cyst-wall and out again at some distance. By firmly tying the threads, necrosis of the constricted bridge of tissue sets in and an internal salivary fistula forms which will functionate like a normal orifice. It is still better to open the cyst from the mouth by means of an incision, or to excise a piece of the wall and then to sew together the margins of the incision in the mucous membrane and in the cyst-wall; in this way a stenosis or a renewed closure of the artificial fistula is prevented. If a dilatation of Steno's duct has been wrongly opened from the cheek, the resulting external fistula must be converted into an internal one by one of the usual methods.

In those rare cases in which there is a cystic dilatation of the excretory duct and no mechanical occlusion or only an imperfect one, good results are obtained by methodically sounding with bougies gradually increasing in size, and systematically emptying and compressing the cyst.

Cysts of the Salivary Glands.—Contrasted with the cysts of the salivary ducts are those of the salivary glands. They are caused by the occlusion of a smaller excretory duct, hence are also retention-cysts.

Pathology.—Pathologically they are generally the result of a chronic interstitial inflammation which leads to proliferation and sclerosis of the connective tissue. It follows that the small excretory ducts will be compressed and occluded in certain places, so that the secretion will accumulate and cause a dilatation of the duct. If the same process goes on in different neighboring ducts, the resulting small cysts will unite and form a larger one. In this way voluminous cysts may form whose lining of cylindrical epithelium, at first well preserved, will gradually be much flattened and in greater part destroyed. The irritation of the growing cyst will set up a reactive proliferation of connective tissue and thus lead to an encapsulation, which is not, however, very marked. It will also be followed by pressure-atrophy of the surrounding gland-tissue, part of which will enter into the formation of the connective-tissue capsule of the cyst.

Cysts of the salivary glands are rather rare, at least as far as the parotid and submaxillary are concerned. The sublingual glands seem to be affected more frequently, for most sublingual cysts termed ranula are to be regarded as retention-cysts of this gland (see Ranula). Only cysts of the parotid and submaxillary will be spoken of here.

In general cysts of the salivary glands remain rather small and reach the size of a hen's egg only exceptionally. They are usually single, less often multiple; though they are most commonly unilocular, distinct septa may be found which prove their origin from a number of smaller cysts. The contents of the cysts are a clear, colorless, stringy fluid, which generally has already lost the characteristic properties of saliva.

Symptoms.—Clinically the salivary gland cysts give symptoms rather late, since they grow slowly and cause disturbance only after they have attained considerable size. Occasionally a more rapid growth is observed owing to increased transudation from the numerous capillaries in walls, and the tumor may only be detected after this sudden enlargem **Diagnosis.**—The diagnosis is easy after the cyst has reached a (siderable size and when it is seated superficially; here one can e fluctuation and sometimes even detect transparency. It is frequently possible to recognize small and deep-seated cysts without an explora puncture, especially when they involve the parotid. One must be car to distinguish between these cysts and cystically degenerated benign malignant tumors. Real tumors, especially those of the mixed ty frequently give such distinct evidences of fluctuation that one is ineli to diagnosticate a cyst; here an exploratory puncture also clears up condition. A case of v. Stubenrauch shows that the infrequent saliv tuberculosis may also appear in the form of a salivary cyst.

Treatment.—Therapeutically puncture, with the injection of tinct of iodine, is indicated. König has achieved good results in this w Injections, drop by drop, of liquefied zinc chloride, and injection; concentrated or of 1 per cent. carbolic acid have also been recommend Simple incision is not advisable; extirpation of the cyst is the sa procedure, but is frequently rendered difficult owing to insuffici encapsulation and abundant hemorrhage. In case of the submaxill gland it is therefore best to extirpate the entire gland. As far as parotid is concerned, König recommends that the injection of tinct of iodine first be given a trial; the cyst should be enucleated only a: this injection has failed.

Other Cystic Structures.—Little is known of other cystic structu of the salivary glands and many observations are questionable. Echi coccus cysts of the parotid have been described by Vieusse,Schuh(Salz and quite recently by Subbotic. A cyst with atheromatous contents large as a good-sized hen's egg, has been observed by Köuig. It seated upon the anterior surface of the parotid and was movable un the skin.

Richet speaks of a dental cyst of the parotid (?) communicating w the mouth.

TUMORS OF THE SALIVARY GLANDS.

Of all the diseases of the salivary glands, their tumors are the m important, and, for the surgeon as well as the pathologist, the m interesting. Despite a large literature there is much to be found h which is not clear and not settled. This applies especially to the called "mixed tumors," which to a certain degree are typical for salivary glands. The term mixed tumor is considered by many, es cially French authors, to refer to the occurrence of both epithelial a connective-tissue elements in one and the same tumor. The oth predominatingly German, theory assumes that the different types cells found in the tumors have one and the same origin, and that t origin is of endothelial nature.

Tumors of the salivary glands may be subdivided as follows:
Connective-tissue tumors:
  Angioma.
  Lymphangioma.
  Lipoma.
  Pure fibroma.
  Pure myxoma.
  Sarcoma.
Mixed tumors.
Epithelial tumors:
  Adenoma.
  Carcinoma.
The tumors of the three large salivary glands are pathologicall
in every way, and the clinical differences are due only to their d
position; hence the tumors of all three glands may be described to

Connective-tissue Tumors.

Angioma.—Angiomata of the salivary glands are rare. In tl
1889 Hartmann collected 9 cases, but not all of these are unquesti
An undoubted case of angioma of the parotid has been obser
Hartmann himself, and another one has been described by Bidc
similar tumor of the submaxillary has been seen by Böckel. The
should not be mistaken for ordinary subcutaneous angiomata,
are located in the neighborhood of the salivary glands, but not
glands themselves. Hence the diagnosis "angioma of the s
glands" is unquestionable only if an involvement of the glanc
has been proved by microscopical examination.

Symptoms.—Clinically the tumors behave just like ordinary
taneous angiomata. Like these they show a tendency to increase 1
and hence demand treatment.

Treatment.—The smaller angiomata are preferably extirpat
in all cases operated upon, the hemorrhage from the salivary
was very considerable, though not dangerous. If the tumor is to
or the child too weak for extirpation, alcohol injections or elec
with long needles penetrating large areas of the angioma are indic

smooth surface may show a lobulated structure; if the cellu
project above the level of the incision, it appears granu
sarcomata are always encapsulated, hence their extirpation
cult.

Spindle-cell sarcomata may also be well circumscribed a
ready enucleation, yet they are not always of this relatively l
acter, especially when spindle and round cells are both pres
latter case and where the tumor is made up of round cell
course is often exceedingly malignant. When involving t
illary gland, they may break through the skin or into the c
mouth.

Diagnosis.—These malignant growths may occasionally
great difficulties in diagnosis; they may especially be mistake
matory processes when they diffuse themselves over the
in a short time, as is usually the case. In a case observed
the direct transition of a chronic inflammatory into a sarcoma
could be followed up microscopically by repeated explorato
Even a histological examination may be unable to distingu
sarcomata of the salivary glands and those developing from
nodes of the parotid and submaxillary region. Concernin
ential diagnosis of malignant tumors of the salivary glands, s

Treatment.—The extirpation of tumors of this kind mus
include a complete removal of the corresponding salivary {
may be very difficult and gives little hope of a permanent

As everywhere else, the most unfavorable form of sar
melanosarcoma. It is occasionally characterized here by a
amount of pigment.

Mixed Tumors.

Mixed tumors are the most important of all the tumors of
glands. They relatively often involve the parotid, less fre
submaxillary. It is not known with certainty whether or no
the sublingual gland. Perhaps some of the sublingual tumo
as adenomata really belong to this group.

Pathology.—Mixed tumors of the salivary glands are ge
encapsulated and their cut surface shows a manifold struc
to cellular, sarcomatous, and carcinomatous portions are fo
tissue and very characteristic inclusions of cartilage, which
abundant that microscopically the tumor may appear like a p
droma. The formation of cysts is rather frequent, calci
ossification less so. The seat of the tumor within the sal
varies; it may develop in its centre and be surrounded on
gland-tissue; it may be placed outside of the gland and cause
upon its surface; or, finally, it may be connected with the glan
of a pedicle. Occasionally the connection is so loose that on
the salivary origin of the tumor. In order to be sure of thi
at any rate find the tumor beneath the parotid fascia in case o

gland. The direction in which the tumor will continue to grow varies with the site of development. For instance, if the tumor starts from the upper and inner glandular portions of the submaxillary gland, the floor of the mouth will project; from the parotid the growth can extend to the pharynx (Périer, Mixter), or it may appear upon the middle of the cheek if it originates from an accessory parotid. In rare cases multiple tumor formations may occur in the parotid as well as in the submaxillary; this explains that a recurrence, also of a benign character, may sometimes appear after the extirpation of a benign form of the tumor.

The nature of mixed tumors is not yet settled. It has already been mentioned that two opposite views are held; according to one the tumors are of connective-tissue origin, according to the other they consist of both epithelial and connective-tissue elements.

The adherents of the first theory, which is supported by Kaufmann, Nasse, and Volkmann, regard the mixed tumors as endotheliomata. They are of the opinion that true epithelial cells do not occur in the tumors, that the epithelial-like strands characteristic of mixed tumors are really the descendants of the endothelial cells and hence of the same class as the fixed connective-tissue, cartilage cells, and mucous cells. Volkmann thinks that the epithelial-like cells can arise from proliferated cartilage cells and mucous cells just as they can be proliferation of endothelial cells, owing to their genetic equivalency; on the other hand, they can also form cartilaginous, mucous, and fibrillary connective tissue.

Opposed to this view there is another, encouraged chiefly by French authors, according to which mixed tumors of the salivary glands contain epithelial as well as connective-tissue elements. Recently this theory has found more adherents, even in Germany. Among these are Wilms and Hinsberg in particular, whose investigations deserve especial attention on account of their embryological basis. It does not lie within the scope of this text-book to discuss these difficult, purely pathological questions with more detail, yet the author cannot fail to refer particularly to the comprehensive investigations of Wilms.

Whether one looks upon the strands of cells in these tumors as endothelial or epithelial, one must confess that the mixed salivary tumors afford much that is in favor of the theory of germinal displacement. With König one has the impression that the cartilaginous or even osseous tissue within the salivary gland is something entirely foreign.

Etiology.—Mixed tumors generally appear during the second and third decades, but their congenital occurrence has been observed, and on the other hand they have been seen to develop in old age. The male sex is affected somewhat more frequently than the female. The left-sided salivary glands are diseased more often than the right. Inheritance has no influence. Injuries and inflammations are regarded as etiological factors; it is particularly stated of the latter that they predispose the salivary glands to tumor formation.

Symptoms.—Clinically the mixed tumors in the large majority of cases are sharply circumscribed and well defined from the surroundings,

Their seat varies according to the part of the gland to which they belong. If they involve the anterior portion of the parotid, the lateral parts of the cheek will stand out; if seated in the middle of the gland, they will surround the external ear from below, elevate the auricle in a characteristic manner, and may even obliterate its lower portion if they are sufficiently large. (Fig. 271.) In another case the tumor may fill the retromaxillary fossa, and extend to the neck, as well as forward over the lower jaw and backward over the sternomastoid (Kaufmann). It has already been mentioned that they may chiefly develop toward the pharynx. If the tumor has its starting point in the submaxillary gland, more or less of it will appear beneath the margin of the jaw in the submaxillary region. (Fig. 272.) A protrusion toward the mouth is rare; if it occurs, an external tumor can be detected at the same time.

FIG. 271.   FIG. 272.

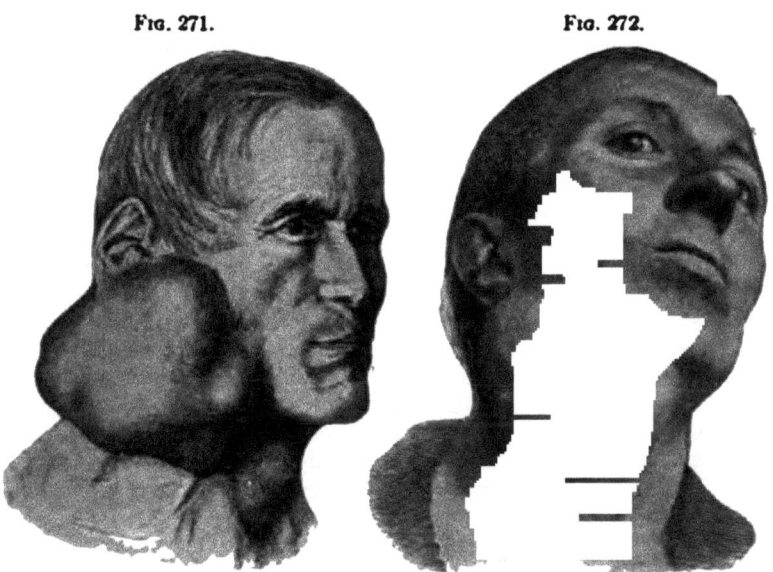

Mixed tumor of the parotid. (After a case in v. Bruns' clinic.)   Mixed tumor of the submaxillary gland. (After a case in v. Bruns' clinic.)

Mixed tumors may attain a very considerable size; about the parotid they have been seen almost as large as a man's head, and about the submaxillary, of the volume of a child's head. The form is rounded, or oval and elongated; the surface is smooth and occasionally lobulated where there is no cartilage, and generally very nodular where there is. The consistence varies. Some mixed tumors, especially those which contain much mucous tissue, are distinctly pseudofluctuating, even when no real softening can as yet be detected macroscopically. On the other hand, tumors with much cartilage have a very firm consistency, which does not, however, seem to be uniform, for besides the cartilaginous portions there will also be soft and almost fluctuating areas, es cially at the summits of the larger eminences. The free mobility of tumor under the skin and upon the deeper parts is characteristic.

The disturbances caused by the tumors are generally slight as l as they have not reached an excessive size and have not changed tl benign character. They are seldom tender on pressure, while sp taneous radiating pains are occasionally complained of. A marl increase of salivary secretion has repeatedly been observed, especia where the submaxillary gland was affected; this salivation can be troublesome that the patients demand an operation for this sympto alone (Rengrueber). Difficulty in chewing and swallowing accompan submaxillary tumors which have spread markedly toward the mou Difficulty in swallowing and breathing was observed in exceptional ca when a submaxillary tumor elevated the floor of the mouth and press the base of the tongue against the posterior pharyngeal wall, or when parotid tumor developed chiefly toward the pharynx. A parotid tum may also compress the auditory meatus and diminish hearing; it c cause facial paralysis, but only when the benign tumors have attain a very considerable size.

All these disturbances are not, however, observed frequently; in ge eral the patients are troubled but little, and there are only two reaso which bring the patient to the surgeon, the disfigurement and the i creased growth which generally comes on after some time. In the fi years the increase in size is extremely slow; in parotid and submaxilla tumors eight years on the average elapsed between the time the tum was first noticed and the operation. The increased growth, developi as it does without known cause, brings the patients to the surgeon mu sooner than the disfigurement, to which they become accustomed. A this acceleration of growth is indeed a symptom which should cau apprehension. Frequently the tumors retain their harmless charact with it, but it also occurs not infrequently that the originally beni tumor suddenly turns exceedingly malignant. It recurs very so and kills the patient in a surprisingly quick time by metastasis in tl lymph-nodes and the inner organs. Besides such secondarily mali nant tumors there are also mixed growths which are malignant fro the start; clinically they are closely allied to pure sarcomata and ca cinomata. It is a remarkable fact that the non-cartilaginous neoplasr show a much higher percentage of malignancy than those which conta cartilage, at least as far as the submaxillary gland is concerned.

Diagnosis.—The general diagnostic characteristics of mixed tumo are not very marked. Their position as well as many other sigr has as little diagnostic value as the age of the patient; but if sever symptoms are present at the same time, one can make a probab diagnosis of benign mixed tumor of the parotid or submaxillar This applies to cases in which a tumor has been evident in the r spective regions for years; where the growth has been slow and h perhaps increased after the tumor had been in existence for son time, and where the examination shows a freely movable growth whic has never been the seat of marked disturbances and which is covered by normal skin, and is neither tender nor spontaneously painful. The diagnosis is certain if the characteristic nodular surface and firm consistence of cartilaginous tumors are present. A symptom of great value for the diagnosis is the free mobility upon the underlying structures; it can even be elicited as a rule with the largest benign growths. Surgeons should never fail to examine tumors of the submaxillary region from the month, since in this way important facts may be learned concerning the relation of the tumor to the salivary gland, and the diagnosis may also be assisted in other ways.

Above all, benign mixed tumors must be differentiated from lymphomata. Of these, only a few rare forms come into consideration here, such as lymphatic tuberculosis, which remains restricted to one lymphnode, and certain glandular hyperplasiæ, which also involve only one gland and which are characterized by a slow, painless course and absence of all tendency to break down. They occur in apparently healthy individuals as a result of long-continued irritation, and since they generally do not attain a considerable size, they are only of importance in the differential diagnosis of the smaller salivary tumors. Finally must be mentioned a rare form of hard, malignant lymphoma described by Riedel. Here there is at first an enlargement of a single, isolated gland, which may possibly be extirpated; the typical symptoms of malignant lymphoma only come on much later.

Besides lymphatic tumors, the following conditions may be mistaken for salivary growths: in the parotid the rare enchondromata of the auditory meatus and lipomata lying upon the parotid; in the submaxillary gland, fibromata of the neck if they involve the submaxillary region.

The differential diagnosis from other salivary diseases includes a few rare tumors, such as adenomata and fibromata, which clinically cannot be distinguished from mixed tumors; and, above all, the cysts. The consistence of many of the tumors may so closely suggest fluctuation that only an exploratory puncture will decide whether or not the surgeon is dealing with a cyst. This refers especially to tumors containing mucous tissue; but in order to simulate fluctuation it is by no means necessary that the mucous parts predominate or that they lead to cyst formation.

The differential diagnosis of the primary or secondary malignant mixed tumor is more difficult than that of the benign tumors of this group. In order to avoid repetition the diagnosis of all malignant tumors will be discussed together under carcinomata.

Prognosis.—The prognosis of mixed tumors is in general a favorable one, but one must always remember that innocent tumors, which in the course of years have slowly increased in size, may suddenly turn malignant and then run a course which could not be more malignant in the most severe type of sarcoma. For submaxillary tumors the author estimates that this phenomenon of sudden malignancy occurs in about 11 per cent. of the cases, hence a more rapid growth of the tumors must always be regarded as an ominous sign. If a benign mixed tumor recurs after it has been extirpated, this in itself is no proof that the tumor has changed its character, for the recurrence has been known to retain the benign character of the original growth. These recurrences find their explanation in that portions of the capsule or of the tumor have remained behind after the operation. It may also happen that there are multiple tumors and that nodules have been overlooked, or finally there may be a certain disposition toward tumor formation on the part of the mother-tissue. But the recurrences after the extirpation of the originally benign tumors may also show a very malignant tendency and may rapidly grow to such dimensions that further operating is impossible. The less common primary malignant mixed tumors have the same prognosis as pure sarcomata or cellular carcinomata, from which they can hardly be distinguished clinically.

Treatment.—The treatment consists in extirpation, which should be performed as early as possible, since one can never guarantee the benign character of the growth. In benign encapsulated tumors the technic is exceedingly simple, but the capsule must always be removed completely with the tumor to guard against recurrence. In case of the parotid the facial nerve should be taken into consideration; it can be avoided in most cases by dividing only the soft parts covering the tumor with a knife down to the capsule, and then dissecting out the growth bluntly with a closed, curved scissors. Where the tumor is surrounded on all sides by parotid tissue, the surgeon must proceed more carefully, and all larger branches of the facial nerve should be lifted off bluntly as soon as they come to view; in such cases it is advisable to carry the incision parallel to the direction of the nerve. In tumors of the submaxillary gland it is desirable to combine the technically simple extirpation of the gland with the removal of the tumor to be certain that all is removed. Malignant mixed tumors require the same treatment as other malignant neoplasms of the salivary glands—that is, the entire gland must be removed even where it is the parotid.

Epithelial Tumors.

Adenoma.—Opinions are still divided as to whether adenomata of the salivary glands occur; some of the more recent authors, as Volkmann, believe that most of these tumors belong to the mixed growths. As opposed to this it must be stated that Nasse has seen 4 pure adenomata of the parotid, and that there can be no doubt as to the correctness of his observations; yet it is probable that many other cases described as adenomata really should be classed among the group of mixed tumors. Adenomata of all three large salivary glands, including the sublingual (Wagner, Nicoladoni), have been observed. Clinically they differ very little from mixed tumors; they generally grow slowly, are encapsulated and of glandular appearance, and occasionally have a remarkably soft consistence, so that their contents exude in masses not unlike granular, boiled rice when the capsule tears. Wölfler observed a peculiar, locally malignant adenoma of the submaxillary gland in a man fifty years old.

The tumor recurred twice, and finally was inoperable on account of its local extension; metastases did not occur and the lymph-nodes were not involved.

Even in the more recent text-books hypertrophy of the salivary glands is still spoken of as a distinct form of tumor. It is very possible that there is a true hypertrophy of these organs, but it is probably not common and most cases described under this name are in all likelihood real tumors or chronic inflammatory processes.

Carcinoma.—Though relatively rare, carcinomata are the most important tumors of the salivary glands, next to the mixed tumors. They

Fig. 273.

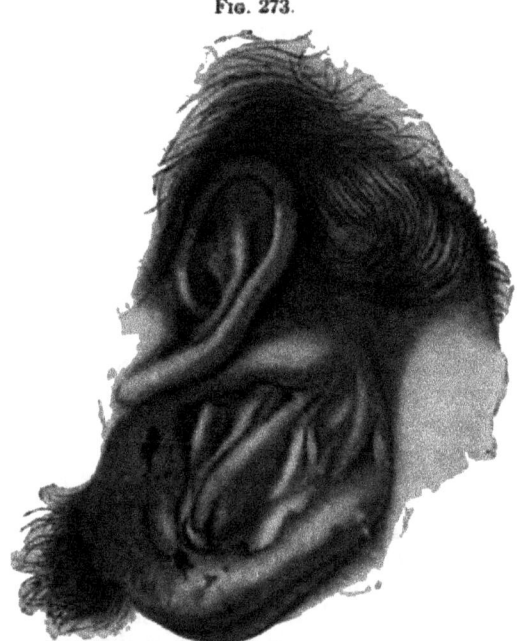

Carcinoma of the parotid in a man aged seventy-six years.

most frequently involve the parotid, considerably less often the submaxillary. Concerning carcinoma of the sublingual gland the opinions are divided, for some authors consider them rare, while others believe that many cancers of the floor of the mouth start from this gland. At any rate there is no clinical difference between carcinomata of the sublingual gland and those of the floor of the mouth, and it will suffice if reference is made to the latter.

Formerly most tumors of the salivary glands were considered to be carcinomata. The great similarity of parts of mixed tumors and carcinomata has already been mentioned. Hence it must be asserted that pathologically a tumor can only be looked upon as a salivary carcinoma if the direct development of the epithelial tabs and strands from t epithelial elements of the gland is evident. It may be difficult for t microscopist to decide whether he is dealing with a primary carcinor of the salivary glands when a carcinoma of the neighborhood exten to the glands or when a malignant mixed tumor of carcinomatous appea ance has diffusely infiltrated them.

According to König, the salivary glands are most often the seat carcinomata rich in cells. At first a few lobules of the gland degenerat these become more and more numerous and turn into masses of cel which extend over the borders of the gland into the neighborhood. Th stroma of these carcinomata is slightly developed; they are medulla in character and show an acinous structure. Tubular carcinomat according to König, develop more from the salivary ducts. They for long tubes lined with cylindrical epithelium; epithelial pearls are foun at their ends and proliferating connective tissue projects warty excres cences into their lumen from without. This gives rise to a structur reminding one of cystosarcoma phyllodes mammæ (O. Weber).

Scirrhus has also been observed to involve the salivary glands beside these cellular forms, which constitute the true medullary carcinomata pathologically it corresponds in every way to that of the breast.

Symptoms.—Clinically it is desirable to distinguish between scirrhu and medullary carcinomata.

Scirrhus of the salivary glands generally develops at an advanced ag and affects men more frequently than women. Clinically it resemble scirrhus of the breast—that is, the tumor formation is less evident tha the cicatricial contraction of the entire neighborhood. In marked ease of scirrhus of the parotid the site of the carcinoma is somewhat sunke and folds of skin radiate to this central depression. This distinct cica tricial contraction probably accounts for the very early development o facial paralysis in scirrhous carcinomata. Besides this "squirrhe atro phique," the French also distinguish a "squirrhe en plaque" in th parotid region. In the latter the skin is affected over a wider area an converted into a hard, leather-like plate. It is analogous to the cance en cuirasse of the breast, and the armor-like induration extends to th neck and the region of the mastoid process, so that a kind of torticolli with marked restriction in the movements of the head follows ($M^i{}_{chaux}$) The lymph-nodes of the neck are affected relatively late in scirrhou cancer of the salivary glands; they generally do not attain a large size but may form a continuous chain from the parotid to the supraclavicula fossa.

The course of the cellular growth, the so-called medullary cancers is quite different. Every now and then quite young individuals suffe from this form of carcinoma, in which the proliferation and tumo formation are the main features. The skin here is not retracted, but pushed outward, and it has a tense, glistening appearance, suggestin an inflammatory process. In a relatively short time it is perforated (Fig. 274), and this is followed by suppuration and occasionally profuse hemorrhage. In contrast to the scirrhus, the tumor is of soft consistence.

The lymph-nodes are involved early; particularly with ulcerating carcinomata they may grow to tumors of considerable size. On the other hand, the facial nerve is involved later than in the scirrhous form.

Disturbances and marked functional derangements are present in all carcinomata, especially in those of the parotid. The facial paralysis in scirrhus of the parotid need not always involve the chief trunk, but may be limited to several branches; it is not always caused by direct destruction of the nerve, since it may also result from compression of cicatricial tissue. Pains are usually present; in general they are more severe in the rapidly proliferating forms, but they may be severe in advanced scirrhus. They may be the main feature of the disease and can become unendurable; they may radiate toward the face, mastoid process, front and back of the neck. Besides this there are disturbances of hearing, difficulty in speaking, chewing, swallowing, and breathing, the latter especially when carcinoma of the parotid or its metastases in the glands extend to the pharynx, and when a carcinoma of the submaxillary spreads chiefly toward the oral cavity. It has already been mentioned that a kind of torticollis may sometimes be observed in scirrhous carcinomata of the parotid.

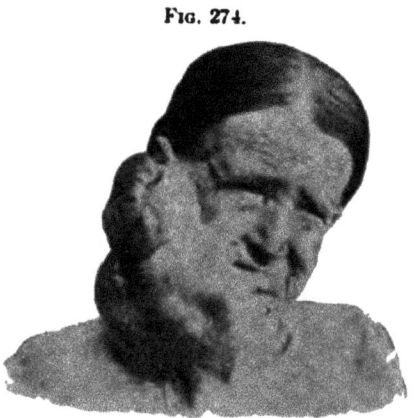

Fig. 274.

Medullary carcinoma of the parotid. (After a case in v. Bruns' clinic.)

Prognosis.—The prognosis of carcinomata of the salivary glands is not good, and permanent cures after operations are rare even in the scirrhous type. In the latter the course of the disease is relatively favorable as far as local extension and involvement of the lymph-nodes are concerned, and many years frequently elapse before the patients die. According to König, there may even be very slowly growing carcinomata in old individuals which involve the facial nerve only later, and which still admit of a partial operation, an extirpation of the diseased part of the parotid. The course is quite different in the encephaloid cancers, which belong to the most malignant class of tumors. They generally kill in several months by rapid local extension, hemorrhage from the ulcerating mass, by quick spreading by way of the lymph-nodes, and by the formation of metastases. The latter are frequently very extensive; in a case of carcinoma of the submaxillary gland observed by Zahn the secondary tumors involved the bones exclusively.

Diagnosis of Malignant Tumors of the Salivary Glands.—The diagnosis of malignant tumors of the salivary glands may be very difficult. This does not, of course, apply to those well-marked and advanced cases

in which an encephaloid carcinoma has perforated the skin and i
proliferating tumor masses project through it, or in which a typi
scirrhus exerts traction on all sides as it shrinks. The diagnosis is di
cult where the process has not yet advanced so far, and it is just in su
cases that an operation is indicated.

First of all, the surgeon must differentiate inflammatory process
especially the "inflammatory tumors" described above and other su
acute and chronic inflammations; furthermore, tuberculous and sypl
litic disease of the salivary glands. A very malignant sarcoma, or
malignant mixed tumor, perhaps even a medullary carcinoma whi
spreads rapidly over the entire gland and becomes adherent to the sl
and surroundings, may impress one clinically as an inflammato
process. Neither age, swelling of the lymph-nodes, nor tenderne
gives a clue as to the one or the other of these affections; at best
facial paralysis occurring in a disease of the parotid can be guarded
employed for the diagnosis of "malignant tumor"; it generally, hov
ever, is only a late symptom of these tumors.

Sometimes it is still more difficult, though less important, to dete
mine if a malignant tumor develops from the salivary glands or no
This refers particularly to lymphosarcomata of the submaxillary, an
above all, the parotid region. König has drawn attention to the dif
culty of this differentiation in particular.

Secondary cancer of the glands is mistaken only on superficial exan
ination. Carcinoma of the submaxillary gland must also be differe
tiated from branchial carcinoma, which for a long time was consider
a submaxillary cancer. In advanced cases both may be difficult
distinguish, but the majority of branchial cancers are not seated so hig
as those of the submaxillary, and where the tumor is extensive tl
history points to the gland as the site of origin.

The differentiation of malignant tumors from inflammatory process
is the most important of all. Certainty can often be obtained only l
means of an exploratory excision.

Treatment.—As soon as the diagnosis of "malignant tumor" is mac
the treatment consists in total extirpation of the salivary gland i
question, in conjunction with removal of the diseased lymph-nodes ar
other secondary foci.

Only in certain rare, exceptional cases is a partial operation pe
mitted in cancer (König), as when a hard, slowly increasing ca
cinoma of the parotid in old people has still left the facial ner
intact. In all other cases the entire salivary gland must be remove
since the entire gland is to be looked upon as infected, as in cance
of other glandular organs. If the submaxillary is affected, the auth
does not hesitate one moment to remove it completely, since this
easy. But in the parotid the surgeon must not only consider the severi
of the lesion, but also the complete paralysis of the facial nerve remaii
ing after the operation, the dangers of this to the eye, and the poss
bility of achieving a permanent cure. One should carefully select th
cases, for one cannot expect to cure permanently a carcinoma of th

parotid which has extended to the mucous membrane of the pharynx, or which has extensively involved the lymph-nodes; if the large vessel and nerve-trunks of the neck are already implicated, the surgeon cannot even expect to remove it radically. Hence he should only operate on the less advanced cases, and should not expose the patients to so severe an operation if no marked advantage can be obtained by it.

TOTAL EXTIRPATION OF THE PAROTID AND SUBMAXILLARY GLAND.

Extirpation of the Parotid Gland.—The extirpation of the parotid gland belongs to the technically difficult operations, but by proceeding slowly and carefully it can be performed without considerable hemorrhage and without much danger. It is advisable to do an extracapsular, and, if possible, a blunt extirpation; if tense cords of tissue must be divided sharply, these should first be ligated if they are suspected to contain vessels, and the knife should be directed against the gland.

If the surgeon does an intracapsular operation, as Liston and Dieffenhach have recommended, it is more difficult to check the hemorrhage from the loose gland-tissue, and a clean, complete extirpation of the gland is impossible. Roser's plan of removing the parotid piecemeal is contrary to modern principles of malignant tumor extirpation.

The skin-incision runs vertically from above downward, directly in front of the tragus; it should be rather extensive. The author begins at about the level of the upper insertion of the auricle and ends 4 to 5 cm. below the angle of the jaw, perhaps still deeper if the parotid reaches far down the neck or if extensive metastases are present in the superficial and deep cervical glands. Adherent portions of the skin are removed in the form of an ellipse. It is advisable to add a horizontal incision to the vertical one, which runs parallel to the zygomatic arch and a finger's breadth below it. It should be carried forward as far as the gland or an accessory parotid extends. In this way a T-shaped incision results. The skin-flaps are dissected off and the entire outer surface of the parotid is exposed. The hemorrhage is occasionally very active; it is carefully checked so that the field of operation remains unobscured.

After exposing the capsule the real extirpation of the gland is begun, preferably at the lower pole, where any lymph-nodes present are removed, the large superficial veins ligated, and the surgeon then proceeds toward the external carotid. The latter is either ligated doubly and divided at once, or a ligature is placed around it, which can be tied in case of more abundant hemorrhage. It is now advisable to free slowly and carefully the gland from above and from the sides (König); this will be easy upon the masseter. The posterior surface is more difficult, since the capsule of the gland is often firmly adherent to the sternomastoid; Faure recommends the removal of a layer of this muscle, so as to avoid opening the capsule. By proceeding downward from above and the sides, and carefully ligating every vessel which is put on the stretch, the gland is rendered more movable; gradually it becomes more and more pediculated, and finally only remains connected with the part of fascia going to the pharynx and with the styloid process Here the surgeon must be particularly careful, since the trunk of the external carotid must be divided, or, if this can be preserved, at least its two terminal branches, the superficial temporal and the internal maxillary; for, though the external carotid may have previously been ligated, it will again be filled with blood.[1] The vessels which have been sacrificed in the course of an extirpation of the parotid are, outside of a few muscular and glandular branches, the venæ jugularis externus, facialis anticus and posticus, the arteria transversa faciei, auricularis posticus, occipitalis, temporalis superficialis, with the anterior auricular branches, the arteria zygomatico-orbitalis, arteria maxillaris internus, and sometimes the external carotid itself. The external carotid and the internal jugular can be saved in every typical extirpation, while the trunk of the facial nerve must be divided.

After the extirpation drain carefully and suture the wound. The after-treatment should pay particular attention to the eye on the side operated upon; it should be kept closed and washed out carefully so as to guard it from the injuries to which it would be exposed if open (facial paralysis).

Extirpation of the Submaxillary Gland.—Extirpation of the sub-maxillary gland is technically much simpler than that of the parotid. An incision is made into the submaxillary region parallel with the margin of the jaw or in a slightly curved direction. Its length depends upon the size of the tumor. The surgeon then passes through the platysma down to the capsule of the gland, frees the lower edge of the gland, and then dissects off tumor and gland from the lower jaw. The facial artery with its accompanying vein is here ligated twice and divided; a labial branch of the facial nerve must generally be sacrificed also. The gland is now bluntly removed from its recess on the inner side of the horizontal ramus of the jaw; while this is being done the excretory duct will become tense and is divided. After separating its mesial connections the tumor and gland are pulled downward; the latter now only hangs with the facial artery as pedicle, and this must be again ligated and divided. The ligation must be done very carefully, for the vessel is divided near the external carotid and readily retracts into the deeper parts. Should the ligature slip off, a very disagreeable hemorrhage would arise. If dealing with malignant tumors which have spread beyond the borders of the gland, the surgeon may have to sacrifice the lingual vessels and the hypoglossal nerve, which describe a curve at the lower margin of the gland, and the lingual nerve, which lies along the upper margin. In these cases the submaxillary and deep cervical lymph-nodes should also be removed.

[1] In order to facilitate the removal of that portion of the parotid lying in the retromandibular fossa, Faure has recommended the resection of a piece about 1 cm. broad from the ascending ramus of the jaw, beginning directly under the insertion of the condylar process and ending 2 cm. above the angle of the jaw.

INJURIES AND DISEASES OF THE JAW.

‹ By Professor Dr. C. SCHLATTER.

CHAPTER XIX.

INJURIES OF THE JAWS.

FRACTURES OF THE UPPER JAW.

If one inspects the upper part of the bony skeleton of the face, it will be noticed that, apart from the nasal structures, the upper jaw and malar bone are the most prominent parts of the bony framework suspended from the base of the skull, and hence most exposed to injuries. Fractures of the malar bone have been discussed in another chapter, and if for symptomatic and therapeutic reasons the author discusses separately fractures of the upper jaw in a more restricted sense, as involving the superior maxillæ alone, he is well aware that the subdivision is somewhat artificial, since both superior maxillæ, the malar bones, the nasal, palate, and lacrymal bones, with their processes, and the ethmoid and sphenoid bones, form, so to speak, an entirety. Though this entire bony framework is subdivided into different parts by a number of suture-lines, these are generally not followed by the course of fractures and fissure; the line of fracture very often runs over several bones, even into the base of the skull.

Fractures of the upper jaw are comparatively rare, for the nose, forehead, malar bone, and lower jaw protect the region of the cheek to a considerable degree from injuries. They are usually direct fractures, hence the result of a force which has acted directly, such as a blow, a thrust, a fall upon the face, and, above all, the kick of a horse. Gunshot injuries of the mouth, especially those inflicted with a suicidal intent, by placing the barrel of the weapon in the mouth, are often accompanied by extensive comminution of the upper jaw. The less common indirect fractures of the upper jaw are seen when the malar bone is driven into the maxillary sinus by a great force or when an injury drives some other bone of the neighborhood into the jaw. Instances have been seen where the lower jaw was driven against the frontal bone, so that the upper jaw was crushed between them, or where a force acting upon the lower jaw drove the smaller arc of the lower jaw into the larger arc of the upper jaw like a wedge, resulting in fracture of the latter.

The most frequent partial fractures of the upper jaw are those the alveolar process. They may be due to a direct blow or fall of the teeth, but much more frequently result from the unskilful extraction of a tooth, especially by means of the tooth-key. The force exerted the latter cannot be well limited, so that it may cause terrible access injuries. Thus the entire alveolar process may be fractured and maxillary sinus opened, and the entire vault of the mouth may detached.

Other partial fractures are those of the frontal process which of accompany nasal fractures, and perforations of the anterior wall of maxillary sinus, the hard palate, and the floor of the orbit, such as caused by sharp objects and projectiles.

The discussion of total fractures of the upper jaw may be prefa by the following observations and investigations, which will aid in understanding of the different forms of fractures:

The meritorious experimental studies of Le Fort on fractures of upper jaw show that there is really a remarkable difference of resista between the bone of the skeleton of the head and those of the h during life or with the soft parts attached; while the former can har be preserved without small lesion of the bones, the latter will o fracture if much force is used. This different behavior depends up the fact that in the unprepared head the brittle portions are everywh surrounded by protecting tissue of great elasticity, while the promin portions consist of firm, hard bone.

The credit of having pointed out that fractures of the upper j behave differently from those of the long hollow bones belongs to Gué In general the surgeon has to deal with long fractures without inj to the soft parts; fracture without dislocation is the rule, displaceme of the fragments the exception. These two facts explain why fract of the upper jaw is frequently not recognized.

Different forms of fractures of the upper jaw may be recogni More recent investigations have discovered definite fracture-lines mor less characteristic. This is of special importance from a forensic po of view.

The most frequent form of fracture is the transverse fracture; it w first studied in detail by Alph. Guérin and bears his name. A numb of clinical and experimental observations have proved that this ty of fracture undoubtedly does exist. The typical transverse fract of Guérin runs backward into the pterygoid process about 1 cm. bel the malar bone and generally on both sides; it results from a sev blow upon the face from before backward, beneath the nostrils, in t median line or somewhat lateral to this. The entire vault of the mou with the teeth may be detached and displaced posteriorly by the h zontal fracture-line; in very marked dislocation the posterior margin the palate may even rest upon the posterior pharyngeal wall and obstr the pharynx. The pterygoid processes are always fractured at the lo of the lower border of the pterygomaxillary fissure—that is, at the po where they offer least resistance. Fissuring and splitting of the pal bones from before backward are not uncommon accessory injuries. In the absence of all dislocation Guérin diagnosticated transverse fracture by the pain which resulted when the inner pterygoid plate was pressed and in several cases by the mobility of the plate. The very first case diagnosticated in this way by Guérin was verified at autopsy.

If the blow acts upon the lower portion of the upper jaw from the side, the fracture takes the direction of the force. If the direction of the force corresponds to the level of the palate, the transverse fracture described above generally results, while a fracture of the pterygoid processes almost always accompanies the transverse fracture where the direction of the force was sagittal; these processes frequently remain intact with a blow from the side.

If the direction of the force is lateral and oblique from above downward, there is a detachment of the alveolar margin with a portion of the jaw whose breadth depends upon the level of the blow.

The observations upon the effects of a blow directed from below upward toward the alveolar process are too few to determine a characteristic type of fracture-lines. In several cases a fissure-line surrounding the malar bone has been found. If the injury is severe and bilateral, the entire median portion of the bony face may be broken off by a fracture-line which runs from the nasal apertures toward the orbits, then symmetrically circumscribes the malar bones, and finally fractures the pterygoid processes at their base. The fracture may be complicated by fissures which split the hard palate from before backward. Even vertical fractures with broad diastases of the upper jaw and hard palate have been observed.

A force acting upon a broad surface from in front, so that both superior maxillar and malar bones are struck, can lead to division of the facial bones from the skull proper. In a case of this kind, accompanied by marked exophthalmos, the author could move the entire median portion of the facial skeleton to and fro laterally in one mass. Another similar fracture was complicated by a broad cleft in the palate, which was closed successfully by four sutures through the palate.

For fractures of the nasal and malar bones and of the skull, complicating fractures of the upper jaw, the reader is referred to the chapter treating of those injuries.

It need hardly be mentioned that comminuted fractures with extensive crushing of the facial bones, such as result from the kick of a horse or the wheels of a wagon, cannot be separated and divided into the classes spoken of above.

Diagnosis.—In most cases of fracture of the upper jaw the symptoms are so distinct that the diagnosis can be made at once despite the swelling of the soft parts, which is generally very marked. Slight degrees of dislocation without disfigurement of the face manifest themselves by the unequal position of the teeth; if there is not even displacement of these, the surgeon generally finds a bloody space between two teeth, hemorrhage from the injured mucous membranes through the mouth and nose, nasal, buccal, and even subconjunctival ecchymoses, swelling of the soft parts, and even emphysema where the maxillary sinus injured.

As in all injuries of the mouth, there is generally salivation. Diagnosis may be rendered difficult if the swelling extends to the pharynx. On palpating with the fingers one frequently recognizes the typical symptoms of a fracture: pain, abnormal mobility, and crepitation. So could a symptom-complex is found by no means in all cases, and the fracture may be obscure. In such cases it is necessary to examine system atically. It is advisable to follow Guérin's suggestion to introduce a finger into the mouth, so that pressure may be exerted upon the inner plate of the pterygoid process. Marked tenderness at this site is sufficient for a diagnosis of horizontal fracture of the upper jaw. Disturbances of sensation must also be looked for. If the fracture-line involves the infraorbital canal, contusion or laceration of the infraorbital nerve may cause anesthesia in the region of the cheek.

The trauma which has caused the fracture of the jaw may also set up severe cerebral symptoms.

Prognosis.—Even in severe comminuted fracture the prognosis is generally favorable beyond expectation. The author has a lasting impression of the healing of such a fracture in a patient brought to Zürich Surgical Clinic for a very extensive comminution of the upper jaw caused by the kick of a horse. Large and small fragments of bone in part only hanging by their periosteum, were lying without order in the swollen and lacerated tissues. The mouth could only be opened with the greatest difficulty and constantly discharged saliva. The patient would not allow the application of a splint to keep two very easily displaceable fragments in position, and left the hospital. The author accidentally met him several weeks later; his comminuted fracture had healed without medical treatment in a remarkably favorable manner with only slight dislocation, although originally the rows of teeth were displaced at least 1 cm. toward each other. The exceptionally favorable prognosis of open fractures of the upper jaw depends upon the slight danger of infection in wounds of the mouth and the abundant vascularization of the mucous membrane and periosteum of the jaw which is unfavorable to the development of necrosis.

Necrosis of bone and injuries of the maxillary sinus naturally delay healing by the formation of fistulæ. A fatal issue is observed almost only in complicating infected injuries of the skull. Hemorrhages generally cease spontaneously or may be checked by packing with iodoform gauze.

Those cases of fracture of the upper jaw received in warfare, in which, according to Hamilton, it was necessary to ligate the carotid artery on account of profuse secondary hemorrhage, belong to the pre-antiseptic period. They were a result of septic infection caused by projectiles of large calibre. To-day the dangers of bleeding to death can no longer be estimated according to these standards.

In simple fractures the patients may chew in from two to three weeks; severe fractures generally heal in from five to eight weeks. The slight degrees of dislocation which remain generally cause no trouble. After fractures of the entire median portion of the facial skeleton the author has seen a lengthening as well as broadening of the middle part of the face. Marked disfigurements can often be improved by dental apparatus. Obstruction of the nasal duct by fragments is fortunately rare; it may give rise to troublesome lachrymal fistulæ.

Treatment.—The treatment of all open fractures of the jaw demands that the month be kept as clean as possible. It should be frequently rinsed with disinfecting solutions (such as potassium chlorate), and where possible it should also be cleansed mechanically. If dealing with a fracture without dislocation, it is sufficient to put the jaw at rest by applying a jaw-bandage around the inferior maxilla and fastening it in the form of a splint to the upper jaw. The patient is not allowed to speak, and receives only fluid nourishment.

If the alveolar process is broken, it is replaced by the fingers until the teeth are placed symmetrically. Loose fragments should be treated as conservatively as possible on account of the good blood-supply of the periosteum. The other dislocation fragments of the jaw can generally also be replaced without difficulty by means of a finger, an elevator, or a sound. It is more difficult to keep the fragments in position than to replace them. A simple ligature around the teeth on both sides of the fracture-line is rarely sufficient, since they become loose in a short time. Splints of gutta-percha which are pressed down upon the replaced row of teeth while warm and which are supposed to keep these in place after they have hardened, are of little use if applied in this primitive way. Taking the impression alone is difficult on account of pain, and frequently they are unbearable on account of the pressure symptoms which develop later and the putrefaction and inflammation which go on beneath them.

In deciding the utility of complicated apparatus for retaining the fragments in place, one must not forget that, as in the case cited, many severe fractures heal exceptionally well without any bandage at all. The act of chewing replaces the fragments rather than displaces them, and too forceful biting, which is harmful, is instinctively avoided by the patient.

The two best-known retention apparatuses are those of Goffre and Gräfe. In both, a splint surrounding the upper jaw is fixed by means of a metal attachment to a hood consisting of metal strips or to a band around the forehead. These devices are easily displaced and cause the patients so much annoyance that they generally must be removed after a short time.

If recourse can be had to a skilful dentist, much can be done in some cases by applying a plate for the gums, which can be fastened to the firm teeth with hooks. In other cases it is advisable to cap the teeth with a caoutchouc-gutta-percha splint or to employ Sauer's method. (See Treatment of Fracture of the Lower Jaw.)

FRACTURES OF THE LOWER JAW.

Owing to the exposed position of the lower jaw it is evident that fi tures more frequently involve this bone than the upper jaw; one r even wonder that they do not occur more often, for they constitute c about 30 per cent. of all fractures. The reason for this immunity lie the exceptional hardness and density of the bone, which makes it e: cially resistant; to this must be added its own mobility and that of head, which considerably weakens the force of a blow.

The infantile lower jaw is only exceptionally fractured, as dur a difficult labor; the great majority—i. e., about nine-tenths—of cases occur in vigorous adults, since these are oftenest exposed injuries.

The most common causes of direct fractures are the same as in upper jaw; the kick of a horse, blows, falls upon the chin, guns injuries, and injuries resulting from the use of the tooth-key. Owing the hardness of the bone the fractured surfaces generally have sh: edges.

The less frequent indirect fractures result from the contraction dilatation of the arch of the jaw by transverse or sagittal pressure. a force acting from the side increases the curvature of the bone, the j breaks at the site of greater flexion, which generally is at the symphy But a second fracture may occur at the point where the force has b: applied, and even a third one at the supporting points of the jaw. a case observed by the author a board in falling struck the angle the jaw. The bone was fractured vertically exactly in the mid of the jaw between the two lower median incisors, also horizontally the point where it was struck—at its angle on the right side. Fractu of the neck of the condyloid process which result from a blow on chin are also indirect. Multiple fractures are comparatively freque according to Hamilton, they constitute about one-third of all cas Simple fissures of the mandible have also been observed; they oc either externally at the site of the injury or more often internally bending fractures. The outer loss of continuity is caused by poin objects acting rapidly so that the bone does not find time to adjust it: to the force; the inner, by blunt objects acting more slowly.

Three groups of fractures of the mandible are distinguished: fractu of the alveolar process, of the body of the jaw, and of its ascendi ramus.

Fractures of the alveolar process are about as common as those the corresponding portion of the upper jaw, since they are due mai: to the same cause: a blow upon the process or the use of the tooth-k Sometimes the fracture manifests itself as a small fragment of b: adhering to an extracted tooth, at other times as a larger fragm: involving several teeth.

Fractures of the body of the lower jaw vary much in seat and for yet certain sites of preference without doubt occur. We can only lo upou the mesial lines of separation, acquired at birth as real fractures of the symphysis, since the cartilage of the symphysis ossifies very early. The rare fractures lying in the region of the symphysis are generally vertical. Fractures at the level or in the neighborhood of the mental foramen, in the region of the canine tooth, are far more frequent than those lying in the median line. The dislocation is usually slight where the fracture is vertical. Most fractures of the body of the bone outside of the symphysis lie beneath the teeth, between which they run perpendicularly. They are oblique fractures and can easily be dislocated in a horizontal or lateral direction, depending upon the muscles which pull upon the fragments. Double and comminuted fractures permit of most displacement. Besides a lateral displacement of the fragments which diminishes the size of the mandibular arch, the surgeon can generally observe a typical dislocation in which the posterior fragment is raised by the masseter and the anterior one depressed by the digastric and the muscles of the chin.

If the middle portion of the mandibular arch is broken off, the fragment may be displaced downward and backward by the action of the geniohyoid, genioglossus, and digastric muscles, so that the tongue falls back and suffocation is imminent.

Disagreeable symptoms occasionally complicate fractures in the region of the molar teeth, owing to injury of the vessels and nerves running in the inferior dental canal. Though the hemorrhage generally stops by itself, patients have been known to bleed to death where no attention was paid to the rupture of the inferior dental artery.

Fractures of the ascending ramus of the jaw are not frequent, since this is protected by thick layers of tissue. The course of the fracture is generally oblique from in front and above, downward and backward. Unless the fracture is bilateral and complicated by a luxation of the condyloid process of the opposite side, it may heal without any dislocation, since both fragments are brought into apposition by the masseter and the pterygoid muscles.

Fracture of the condyloid process almost always involves its neck. It has already been stated that there may be indirect fractures resulting from a blow upon the chin, and also from a force with a lateral direction, when the neck of the condyloid process of the opposite side is broken. The dislocation in this form of fracture is characteristic in that chin and jaw are pulled toward the injured side especially by the internal pterygoid muscle of the opposite side. In dislocation of the jaw, on the other hand, the chin will point toward the normal side. These fractures may be accompanied by fractures of the glenoid cavity, and even by fractures of the base of the skull.

If both condyloid processes break off, the whole lower jaw will be pushed upward and backward and the lower teeth will lie far behind the upper.

The coronoid process can only be broken off by a direct blow. Fractures of this kind are rare, and are always accompanied by other fractures, as of the malar bone, upper jaw, or the skull.

Diagnosis.—The symptoms of fracture of the lower jaw are gene
so marked that a diagnosis is rarely difficult. Pain is the most con
of all the signs of fracture. It is increased by every movement of
jaw, and chewing and talking are avoided. Profuse salivation is pr
as in fractures of the upper jaw, so that the dribbling of saliva an
the patient to a marked degree. At first the saliva is generally m
with blood, for in the majority of cases the fractures are compo
The tear in the mucous membrane can generally be seen when the m
is opened; at the same time the unequal position of the teeth att
attention, so that a diagnosis is frequently possible by mere inspec
Palpation, though sometimes superfluous, will elicit crepitation
abnormal mobility. Fractures of the symphysis without disloca
are evident by pain on pressure and motion. In doubtful cases
entire mandibular arch can be palpated with two fingers to detern
if abnormal mobility is present. Fractures of the ascending ramus

Fig. 275.

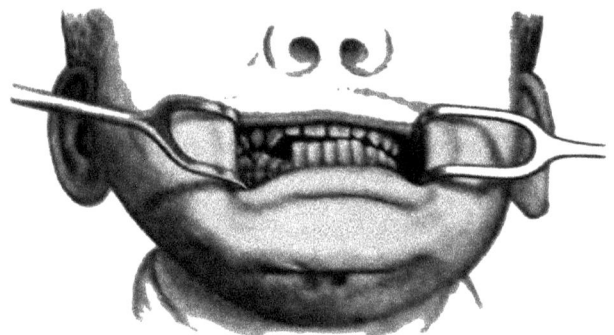

Fracture of the jaw, with deformity. Suture of bone from mouth.

best be felt from within the mouth; they manifest themselves by s
ing and marked tenderness on pressure. In fractures of the ned
the condyloid process there is a slight depression in front of the exte
auditory meatus because the condyle is dislocated toward the fixing
inward owing to the pull of the external pterygoid muscle; besides (
the somewhat prominent and readily palpable condyle does not fil
the motions of the jaw.

Fractures of the coronoid process can only be suspected from the p
elicited by palpating it from the mouth and when the jaw is mo
extensively.

Prognosis.—The prognosis of fractures of the lower jaw is usual
favorable. Simple fractures without much laceration of the g
generally heal within from four to six weeks with very slight diffor
which may manifest itself in an irregularity of the teeth; even se
upon fractures run a remarkably favorable course in contrast to si
injuries of other bones. Death as a result of septic infection of t

wounds is exceedingly rare. In comminuted fractures the course may naturally be very much prolonged by the protracted formation of sequestra owing to ostitis. It must be emphasized that pseudarthroses are rare after fractures of the lower jaw, despite the difficulty in firmly immobilizing the bone (according to Norris, 2 cases in 150; according to the statistics of Muhlenberg and Berenger-Féraud, they form only about 2 per cent. of all pseudarthroses observed). Most cases of con-nective-tissue union resulted from gunshot injuries or were complicated by sequestra. The abundant formation of callus is due to the rich blood-supply of the periosteum, and probably also to the constant irri-tation which the imperfectly approximated fractured surfaces exert upon each other.

Permanent disturbances on the part of the inferior dental nerve, such as severe attacks of neuralgia, anæsthesia of the corresponding half of the lower lip, and paralyses of the quadratus and triangularis menti, are also rare (Malgaigne with his rich experience has not seen a single case of this kind) and generally accompany only those fractures which lie behind the mental foramen. Most of these symptoms dis-appear spontaneously. They are probably due to the pressure exerted by a hemorrhage in the inferior dental canal; rarely obstinate attacks of neuralgia require an operative exposure of the site of compression. In a few cases atrophy of half of the jaw has been observed after a fracture; this was probably due to diminished nutrition from occlusion of the inferior dental artery.

In the rare fracture of the coronoid process the union is never bony, but only fibrous, since the temporal muscle raises the broken fragment and thus causes a wide separation. The act of mastication is interfered with but little, however, since the masseter and pterygoid muscles compensate for the action of the temporal.

Treatment.—The treatment of fracture of the lower jaw may be very simple where there are no lacerations of the mucous membrane and no particular tendency to dislocation; a sling or merely a piece of cloth around the chin suffices to put the jaw at rest. The use of fluid and later soft food generally causes no difficulty; the use of a feeding-cup, or a glass or stomach-tube is only rarely necessary.

Since most fractures are open, the utmost care must be exercised to clean and disinfect the mouth as far as this is possible. It should be irrigated as well as rinsed frequently, especially after meals, with antiseptic mouth-washes (solutions of potassium chlorate or perman-ganate, salicylic acid, etc.).

With the exception of fracture of the condyloid process, it is generally not difficult to set the bony fragments, even where the chin is typically dislocated downward and backward in double fracture. It generally falls easily and rapidly into its normal position if the necessary pressure is exerted by the fingers grasping the mandibular arch from within and without. The number of cases in which a replacement is impossible, or in which this requires a division of the muscles inserted into the fragment, is small.

Condylar fractures, in which the broken articular surface is pu
forward and inward by the external pterygoid muscle, are set accor
to the suggestion of Ribes, by first pulling the jaw forward and
pressing the condyle from within outward, by the finger placed u
the upper, lateral wall of the pharynx.

It is much more difficult and troublesome to keep the fragment
place. If a well-applied jaw-bandage does not answer, little more
be expected from a ligature placed around the teeth bordering
fracture-line, such as Hippocrates recommended. The author has l
satisfied with its results in but a single one of the cases treated by
in this way. With much experience he finds that a silk threa
insufficient, and that silver or gold wire frequently cannot be borne at
the neck of the tooth, and that in addition the fixed teeth are ea
loosened. One of the most modern methods is constructed on
principle of this ancient method: it is the union of the fragments v
the rings first suggested by Angle, and then modified by Löhers.
author discusses this method first on account of its exceeding simplic
it enables every surgeon to apply a well-fitting support to the jaw with
special dental training.

The accompanying illustration shows the clamps of Löhers. On
lingual side is a small screw, by means of which the device may
adjusted, and which applies
metal ring firmly to the crown
the tooth. A tube is soldered
the facial side of the ring. A r
is fixed to a firm tooth to the ri
and to the left of the fractu
Then a thick wire of soft silver
nickel is passed through the su
tubes on both sides, and its en
fixed by being bent over shar
behind the tube. Finally,
middle of the wire in the nei
borhood of the fracture is grasp
with a flat forceps and turned l
a screw until the dislocation is c
rected completely. In order
apply these rings there must
firm teeth in the neighborhood
the fracture. The author will
discuss the modification of this method where there are larger g
between the teeth, but refers to the publication of Ribe, since the b
surgeon will hardly attempt to solder on the leaden strips which brie
over the gap.

Angle places strips of platinum or German silver around the te
in the form of a sling and fastens them with screws. A wire is pas
through the sheaths, which are soldered to the margins in front; it
shortened by pulling on the screw until the fractured ends are in co

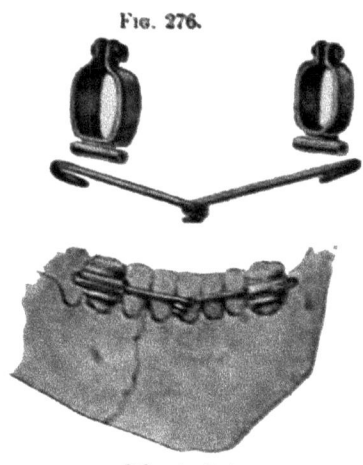

Fig. 276.

Löhers' splint.

tation; or else metal buttons are fixed to the strips and these surrounded by flexible wire in the form of a figure 8.

Sauer's first dressing has also been constructed for the use of the ordinary practitioner. (Fig. 277.) It consists of a tin-plated wire of iron or aluminum bronze 2 mm. thick, which is bent as near as possible to conform to the normal lower jaw without taking an impression. The intact upper jaw will serve as an approximate model. Posteriorly the wire should reach only to the middle of the second molar tooth, since otherwise it will easily cause pressure-gangrene. The wire is then placed against the neck of the teeth and fastened by turns of a flexible wire.

Fɪɢ. 277.

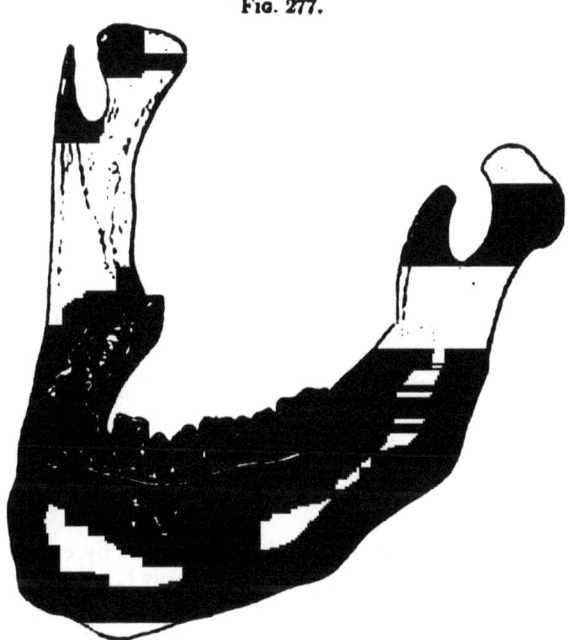

Sauer's splint.

One does not always succeed in overcoming the more marked dislocations of the fractured ends with the first dressing. Absolutely perfect adjustment occurs after a time; the upper jaw usually corrects slight irregularities in the act of mastication. By the end of the fourth week the surgeon may try to do without the splint.

At this place must be mentioned the exceedingly simple temporary splint of Claud Martin, of Lyon. Fig. 278 shows that it consists of three silver wires which approximately possess the form of the dental arch, and which are connected with each other at certain intervals by transverse wires. They can be kept on hand, and may be easily given the desired shape, since they are very flexible. The apparatus is placed

upon the replaced row of teeth and fastened to the teeth with silk th
The middle splint resting upon the masticating surface prevent
annoying slipping of the apparatus and avoids pressure upon the g
it thus removes an objection common to most other splints.

If the ordinary practitioner does not obtain a satisfactory result
the aid of these simple methods and is obliged to depend upon his
efforts, he will utilize one or another of the methods which are g
in the text-books only, and will finally abandon the task and suture
bone. For this is a method of fixation which does not fail, and w
none of the others equal in efficiency; besides, it is easily done.
holes may be drilled on both sides of the fracture without pain by m
of a 1 per cent. cocaine-eucaine solution. It is advisable to place
holes some distance beneath the teeth, if necessary after the soft p
have been dissected off somewhat, so as to avoid coming into con
with the roots of the teeth. The danger which dentists occasion
speak of, even where strict asepsis was observed during the sutu

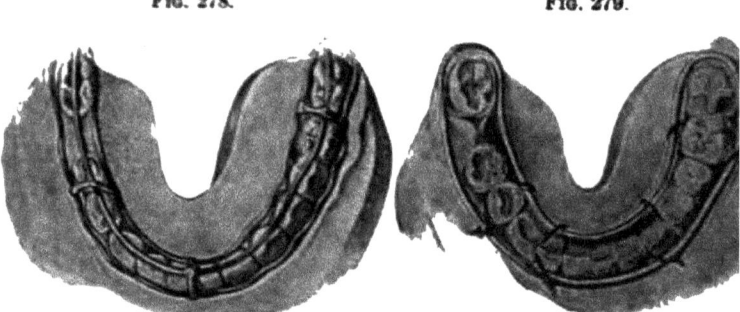

Fig. 278.   Fig. 279.

Martin's splint.   Hammond's splint.

and in the after-treatment, cannot be considered by experienced
geons, who are frequently in the position to apply bone sutures in pa
resections of the jaw. Nevertheless, in the treatment of easily disloc
fractures of the jaw the surgeon unhesitatingly admits the superio
of the dentist with his modern and perfected technical methods. '
latter is indeed in a position to obtain the same result in a more conse
tive way by means of skilfully constructed appliances.

Dental splints are most satisfactorily made of metal for many reas
for they leave the masticating surface of the jaw exposed and do
decompose. They must be hammered into shape very accurately (
plaster-of-Paris casts. Their accurate apposition to the teeth al
guarantees a good hold; besides they are generally fastened by me
of several thin wire loops running between the teeth to prevent tl
from falling out during sleep.

The first splint of the kind was described by Hammond in 1!
Sauer has perfected the method by constructing his parted wire dress
which is especially indicated for treating widely dislocated fragm

which can only be replaced gradually. If the dislocation is not corrected by the wire appliance alone, it is advisable to apply an oblique splint to the much displaced fragment, since the upper teeth will force it into its normal position when biting.

In suitable cases the fragments may be secured with a bridge of gold wire, by crown-work.

From a surgical point of view, metal splints undoubtedly find most favor, since they do not interfere with attempts to keep the mouth clean. For technical reasons the India-rubber and gutta-percha appliances cannot be done away with altogether. The pressure of the teeth is not only a requisite in the rubber and rubber-gutta-percha splints, recommended first by Henry Weber and then by Suersen, Haun, and others, but they may be better tolerated at first, since the metal splints are not very exactly fitted and are often painful. But after these appliances have been in place for some time, so much putrefaction and stagnation of

FIG. 280.

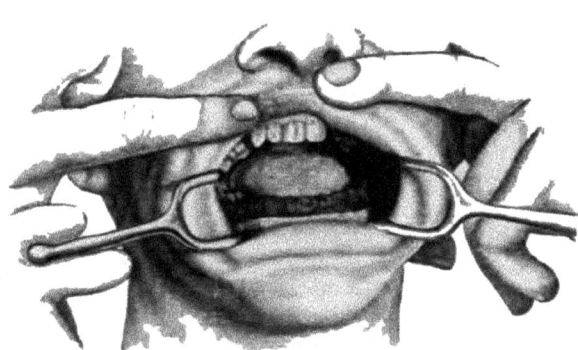

Dental splint in place.

decomposed products occurs, especially where gutta-percha has been used, that this material must be condemned from a surgical standpoint, in view of the fact that most fractures are compound. Even Martin's permanent dressing, so suggestive on account of its delicate workmanship, is not entirely free from this objection. It is made of metal, and caps over only the lateral surface of the teeth, so that the masticating and cutting surfaces are exposed.

Warnekros overcame this lack of asepsis by constructing appliances which can be removed so that the neighborhood of the fracture can be cleaned every few days. Even here it would be an advantage if this troublesome cleansing, possible only at long intervals, could be done away with by the construction of metal splints which do not cause pain while in place.

The different methods by means of which extension is applied to the lower jaw require rest in bed or a plaster-of-Paris bandage acting as support, and they probably never will meet with much favor in eyes of the surgeon or patient.

Fractures of the ascending ramus and the condylar process can erally only be managed with bandages (funda maxillæ,. capistrum necessary with pressure-pads); ceptionally a suitable splint be of value in the former. In treatment of fractures of the lo jaw one must individualize to great extent, and the method cussed must be modified and co bined to suit individual cases.

In imperfectly healed fracture late treatment with suitable spli may be successful.

The most rational way of de ing with pseudarthroses is by fre ening the surface and suturing bone.

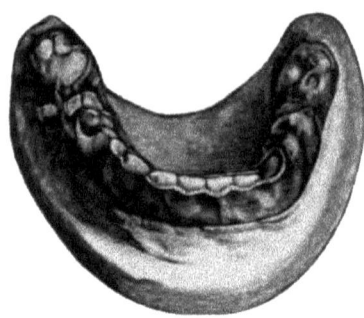

Fig. 281.

Dental splint applied to cast.

Loose sequestra should be removed if possible from the mouth. scesses are incised early and allowed to drain into the mouth if th communicate with it.

DISLOCATIONS OF THE LOWER JAW.

By the insertion of a meniscus the articulation of the jaw form kind of double joint which is enclosed by a comparatively wide ca sule. As a detailed description of the complicated mechanism of t joint would lead us too far, the author will only remark that centre of rotation of the articulations does not lie within the latt as is the case in other bones, but in an axis which lies in the region both lingulæ. In opening the mouth, motion first takes place betwe the head of the joint and the intra-articular disc or cartilage; upon wic excursions, however, both the head of the joint and the meniscus mo upon the tubercle of the joint (tuberculum articulæ). If the mouth opened immoderately, the head of the jaw, together with the menisc slips forward beyond the articular tubercle and remains fixed in th position. This is not caused, however, as Nélaton believed, by a hooki of the coronoid process in front of the anterior border of the malar bon but by the tubercle itself; later it is caused also by the contraction of t muscles, particularly the masseter and temporal, and the stretching the sphenomaxillary and stylomaxillary ligaments. This *displaceme forward of the head of the joint is the typical form of dislocation of t jaw.* In young children this does not occur, as in early childhood t tubercle of the joint is absent and the ascending ramus of the jaw placed at a more obtuse angle with the arch of the jaw than in th adult, whereby a displacement forward of the head of the joint is re dered more difficult. For the same reason the senile joint is less liab to be dislocated. The frequent occurrence of this dislocation among women—four times more frequently than in men, according to Krönlein —is readily explained by a shallower development of the articulation, with a less perfectly developed articular tubercle, in the female.

Owing, moreover, to the wide articular capsule, dislocations of the jaw are peculiar in so far as they occur without tearing the former. Typical dislocations of the jaw are usually *intracapsular.*

Bilateral dislocation is more frequent than unilateral. According to Hamilton, two of three cases are bilateral.

Dislocation is generally caused by opening the mouth too widely. This may be produced actively, by muscular exertion, as, for example, in yawning, laughing, screaming, or vomiting, or the jaw may be put into an abnormal position passively either by violence acting from without or through the mouth, as, for example, by inserting a large morsel of food. Violence from the side, as a blow upon the side of the face, usually leads to unilateral dislocation. Dislocations of the jaw during the extraction of teeth are not infrequent occurrences. The author has observed dislocation of the jaw produced by the extraction of a tooth which always recurred with subsequent extraction of teeth from the lower jaw.

Symptoms.—The symptoms of dislocation forward are so noticeable that the patient usually makes the diagnosis himself. The most conspicuous feature in unilateral and bilateral dislocation is the *widely opened mouth* and *fixation of the lower jaw* in this position, and, at the same time, the *projection of the lower teeth beyond the line of the upper teeth.* The patient is absolutely incapable of closing his mouth. On account of this abnormally fixed position, chewing is impossible, speaking is decidedly difficult, and an annoying flow of saliva is produced. Particularly in bilateral dislocation the masseter can frequently be noticed projecting in relief from the flattened and elongated region of the cheek. If the region of the joint be palpated, a distinct gap is felt in front of the tragus at the site of the glenoid cavity; in front of the articular tubercle, however, beneath the malar bone can be felt the displaced head of the joint. In *unilateral dislocation* these symptoms are to be found only in the region of the joint on the affected side; accordingly the *chin is displaced toward the sound side,* which, as was mentioned above, is an important sign in the differential diagnosis from fracture of the jaw. For the rest, there is the same locking of the jaw as in bilateral dislocation, though not so well marked. In most cases pain is severe only in the beginning. If the dislocated jaw is not reduced, motion subsequently becomes more free through a loosening of the capsule. At the same time the conditions which subsequently exist are very annoying, for the only teeth that can be brought into contact are the last molar; thus, chewing is hardly possible.

Treatment.—The treatment requires that the dislocated head of the jaw be forced under the prominence of the articular tubercle and then pressed back, whereby closure is again rendered possible. In recent dislocations reduction is easily accomplished in the majority of cases. Occasionally, however, attempts at reduction meet with considerable difficulty even under anæsthesia. In older dislocations the adhes of the head of the jaw must first be torn by forcible movements.

Reduction is best accomplished in the following manner: The thum well wrapped in a cloth, are inserted into the mouth and laid upon molar teeth on each side, and with the remaining fingers the lower is grasped from without and below. Thereupon the last molar te are pressed downward and at the same time backward with the thum while the remaining fingers raise up the chin. By this lever-like mo it is usually possible, even at the first attempt, to push the heads of articulations beneath and behind the articular tubercles. If, in case bilateral dislocation, any difficulty be met, the head of the articulat of one side is first replaced and then that of the opposite side. At tin pressure upon the coronoid processes, with the thumbs inserted into mouth, easily brings about reduction. Frequently also, direct press backward upon the head of the jaw, at the same time that the lever-l motions are carried out, will effect a speedy reduction. In other ca cork stoppers or wooden wedges placed between the posterior mo teeth, serving as a fulcrum, offer greater leverage for the jaw and fac tate reduction. For those rare cases of irreducible dislocation of the j the operative removal of the condyloid processes has been recommend Kramer has recently referred to the observation of Maisonneuve, tl the principal impediment in reducing a dislocated jaw lies in the abn mal tension of muscles and ligaments, and he has seen good results foll division of the external lateral ligament, together with the masseter a external pterygoid muscles, when the latter have been greatly stretch

Careful after-treatment is of the greatest value, as there is a marl tendency for dislocations to recur or a so-called *habitual dislocation* develop. For at least one week the lower jaw should be immobili by a bandage (funda). Permanent results are not possible. Genera nothing can be done in the case of habitual dislocations. They ha this advantage, however, that they are generally easy to replace. Fo long time the author had an old woman under treatment who for ye woke every morning to find her jaw dislocated. Each day her h band had reduced it. It was only after his death that she applied the surgical polyclinic for assistance.

Besides the above-described typical *forward dislocation of the ja* there occurs very rarely a dislocation *backward*. In this form the artic lar process glides over the small tympanic tubercle which closes t articular fossa behind and reaches the tympanico-stylomastoid fos which is, however, developed in the female only sufficiently to recei the head of the articulation. According to Thiem, in forcibly closi the teeth the temporal muscle produced dislocation of the jaw backwa In this form of dislocation the mouth is tightly closed, the teeth of t lower jaw rest behind those of the upper jaw, and the condyloid proce can be felt beneath the external auditory meatus in front of the masto process. Reduction is accomplished by forcibly opening the mou under anæsthesia, or by first pressing the lower jaw backward, th downward, and bringing it forward.

CHAPTER XX.

DISEASES OF THE JAWS.

ACTINOMYCOSIS OF THE JAW.

ACTINOMYCOSIS is undoubtedly the most frequent chronic infectious disease of the jaw. This affection is described in detail elsewhere under Diseases of the Face, the Salivary Glands, and the Mouth, but must be referred to again at this place, since the maxillary bones are the site of preference not only of the secondary manifestations of actinomycosis, but also of the less common primary focus of infection.

In actinomycosis of animals as well as of man the surgeon is dealing with an infection coming directly or indirectly from a plant infected by a fungus. Yet the most recent investigations have shown that the various pathological manifestations known as actinomycosis do not depend, as was formerly believed, upon a single specific ray-fungus. An accurate bacteriological examination by Silberschmidt, of several cases of actinomycosis of the upper jaw observed at the Zurich Surgical Clinic and Dispensary, showed that not a single one of the isolated incitors of the disease corresponded morphologically to the fungus described accurately by Boström as the sole cause of actinomycosis in man and animals. In the same way the cultures differed from the actinomyces described by Wolff and Israel. A number of different micro-organisms belonging to the class of *Actinomycetes* are capable of giving rise to the typical pathological picture. Mixed infections are exceptional in human actinomycosis.

From the fact that actinomycosis in animals and man involves most frequently the parts adjacent to the month it is permissible to conclude that food plays a part in the etiology of the disease. It is believed that minor injuries of the oral mucous membrane allow the fungus to enter. Boström has even proved the close relation which the introduction of barley-grains has to the affection among animals. A large number of observations point to the same mode of infection in man. But in many cases the etiology of the disease remains obscure.

The surgeon can hardly do otherwise than to assume the ubiquitous presence of the germ, and that it may retain its vitality upon inorganic material. Among others, the interesting observations of O. Wyss and Silberschmidt favor these views. These authors found peculiar struc-tures, the size of a pinhead, upon the inner side of an egg-shell. Micro-scopical and cultural examination showed that these consisted of typical threads with long branches like bovine actinomyces. The egg, still well preserved, had been kept on straw for five months, and during this time the micro-organisms had probably penetrated the shell.

Transmission of the infection from diseased animals to man (man to man probably does not occur.

Formerly the mistake was made of looking upon actinomycoti tions of the jaw as primary bone infections, until more accurate of tions showed that in most cases there is a primary infection of t parts, with infiltration of these instead of the supposed bone tume the bone is diseased, it is affected only secondarily. To-day the of view, that a primary actinomycosis of the jaw does not occur at a its supporters. Israel's opinion, that carious teeth play an imp part in jaw infections, is doubted more and more at present. seems to have received valuable support from a recent observa Silberschmidt, who obtained cultures of actinomycosis from the co of the opened root-canal of a carious tooth. Yet even in this c infection from the edge of the gums or from the alveolar peric cannot be strictly excluded. The old discussion as to whether the sitie infection finds its way through the teeth, around the tooth, means of the circulation by metastasis, is an idle one for the surg most cases. It is a fact that the upper as well as the lower jaw n destroyed to a marked degree by the ray-fungus.

In by far the largest number of cases of infection from the al margin or the gum of the lower jaw the process extends to the sub lary or submental region, or to the tissues of the cheek, where the acteristic, diffuse, slightly reddened and but little tender swellin first doughy and later board-like, develop. In other cases th an entirely different pathological picture: a swelling appears i region of a carious tooth or in the gap left by an extracted which looks very much like a gum-boil of an acutely infectious n and differs from this only by its slower growth and less marked t ness. Gradually the swelling breaks down externally or towar mouth.

In some cases the infiltration is not restricted to the region of th but extends downward along the sternomastoid to the clavicle or the ascending ramus of the jaw to the base of the skull. Met glandular swellings are not common in actinomycosis, since the in tion does not spread by way of the lymph-tracts, but by continuit a girl affected with primary actinomycosis of the lower jaw the a could follow the extension of the disease to the other side of the he well as upward and downward; one abscess after another develop succession until the patient died of actinomycosis of the base of the and meningitis, after having been ill two years.

The lower jaw itself can participate in the disease in different Periosteal changes constitute the mildest forms; the periosteum is ened or even destroyed by secondary inflammation, and in the case there may be a separation of small sequestra. In other cases lous tracts run from the gum or a diseased tooth into the depths, they end in a cavity filled with very vascular granulations. The around these cavities is often so rotten that pressure with the fi elicits crepitation. New fistulous canals run from the cavities int surrounding soft parts; in the cavities themselves there often are loose sequestra (cases of Février, Murphy, and Israel).

The third type of jaw affection, which begins centrally in animals and gives rise to a pathological picture resembling a myeloid sarcoma, in man occurs in a less characteristic manner (cases of Guermonprez, Ducor, Poncet, Legrain).

Actinomycosis of the upper jaw generally pursues a more serious and rapid course. The process here generally begins with toothache, loosening of the teeth, and tumefaction at the alveolar process. Gradually an abscess, fistulæ, and bone-necrosis form, but a reaction on the part of the bone does not occur, and there is slight tendency toward the formation of osteophytes or the encapsulation of the tissues, so that the infections find all portals opened. The maxillary sinus is easily affected, the base of the skull much endangered, and the surrounding muscles and soft parts are permeated, so the trismus and disturbance of nutrition occur owing to the infiltration of the muscles of mastication, and gravitation abscesses into the posterior mediastinum with sometimes even erosions of the vertebræ, owing to involvement of the prevertebral connective tissue.

Diagnosis.—How different the symptoms and course of the disease may be is evident from the popular distinction of actinomycosis from pseudoactinomycosis. The patients generally notice first the thickening of the gums or of the alveolar margin; then an infiltration appears at the angle of the jaw or the cheek. It is first doughy, later board-like in consistence, and the course is exceedingly protracted, for there may be no changes for a long time Finally, several areas soften and suppurate. The pus is scant in amount, thick, and often of chocolate color, and in it one may often detect the characteristic yellow granules with the naked eye. They vary in size from that of a grain of sand to that of a pinhead, and under the microscope will be found to consist of threads of mycelia, partly with club-shaped ends.

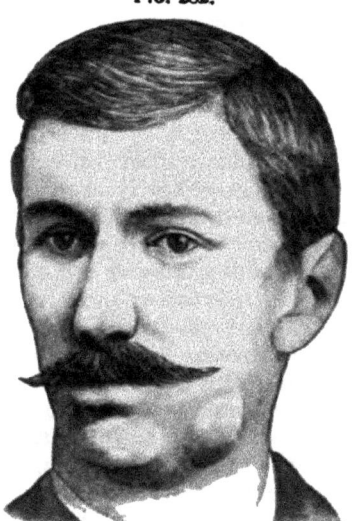

Fig. 282.

Actinomycosis of lower jaw. Clinical course like a recurring dental abscess.

In other instances the disease runs a course very much like the common recurring dental abscess. According to the author's personal experience, these cases are not rare. In rather rapid succession there is a slight toothache, a gum-boil, or external suppuration, so that, as in Fig. 282, there is not the slightest reason for a diagnosis of actinomycosis from the external appearance.

Even the direct microscopical examination of the pus or of se of the tissue does not always lead to a diagnosis. Cultures mu made to detect the germs of the disease. A few aërobic and anaë agar and bouillon cultures are sufficient.

This changeable clinical picture can be readily explained if assumed that several varieties of actinomyces, instead of one sp one, can cause the disease. This may also explain the peculiar that the iodides act almost as specifics in some cases, while in o they have no effect at all.

Prognosis.—In general the prognosis of actinomycosis is unfavo on account of the tendency of the disease to spread. Involveme the upper jaw is particularly feared on account of the ease with v it spreads to the base of the skull. On the other hand, it must n forgotten that actinomycosis of the face may heal spontaneously thr suppuration, and that the iodide treatment is often followed by rem able results in localized affections of the jaw.

Treatment.—In some places an almost specific action upon ac mycosis is ascribed to potassium iodide. It is given internally in doses of from 2.5 to 6 grams (45 to 90 grains), to be increased e day; or a 1 to 2 per cent. solution is injected parenchymatously (e eight days the contents of two to four Pravaz syringes, or twice a one to two syringefuls).

The author has seen little benefit from the internal use of potas iodide; the parenchymatous injections have been followed in par surprising results, in part they failed completely. Poncet consi potassium iodide indicated only in recent cases, during the stage induration and where the process does not extend deeply. In cases it is proper to try the drug first, and to operate only if it proved without effect. Even in a case of actinomycotic infiltr extending superficially over a large surface the author has seen disease recede against expectation after injections of potassium io

In from two to three weeks one will be able to decide upon the v of the iodide treatment; if it has proved useless, one must resort tc knife, sharp spoon, or thermocautery. In general one should not ex benefit from potassium iodide in extensive affections; it is better to have resource to operative treatment at once or to a combinatio the latter with potassium iodide.

A complete excision of the diseased area by incisions in the hea tissue, such as would promise a complete cure, is not often poss Generally all that is accomplished is the incision and drainage abscesses and fistulous tracts with curetting and thermocauterisatio diseased tissues and removal of sequestra.

TUBERCULOSIS OF THE MAXILLARY BONES.

Tuberculous affections of the maxillary bones are rather rare; t appear most frequently in the form of a tuberculous periostitis or os of the orbital margin of the upper jaw or at the junction of the malar bone with the upper jaw. In children tuberculous foci occur here which are exceedingly typical in their localization, as well as in their course and final result. Generally after an acute infectious disease which has run its course, particularly measles, a swelling develops at the orbital margin or at the malar process of the upper jaw, in conjunction with other scrofulous symptoms. Gradually this softens and forms an abscess, and a protracted suppurating fistula with sequestration results. Finally, a marked retraction of the skin of the lower lid into the scar of the fistula remains. In such cases it is well to expose and scrape out the carious focus as soon as possible, so as to avoid extreme ectropion.

Tuberculous affection of the nasal and palate processes of the upper jaw in young children has been repeatedly wrongly described as disease of the maxillary sinus. Such diagnoses do not hold for embryological reasons.

Tuberculosis of the alveolar processes has been observed repeatedly; Zauby has collected about 40 cases of this kind. The infection gains entrance through the spaces between the teeth and gums and by way of carious teeth. Wounds following the extraction of teeth also permit the infection to enter readily, especially in phthisis. The tuberculous involvement of the teeth is therefore as a rule a secondary affection of individuals otherwise tuberculous; undoubtedly, however, it may occur primarily. At first one finds a painful swelling and ulceration of the gum, which bleeds readily; later the roots of the teeth are exposed and the teeth fall out, and parts of the jaw may become necrotic. Slight pain and much salivation accompany the process.

The diagnosis is generally easy; if there are any difficulties, a microscopical and bacteriological examination of small excised pieces of tissue settles all doubt.

The prognosis is serious, since the disease is generally accompanied by pulmonary phthisis. Otherwise local surgical treatment promises good results. It consists of removing the suspicious tissue, curetting, and cauterizing with lactic acid.

The rare occurrence of tuberculous inflammations of the body of the jaw is explained by the infrequency of primary tuberculous foci upon the gums and in the month.

Tuberculosis of the lower jaw must be discussed separately on account of its malignant course. Etiologically, two classes may be distinguished: those which begin primarily in or upon the body, and those which extend to the body secondarily from the mucous membrane or the alveolar margin.

The cases observed of primary tuberculosis of the jaw leave the surgeon completely in the dark as to how this originates. It is true that the patients are generally tainted by heredity, but external causes, such as trauma or exposure to cold, are not mentioned. It is impossible to decide if the tubercle bacilli reach the site by way of the circulation or directly from the teeth or the gums. The tuberculous lesion is generally located

in the lower margin of the horizontal portion of the mandible, espe
in the region of the chin or the angle of the jaw; but the
ramus can also be involved primarily.   The disease manifests itsel
as a hard diffuse swelling of the affected part of the jaw.   The pr
not marked; the patients have a good appetite and are not fevr

Fig. 283.

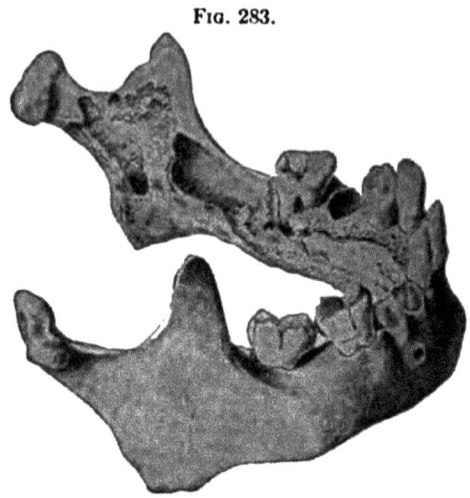

and as a rule they only consult the physician when the trismus, w
appears early, will not disappear, or when, after months, softer
occurs in some part of the swelling.   Incisions and extraction of ne
boring teeth, which are wrongly looked upon as the cause, prove witl
effect.   A sound introduced into the incision or the cavity of the tr
                                                        l sequestr
Despite energetic removal of the foei, or even resection of the mandi
recurrence follows recurrence, one complication is added to the ot
and new fistula and large swellings of the lymph-nodes of the neck
back develop; the process creeps to the glenoid cavity, the audi
meatus, and even into the base of the skull.   After a duration of sev
years the disease generally ends fatally.

Secondary tuberculosis of the jaw differs from the primary form
described chiefly in that it takes its origin from affections of the te
Hence it begins with severe toothache, purulent periostitis, and m
marked general disturbances.   Its later course is accompanied by
formation of fistulæ in the jaw and glandular swelling; it resembles
same stage of the primary disease, but the prognosis seems to be sor
what more favorable.

The diagnosis can always be made definitely in the second stage,
in the first there may be some difficulty, and other tumefactions, sarcor
actinomycosis, and syphilis must be excluded.   Carcinoma hardly co

into consideration, since it almost always affects the lower jaw secondarily from foci in the surrounding skin, mucous membrane, or glands. Besides, carcinoma always appears after the fortieth year, tuberculosis before that age.

In the beginning it is not easy to distinguish tuberculosis from sarcoma of the lower jaw, especially its myeloid form, which is relatively frequent. While tuberculosis runs a protracted course, a sarcoma generally grows rapidly and tends to break through the bone, so that the palpating finger soon makes out a thin shell of bone which can readily be pressed in. Large hard metastases in the lymph-nodes are absent in sarcoma, and fistulæ do not occur in the later stages. In doubtful cases the diagnosis can be made by an exploratory excision or by the reaction of the organism to tuberculin injections.

Tuberculosis of the lower jaw may most readily be mistaken for actinomycosis. The character of the pus discharging from the fistulæ (see Actinomycosis of the Jaw) and the behavior of the lymph-nodes aid in the differential diagnosis. In actinomycosis the latter generally remains unchanged, while in tuberculosis glandular swelling belongs to the clinical picture.

Syphilis of the lower jaw is rare; it manifests itself in firm swellings, and is generally accompanied by other characteristic symptoms of the disease (see Diagnosis of Syphilis).

The necessity of primary radical therapy is evident from the results seen in those cases that have been treated by insufficient measures or not at all. This treatment should be radical even if an early resection is necessary to remove completely the diseased foci. Simple curetting does not suffice, and the hammer and chisel must be employed for quite some distance into the healthy bone. Extensive resections interfere with the function of the jaw, but the many scars and fistulæ after conservative treatment bring about a much worse cosmetic result. Losses of continuity in the mandibular arch may be corrected by mechanical appliances (see Resection of the Lower Jaw). A tonic general treatment should assist the local.

SYPHILIS OF THE JAW.

The author refers to the section on Syphilis of the Month concerning the observations of Fournier, Ritter, and Miller upon the primary syphilitic lesion of the gum and the dangers of transmitting syphilitic virus by dental instruments.

The affections of the jaw belong exclusively to the tertiary stage of syphilis.

The disease shows itself in the lower jaw chiefly in the form of gummatous periostitis and exostoses, which prefer the outer side of the jaw and its angle. The periostitis is more often circumscribed than diffuse, and appears as rounded, smooth, hard, insensitive swellings upon the buccal side of the jaw. They generally resolve or develop into exostoses;

disintegration with necrosis of bone and rupture with discharge o externally or into the mouth is less common.

The diffuse gummatous periostitis has a much worse prognosis the circumscribed owing to protracted suppuration, extensive nec and danger of sepsis.

Rostan and Fournier have observed paralysis of the inferior d nerve as a result of syphilitic exostoses in the region of the mental men.

The hard palate as well as the soft palate is a site of preference *excellence* for tertiary syphilitic disease. Besides the ordinary gumma swellings and syphilitic ulcers, the hard palate is very often the se syphilitic disease of the bone. This disease begins as a roun nodular swelling which softens and breaks down later, and leac necrosis and perforation of the palate. Extension of the syphilitic pro from the nasal cavities to the mouth seems probable, from the pr ence of the disease for the nasal portions of the upper jaw (see Syp of the Nose). In severe cases the framework of the jaw is destro and in addition the base of the skull is affected, so that a meningit imminent. Large perforations into the nasal cavities are followec annoying passage of food into the nose and marked disturbance speech.

In most cases this chronic infectious disease, with its mani courses, can be diagnosticated easily by the personal history, l examination, and other symptoms of the affection. If, however, symptoms of syphilis have preceded the condition, it may easily be i taken for tuberculosis, and even the most experienced specialist i find it impossible to differentiate the two.

Theoretically it has been recommended to examine the granulati for tubercle bacilli and to inoculate animals, but practically this is ra satisfactory. There are much simpler diagnostic aids of inestima value in tuberculin injections, and, above all, in the specific actioi potassium iodide in Ines.

Treatment.—The rule for treating syphilitic affections of the jai to give potassium iodide at once, from 3 to 4 grams (45 to 60 gra as an average daily dose; in imminent perforation of the palate, e 5 to 8 grams (75 to 120 grains) are necessary to combat the desti tive process. The risk of setting up a mild transient iodism is no be considered in view of the impending necrosis of the jaw, which leave its mark permanently.

It is better not to use mercury at all, since it is less efficient and mi cause salivation.

A local treatment, consisting of frequently rinsing the mouth v antiseptic fluids, is appropriate. Where there is retention of pus i gangrene, the surgeon must incise early, drain off the secretions, i extract sequestra if necessary. Small defects of the hard palate covered by plastic operations; large ones are better closed by mechan appliances, for the cicatricial changes in the flap of mucous membr and periosteum and its poorly nourished conditions will frequently l vent a plastic repair. The obturator should be applied as early as possible, since the passage of food and saliva through the perforation causes continual irritation.

PHOSPHORUS NECROSIS (PHOSPHORUS PERIOSTITIS).

As early as 1867 Thiersch cherished the hope that this terrible trade disease would soon be a matter of medical history, and since that time the same expectation has been repeatedly expressed in the literature on phosphorus necrosis. To-day, at the beginning of the twentieth century, this has not been realized despite all sanitary direction and precautions.

From the author's personal inquiries he can confirm the very recent statement of v. Stubenrauch, that necrosis of the jaw still occurs even in factories which deny the presence of poisoning among their workmen. After repeated fruitless attempts to control the evil by stringent hygienic regulations, Switzerland has prohibited by statute the manufacture, import, export, and sale of matches made with yellow phosphorus; and it is to be hoped that other countries will protect workers with phosphorus by like enactments. The lower classes unwillingly part with matches which can be so easily ignited on almost any surface. Even if the use of matches made of yellow phosphorus should be discontinued, the disease would not disappear. Quite recently it has occurred in other industries in which phosphorus is employed, such as phosphorus-bronze foundries and Swedish match factories, where amorphous phosphorus contaminated with yellow phosphorus is used.

According to statistics from 2 to 5 per cent. of workers with phosphorus suffer from necrosis of the jaw. Since laborers who work exclusively with phosphorus were mostly affected, it was easy to look upon the latter as the cause of the disease. By excellent clinical and experimental work v. Bibra and Geist have proved that the affection of the jaw occurring in match factory employés is to be ascribed to phosphorus alone, and especially to the vapors of phosphorus. Formerly arsenic, sulphur fumes, and ozone were wrongly ascribed as causes. The fumes of phosphorus are chiefly given off in the drying chamber of match factories. Hence dipping the matches into the mass containing the phosphorus, drying them, and finally removing the dried matches from the chamber and packing them into boxes, are particularly dangerous occupations. Those workmen who dip the wood into the glue-like mass are affected most early and frequently, since the warm mass fumes considerably. But phosphorus may also be dissolved in gum arabic or tragacanth, and since phosphorus masses prepared in this way are used cold for dipping, the latter method is much less dangerous and is therefore prescribed by law in most countries.

Abundant clinical observations, with studies on anatomical preparation, have explained the pathological changes and the course of the disease, but the manner in which the fumes of phosphorus bring about the initial change in the bone remains unknown, despite numerous experimental investigation. It is especially important to determine the former act directly and locally upon the same which later become necrotic, or if they first affect the body generally. In the latter case general disease would subsequently arise in the jaws, where the free inflammatory conditions following dental caries would find the bone less resistant owing to the constitutional disorder.

The theory that the fumes of phosphorus act locally seems probable in view of the fact that only the jaw is primarily affected by phosphorus necrosis. The valuable experimental studies of Wegner form the support for this theory. The latter found that if rabbits are exposed to the fumes of phosphorus for a long period in a closed place, some develop necrosis of the jaw, but the majority remain well. The jaw is, however, certain to appear if small pieces of periosteum with mucous membrane are removed from the jaws of the exposed animals. If the fumes excite an ossifying periostitis at other sites where the bone is bared of periosteum, as in the tibia, this only occurs when the natural tendency toward healing is interfered with by continued periostitis laceration. Changes in the bones of the jaw were never found when the animals received phosphorus by the mouth.

It must be emphasized here that a process identical to that seen in man could not be induced in any of the animals experimented upon. Necrosis of the jaw which progress continuously until the entire jaw is destroyed, such as are seen in man, do not occur in animals.

But the experiments of Wegner can also be interpreted in favor of general intoxication in which point of minor resistance is created by baring of a piece of bone. This latter theory is supported by clinical observations which have given evidence of the peculiar fact that workmen who have relinquished their occupation in match factories a long time may develop a late necrosis of the jaw without symptoms of phosphorus-poisoning in the interval. The author will only mention the case of necrosis observed by Kosinski, for which no other cause could be determined except that the patient had worked in a match factory twelve years previously; in the interval the patient had always been well.

In connection with the jaw affection in man there are a number of objections to the law of the local action of the phosphorus fumes, based upon animal experiments. The first investigators were of the opinion that carious teeth or recent gaps between the teeth are necessary to up the lesion of the jaw. With a greater experience, however, it was found that workmen with carious teeth can be exposed to the evil influences for years with impunity. Of course, those with defective teeth are affected more easily than those with normal teeth, according to I at least three times as often. Nevertheless, individuals with perfect healthy teeth are not rarely attacked by the disease.

V. Stubenrauch and others are opposed to the theory of the local action of the fumes, and warmly support the belief that the phosphorus enters the blood by way of the pulmonary circulation. The author may agree with v. Stubenrauch when he estimates that the amount of phosphorus which can enter through carious teeth in a given space of time only an exceedingly small fraction of the amount which reaches the blood by way of the pulmonary circulation. The author must also confess that parts of the bone protected against the action of the fumes, particularly the ascending rami, would probably not be involved if inhalation of the fumes locally irritates the periosteum. But the ascending rami are just the place where enormous osteophytes do occur.

Schuchardt is also of the opinion that the phosphorus first causes a general disease of the skeleton which brings about the necrosis by being brought in contact with bacterial infection. A certain disposition to necrosis on the part of the jaw-bones must be assumed for this theory. His explanation of the predisposing skeletal disease is not, however, free from objections; it is supposed to manifest itself in softness and brittleness of the bone, analogous to rhachitis.

Stockmann bacteriologically examined the pus of 6 cases of phosphorus necrosis of the jaw and found tubercle bacilli in all. He therefore looks upon phosphorus-necrosis as a tuberculous necrosis; he believes that further proof is to be found in the fact that pulmonary tuberculosis or tuberculosis of other organs is present in most fatal cases. Histological examination of the diseased bone does not, however, support the view of Stockmann, for in none of the preparations can pathological changes characteristic of tuberculosis be found. Besides, only a fraction of those succumbing after necrosis of the jaw die of tuberculosis.

Kocher is also of the opinion that irritation of bone-forming tissue is not the first action of phosphorus; he inclines toward Ackermann's explanation that cell-necrosis and hyaline degeneration of the vessel-walls are the changes which appear first and which predispose to necrosis.

At any rate, the causation of phosphorus-necrosis depends upon two factors: the influence of phosphorus and an infection manifesting itself as suppurative inflammation. Without sepsis there will be no necrosis. It is impossible at present to decide definitely whether phosphorus acts through the intact gums, or whether it passes through carious teeth or the gaps between the teeth, or finally whether it enters by way of the circulation. Yet the theory of v. Stubenrauch seems probable. According to it, the phosphorus reaching the jaw by way of the blood sets up primary changes, presumably in the marrow, which bring about a deposit in bone in the interior of the jaw. These changes, however, remain latent as long as the bone is not infected. The periostitis of the jaw, whose products are deposited upon the diseased bone as massive osteophytes, occurs only as a result of suppurative infection of the bone or periosteum. This infection generally starts from the cavities of carious teeth, and secondarily renders the bone, modified by the phosphorus, necrotic.

Among other etiological discussions, the chief interest centres around the question as to how long on the average one must be exposed to the influence of the fumes before the disease will make its appearance. This is not easy to answer, since the onset is not acute. The disease generally begins with mild toothache only, so that one generally gets a meagre personal history. The time from the entrance into the factory to the

development of the disease fluctuates exceedingly, for it depends c
upon the hygienic conditions in the factory, the solvent used for the
phorus (see above), and the cleanliness and care of the work
Rydygier speaks of a girl who showed the first symptoms of the di
after three weeks, though she had no defective teeth before begi
work. Schultz refers to a laborer who was exposed to the fume
thirty years without being affected. From many observations Hirt
tions five years as an average.

Age and sex do not seem to have any particular influence upo
disease. If statistics show that more women and young person
affected than men, this finds a simple explanation in the fact that
places chiefly employ women and children to do the work.

It is easy to understand that tuberculosis and anæmia predispo
the disease, since they render the patients less resistant. Pregnanc
the puerperal state may also act in the same way.

The lower jaw is affected considerably more than the upper; acco
to Hirt the average relation is as 5 to 3; according to Thiersch, 9
This probably has the same cause as the greater frequency of affe
of the teeth at the lower jaw. The teeth here are surrounded mo
saliva and exposed to a greater degree to deleterious substances
those of the upper jaw.

With a different conception of the etiology, the interpretation c
pathological changes in phosphorus-necrosis has also undergo
change. The theory that the periosteum is primarily diseased c
to a specific inflammation caused by the phosphorus, and that this
phorus periostitis secondarily involves the bone and sets up a nec
may be discarded. If the periosteum really were irritated by the
phorus, an extensive regeneration of bone would be observed after
operations; but in many cases this is absent, and the intense irrit
which the suppuration exercises must be looked upon as the cau
the energetic regeneration of bone. This is most marked if suppur
has been present before the operation; if this is not the case, it is
scant or absent entirely, even where the periosteum is spared altog
after resection of the lower jaw.

In the early stage v. Stubenrauch states that the main bone lesi
phosphorus-necrosis is a deposit of bone in the interior, while in
later stage it is a lacunar absorption of the bone. Since the de
leads to sclerosis, the jaw is at first hard and sclerotic, and sine
absorption renders it worm-eaten, it later becomes brittle. The de
is due to irritation on the part of the phosphorus or to an inflamm
process in the marrow; the absorption results from the infection. 1
these processes go on in the interior of the jaw, the periosteum, a:
slowly raised from the bone by the suppuration, forms new bone.
entire case of new bone may even develop, which can imperfectly re
the necrotic jaw. (See Fig. 284.)

The osteophytes only rarely cover the entire bone uniformly; the
generally developed most at the under side of the lower jaw, whil
alveolar margin is almost always completely free. If the pus ret

in contact with the osteophytes very long, even these deposits may be destroyed by suppuration, and permanent bone appears.

Owing to its peculiar anatomical structure, the upper jaw is only rarely regenerated as completely as the lower.

Symptoms.—The first symptom, common to all cases of phosphorus-necrosis, is toothache, generally starting from a defective tooth. The pain is generally slight, and intermits for long periods. After an interval of more or less duration the next symptoms appear as a swelling upon the jaw and gum and a loosening of the teeth; suppuration with a most

FIG. 284.

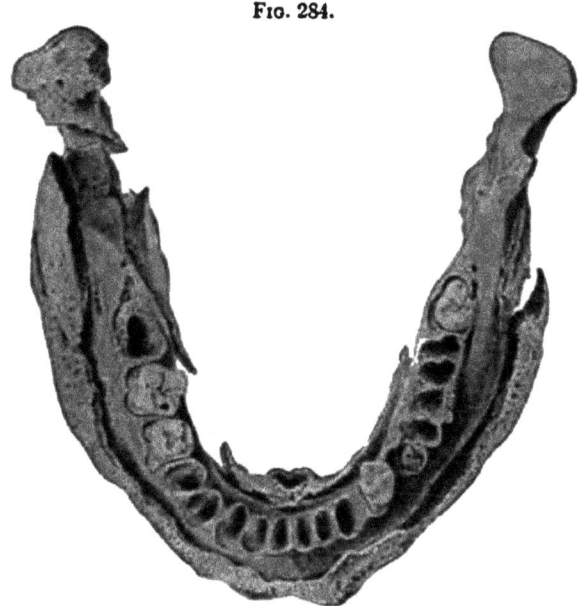

Phosphorus necrosis of lower jaw.

disgusting odor is detected, and the clinical picture of a gum-boil develops. Temporary improvement may follow if the tooth is extracted or the periostitic abscess incised; but soon pain and the formation of abscesses and fistulæ begins anew, and the pus is converted into a stinking fluid mixed with blood. During the later stages the face is changed in a characteristic way: it is much swollen over the inflamed areas, and the skin is tense and not discolored or of a livid red. The general condition of the patients becomes worse and worse, owing to the pain, the difficulty in chewing food, and the foul pus which passes into the stomach. Frequently the condition is complicated by pulmonary disease. With a very chronic course the temperature may be normal or there may occasionally be periods of fever.

The disease generally runs a somewhat milder course in the upper jaw, since the inflammatory secretions discharge more readily; on the

other hand, the danger of extension is greater than with the lower j
and the vomer, orbits, sphenoid and malar bones and even the b
have been affected.

Two, three, or more years pass until a large piece of the jaw
separated sufficiently to be thrown off spontaneously. After this :
puration generally decreases rapidly. Gaps in the new case of b
will be filled in by granulations and connective tissue, and in necr
of the lower jaw under the most favorable conditions a movable b
arch may result (Fig. 284), which replaces the destroyed bone n
in a cosmetic than in a functional way. In the majority of cases n
or less marked deformity remains.

Prognosis.—The prognosis of the disease is much better than
merly, since sanitary police regulations at once remove the affer
individual from his harmful surroundings. According to Trelat,
mortality of the cases observed formerly amounted to nearly 50

FIG. 285.

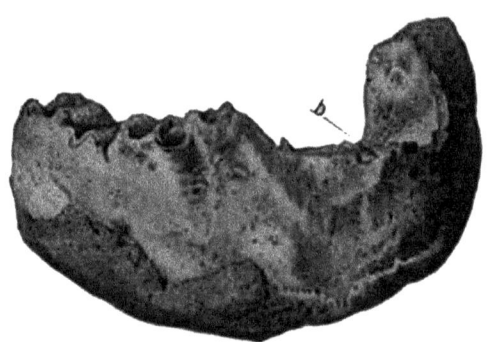

Phosphorus necrosis of the lower jaw in a man aged thirty-eight years. *b.* Defect caused
the operation.

cent. Death is caused directly by any one of a number of complicatic
such as amyloid degeneration of the abdominal organs, nephritis, ǀ
monary phthisis, infection of the base of the skull.

Treatment.—The inadequacy of prophylaxis by sanitary police re
lations has been referred to at the beginning of the chapter. If
match industry, which employs phosphorus, cannot be forbidden a
gether, the prophylaxis should at least demand the following:

Sick or weakly individuals suffering from carious teeth or tuber
losis should not be allowed to take part in the work. The worksh
should be thoroughly ventilated, and on entering and leaving the clot
must be . changed, the hands washed, and the mouth rinsed. ꟾ
employés should not eat where they work. The rooms where pɦ
phorus mass is prepared and where the matches are dipped, dried, ɩ
packed, must be kept isolated from the rest of the factory.

The cases may be treated in three different ways. An early, sub-periosteal, and a subosteophytic resection, and expectative method are distinguished.

Fig. 286.

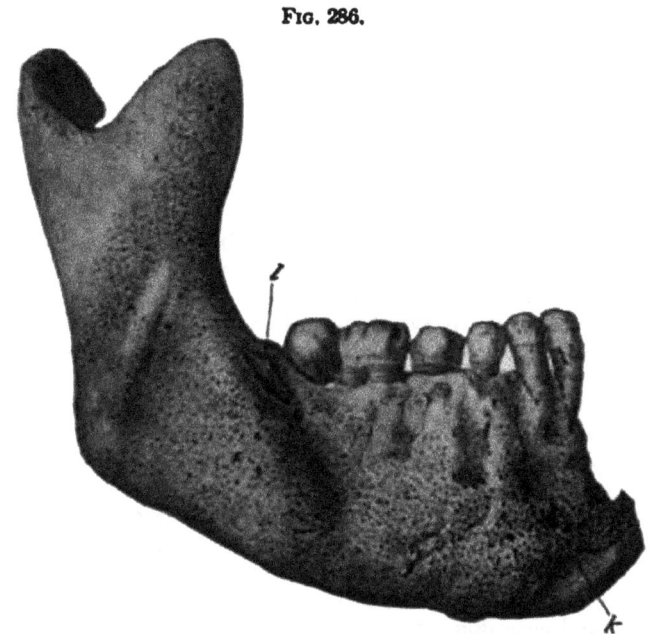

Phosphorus necrosis of the lower jaw in a woman aged twenty-five years. *k.* Beginning line of demarcation. *l.* Small cloaca with cortical sequestrum.

Fig. 287.

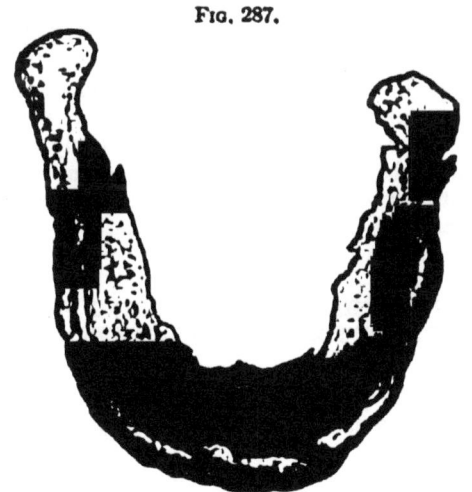

Total necrosis of the lower jaw.

The propriety of the third method lies especially in its good cosme result. But in most cases the new formation is too incomplete a uncertain to justify the protracted suppuration with its dangers a pain. A few brilliant cases, which, however, were the exception, ha blinded criticism. The subosteophytic method has the great disadva tage of obliging one to keep the case under constant observation, sin one must wait for the demarcation of the necrotic tissue. The lat generally goes on so slowly that the disease continues on the avera for at least one and a half years. The entire lower jaw is genera destroyed by this method in any event.

Recently the early subperiosteal resection has found most fav The objections were that it did not cure, since the process spre and a regeneration of bone did not occur, but these objections pro not valid on close observation. If one operates boldly in the healt tissue, one can indeed check the advance of the disease. Since t entire jaw is almost always destroyed in necrosis, one more read decides upon a total resection of one or both halves of the jaw. T cure is rapid and complete in proportion to how early and radical operate. In some cases it may be of advantage to resect the hal separately after a longer interval.

In phosphorus-necrosis Bogdanik extirpates if possible the entire j in one sitting. He removes it from the mouth without any exten incision, and says he gets much better cosmetic and functional resu than with partial resections. This method suggested itself to him the constant deviation of the remaining piece, and by the fact that t remaining bone soon becomes affected after partial resection.

The second objection against early resection, that no regeneration bone follows, does not hold, provided the periosteum is spared during t operation.

INFLAMMATIONS OF THE JAW IN TABES.

Trophic changes in the jaws may occur in all stages of tabes dorsal and may even be the first symptom. They are characteristic in th they begin with loosening and falling out of perfectly healthy teeth a with anæsthesia of the adjacent portions of the gum. In some of t cases they eventually lead to atrophy of the jaw, in others to rath painless suppuration with necrosis of the bone.

INFLAMMATION OF THE BONES OCCURRING AMONG WORKE IN MOTHER-OF-PEARL (PEARL-CARVERS' BONES).

As occasionally the jaws are affected by this rather rare, thou extremely peculiar, disease of the bones, its important clinical featur will be briefly described here.

In the year 1870 Englisch called attention to a group of symptoi characteristic of this disease, and showed that the latter attacked on a certain class of workers, namely, mother-of-pearl carvers, that it occurred only in individuals about the time of puberty, and that it had an absolutely characteristic onset and course. A mother-of-pearl carver is suddenly seized with violent tearing pains in one of his bones. A swelling regularly develops at the diaphysis of the bone, usually close to the boundary between epiphysis and diaphysis. This swelling involves the overlying soft parts and, pathologically considered, consists of an osteomyelitis followed by ostitis and periostitis. During the initial stage pain is not increased by pressure upon the affected bone, but as soon as the swelling has developed the slightest touch is extremely painful.

Gussenbauer found slight fever in the 6 cases from Billroth's clinic. The pain and swelling of the bone gradually recede until the latter has reached its normal size. Quite exceptionally an abscess is formed. Should the patient resume his accustomed occupation, however, a fresh attack as a rule sets in.

In one of Gussenbauer's cases and in both of Fischer's the jaw was the seat of the disease. Gussenbauer's patient was fifteen years old, and had been for three years a mother-of-pearl carver. The right half of his lower jaw had been previously affected six times in a similar manner. He showed considerable swelling, extending from the articulation of the jaw to the first incisor tooth, where it was sharply bounded by a steep ascending ridge in the periosteum.

Gussenbauer believes that conchiolin is the cause of this recurrent inflammation of bones. This is an inorganic substance present in the innermost layer of the shell of the pearl oyster, *Avicula margaritifera*. and he believes that, like other kinds of dust, this enters the circulation, and collects in the capillaries of the bone-marrow on account of a slowing of the blood-current, producing embolism, at first only of the capillaries in the diaphysis, finally also of the smaller arteries, thus leading to an infarction. At present there is no positive proof of this hypothesis.

The prognosis of the disease is favorable provided the patient relinquishes his occupation.

Treatment consists of the application of moist heat and remedies aiding absorption.

PERIOSTITIS, OSTITIS, OSTEOMYELITIS, AND NECROSIS OF THE JAW.

The usual course of inflammatory processes of the jaw suggests the above heading for this section. As in the ease of inflammation of other bones, one does not find in many cases a sharply defined periostitis, ostitis, or osteomyelitis. Very frequently, owing to the intimate relations of the layers of bone, inflammation may extend either from without or within to other portions of the bone. This applies to *periostitis*, which frequently results from carious teeth. It may be mentioned here, how-

ever, that traumatism, accidental or surgical in character, prod
injury of the mucous membrane, may be the cause of inflammati
the periosteum; also constitutional diseases (scurvy), infectious di:
(typhoid), particularly the exanthemata (scarlatina, measles, small
The latter forms have been observed, generally in children at ɪ
the fifth year, so that the development of the teeth must be conced
have a predisposing influence.

At the time of the second dentition inflammations of the ja'
not infrequently observed without concomitant general diseases.
the eruption of the wisdom teeth is popularly feared on accou
the frequent secondary inflammatory manifestations in the jaw ‹
are almost always due to infection.

As the lower jaw is more continuously exposed to injurious influ
than the upper jaw, its diseases are more frequent and obst
Inflammation of the lower jaw may be dangerous for the reasor
it frequently extends downward to the larynx.

If, following an abscess resulting from periostitis of the alɪ
process, the periosteum remains detached for any length of timɪ

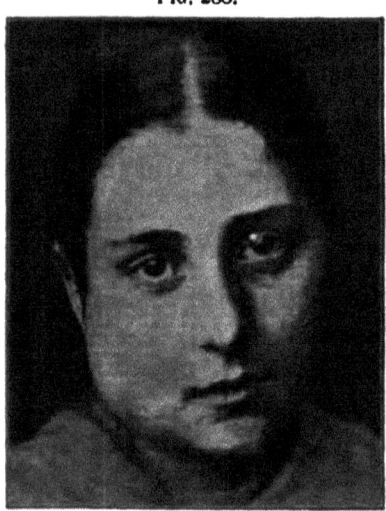

Fig. 288.

Periostitis of the lower jaw.

to any great extent, a small pɪ
of the bone may undergo nec
Such formation of a sequestrɪ
the jaw can usually be avoid
early incision.

Besides the usual patholɪ
forms of periostitis, simple
purulent and *purulent*, ther
mains a third, though rathei
form, *periostitis ossificans*.
immense broadening of the
lower portion of the face ol
fifteen-year-old girl, shown in
288, is the result of a slowl
veloping ossifying periostitis :
lating exactly the course of ɪ
coma. Three months befori
mission to the hospital the pɪ
noticed for the first time tha
right cheek was slightly swɪ
The teeth of the right lowei
were absolutely sound, tootl
had never occurred; during the growth of the tumor, however, then
occasionally pain in the right ear. The tumor was hard, scarcely sen:
to pressure, extending from the anterior border of the masseter p
riorly over the ascending ramus of the jaw, but limited exactly tɪ
outer and inferior surface of the maxilla. No abnormality coul
felt through the buccal cavity. Cutting down on the tumor it was fɪ
that the swelling of the jaw was composed of soft, spongy bone-ti
deposited upon the hard bony shell of the lower jaw in a layer ɪ

2 cm. thick, which could easily be removed with a sharp spoon. The shape of the maxilla was not changed.

As bone, in its strictest sense, is composed largely of inorganic substance, it is only possible to speak of an ostitis in the sense that the Haversian canals are the seat of inflammation. The latter condition possesses little significance, however, compared with periostitis or osteomyelitis, which nearly always precedes it, so that it will be sufficient to discuss these two principal kinds of inflammation. Reference will be made here only to the Haversian canals as agents between inflammations of the periosteum and inflammation of the bone-marrow.

Osteomyelitis is caused either by an infection extending from without to the medullary spaces, or it is of so-called idiopathic origin—*i. e.*, originating in the circulation.

The first manner of infection is easily conceivable in injuries of the jaws, principally compound fractures, as a result of which the bone-marrow is exposed. It is more difficult, however, to come to a conclusion regarding the extremely important practical question as to whether the extraction of teeth within an inflamed area is capable of bringing about the serious clinical picture of osteomyelitis. Admitting this path of infection, it is surprising that with the innumerable extractions of teeth, which are done generally without any aseptic precautions, inflammation of the marrow, with necrosis, does not take place more frequently. Based upon this consideration, it is maintained that in most cases in which osteomyelitis has been observed after the extraction of teeth, the former had existed when extraction was done.

The author's experience would support the old conception of Huster regarding the danger of extracting teeth in the presence of inflammatory conditions. Accordingly, the author proceeds very cautiously in such cases. In a case of periostitis of the superior maxilla which was running a slow benign course, the extraction of a tooth was followed by infection, with high temperature, putrefaction, and subsequent necrosis of the bone, and extensive drainage and removal of the sequestrum were rendered necessary. As favoring the view that there is less danger of infection in the extraction of teeth under ordinary circumstances, it may be maintained that an inflamed area, with dilated bloodvessels and hyperæmia offers conditions more favorable for absorption than does a normal alveolar process, and that in case of purulent inflammation of the alveolar region there are surely present virulent germs which would not find their way into the cavity of the mouth under ordinary circumstances.

The solution of this problem lies probably in the proper after-treatment. General fundamental surgical principles would compel the surgeon to act here according to the old rule, *Ubi pus ibi evacua*, and to proceed in a similar manner as in the case of inflammation of other bones—*i. e.*, to remove the sequestrum; one would hardly do anything else in case of a tooth bathed with pus. In case of the jaw such a procedure is not only permissible, but even imperative, provided that the after-treatment of the resulting wound of the bone be carried out as

carefully as it would be in the case of any other bone. The opera
should not end with the extraction of the tooth. The latter proceed
should be followed by thorough irrigation of the cavity of the tooth v
antiseptic solutions (as, for example, 2 per cent. solution of carb
acid), and subsequent packing with iodoform gauze.

Idiopathic osteomyelitis (infection of the bone-marrow through
circulation) is rarely observed as a single focus of inflammation.
usually occurs in connection with medullary inflammation of other bo
and usually in young individuals. The lower jaw is more freque
the seat of disease than the upper. Regarding the latter, the syr
toms in the beginning may be characteristic of empyema of the maxill
sinus, and may lead to confusion. Fig. 289 shows the lower jaw o

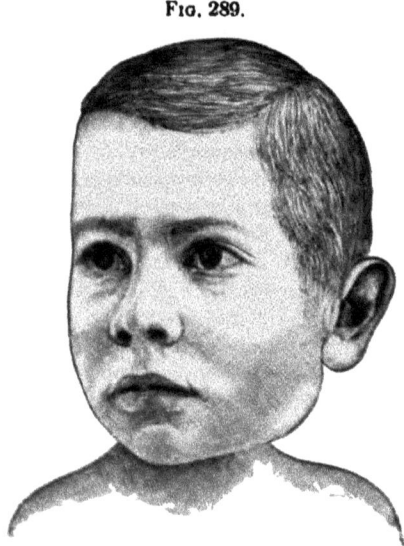

FIG. 289.

Osteomyelitis of lower jaw.

seven-year-old boy affected v
osteomyelitis. He had first :
fered from acute myelitis of
left hip-bone as a result
trauma, and during conva
cence, fully half a year later
showed this metastasis in
jaw. The swelling of the lo
jaw developed slowly, and in
beginning was painless and
accompanied by fever. It '
not until after a number
weeks, when œdema of the
cheek had extended to the ʃ
that severe pain of the lo
jaw set in, accompanied by ʃ
mus and high temperature v
delirium. In the course of a
days all manifestations dis
peared without suppuration. :
at the present time the boy, h
ing fully recovered in all ol
respects, bears only the thick

ing of the jaw shown in the illustration. This one example points
a fact which has frequently been confirmed, that acute osteomyel
of the jaw does not always follow the lightning course of acute infl
mation of the marrow of other bones, but frequently produces mil
symptoms in the form of a so-called osteomyelitis sicca. In ol
cases, however, it is true, in spite of its local character, that the cor
is accompanied by severe general manifestations, with suppurat
and early loosening of the teeth. Contrary to expectation, the la
are frequently capable of being preserved, and after the process
terminated become firmly reunited.

Diffuse osteomyelitis affecting the lower jaw shows the rapid cor
of the disease in a marked form. Following severe chills, the tempe
ture may reach 104° F., or higher. Œdema of the soft parts become

extensive that the head is deformed to a terrible degree. The swelling into the buccal cavity, which frequently prevents the taking of nourishment, is generally of no significance, as the patients almost always succumb rapidly as a result of general septic manifestation. In addition, extension of this infection to the meninges and brain is imminent. Under the most favorable circumstances total necrosis, or almost total necrosis, is to be expected.

The rational treatment must in the first place seek to provide rapid evacuation of pus and attempt to prevent extensive separation of periosteum and subsequent necrosis. This can be accomplished only by early free incision to the bone from without. If the incision be made along the lower border of the jaw, it produces only slight deformity. Incision from the buccal cavity is useless. Owing to the fact that ankylosis of the jaw is liable to complicate this disease, immobilizing bandages for the jaw should be soon discarded. If the general condition is good, and there is only a small amount of suppuration, removal of the sequestrum may be delayed until the necrotic fragments of bone have been loosened. The expectant method of treatment possesses the advantage that a new layer of bone can be formed from the osteophytes. If the sequestrum can be removed through the buccal cavity, this method is to be preferred to sequestrotomy from without. The latter, however, is generally rendered necessary by existing circumstances.

More extensive defects of bone which exist after the sequestrum has been expelled, particularly if located in the upper jaw, may be successfully repaired by mechanical means.

TUMORS OF THE JAW.

Statistics covering all benign and malignant tumors of the jaw show that the upper and lower are equally predisposed to disease. Of the different kinds of tumors, carcinoma and sarcoma are the most prevalent. Examination of the latest compilation of tumors of the upper jaw shows that among approximately 750 cases there were nearly 400 carcinomata, as against 300 sarcomata (including epulis). While carcinoma more frequently affects the male sex, sarcoma appears to have a predilection for the female sex.

It is practical to consider separately tumors of the gums and alveolar process and tumors of the body of the jaw.

Tumors of the Gums and Alveolar Process.

Consideration of a number of extremely rare tumors of the alveolar process of the jaw, such as angioma and cirsoid aneurysm of the dental artery, may be omitted here; also those proliferations of the gums, called polypi, which grow from the margin of the gums into the cavities of teeth destroyed by caries, or which have been caused by irritating dental appliances, as they have little surgical interest. A clip of the scissors quickly and effectually removes them.

The real tumors of the gums, more or less pedunculated, originati principally in the gaps between the teeth, have from ancient times bo: the name *epulis*. This term has a purely topographical significan being derived from the Greek ἐπι (on) and οὖλις (the gums), and me:

FIG. 290.

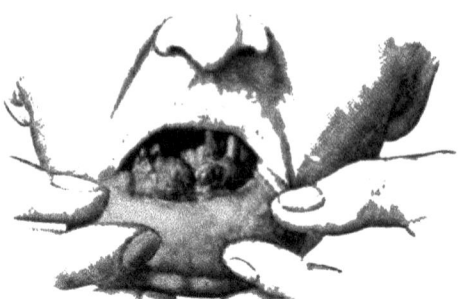

Sarcomatous epulis in a woman aged fifty-six years.

nothing more. It is applied to a tumor which is attached to the gu: in distinction to *parulis*. They are bright-red proliferations of the s: of a cherry or walnut or larger, painless provided the jaw is not involv They frequently extend by a broad base over the edges of a number alveoli, and are followed by loose ing of the affected teeth. Their s face generally shows impressions teeth.

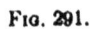

FIG. 291.

The histological character epulis tumors varies considerab Usually it is that of a *sarcoma*, w spindle cells or very frequently wi giant-cell structure—that is, a s coma giganto-cellulare. Frequent however, one finds upon microseo; cal examination a more harml: *fibroma*, characterized by dense co nective tissue. Both these forms new growth explain the frequent c currence of these tumors in the la: years of childhood, at the time puberty, and in middle age. Mc rarely there are found myxomato

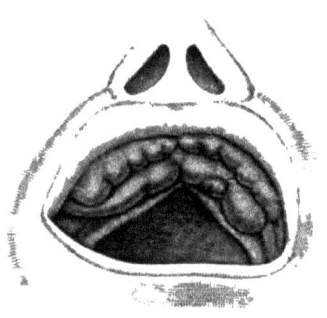

Lobulated fibroma of the gums from irritation of a dental plate.

or osteoid forms. In more advanced age carcinomatous new growt may occur at the edge of the jaws in the form of epulis. They ha been observed even in childhood.

The starting point of these tumors is the periosteum of the alveol process or the connective tissue of the alveolar portion of the ja Frequently their occurrence may be referred to local irritation.

PLATE XII.

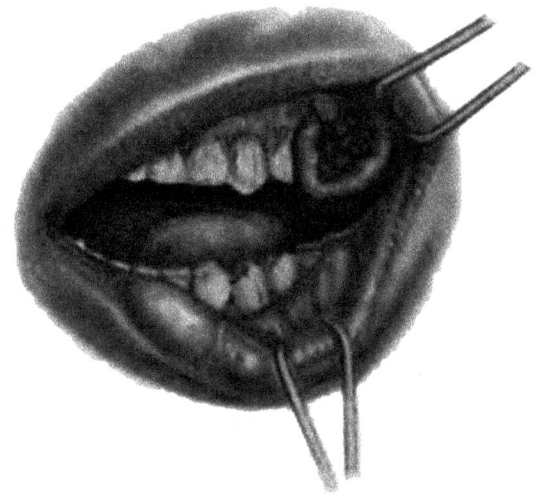

Epulis. (Grünwald.)

nosis.—The diagnosis of the kind of tumor depends, in the first
upon its consistence. Sarcoma is of a softer character than
a; consequently it bleeds more easily than the latter. It shows
rapid growth in general and is more liable to involve the bone

FIG. 292.

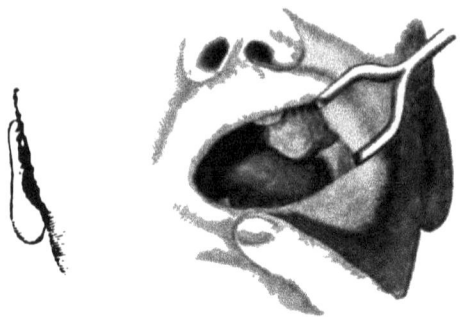

Fibroma epulis of the upper gum from a woman aged twenty-eight years.

he benign fibroma, which only acts by producing pressure. Dis-
the glands is rare in case of sarcoma.
inomatous epulis occurs principally in older individuals, and
lly in the region of the posterior molar and wisdom teeth, which,
ted by caries, frequently subject the mucous membrane to chronic

FIG. 293.

Epulis.

on. It easily ulcerates, extends rapidly to the jaw, and is fol-
by metastases of the glands.
tment.—In all cases the treatment should be radical, not simply
noval of the growth with scissors, as is too often the case. Even

the benign forms recur after such an incomplete operation. It is alwa necessary to remove the underlying bone, and often the teeth in conne tion with it. If the disease has involved the alveolar process or the ji only, extensive resection through healthy bone suffices. Beside t different bone-saws, bone-scissors and gouge-forceps are useful. T hemorrhage is usually profuse. It is controlled by packing with iodofoi gauze; at times the cautery is necessary.

Tumors of the Body of the Jaw.

First will be discussed those new growths of the body of the jaw t occurrence of which depends directly upon some disturbance in t development of the teeth. They are *odontomata* and *follicular dental cys*

Odontoma.—Broca has given the name odontoma to tumors whi are made up of tissue like the teeth either during the time of th development or later. As a cause of this increased growth some ir tation caused by disturbances in the development of the dental follicl must be assumed.

Odontomata are divided, according to the stage of development the dental follicles in which they occur, into embryoplastic, odont plastic, and those occurring at the period of crown- and root-formatio

FIG. 294.

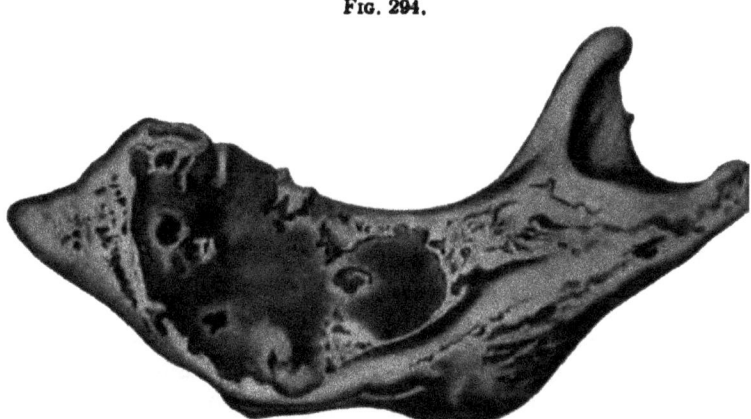

Odontoma of the lower jaw.

If a tumor develops in the dental sac at a time when the latter composed of mucous tissue, only a pure myxoma results. If connect tissue takes part in the hyperplasia, as is frequently the case, the results a fibrous odontoma. During the second or odontoplastic peri of development soft fibrous tumors are liable to occur, with, howev a tendency to eburnation, particularly during advanced stages of dev opment.

The crown odontoma, belonging to the third period of developme are bony tumors, owing to the fact that they contain dentine and enam

They are irregular in outline and attached to the neck of the tooth. Root odontomata are characterized by layers of cement-substance which never contains enamel.

This histological classification of odontomata is not accepted by all investigators. Some of these tumors have been described as benign epithelioma (epithéliome adamantins).

Diagnosis.—The diagnosis of soft odontoma is frequently very difficult, for confusion with other tumors of the jaw, such as cysts, fibroids, and particularly sarcoma, is likely. The slow growth of a tumor, however, its freedom from pain, with an irregular surface, render a probable diagnosis possible in many cases. The diagnosis can be made with certainty only by operative exposure of the tumor. For-

FIG. 295.

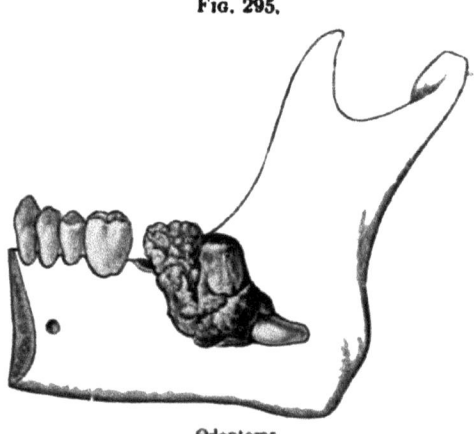

Odontoma.

tunately, this is indicated in the case of all tumors entering into differential diagnosis. The operation shows a soft tissue, characterized frequently by included masses of cement or dentine, sharply defined from the bone and occasionally encapsulated.

The hard odontomata, which occur more frequently, do not as a rule occasion confusion, particularly if Broca's rule is borne in mind, that any new growth of the jaw which occurs after complete development of the teeth is certainly not an odontoma. In the great majority of cases the permanent molar teeth, particularly the wisdom teeth, are the seat of the lesion.

Broca calls attention, moreover, to the fact that odontoma, as opposed to dental cyst, is characterized by a swelling on the outer as well as on the inner side of the jaw, and that it frequently involves the alveolar border, while dental cysts have a tendency to develop toward the outer side of the jaw at some distance from the alveolar border.

Prognosis.—The generally favorable prognosis of odontoma is subject to certain limitations in so far as a benign tumor may in its subsequent course lead to inflammatory and necrotic processes in the bone.

Treatment.—The treatment consists in radical removal of the tumor which can generally be easily accomplished under local anæsthesi owing to the tendency of these tumors to be sharply circumscribed When they are larger, or inflammatory conditions are present, thei removal may necessitate general anæsthesia. Different routes must h employed in these operations. Crown odontomata can usually b removed through the month after incising the mucous membrane o after partial resection of the alveolar border. When an odontoma i more deeply embedded in the bone, exposure of the respective portio of the jaw from without can hardly be avoided. Total resection of th jaw is hardly ever necessary.

Follicular Dental Cysts.—These occur as a result of disturbanc in the development of the dental sac, and, with the exception of th wisdom teeth, can therefore occur only during the early years of life Cystic degeneration may, however, occur even when the dental sac i properly placed, but usually irritation of a tooth abnormally placed which does not break through the bony covering, leads to cystic dila tation of the lining of the sac.

Fig. 296.

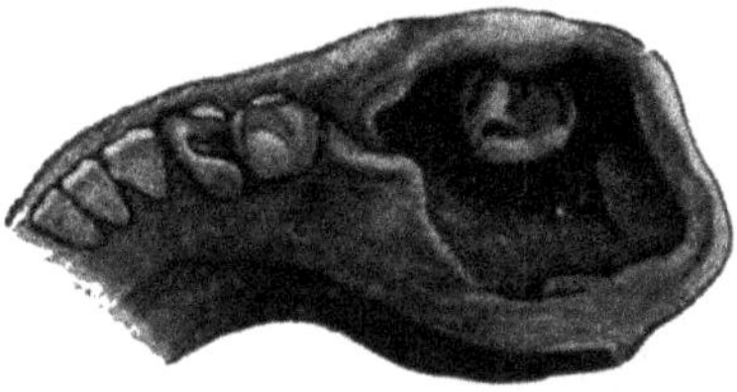

Dental cyst of the lower jaw in a boy aged fourteen years.

Accordingly, in every case of follicular cyst a tooth ought to h missing from the mouth and be found within the cyst, if not in a full; developed condition, at least in the form of a rudimentary tooth; bu exceptionally cysts originate from erratic tooth germs. The epithelia lining of the inner wall of the cyst must be considered the remains o the dental follicle. Such tumors are more frequently met with in th lower jaw than in the upper. They produce thin-walled swellings o the bone which may protrude principally at the weaker outer surfac of the jaw. In the upper jaw the cysts may even grow into the maxillar sinus. The contents are usually a serous, somewhat mucoid fluid. I rare cases the latter becomes purulent and produces severe inflammatio of the jaw.

Diagnosis.—The diagnosis is based principally upon the extraordi narily slow growth of a round, painless tumor, the tendency to develo toward the outer surface of the jaw, and upon the subsequently devel oping, yielding character of the wall, which is frequently felt as parchment-like crackling. Exploratory puncture or an *x*-ray exposur might contribute to the certainty of the diagnosis.

Treatment.—The treatment consists in the removal of the outer wall of the cyst, which, on account of the thinness of the bone, can usually be accomplished through the mouth with a pair of strong scissors. The remainder of the cyst gradually diminishes in size without further treatment, and disappears almost entirely.

Cystoma of the Jaw.—Beside follicular cysts, there occur in the jaw a number of other unilocular and multilocular cystic tumors of dental and paradental origin. Some of them originate in inclusions of the epithelium of the mouth within the substance of the jaw. The manner of occurrence may explain the frequent mixed forms of cysts with solid tissue new growths as a result of a process of cystic degeneration and cellular proliferation.

Fig. 297.

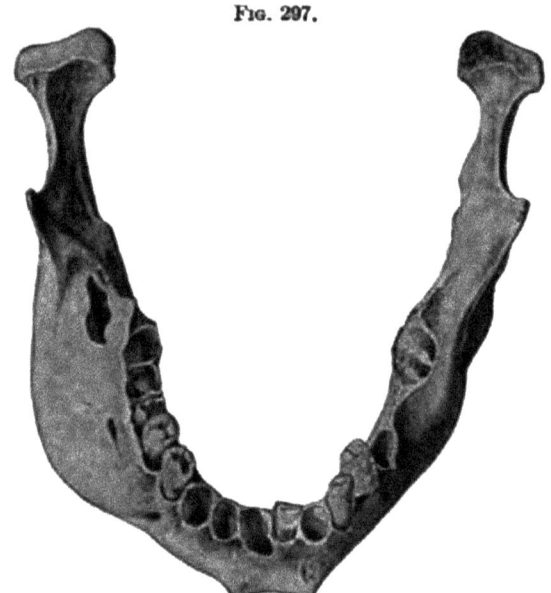

Dental cyst, lower jaw.

The so-called *periosteal cysts* are caused by periostitis of the root, and are, therefore, of inflammatory origin. The inflammatory processes at the apex of the root of a tooth may cause the accumulation of a slightly turbid fluid exudate, which brings about a separation of the periosteum of the root of the tooth, and which is followed by the gradual development of small cystic cavities. As these kinds of cysts originate in carious teeth, they are generally observed only in adults, more frequently in the molar and bicuspid teeth than those situated anteriorly. They also frequently involve the maxillary sinus.

Diagnosis and Treatment.—In regard to diagnosis and treatment, the reader is referred to the discussion on follicular cysts. In the periosteal forms the diseased root should in all cases be removed at the san time. Large and multilocular cysts may demand total resection of tl jaw.

Connective-tissue Tumors of the Jaw.

The group of connective-tissue tumors is represented in the jaw on by fibromata. Myxomata are rarely found pure, but generally as mixt fibrous tumors. They are distinguished symptomatically from the pui forms by their softer consistency. In other respects they do not deman special discussion. Only two cases of lipoma are known; both occurre in the upper jaw.

Fibroma.—This occurs usually in youth, more frequently in the upp than in the lower jaw. Apparently traumatic irritation of the tee plays an etiological part. According to their point of origin, the: tumors are distinguished as *periosteal* and *osteal* (or central) fibromat The former, originating in the periosteum, are more rare. They ha\

FIG. 298.

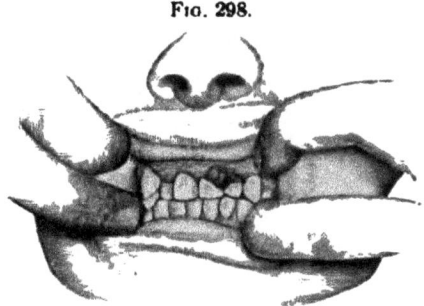

Small fibroma of gum.

been discussed in part above as epulis tumors. Those occurring in th body of the jaw are at first freely attached to the surface of the bone i the form of rounded or lobular tumors, but may later develop into larg growths, and by means of pressure bring about disappearance of th bone lamellæ.

The osteal or central fibromata originate in the interior of the ja from some connective-tissue portion of the medullary tissue of th Haversian canals, the vessels, the nerves, or the peridontium, and ai surrounded by a shell-like covering of bone. The tumor, as it increase in size, gradually breaks through the bone, and may later cause th cheek to protrude or may project out of the mouth, and, in case the upper jaw, penetrate into the maxillary sinus.

The consistence of these growths is variable. Generally they for1 dense tumors. They may, however, become soft or bone-like, according 1 the abundance of vessels and the deposit of lime, cartilage, or bone-tissu

Diagnosis.—The diagnosis of periosteal fibroma is readily made b the firm consistence and slow growth of the tumor in a young subjee and eventually by exploratory incision. Central fibroma, on the contrary, is hardly recognizable in its initial stages, for the only noticeable feature is a swelling of the jaw, which is only exceptionally accompanied by pain, as in case of compression of a nerve. It is only when the tumor breaks through that its firm, nodular character, absence of adhesion with the surrounding tissues, and the absence of swelling of the lymph-glands lead to the conclusion of a benign tumor.

Prognosis.—The prognosis is generally favorable; at the same time, a certain reserve is advisable on account of a possible sarcomatous change in the new growth.

Fig. 299.

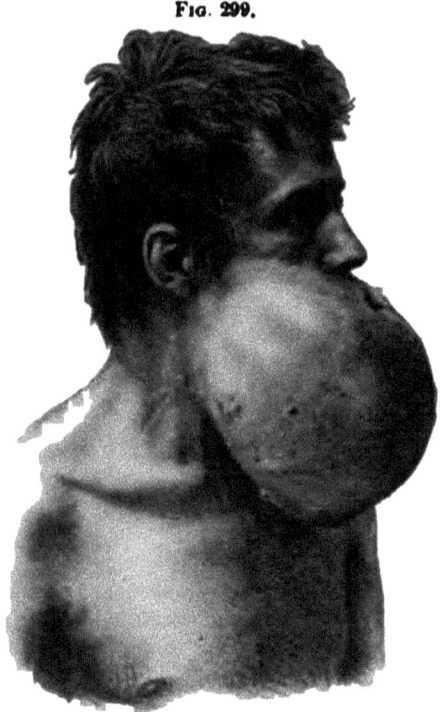

Alveola cystoma.

Treatment.—The treatment consists in the operative removal of the tumor, with the layer of periosteum or bone forming the starting point. In the case of central fibroma total resection of the jaw may become necessary.

Chondroma of the Jaw.—Clinically, chondroma is very similar to fibroma of the jaw, but it occurs much more infrequently than the latter. These growths are also divided into tumors originating in the periosteum, perichondromata or ecchondromata, and those originating in the interior of the jaw, enchondromata. This distinction has little

practical value.   It has been maintained that enchondroma occu
principally in the lower jaw and ecchondroma in the upper jaw.
the lower jaw, which is more frequently affected by this form of n(

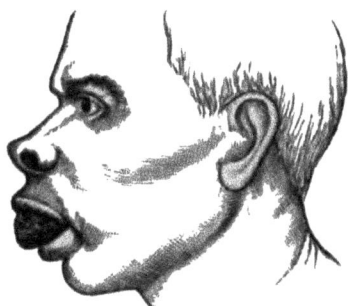

FIG. 300.

Enchondroma of the upper jaw.

growth than the upper, there a
developed hard nodular tumo
gradually involving the entire bo
and proliferating outward.   T
points of origin in the upper ji
are enumerated in the order of th(
frequency: alveolar process, the a
terior surface, the maxillary sim
the nasal process, the hard palat
and the outer wall of the nasal cavil
At these sites chondromata may d
velop into shapeless tumors, di
figuring the face and threatenii
even the orbital and cranial cavitie
Young individuals are more fr
quently attacked by the di
ease.   Histologically it
either a pure hyaline cho
droma, fibrochondroma, (
ossifying chondroma. The:
forms of new growth fr
quently require one and tw
decades for their develoj
ment.

FIG. 301.

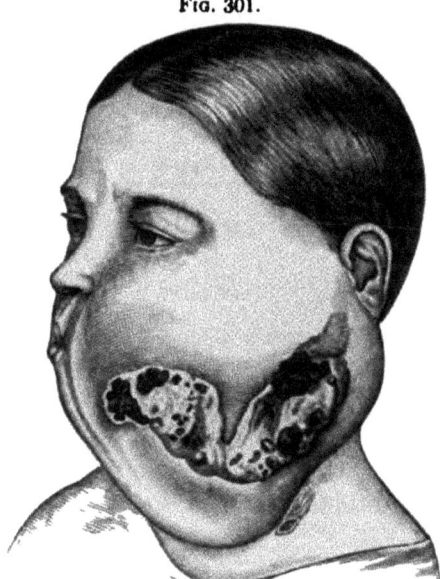

Exostosis of the lower jaw in a woman aged twenty-seven
years; duration, thirteen years.

Osteoma.—The few ne
growths that have been d
scribed as diffuse hypero
toses possess little practic:
interest, as, on account (
their slow growth and sligl
disturbance they seldo(
become the objects of su
gical interference.   The a'
thor has referred above '
the *development of exostos*
in the course of the gre
variety of inflammatory pr
cesses of the jaw.
Hard osteoma is not i
frequently observed in tl

frontal sinus, orbital cavity, and nasal process of the frontal bon
From this point it may extend to the jaw.   On the other hand, it m:
originate from within the interior of the jaw.   Osteoma usually cal
for surgical aid, not so much on account of cosmetic and function
disturbances, as by the effects of pressure upon nerves, vessels, nas

passages, tear-ducts, orbital cavities, even the base of the skull and the cranial cavity.

Diagnosis.—The diagnosis is possible in those cases only in which a chondroma or osteoma is situated at the surface. The great hardness of a tumor, its firm attachment to the jaw, and its slow growth would determine the probably benign, chondral or osteal character of a new growth. An exact histological or even genetic diagnosis can, however, be arrived at only by operative exposure of the tumor.

Treatment.—If the symptoms caused by an osteoma render its operative removal necessary, the resection must include healthy bone in order to avoid recurrence. In this way the great and often surprising difficulties which eburnated portions of bone offer to instruments can be avoided.

FIG. 302.

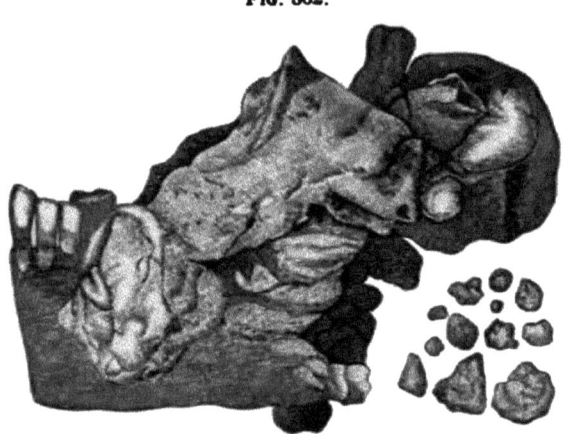

Excised lower jaw with exostosis; two-thirds natural size.

Sarcoma of the Jaw.—If one very properly includes sarcomatous epulis among sarcomata of the jaw, these new growths constitute the most frequent tumor of the lower jaw, and—as the introductory remarks indicate—in the upper jaw they would not be found so far behind carcinoma in frequency as one might be led to believe by earlier statistics, which do not include epulis.

Sarcoma is usually a disease of youth; the average age of the author's patients was thirty-five years. Old age, however, is not exempt.

Regarding the etiology, it can only be said that, according to the author's observations, a coincidence of sarcoma with caries of the teeth and inflammatory conditions of the gums is conspicuously frequent.

The majority of sarcomatous new growths are observed in the alveolar processes, particularly in the anterior portion of the latter in the region of the incisor and canine teeth.

Sarcomata are divided into those originating in the periosteum and those originating in the bone-marrow, or periosteal and myelogenous growths. Histologically they are at times spindle-cell or giant-cell sar-

comata, at times small-cell new growths, frequently mixed tumors, wi
mxyoma, enchondroma, and angioma, not infrequently also cys
tumors. There are several observations of melanotic tumors. T
above classification, which considers the point of origin, coincides larg
with the clinical division into *hard* and *soft* sarcoma. This has a din
bearing also on the prognosis, and above all on the treatment. Tum
originating in the periosteum usually have a firm consistence and purs
a benign course. Sarcomata proliferating from the marrow and causi
swelling of the bone are soft tumors, and are among the most maligns
of neoplasms.

Fig. 303.

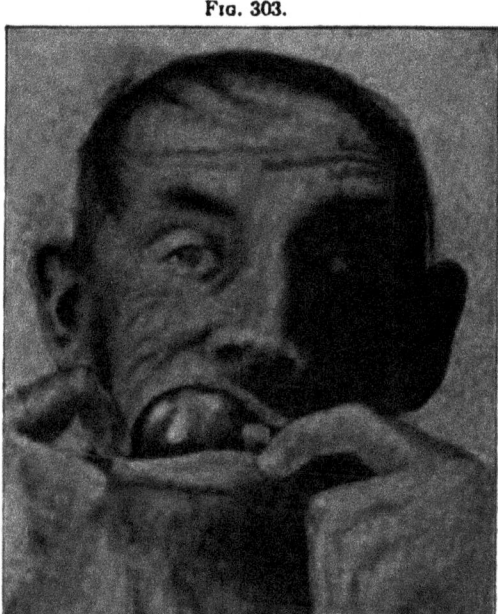

Periosteal sarcoma.

Periosteal sarcomata have a peculiar radiate structure and occasional
contain certain trabeculæ of bone showing a distinctly stellate arrang
ment. They are hard tumors, attached to the bone, but extending in ;
directions. In the upper jaw they are very liable to involve the maxilla
sinus. In the lower jaw, not only the body, but the angle of the ja
also is frequently the seat of the lesion.

The tissue composing *myelogenous sarcoma* is usually very rich in cel
containing little intercellular substance, and for this reason it has receive
the name medullary sponge (Markschwämme). The consistence ar
color vary according to the kind of growth, and according to the number
vessels. Usually the tissues are of a reddish-brown or a grayish-red colo

If softening or cystic change occurs in a tumor, there may be four
in the cysts a bloody or serosanguinous fluid, resulting from ruj

ture of vessels. Occasionally there have been observed in such cysts gelatinous and semisolid masses which had resulted from mucous and fatty changes in the elements of a sarcoma. In the beginning a myelogenous sarcoma is covered by the outer shell of bone. It rapidly grows in all directions, breaks through the bone, and appears within the region of the month and check as a tumor, frequently of enormous size, which finally undergoes ulceration. In the upper jaw these forms are very liable to develop toward the maxillary sinus; at times they attack the orbital cavity, the nasal passages, the pharynx, even the base of the skull. In general, however, there is no tendency in case of sarcoma of the upper jaw to extend very early into the adjacent regions. For this reason any manifestations on the part of neighboring organs do not set in until late, and pain is generally considerably less intense than that of carcinoma.

Diagnosis.—The diagnosis of hard periosteal sarcoma which develops at the surface of the jaw from the onset does not occasion any great difficulty. These tumors begin to develop as small, hard, usually round nodules upon the outer or inner surface of the lower jaw. In general they cause only slight pain, and their serious nature is brought to notice only by their growth, the loosening of the teeth, and the difficulty in chewing and speaking. In doubtful cases microscopical examination of portions of the tumor obtained by exploratory excision will clear up the situation. In distinction to tumors these new growths are characterized by their rapidity of growth. At times, however, they at first remain for a long time unchanged, and then suddenly increase rapidly.

The early diagnosis of the *myelogenous* forms is more difficult. In the upper jaw these new growths frequently are masked by the symptoms of the sinus affection. In the lower jaw the bony wall, being slow to yield, obscures the onset of the disease. Only the swelling of the jaw and the breaking through of the tumor explain the dull pains which have frequently been felt in the interior of the jaw for some time. In this way tumors the size of an apple or a child's head frequently develop in the inferior maxilla. In the upper jaw a swelling and diminished resistance of the thinned-out anterior wall of the sinus frequently becomes evident by a parchment-like crackling. They are usually followed by symptoms of obstruction of the nasal passages and palate. Swelling of the adjacent *lymph-glands* was noted by the author in 5 out of 33 cases. Metastases of the submaxillary glands were seen in only 2 instances. In one case the glands could be discovered only at the time of operation owing to their deep situation.

Fig. 304.

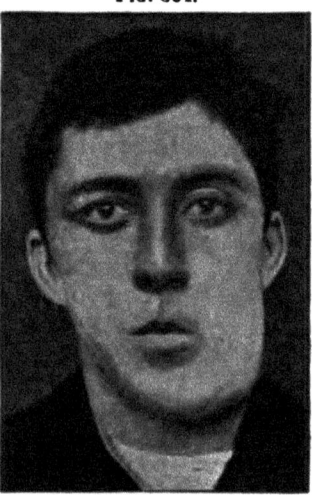
Myelogenous sarcoma.

Prognosis.—It is hardly necessary, after what has been stated ab
to emphasize that the prognosis is decidedly worse in myelogen

Fig. 305.

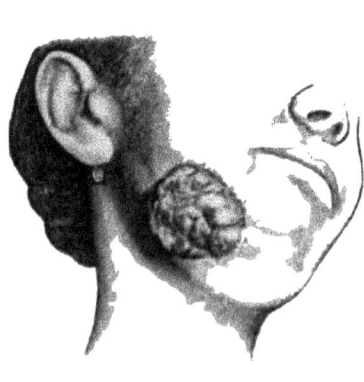

Rapidly growing round-cell sarcoma of the
lower jaw in a pregnant woman.

Fig. 306.

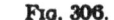
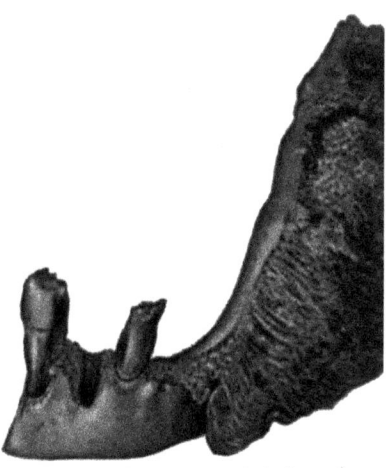

Osteosarcoma of the lower jaw.

Fig. 307.

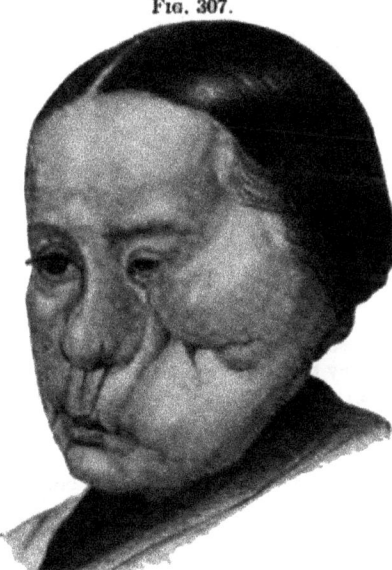

Recurrent spindle-cell sarcoma in the region of the
external angle of the eye in a woman aged fifty-
seven years.

soft sarcoma than in the h
periosteal forms. Epulis off
generally a more favorable pr
nosis, provided it is not sim
removed with a knife or sciss
but by resection of the disea
portion of the alveolar proc
On the other hand, sarcoma
the body of the jaw is not I
malignant than carcinoma,
cept for the fact possibly t
it grows more slowly and d
not traverse the body-wall
quickly. Information rega
ing the dangers of operat
interference and its perman
results is given in the chapter
Operations on the Jaw.

A rare benign form of ep
may be mentioned here, wh
is histologically similar to
giant-cell sarcoma *epulis* iss
osseuse encystée. It leaves
alveolar edge itself intact,
breaks through the walls of the jaw; in the case of the upper jaw, the si
of the jaw also, and makes its appearance on the cheek and on the gu

Treatment.—In carrying out the treatment, the exceedingly great danger of recurrence should be kept in mind, and for this reason one should always proceed boldly into the sound tissues. Unfortunately, periosteal tumors in their early stages are frequently removed by physieiaus without surgical training, so that recurrences requiring extensive surgical interference are certain to follow. Only those forms of sarcoma attached to the alveolar process and well circumscribed justify a partial resection; in nearly all other cases, particularly in the myelogenous forms, a total resection of the diseased portion of the jaw, carried well into healthy tissue, offers the only prospect of recovery. While in tumors of the lower jaw it is possible to proceed without hindrance and to replace the resected portion by mechanical measures, in case of the upper jaw involvement of the base of the skull frequently compels an attempt to remove the tumor to be abandoned.

Fig. 308.

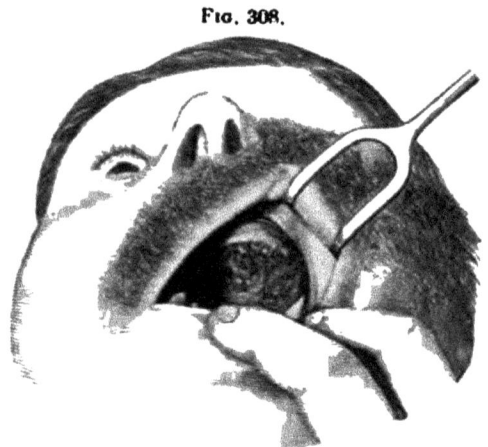

Epithelioma of superior maxilla.

Carcinoma of the Jaw.—These tumors, which belong to well-advanced or old age are either primary tumors originating in the epithelium of the jaw or secondary new growths extending to the jaw from the neighboring structures—lips, parotid, tongue, floor of the mouth, or submaxillary lymph-glands. The primary forms have their origin not only in the epithelium of the mucous membrane and the glands embedded in the latter or in the maxillary sinus, but also on those paradental epithelial indentations which were mentioned in the etiology of cysts of the jaw. The average age of the author's patients at the time of admission to the hospital was 56.4 years; the youngest patient was thirty-nine years, the oldest in his eightieth year. Carcinoma occurred much more frequently in the upper jaw; for 26 cases of carcinoma of the upper jaw there were only 2 in the lower jaw. It is true that in this calculation it was necessary to include under carcinoma of the upper jaw carcinoma

of the nasal cavity, because a local distinction is frequently impossi
In nearly all cases of central carcinoma of the upper jaw the correspc
ing nasal cavity is affected, and it is impossible to determine subseque
whether the process originated in the mucous membrane of the nos
in the mucous membrane of the maxillary sinus.

In the material observed by the author there was an hereditary
deney in one-fifth of the cases. In a high percentage, acute and chm
diseases of the teeth and gums preceded the development of carcino
Smoking may be put down as a further etiological factor. In twi
the author's cases a carcinomatous ulcer developed beneath the p
of artificial teeth, which observation would speak in favor of traum
origin of the disease. Even syphilitic soil predisposes to carcinomat
disease.

Fig. 309.

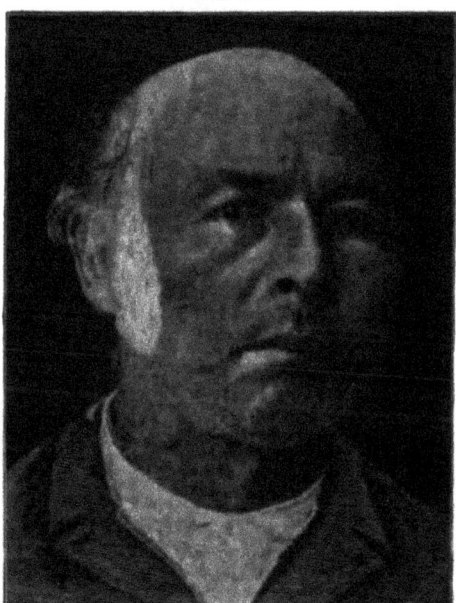

Swelling of upper jaw, due to beginning carcinoma.

Finally may be mentioned two further cases from the author's cl
which would show that carcinomatous disease of the jaw was proba
of a metastatic nature. The first observation is that of a woman, si
years old, who was operated upon for carcinoma of the left breast.
year and three-quarters later she presented herself at the clinic, with
local recurrence, but with a central carcinoma of the left half of the lo
jaw. In the second case four and a half years after removal of the
breast for carcinoma there developed, besides a local recurrence, a
cinoma of the left maxillary sinus. The ease mentioned first is als

proof that cancerous disease of the lower jaw occasionally, though rarely, originates in the body of the jaw.

In the upper jaw the most frequent point of origin of the disease is the mucous lining of the maxillary sinus and the nasal cavity. Of the author's 28 cases, 17 belonged to this category; 6 times carcinoma originated in the alveolar process, and twice in the hard palate. In the body of the jaw the soft, spongy medullary carcinoma is generally observed.

Symptoms.—The most frequent and at the same time the *first symptom* is *pain*. The latter is not characterized by location or intensity.

FIG. 310.

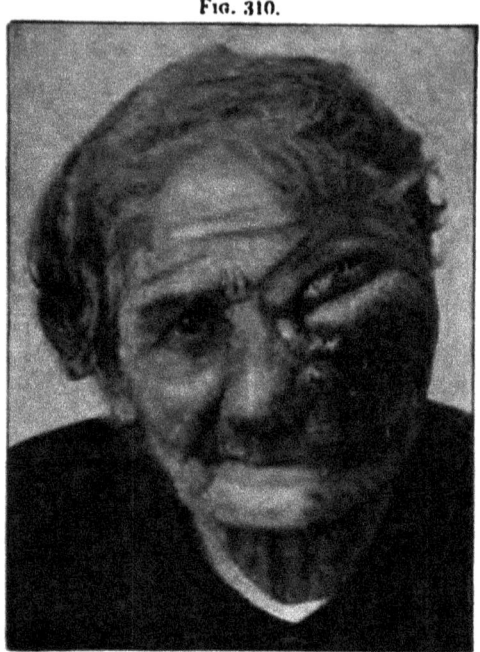

Ulcerating carcinoma of left upper jaw.

Sometimes it occurs as violent toothache; at other times as a dull pain in one-half of the face which occasionally radiates to the ear, neck, or back of the head. In carcinoma of the upper jaw a relatively frequent and early additional symptom is *obstruction of one nasal passage*. Upon digital examination through the mouth the region of the posterior nares and the nasopharynx is filled with soft, gelatinous tumor masses. It is easy to understand therefore why many patients are at first treated by dentists and nose specialists. Unfortunately, while the teeth are extracted and polypi removed, nothing is accomplished and the favorable opportunity for the thorough operative excision of this dangerous disease is lost. The new growth is rendered more con-

spicuous by the swelling of the *respective half of the face*, the enlai
ment and broadening of the corresponding half of the nose, and by
thinning of the anterior wall of the sinus, the latter frequently givin
parchment-like crackling upon palpation. If the bone has been entir
destroyed by the tumor, there is felt beneath the soft parts of the che
or of the hard palate a soft, elastic, frequently pseudofluctuating tum
which may lead to the diagnosis of dental abscess or emphysema of
maxillary sinus, and has frequently led a physician to make an incisi
with the result that blood, instead of pus, was evacuated. The appe
ance of the skin of the cheek varies. At first there are no changes; la
it becomes adherent, more or less infiltrated, reddish or bluish-red
color; and finally, though rarely, the tumor breaks through and und
goes ulceration, as shown in Fig. 310.

In addition, there are found manifestations of compression on the p
of neighboring organs, as the tear-ducts and the orbital cavity. T
obstruction of the nasal tear-ducts causes the annoying manifestatic
of dacryostenosis. In more than one-half of the author's cases t
orbital cavity was involved. There was observed fixation, dislocatic
or protrusion of the eyeball. In one case the latter seemed to be co
pletely dislocated out of the orbital cavity. Frequently, increased t
sion of the ball could be confirmed, but it was not destroyed in a sin
case. Further, there was observed in the eye dilatation and slugg
reaction of the pupil, and upon ophthalmoscopic examination the reti
veins were markedly engorged and tortuous; there were hemorrhage ii
the retina, neuritis, and atrophy of the optic nerve. Vision was w
preserved in some cases; in others it was diminished or lost. In o
case, with right-sided inoperable carcinoma of the upper jaw which h
probably broken through into the cranial cavity, there was observ
bilateral amaurosis as a result of total atrophy of both optic nerves.

Involvement of the maxillary articulation or the muscles of mastic
tion produces ankylosis of the jaw.

Medullary carcinoma situated upon the alveolar process of the upf
jaw or the hard palate is usually very soft and commences as a sm
nodule or easily bleeding, hard, deeply clefted ulcer, and extends rapic
over the mucous membrane of the cheek and cavity of the upper ja
destroying the tissues in its progress, so that one soon finds the sai
clinical picture as presented by primary carcinoma of the maxilla
sinus.

Besides these soft medullary tumors, there occur more infrequen
ulcerating forms or hard carcinomata which grow more slowly.

Not only in carcinoma of the alveolar process of the upper jaw, t
also in the above-mentioned central carcinoma of the lower jaw, t
author has observed complete sequestration of the diseased portion
bone.

Besides the general carcinomatous cachexia, the local disturbanc
such as interference with mastication, the fetor, constant flow of sali
loss of sleep on account of the pain, at times also profuse hemorrha
from mouth and nose, cause exhaustion. In the author's cases t

average duration of the disease from the onset of the first symptoms
until admission to the hospital was 4.8 months.

In carcinoma of the lower jaw the submaxillary lymph-glands are
involved early. In carcinoma of the upper jaw surprisingly few metastases of lymphatic glands are found. Some of the latter escape notice,
however, because carcinoma-
tous infection follows a deep
course along the internal maxillary artery and the internal
carotid, attacking the deeper
lymph-glands. In all the cases
of prop₁₊ₗₑₜᵢₖ ligation of the
carotid for resection of the upper jaw that have been published, diseased lymph-glands
were repeatedly and unexpectedly found at the division of the
carotid.

Diagnosis.—As the symptomatology has been so thoroughly discussed, it is not necessary
to take up in detail the diagnosis of carcinoma. As opposed
to sarcoma, these tumors possess the following characteristic
qualities: they usually occur in
old age, developing more frequently in the upper than in
the lower jaw, are more painful,
grow more rapidly, and in their
progress spare the surrounding tissues even less than sarcoma. In the lower jaw they

Fig. 311.

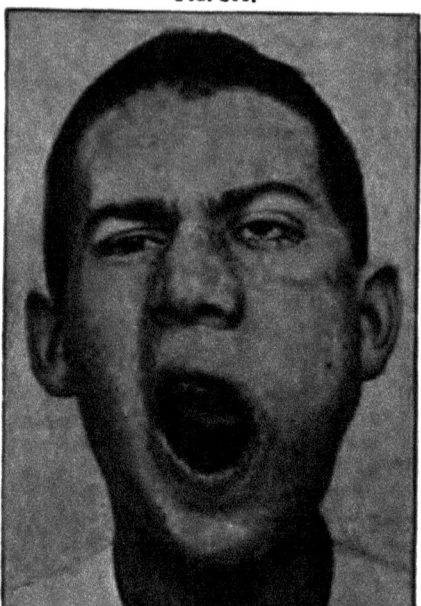

Retromaxillary fibroma.

are more frequently accompanied by metastases of the lymph-glands.
As in a large number of cases the orbital cavity is involved, the change
in position of the eyeball and the manifestations of compression and
stasis in its fundus might lead to the suspicion of the presence of a
retrobulbar tumor, the most important sign of which is a unilateral,
constantly increasing protrusion of the eyeball. The differential diagnosis between tumors of the jaw and retrobulbar tumor of primary
origin will seldom cause any serious difficulty, because, at that stage
in the development of a neoplasm of the jaw in which the orbital cavity
is affected, other local symptoms will always have become manifest.

Prognosis.—The prognosis of carcinoma, which is on the whole a
gloomy one, varies according to the structure, location, and extent of
the process. It is comparatively good in disease of the alveolar process.
In carcinoma of the body of the jaw immediate and thorough resection
of all diseased tissues may offer some hope of a cure. In the chapter

treating on operations on the jaw it will be shown what little prospe there is of permanent recovery.

Retromaxillary Tumors.—Excluding the group of nasopharyng polypi whose root and branches are limited to the nasopharynx, or those severe forms of tumor situated behind the superior maxilla w be described which v. Langenbeck has called retromaxillary tumo These growths originate either in the roof of the pharynx, sending process from this point through the sphenopalatine foramen into t sphenomaxillary fossa, or they originate in the pterygopalatine for and send processes into the pharynx and the sphenomaxillary fos In the majority of cases they are *fibrous tumors,* and are obser almost exclusively in young males. Cavernous angioma, sarcoma, a carcinoma do, however, occur. Fibromata show the most typi symptoms, growing in the direction of least resistance; their masses the nasal cavity, causing a slight swelling of the cheek brought abo by that portion of the tumor growing out of the sphenomaxillary fos They cause the temporal region to be enlarged, approaching the lat beneath the zygomatic arch. In a like manner they affeet the regi of the glossopalatine arch and produce a protrusion of the eyeball a result of pressure exerted from the pterygopalatine fossa upon t sphenomaxillary orbital fissure and the orbital cavity. If no maligna degeneration of the tumor is present, the alveolar process and ha palate remain intact. Particularly characteristic and diagnostically ve important is the hour-glass-shaped swelling in the temporal region abo and below the zygomatic arch, while the latter remains distinc definable.

In accordance with their destructive progress, sarcomatous or carcir matous tumors show a less distinct clinical picture. Initial sympton that the author has observed a long time before any tumor could seen or felt from without, were dull headaches and pain in one maxilla articulation during mastication, with manifestations of compression a displacement on the part of neighboring organs, partienlarly exop thalmos, but also ptosis, diplopia, fixation of the eyeball, choked dis optic nerve neuritis, diminution in power of vision, and even to amaurosis. Obstruction of the nasal passages is occasionally preced by increased secretion and hemorrhage.

Even fibroma may undergo secondary adhesions and cause seconda perforation of neighboring bones. Perforating the thin nasal wall the maxillary sinus, it may grow into the latter from the nose, beginning in the pharynx, become adherent to the base of the sku penetrate into the sphenoidal sinus, and perforate the base of the sku

Confusion of retromaxillary exophthalmos and the rest of the mai festations on the part of the eye with those caused by orbital tume can probably always be avoided if in doubtful cases the nasophary is subjected to a careful examination.

Prognosis.—From the above symptomatology it will be seen th independent of malignant carcinomatous and sarcomatous forms, t prognosis of retromaxillary tumors is very serious on account of th threatening tendency to involve the base of the skull and because of hemorrhage. In order to form a correct opinion of the disease it is of the greatest significance to keep in mind that polypus of the nasopharynx, a disease belonging to the period of adolescence, shows a tendency to atrophy after the twenty-fifth year. Occasionally, gradual spontaneous disappearance of these tumors has also been observed.

Treatment.—Three methods of extirpating these tumors are employed at the present time. The oldest and most radical method is that of v. Langenbeck. By means of a temporary resection of

FIG. 312.

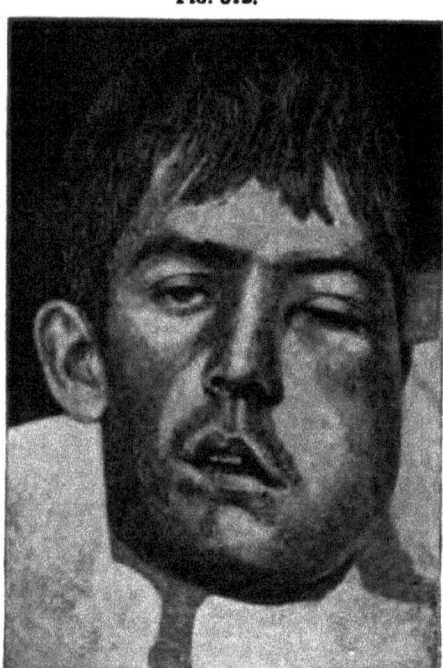

Retromaxillary fibroma.

the superior maxilla (see Operations on the Jaw) he provides access to the root and branches of the tumor in order to remove the latter completely and to cauterize the base of origin with the actual cautery. Though this bold operation is a rational one, it is also dangerous. It cannot be sufficiently emphasized that this operation is one of the bloodiest in surgical technic, and that the danger of death from hemorrhage upon the operating-table is great. Lincoln's statistics show that in thirty-nine such operations death took place eight times during or immediately after the operation. In using the saw it is impossible to avoid injuring these tumors, which are frequently very vascular and cavern-

ous. It is of advantage to proceed with Gigli's wire saw, to wl
reference will again be made in a subsequent section.

On account of the great danger of hemorrhage in v. Langenbe
method, and because the tendency of the tumor to recur disappe
toward the end of adolescence, v. Bruns refrains from removing
tumor in continuity and in one step. He resects the nasopharyng
portion through the existing passages with the galvanocaustic loop,
galvanocautèry, or electrolysis. The retromaxillary portion he remo
by means of a temporary resection of the zygoma. Even in the seve
cases of retromaxillary nasopharyngeal fibroid, with extensive tum
of the temple, cheek, and orbital cavity, complete cure without deforn
can be brought about. The temporary resection of the malar is carn
out in a different manner, according to whether the orbital cavity
free or occupied by a process of the tumor. If the tumor occupies
temporal fossa and cheek and the orbital cavity is free, the skin-incis
is carried, according to v. Bruns' suggestion, behind the outer angle
the eye, somewhat obliquely, from behind and above, forward a
downward. It should commence at the upper margin of the tempc
fossa and end in a slight curve backward, a little above the level of
angle of the month. From this vertical incision a horizontal incis
is carried along the superior border of the zygoma. Both incisions
carried to the bone. The body of the zygoma is divided in line w
the first incision by means of a pointed saw, and in the horizon
incision the posterior end of the zygomatic arch is divided with a chi:
The lower flap, together with the zygomatic arch and masseter, is folc
down and outward, the upper flap is folded up and outward, whereup
the tumor can be enucleated from the sphenomaxillary fossa in cc
tinuity, and can be followed up to its pedicle in the sphenopalati
fissure.

If the orbital cavity is occupied by a process of the tumor, the ent
malar bone, together with its orbital portion, is folded up. A verti
incision, beginning 1 cm. behind the angle of the eye, is carried do
in a curve, with its convexity forward. A second horizontal incisi
runs from the outer angle of the eye along the superior border of t
zygomatic arch nearly to the outer ear. With pointed saw and a chi
the bone is divided at three points—at the junction of the malar w
the frontal in a horizontal direction; at the junction of the super
maxilla through the sphenomaxillary fissure in a vertical direction; at
finally, at the posterior end of the zygomatic arch. The whole ma
bone can now be folded up, whereupon the tumor filling the floor
the orbital cavity and sphenomaxillary fossa is made directly accessil

The most conservative method is undoubtedly the treatment of th
tumors by electrolysis, and is well worth while attempting. A Voltol
loop carried around the tumor is connected with the negative po
According to Schmidthinssen, the positive pole should be attached to
lowest portion of the tumor by means of a hook. Seven or eight sittin
of twenty minutes' duration each ought to be sufficient to free a pati
from a fibroma.

DISEASES OF THE TEMPOROMAXILLARY ARTICULATION.

Inflammations of the maxillary articulation are comparatively rare, probably for the reason that on account of its position the joint is protected from trauma, the principal etiological factor in joint-inflammations. In infectious diseases, particularly articular rheumatism, the maxillary articulation is occasionally involved; not infrequently also in gonorrhœa. Among chronic infectious diseases which may affect this joint may be mentioned tuberculosis and actinomycosis. There occur, further, inflammations that have extended from the jaw or temporal bone from the surrounding soft parts, principally the parotid, and inflammations of metastatic character. Finally, in old individuals, the occurrence of arthritis deformans must be considered.

FIG. 313.

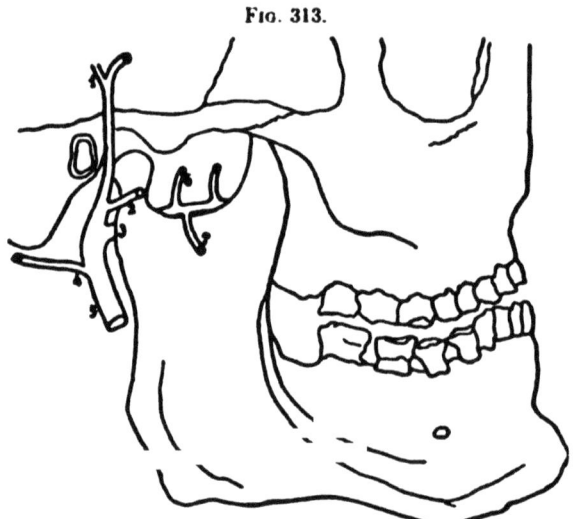

Plan of the internal maxillary artery and its branches : 1, superf. temporal; 2, transverse facial; 3, internal maxillary; 4, postauricular; 5, ext. carotid; 6, mid. meningeal; 7, inf. dental.

Symptoms.—The symptoms of acute non-purulent inflammations are the general ones—i. e., swelling, pain, and disturbance of function. The patient carefully avoids opening his mouth and chewing. In acute purulent arthritis these manifestations occur to a more marked degree, and are accompanied by redness in the region of the joint and a rise of temperature. In case of infected injuries the process is liable to extend to the cavity of the skull. Frequently pus seeks an outlet by spontaneous perforation into the auditory canal. After recovery from purulent inflammation there is always ankylosis of the joint.

Chronic inflammation of the maxillary articulation, whether of rheumatic or infectious origin or the result of undue exertion on the part of the joint or of an arthritis deformans, is usually betrayed by friction-

sounds elicited by moving the jaw. This crackling sound occurs tc
most annoying degree after the jaw has been at rest for a long tim(
    Treatment.—The treatment must consider in the first place t
etiology. In chronic forms iodine applied in various ways is the pri
eipal remedy employed, though occasionally moist heat may also bri
about relief. More frequently the surgeon is called upon to treat, r.
the inflammation itself, but its effect, namely, ankylosis of the artic
lation of the jaw.
    Articular ankylosis has been observed in earliest childhood, probal
as the result of injuries during delivery. Unlike most other forms
ankylosis, these forms do not show connective-tissue adhesions, h
bony union, and are particularly serious for the reason that the j(
which has sustained loss of function is markedly retarded in develo
ment, and the receding chin gives the face a kind of "bird profil(
(Vogelgesicht). Similar disturbances follow arthritis occurring duri
the age of development, and which originates in the parotid, midc
ear, or the lower jaw. Fig. 314 shows a young man who suffered fro

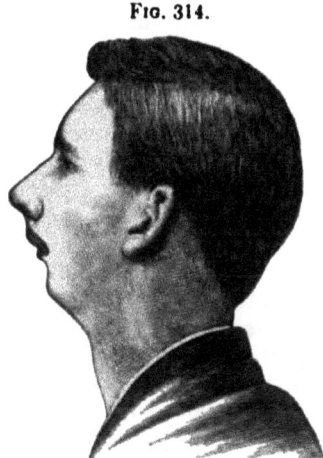

Fio. 314.

Impaired development of jaw, due to
osteomyelitis and arthritis.

osteomyelitis of the lower jaw wh(
six years old. As a result of this I
acquired arthritis of the maxillary a
ticulation, with conseqnent impair(
development of the lower jaw.
    Besides true or articular ankylos
there also' occurs a so-called false a!
kylosis caused by *cicatricial* or *mu*
cular contraction after defects of tl
soft parts of the cheeks—burns, col
tused wounds, and ulcerations, as, f(
example, noma and ulcerative stom:
titis. Muscular ankylosis is only rare
primary; myositis, most often contra
ture of muscles, is an accompanyir
manifestation of cicatricial contractio
    In ankylosis of *one* maxillary artic
lation, the surgeon generally, thou(
not always, finds loss of motion
the other.

    In order to make a diagnosis it is necessary to determine clearly tl
etiology of the disease, its location, and the manner and degree
ankylosis, by a careful inquiry into the history and a thorough exan
ination. In making the latter it is usually impossible to avoid forcib
opening the jaws with a speculum under an anæsthetic.
    In some cases the treatment may be prophylactic by attempting
prevent the extension of inflammatory process to the joint from adjace
regions, avoiding cicatricial contraction by plastic operations, and I
not immobilizing the joint for too long a time, as has been remark(
in the treatment of fractures of the jaw.
    In extensive connective-tissue ankylosis resulting from cicatricial co

traction, simple subcutaneous or submucous incision of the scar is seldom successful, and almost always results in a new scar. In such cases, with extensive defects of the cheek, Gussenhauer has taken a flap from the cervical region and sutured it into the defect with the cutaneous surface turned in. Bardenheuer took a flap from the frontal region. The outer surface of the flap was covered with a graft.

In cicatricial ankylosis, as well as in arthritic ankylosis, of connective-tissue formation, *mechanical dilatation* should first be tried. Sudden tears are usually followed by swelling of the joint, which again requires a long period of rest. *Slow methodical dilatation* of the jaw is more to the purpose. For these systematic attempts at dilatation simple wooden wedges are applicable, or wooden or ivory conical bolts, with spiral grooves running from the apex to the base, into which the edges of the teeth rest when the instrument is passed into the mouth. If this methodical dilatation does not produce sufficient mobility, it is necessary to reset the head of the articulation through the temporal region or to make a false joint in front of the ankylosed head of the jaw. Proceeding according to Esmarch and Rizzoli's method, the jaw is simply divided transversely in front of the adherent scar, or, better still, in order to prevent reunion, a wedge-shaped piece with its base downward is resected. According to Helferich's suggestion, reunion may be more effectually prevented by interposing *muscle* between the divided fragments. After resecting a fairly large piece of bone, Helferich constructs a flap about two fingers wide from the entire thickness of the temporal muscle, with its base placed downward, and after resecting a piece of the malar bone turns this flap down and carefully implants its apex into the gap between the two fragments of bone, attaching it to the edges of the gap by two sutures. Rochet recommends resecting a portion of the ascending ramus of the lower jaw and interposing a flap from the masseter. In the same way v. Mikulicz draws forward a flap from the masseter, thus avoiding the resection of part of the zygomatic arch.

In order to expose the site of resection, which should be placed as near the head of the articulation as possible, provided the scar-tissue permits it, König carries an incision parallel with the inferior border of the zygomatic arch as far as the bone. To this he adds a second, running vertically from the end of the first, which divides only the skin. In order to avoid the branches of the facial nerve, Grieg recommends an incision at a level with the supraorbital ridge, running posteriorly above the malar bone nearly to the auditory canal; here it is prolonged downward about a finger breadth in front of the latter to the level of the lobe of the ear. The flap thus outlined is turned downward and forward, the superficial temporal artery divided, after transfixion if necessary, the fascia of the masseter divided along the bone, and turned down with the parotid. It is then possible to free the jaw, beginning at the head of the articulation, and to cut through the neck transversely.

The internal maxillary artery and the facial nerve are less exposed to danger by Küster's incision placed upon the posterior surface of the ascending ramus of the jaw, from which the soft parts are dissected away from the internal and external surface of the jaw. It is true access provided by this method is not so free as in the methods described.

It is difficult at times to decide which one of the maxillary articula has been destroyed, so that one must be prepared to operate upon sides of the jaw.

The prognosis is worse in those cases in which bony union e: not only in the region of the joint, but also between the coronoid pr and the zygomatic arch, as a result of which a false joint would to be placed too far forward to give a good result.

Von Bergmann successfully attempted to improve the deformi the receding chin by extensive resection of all processes, includin coronoid process, and by subsequent displacement forward of the e jaw, the latter being accomplished by an artificial dental apparati

CHAPTER XXI.

OPERATIONS ON THE JAWS.

RESECTION OF THE LOWER JAW.

IN the lower jaw are distinguished *partial resection*, without complete solution of continuity, of the arch of the jaw; and *total resection*, in which the arch of the jaw is completely divided to a greater or less extent. If in the latter operation the articular portion be also removed, it is known as a *disarticulation*. In contrast to this operation, which produces a permanent defect, there is *temporary resection of the jaw*, by means of which access is obtained to the posterior portion of the buccal cavity, and the anterior pharyngeal region.

It is advisable in all operations upon the jaw to place the patient in a half-sitting posture, with head bent forward, in order to prevent the aspiration of blood.

Partial resections, which involve only the alveolar process, or possibly also a portion of the body of the jaw, can as a rule be easily carried out through the month by means of strong bone-shears or gouge-forceps. In some cases the operation can be carried out under local anæsthesia by means of subperiosteal injections of a 1 per cent. eucaine-cocaine solution. Division of an angle of the mouth is rarely necessary, for in most affections involving the lateral portions of the jaw the opening of the mouth can be drawn sufficiently to one side with retractors. Hemorrhage following these operations can always be controlled by packing with iodoform gauze, even if at first it is considerable in amount. The retention of gauze-tampons in the wedge-shaped defects is frequently difficult. If the mouth is disinfected with antiseptic mouth-washes, it is unnecessary to continue packing for any length of time.

In **complete resections** an attempt should be made to preserve the edge of periosteum, and with this purpose in view the bone should be cut subperiosteally. In case of malignant tumors such consideration is naturally impossible. According to the location of the portion to be resected, the operation is carried out either without any skin-incision, by dividing the lower lip in the median line, by dividing the soft parts along the inferior border of the jaw, or by combining the above methods. The central portions of the body of the jaw may be rendered accessible by dissecting the lower lip away from the jaw until the soft portion of the chin can be pushed back beneath the bone. The operation by means of the median incision possesses the advantage of simplicity and minimum cosmetic disfigurement. By this incision the lower lip is divided to beneath the chin or as far as the hyoid bone, and in this way

ample room is provided for operations upon the middle portions of t
jaw.

Before dividing the genioglossal and geniohyoid muscles, which a
inserted into the middle portion, or before sawing through the bone
this site, a strong ligature should be passed through the fleshy porti
of the tongue, and the latter held by this loop. For in some cases,
soon as these muscle insertions are divided there is a sudden danger
suffocation, owing to the tongue falling back and closing the entran
to the larynx.

Where it is necessary to resect in the region of the angle or ascendi
ramus of the jaw it is advisable to proceed from the border of the bor
In order to avoid injuring the branches of the facial artery the incisi
of the soft parts should not be carried exactly over the border of t
jaw, but somewhat beneath the chin. From this incision the periosteu
is dissected up on either side as far as the teeth.

For dividing bone Gigli's wire saws are practicable; they have to
large extent taken the place of narrow-bladed saws, and almost caus
chain-saws to be discarded from the surgical instrumentarium. Hemo
rhage from the vessels of the central canal is usually considerable, b
can easily be stopped by strips of iodoform gauze packed into the lum
of the canal. In some cases the mucous membrane of the tongue c
be subsequently united to the skin of the cheek and lip by suture
making primary closure of the resection wound possible.

In *disarticulation* of one-half of the jaw the incision through the so
parts is carried from the inferior border of the bone along the posteri
border of the ascending ramus as far as the lobe of the ear, stoppi
here, however, in order to spare the parotid and the facial nerve.
conditions permit, after subperiosteal exposure of the bone the ant
rior line of resection is carried through the bone in order to allow tl
respective half of the jaw to be pulled down and thus to facilitate tl
dissection of the soft parts. After the muscles and mucous membrai
have been divided, the respective half of the jaw can be pulled dow
sufficiently far to render the coronoid process visible and palpable. Tl
point of the latter should be divided with a pair of strong forceps, th
severing the insertion of the temporal muscle. In order to enucleate tl
head and neck of the jaw several rotary movements are made with tl
loosened bone, the joint-capsule and external pterygoid muscle tor
through, and any injury of the internal maxillary artery avoided.

Total resection of the entire lower jaw consists of the combine
resection of each half.

A very important feature in the technic of resection is the *immedia
artificial replacement of the resected portion of the jaw whenever there
solution of continuity.* Unless this is done, the patient is placed in
most unfortunate condition; he suffers not only from difficulty in chev
ing, swallowing, and speaking, annoying flow of saliva, disfiguremei
of the face through a sinking in of the chin, and a constant danger
suffocation on account of the tendency of the tongue to fall back; h
condition is rendered serious through a secondary displacement of th

stumps of the jaw. By retraction of the muscles and of the cicatrix the stumps of the jaw are drawn inward in a surprisingly short time. Thus they cause the cavity of the mouth to become narrower, press upon the tongue, and by constant irritation produce ulceration. Lallemand reports a case in which a space only 2 cm. wide remained between the approximated stumps. These unfortunate secondary conditions naturally led to the application of various artificial devices. Some of these were only cosmetic, but others effected a functional improvement.

The cases are rare in which the defect can be bridged over by an osteoplastic operation, using material taken from the remaining portion of the jaw. Even portions of other bones, as the femur, clavicle, and frontal bones, have been used to fill up the gap in the arch of the jaw. In endeavoring to correct the evil results of resection two Berlin dentists, Süersen and Sauer, gained great distinction. Sauer's

Fig. 315.

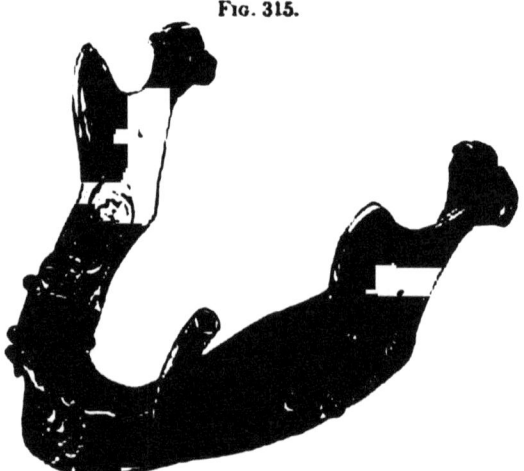

Martin's artificial jaw.

resection-bandages cause the muscles of mastication to force apart gradually the approximated bone-stumps. At the outer side of the teeth of the stump of the lower jaw a metal plate is fastened with wire. This metal plate is directed upward and outward, and even when the mouth is opened it projects beyond the line of the upper teeth. In the act of chewing the teeth of the upper jaw strike upon this inclined plane, and thus produce a separating action upon the stumps of the lower jaw. This secondary method of correction may bring about satisfactory results in single instances, but in other cases it fails completely, and is so tedious that it requires almost an extraordinary patience on the part of the physician and patient. It is easier here, as elsewhere, to prevent the evil than to cure it.

A surgeon and dentist of Lyons, C. Martin, was the first to attempt replacing the resected portion of the jaw by a "Prothèse immédiate,"

and as early as 1889 appeared publicly with a series of brilliant ɪ
in cases that had been observed for years.

Martin constructs an artificial jaw from gutta-percha (Fig. 315),
attachment of the latter to the stump of the jaw constitutes a s
the operation itself. By means of nails and screws the lateral proj
metal plates of the gutta-percha splint are fastened to the stumps
jaw. As gutta-percha can be readily cut, the size of the artificiɪ
can be accurately fashioned at the time of operation to meet the eɪ
conditions. This provisional apparatus remains in place througho
entire period of wound repair. It is traversed by a system of chɪ
which allow the wound surface to be cleansed at all times by inj

FIG. 316.

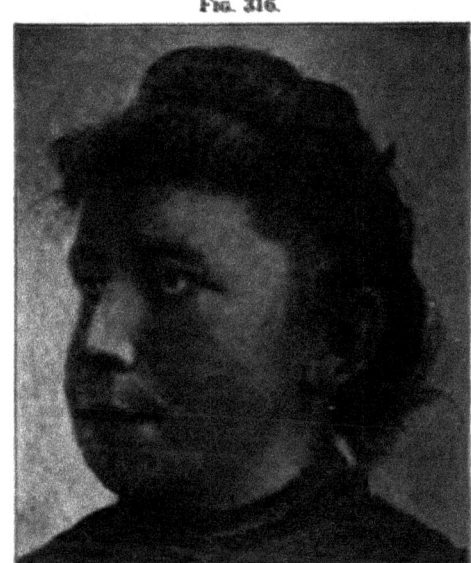

Martin's artificial jaw applied.　Patient eight years after resection of 10 cm. of lower ɪ

disinfectant solutions. After cicatrization has become compleɪ
provisional splint, designed to support the bones and soft pɪ
removed and a permanent artificial piece, provided with teeth, is inɪ
This can be easily removed at any time in order to be cleansed.

In the case of the eighteen-year-old girl shown in Fig. 316, the ɪ
resected a portion of the arch of the jaw 10 cm. long, eight yeaɪ
on account of myelogenous sarcoma of the lower jaw, and apɪ
Martin splint immediately after the operation. Insertion of a perɪ
artificial piece followed a few weeks later. After every meal thiɪ
can be removed by the girl herself, cleansed and reinserted. Siɪ
operation this artificial lower jaw had to be replaced four times in a
ance with the increased growth of the rest of the skeleton—i. e., a
size had to be made. The cosmetic and functional result is at the ɪ

time excellent, the girl having remained free from recurrence. The region of the mouth and chin does not show the slightest changes, with

Fig. 317.

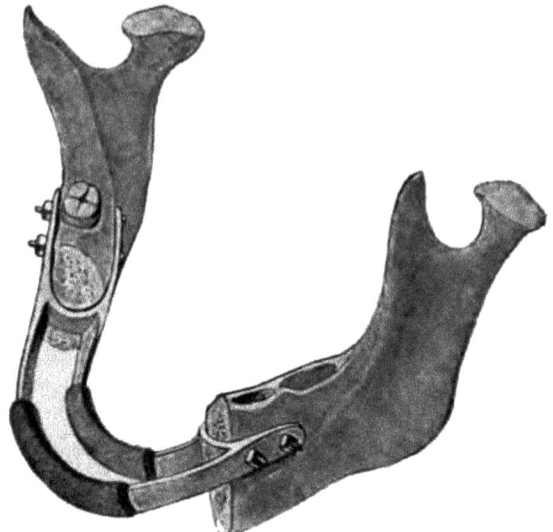

Bünnecken's artificial jaw.

Fig. 318.

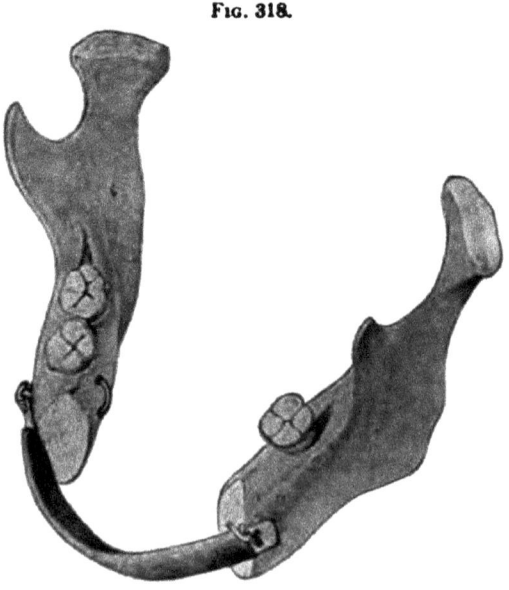

Partsch's artificial jaw.

the exception of a fine linear scar in the submental region; neither sp
nor the act of mastication is impaired.   The gitl is able to bite thro
an apple with the artificial jaw.

The greatest disadvantage of the Martin splint is the fact that
surgeon is dependent upon the dentist.   Bönnecken, Partsch, and S
pany have recommended metal splints, principally for antiseptic reas
These are shown in Figs. 317 to 319.

It would certainly be an advantage if gutta-percha splints coulc
replaced by metal ones which fulfilled the same purpose, but, as fa
material is concerned, the surgeon requires a splint that can be fi
by himself at the time of operation, according to the defect which res

FIG. 319.

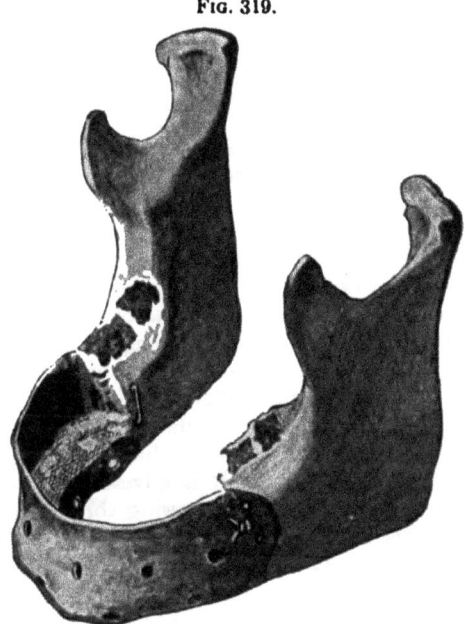

Stoppany's artificial jaw.

from resection.   In an emergency the author has fastened a simple
plate to the stumps of the jaw, to fit the defect, and even with this pri
tive method has obtained satisfactory results.

The above conditions are fulfilled by Partsch's and by Stoppar
aluminum splint.   The author has preferred the latter principally
the reason that it attempts to support the chin.   This lack of supp
for the soft parts of the chin is a defect that the author has obser
in employing various forms of splints.   Even with the fixation sutu
applied to the chin and to the splint he has been unable to combat
condition.   The best results are obtained with large splints which stre
the soft parts to a sufficient degree.   Stoppany's splint possesses adv

tages in so far as it allows easy cleaning and inspection of the wound surfaces and renders it possible to take an impression for a permanent splint without removing the "Prothèse immédiate," which might entail serious consequences even if for a short time only.

The provisional splint should, if possible, be replaced by a permanent one as early as the third week.

Temporary or osteoplastic resection of the lower jaw was first carried out and recommended by Roux and later by Sédillot as a preliminary operation for exposing the floor of the mouth, base of the tongue, and the anterior pharyngeal region. It is carried out either in the median line or in front of the ascending ramus of the jaw (B. v. Langenbeck). For exposing the region in front of the isthmus of the fauces, the *median division* of the lower lip and jaw, as described above, is applicable. The point of a strong sharp steel hook is inserted into the lumen of the central canal on either side, which usually bleeds considerably. By forcibly pulling apart the two halves of the jaw hemorrhage can be controlled. This preliminary operation offers surprisingly free access to the cavity of the mouth and obviates the danger of aspiration. By means of silver sutures accurately applied the two halves of the jaw can be so firmly reunited that the function of the jaw is only temporarily and slightly disturbed.

Access to tumors behind the isthmus of the fauces or the lateral portions of the tongue is obtained by v. Langenbeck's method of dividing the jaw in front of the *ascending ramus* of the jaw. After division of the soft parts, in a vertical line beginning at the angle of the mouth, the saw-cut is carried from behind and inward, forward and outward, because of the tendency of the posterior end of the jaw to be displaced inward and upward, which can in this way be prevented. Kocher places the incision of the soft parts in a line running from the mastoid process toward the hyoid bone. It is advisable to drill the holes for the subsequent wire sutures before sawing through the jaw, because the intact jaw offers better resistance to the drill than the half jaw that has been rendered mobile.

RESECTION OF THE UPPER JAW.

In the upper jaw, surgeons also distinguish *partial resection*, involving the alveolar process and the adjacent palate, *total resection* of one or both *sides*, and *temporary* or *osteoplastic* resection.

Partial resection of the alveolar process is carried out with strong bone-shears and gouge-forceps, after extraction of the teeth situated in the line of resection, in a similar manner to resection of the lower jaw. Chisel and mallet may also be used, as the portions of bone to be removed are more firmly placed than in the lower jaw. The author has used Gigli's wire saw to great advantage in this situation. Hemorrhage can usually be rapidly controlled with iodoform gauze. If the cavity of the month be carefully cleansed with antiseptic mouth-washes, the wounds generally skin over rapidly. It is difficult to draw conclusions from the widely different views held at the present tin regard to *total resection of the upper* jaw and at the same time do tice to all the opinions expressed. Gensoul first performed this of tion in the year 1827. How little the antiseptic era influenced prognosis of this operation is shown by a comparison of Rabe's Krönlein's compilations. The former collected 606 cases of m operations upon the upper jaw between the years 1827 and 1873, found a mortality of 18.4 per cent., while Krönlein calculated a 1 tality of 21.5 per cent. from 158 total resections taken from the t septic period 1870 to 1897. König estimates the mortality at abou per cent. In his most recent communications Krönlein has conclusi shown where the cause of failure in these recent cases should be looked Instead of the former danger from accidental wound infection, there at the present time diseases of the air-passages, suffocation, putrid (fe bronchitis, pleuro- and bronchopneumonia. More than one-half o deaths after this operation are referable to these complications. K lein considers most of these diseases to be the results of aspiration du anæsthesia, and supports his opinion with the surprisingly good res in his own cases, which were operated upon under more or less sug tive anæsthesia, and show a mortality of only 2.8 per cent. At present time this has been carried to such a degree that the u injection of from 0.01 gram (⅙ grain) to not more than 0.015 g (¼ grain) of morphine is given before the operation, and at the be ning of the operation only a few whiffs of ether, which act more suggestion. The entire operation is carried out *without anæsthesia* Heuter suggested in the year 1867.

That aspiration of blood has always been a complication dreaded surgeons is shown by the early proposals, frequently carried out at present time, to perform the operation after *prophylactic tracheoto* and *tamponing* of the trachea or with *the head dependent*. It is 1 properly urged against *prophylactic* tracheotomy that on account of danger it is by no means a trifling procedure, and that it deprives patient of the possibility of expelling mucus and secretions by exp tion. Martens reports over 28 per cent. of deaths in patients upon wl prophylactic tracheotomy was performed with insertion of Tremle burg's tampon cannula. The operation with dependent head, accord to Rose, was not practicable for the reason principally that the fiel operation is extremely inaccessible and the loss of blood considerabl

A more favorable reception than that accorded the above two meth seems recently to have been extended to a prophylactic operation wl does not purpose preventing a large amount of blood from entering air-passages, but is intended to lessen hemorrhage as much as poss by *preliminary ligation* of the carotid. The author finds opinions o' whelmingly in favor of this preliminary operation (Reyher, v. Les Bryant, Schönborn, Kocher, Schlatter, and Fritz König from v. B(mann's clinic). This ligation is strongly recommended in all ance patients that have become exhausted by hemorrhage and cachexia, 1 vided they do not suffer from diseases of the vessels, particularly arterio-sclerosis. This allows the operator to be humane without being obliged to subject the patient to greater risk.

In regard to the manner and site of ligation, there is still a difference of opinion. *In the great majority of cases ligation of the external carotid alone is sufficient;* this may be permanent, and if carried out aseptically is not dangerous. On account of possible effects upon the brain ligation of the common carotid should be carried out in exceptional cases only. The latter operation appears to be less dangerous in the form of a temporary constriction than as a permanent ligation.

Numerous reasons have led the author to recommend the exposure of the bifurcation of the carotid, and to carry out ligation of the external carotid from this incision prolonged upward. For in one case the effect of ligation of the external carotid was insufficient, and it was only by ligation of the internal carotid, which had been exposed by the incision over the bifurcation, that hemorrhage was diminished. Several other cases (v. Lesser, Schönborn, Schlatter) showed that at the bifurcation of the common carotid lymph-glands are found which could not be diagnosticated from the surface. For the formation of metastases follows the lymph-tracts of the internal maxillary and external carotid (arteries) toward the bifurcation. In malignant tumors of the upper jaw glandular enlargement in the submaxillary region is rare. Fritz König prefers preliminary ligation of the external carotid above the superior thyroid artery between the latter and the lingual artery because he fears the collateral circulation through the thyroid. In one case he observed secondary hemorrhage from the soft parts of the cheek twenty minutes after ligation of the external carotid just above the bifurcation. This suggestion of König can be accepted without sacrificing the advantages of exposure of the bifurcation if ligation be performed by prolonging the above incision of the soft parts. It may be remarked, however, in regard to the much disputed assumption of an anastomosis between the two superior thyroid arteries, that the existence of the latter is strenuously denied by anatomists of the present day, and that it would be more reasonable to conclude that secondary hemorrhage comes from the vascular system of the opposite side of the head. Further, on account of the small space between these arteries and the frequent anomalies of vessels, ligation between the superior thyroid and lingual arteries is decidedly more difficult than ligation immediately above the bifurcation of the carotid.

In the endeavor to reduce loss of blood, and aspiration pneumonia, to a minimum, Stein goes a step further. He proposes to operate with the head in the dependent position after ligation of the external carotid. In this way he prevents absolutely the entrance of blood into the air-passages.

Regarding the *technic of resection of the upper jaw,* it may be stated, in the first place, that the operation upon the bone is in general and in detail the same in all the methods. The differences lie principally in the form of incision through the soft parts.

The most important forms of incisions are those of Velpeau, Langenbeck, and that of Dieffenback modified by Kocher, and Wel Velpeau's incision is a curved one from the base of the malar b to the angle of the mouth. In most cases this form of incision is satisfactory because it exposes too little of those regions which are frequently the site of carcinoma, namely, the infraorbital ridge, orbital plate, and the region of the ethmoid, and because in additio extensively injures Steno's duct, and almost all branches of the fa nerve.

Where a tumor extends well into the region of the malar bone, Langenbeck's incision, extending in a crescent from the malar bone the ala of the nose without dividing the upper lip, provides suffici space and offers a satisfactory cosmetic result because the continuity the upper lip is not affected. But by this incision also the upper fa branches are divided so that the mouth remains crooked. The t view of the relations, and the freest access to the entire body of upper jaw is, without doubt, provided by Weber's modification

FIG. 320.   FIG. 321.   FIG. 322.   FIG. 323.

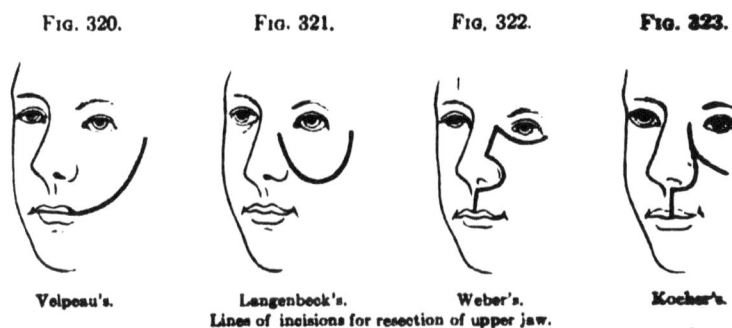

Velpeau's.   Langenbeck's.   Weber's.   Kocher's.
Lines of incisions for resection of upper jaw.

Dieffenback's incision. The incision should begin below the inner an of the eye, pass down beside the nose around the ala to beneath t septum, from which point the upper lip is divided through the mid or to one side of the raphe. If this incision does not allow of suffici inspection, an additional horizontal incision is carried along the inf orbital ridge. Unfortunately this excellent method, which spares t branches of the facial nerve more than any other, has this disadvanta that the angle of the flap occasionally becomes necrotic, and repair the defect by granulation predisposes to the formation of ectropion the lower eyelid. Kocher makes an incision similar to that of Web and adds to this a horizontal incision running from the inferior bor of the orbicularis oculi muscle over the attachment of the superior qu ratus muscle of the lip (boundary between region of the upper and low facial). The flap formed by these two incisions through the soft pa is dissected from the underlying bone until the anterior surface of t jaw is exposed. It is frequently impossible to proceed directly over t bone, owing to the involvement of the periosteum and soft parts.

For the purpose of dividing the bone, narrow-bladed saws, strong bone-shears, or a chisel and mallet, may be employed. The author prefers Gigli's wire saw to all these instruments; the latter render the entire technic of the operation more delicate, as the slender wires armed with needles can readily be passed around the portions of bone to be divided, without producing extensive injury of the soft parts; and furthermore, during the act of sawing, the tumor masses which bleed easily are not injured, as is the case with narrow-bladed saws. The first step in the removal of the bone is to push back the periosteum at the floor of the orbital cavity as far as the sphenomaxillary fissure, during which proceeding the eyeball should be protected by a spatula-like instrument and pressed upward. Into the fissure is passed a half-curved needle

Fig. 324.

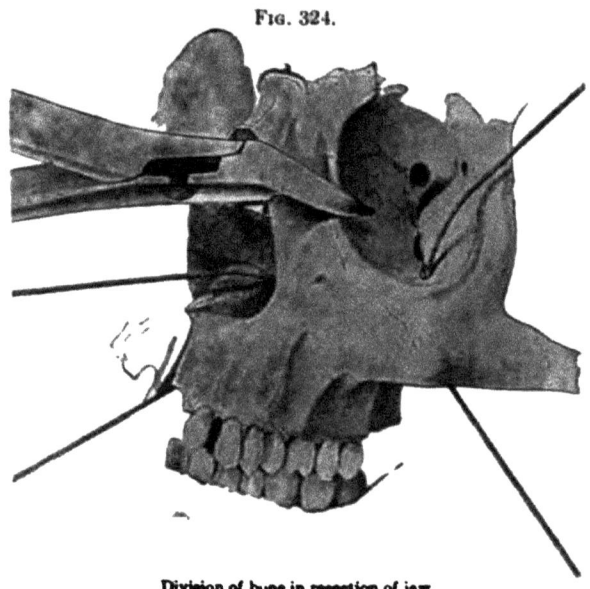

Division of bone in resection of jaw.

connected with the wire saw; from this point it is passed along the posterior surface of the malar bone until it re-emerges in the malar fossa. In this plane the malar bone is sawn through. (See Fig. 324.) The second step is the division of the articulation of the upper jaw, with the nasal and frontal bones. This is most simply done with bone-shears. With these one should cut from the anterior orifice of the nose as far as the sphenomaxillary fissure. The third step is the division of the hard palate with the saw. At the end of the entire operation the palatal flap hanging down from the middle of the roof of the mouth is again sutured to the buccal mucous membrane. If, however, the mucoperiosteal covering of the palatal arch can no longer be preserved, it is divided in the median line, and the soft palate divided from the hard

palate by a transverse incision. After extracting one of the upper midd
incisor teeth, the hard palate is cut through either with a narrow-blade
saw carried from the cavity of the mouth toward the nasal cavity, (
in some cases, better still, with a wire saw which is brought through tl
nose with a curved probe or by means of a Bellocque tube. Frequent
it is advisable to force a drainage trocar from the nose into the cavit
of the month, at the posterior border of the hard palate, and to pa
the wire saw through this opening around the palatal plate. Finall;
a broad elevator is inserted into the saw-cut in the malar bone, in orde
to loosen the jaw, which is still attached to the palatal bone. The ja
is then grasped with a pair of strong toothed bone-forceps and twisted or
with a jerk. In order to control the first hemorrhage an iodoform gau
tampon is quickly packed into the wound; in case any branches of th
internal maxillary artery are spurting they can as a rule be readily caugl
and tied. As a rule fragments of tumor still remain, which must subse
quently be removed with a sharp spoon and bone-shears. As malignar
tumors frequently proliferate into the orbital cavity without causing an
manifestations on the part of the eyeball, it is advisable in the case (
extensive tumors, before beginning the resection, to obtain the patient'
consent to a *removal of the eyeball* if the latter operation should prov
necessary.

Defects of the skin of the cheek are covered by skin-flaps taken from
the temporal or frontal regions. (See meloplastic.)

It is advisable to keep the cavity of the wound filled for from six t
eight days with a strip of iodoform gauze, the end of which is brough
out through the nostril of the side operated upon. In case the mucou
membrane of the hard palate was removed at the same time, the tampo
can usually be held in place by fixation sutures. The repair of the woun
cavity proceeds rapidly, with contraction of the soft parts of the cheel

In those rare cases in which the bony palate is not diseased, the uppe
jaw, exposed by v. Langenbeck's skin incision, is sawn from the alveola
process by an incision running transversely above the roots of the teetl

The intrabuccal methods of resection of the upper jaw, recently pro
posed, have not found very extensive employment. They do not provid
the necessary view of the usually very extensive field of operation.

For the *resection of both halves of the upper jaw* Heyfelder, who wa
the first to perform this operation, in 1841, chose an incision similar t
that of Velpeau's method, running from the external angle of the ey
on each side to the angles of the month. By this procedure the entir
face as far as the orbital cavities is dissected away. The nasal processe
are divided transversely from one orbit to the other, and the mala
articulation divided on either side, the palate not requiring division
With the median incision of Dieffenback, running through the middl
of the nose, with the addition of transverse incisions extending fron
the latter to both inner angles of the eyes, one can provide sufficien
access for the removal of both upper jaws.

The cosmetic and functional disturbances which remain after exten
sive resection of the upper jaw may in some cases be quite considerabl

and demand plastic restoration of the defect. If the skin of the cheek should have to be removed, an attempt at covering the latter defect should be made by means of skin-flaps taken from the frontal or cervical region, or the region of the cheek. The most appreciable loss is that of the hard palate, on account of the wide communication produced between the nasal cavity and that of the mouth. Bardenheuer uses the nasal septum to cover the defect of the hard palate. The former is detached from the anterior portion of the frame of the nose and the base of the skull, and turned upon its attachment as on a hinge until it assumes a horizontal position. Its edges are united with the soft palate on one side and the edge of mucous membrane of the buccal flap on the other.

Another annoying deformity is caused by the dislocation downward of the eyeball and the sinking down of the lower lid. Fr. König seeks to prevent this deformity at the time of resection, by providing support for the eyeball by a flap taken from the temporal muscle. From the attachment of the temporal muscle to the lower jaw he takes a strip of muscle, a half finger in breadth, in connection with a piece of the anterior border of the coronoid process of the mandibula (inferior maxilla), which he chisels away as far as the horizontal ramus; he then carries this piece transversely below and around the eyeball toward the nasal wall of the cavity of the mouth, where it is fastened to the remains of the frontal process of the upper jaw.

Where defects of the jaws can be satisfactorily covered by natural means, this form of plastic secondary operation is always preferable to artificial splints. But in most cases the results obtained under great difficulties are only moderate and easily excelled by results obtained with modern dental appliances. In a patient in whom the author removed the entire right upper jaw and part of the left, five years ago, the splint had to restore the entire hard palate on the right side and part of it on the left, also support the eyeball, which was prolapsed, and in addition, owing to retraction forward of the soft palate, had to hold an obturator. The results obtained with this splint, which has been worn without annoyance, are excellent. The nasal cavity is completely cut off from the cavity of the mouth. Diplopia, caused by prolapse of the eyeball, has been remedied by the process of the splint; the halting speech produced by retraction forward of the soft palate has become perfect through the use of the obturator.

In noting the permanent effects of these operative procedures, it is found that the results are decidedly unsatisfactory. At the Zürich Surgical Clinic the author observed recurrences after an average of 3.9 months in all cases of malignant tumor involving the entire jaw. Küster recorded no permanent results. In the Erlangen statistics 1 permanent cure was recorded in 17 cases. In the Greifswald statistics, of 17 cases there was not one permanent cure. Estlander found 10 recurrences in 12 operations. In the Göttingen clinic, of 74 total resections with 23 deaths, Martens found 16 permanent cures. Stein has recently reported from v. Bergmann's clinic that of 13 resections for carcinoma of the upper jaw, between 1890 and 1900, not one of those whose record was obtain-

able is living at the present time. After total resection of the u[
jaw on account of carcinoma recurrence took place on an average a[
3.6 months after the operation, while death usually took place a
thirteen months. The prognosis is more favorable in cases of sarco
Of 11 cases undergoing resection (total), 8 are living to-day; of th
2 are suffering from a recurrence, and 6 are entirely well. The permai
cures, in 47 cases of total resection at the Berlin Surgical Clinic, S
estimates at 12.6 per cent. of all cases. Cases of partial resection l
shown permanent cure for at least three years in 50 per cent. of
cases.

Osteoplastic resection of the upper jaw purposes a tempo[
exposure of the base of the skull together with any tumors origina[
from the latter, and is carried out either from the *face* or through
mouth. The introduction of this operation is due to the genius o
Langenbeck. The latter chose the facial route, and proceeded as follo

FIG. 325.   FIG. 326.

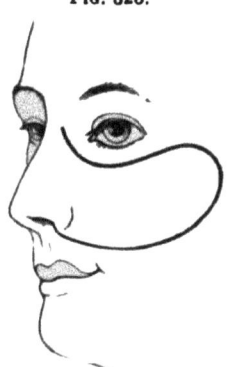

Skin incision for osteoplastic resection
of upper jaw.

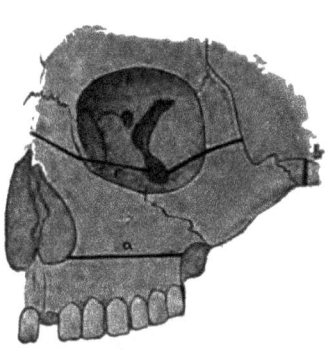

Line of bone division in osteoplastic resecti[
of upper jaw.

The skin-incision is carried from the inner angle of one eye along
infraorbital ridge as far as the middle of the zygomatic arch; from t
point it is carried in a loop curving downward and turning back as
as the outer angle of the nostril. The soft parts are not dissected ba
but turned inward, together with the bone, after the latter has b
divided. After dividing the origin of the masseter from the infe[
border of the malar bone the index finger or an elevator is inserted i
the pterygopalatine fossa, and with this guide a narrow-bladed saw
passed in the direction of the pharynx, where the point of the saw
caught by the index finger of the opposite hand, passed into the phar[
through the mouth. The upper jaw is now cut through horizont[
with the saw above the alveolar process as far as the apertura p[
formis. (See Fig. 326, *a.*) In this way the upper jaw is freed fr
below. Externally this is accomplished by freeing the outer angle
the orbit and the angle between the temporal and frontal process of

malar bone from the soft parts, beginning at the skin-incision along the infraorbital ridge, and by sawing through the middle of the zygomatic arch. (See Fig. 326, *b.*) The superior connection of the jaw is severed by dividing the frontal process of the malar bone as far as the spheno-maxillary fissure, and by dividing the orbital plate of the upper jaw, avoiding the nasal duct. (Fig. 326, *c.*) By means of an elevator inserted under the malar bone the portion of upper jaw outlined by the 'saw-cuts can be turned toward the median line. In so doing the articulations between nasal bones and upper jaw are usually broken. The tumor thus exposed can be raised out of the pterygopalatine fossa and its pedicle divided from the base of the skull with a knife, scissors, or thermocautery. Finally the jaw is turned back and secured in its former position by carefully applied skin sutures.

In order not to divide branches of the facial nerve, O. Weber places the base of the bone and soft-part flap at the zygomatic arch instead of at the nose, so that the upper jaw can be turned outward. The saw-cuts are the same as in the above method. The bone is broken along the articulation between the malar bone and the zygomatic process of the temporal bone.

Beside these facial methods of osteoplastic resection, various *oral* methods have come to be employed for the reason principally of allowing freer inspection. These methods consist in either a temporary division of the hard palate, or an attempt to turn down the palatal plate, together with the alveolar process, toward the cavity of the mouth (Hugier), or in turning out both halves of the upper jaw toward either side (Kocher). The former method has been developed particularly by Gussenbauer. He divides the mucoperiosteal covering of the hard palate in the median line, dissects it away on either side as far as the alveolar processes, removes the palatal processes and palatal bones, and after extirpation of the pharyngeal tumor reunites the two lateral flaps of the covering of the palate.

Kocher chisels through both halves of the upper jaw above the alveolar border, after having split the upper lip. He then chisels through the hard palate in the median line, and turns out the two horizontal halves of the upper jaw with a strong jerk. In spite of employing all the prophylactic measures discussed above, this operation is a very bloody one and has not been generally employed.

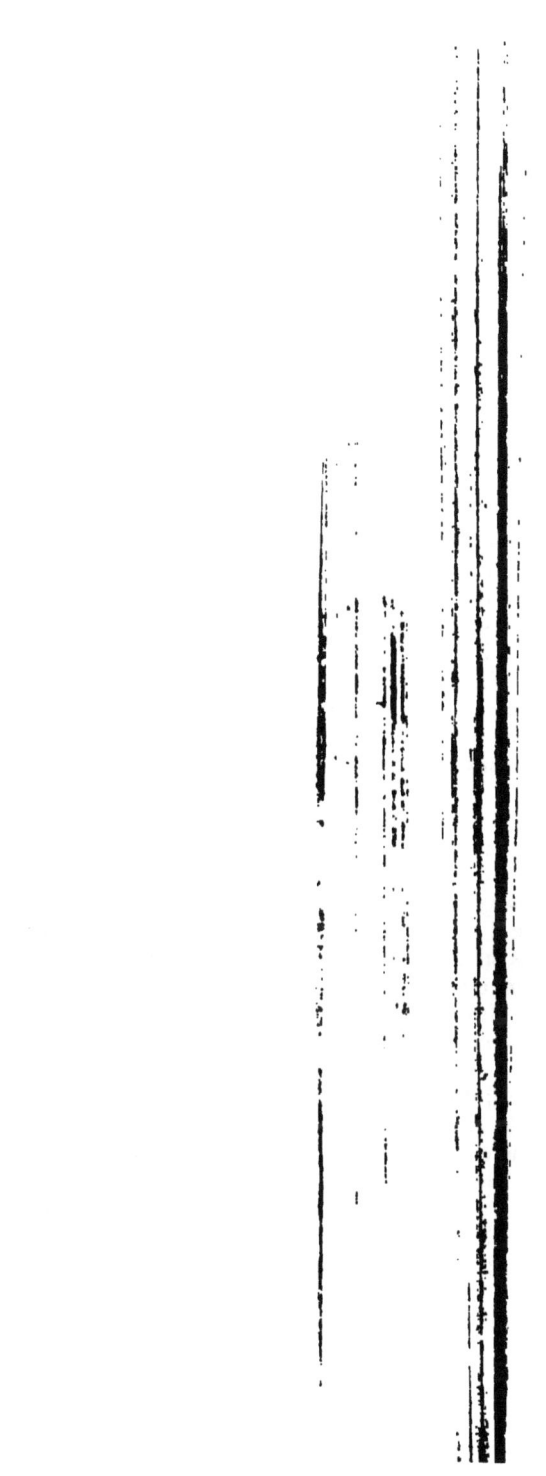

MALFORMATIONS, INJURIES, AND SURGICAL DISEASES OF THE NOSE AND ITS ADJACENT TISSUES.

By Prof. W. KÜMMEL.

Anatomical Remarks.—In the following description, in accordance with the plan of this work, only such subjects are discussed as possess general surgical interest. At the outset a few remarks will be made in regard to the anatomical relations of the interior of the nose which are of importance in conducting examinations.

In front of the anterior extremity of both inferior turbinated bones is situated the most accessible portion of the nose. The lower portion of the latter, the vestibule, is divided from the atrium of the middle meatus by a low swelling on the lateral wall of the nose (Schwalbe). The inferior turbinated bone lies nearest the anterior nares and is most accessible for examination. It projects slightly from the lateral walls of the nose, immediately behind the nostril, and extends backward, gradually projecting more toward the median line, to terminate in a club-shaped or frequently a nodular swelling. Its free border extends almost horizontally. Its line of attachment lies somewhat higher and almost follows the line of a quadrant with convexity outward. The line of attachment of the middle turbinated bone generally forms a right angle, with a short anterior ascending leg and a long posterior descending leg. The free portion (operculum), better developed than that of the other turbinated bones, usually projects beyond a line joining the extremities of its line of attachment, and in this way it covers a portion of the lateral wall of the nose. Here, close behind the anterior extremity of the middle turbinated bone, lies the "hiatus semilunaris," or according to the new nomenclature "infundibulum ethmoidale," a crescent-shaped depression of the mucous membrane. Immediately above and behind the hiatus and behind the attachment of the middle turbinate is an oval prominence, the ethmoidal bulla. In the anterior superior portion of the hiatus is the opening of the nasofrontal duct of the frontal sinus; in the posterior portion is situated that of the maxillary sinus. Close behind the hiatus there is frequently found, but only in older individuals, a second opening into the maxillary sinus. The opening of the middle ethmoidal cells usually lies just above or below the attachment of the middle turbinated bone, that of the posterior ethmoidal cells is occasionally placed above the superior meatus. The opening of the sphenoidal sinus is situated

(735)

in the most posterior superior portion of the superior meatus, near roof. It is directed anteriorly, but in spite of this fact it can b s from in front only when the middle turbinated bone, and particula its posterior portion, is at some distance from the septum. The frequ variations in the region of attachment of the middle turbinated bone due principally to the difference in development of the ethmoidal ce The latter penetrate to a variable distance into the turbinated bone it and occasionally transform it into a shell of bone, thus preventing ab lutely inspection and the entrance of instruments into the openings the other accessory cavities.

The *nasal septum* is very rarely situated in the median line througho its whole extent, being more often deflected to one side or the other. consists of three rigid portions and a membranous portion. From anterior nasal spine the vomer extends obliquely upward and backwa in order to be attached beneath the sphenoid sinus to the body of tl bone. About 1 cm. behind this superior point of attachment its poster border runs downward, almost vertically in the adult, very obliqu in children, and almost horizontally in the newborn. To the obliq anterior or relatively superior border, at its superior posterior porti is attached the thin perpendicular plate of the ethmoid. The anteri border of the latter is generally notched, and terminates about the mid of the anterior border of the vomer. Between these two lamellæ of bo which form a right angle opening anteriorly, lies the cartilaginous septu the triangular cartilage ("cartilago quadrangularis"). The anteri border of this cartilaginous plate rises from the anterior nasal spine at angle of nearly 30 degrees and extends upward and forward. It c readily be felt from without by pressing with the finger against t septum from below. As a rule it projects further on one side th on the other. The remaining portion of the septum, which is almo triangular in shape, is membranous.

The space between the floor of the nose and the level of the midd turbinated bone represents the respiratory portion ("pars respiratoria' the overlying space the olfactory portion ("pars olfactoria"). Und moderately good circumstances in examining from in front the enti respiratory portion is visible. It is impossible to see any great part the olfactory region unless there is extensive destruction or atrophy the middle turbinated bone. In the living subject the superior tu binated bone is hardly even visible from in front. It is of little or surgical significance.

Methods of Examination.—The principal requirement in examin tions of the nasal cavity is proper illumination. The rays of light mu fall in the same direction as the line of sight, as otherwise the numero bony processes within such a narrow cavity would produce too ma confusing shadows. As the best illumination, sunlight, reflected by perforated mirror, is frequently not obtainable, and the surgeon must most cases be satisfied with artificial sources of light. Any well-burnii lamp can be employed. The red rays present in many kinds of lig cause little disturbance here, as red tones predominate in the nas cavity. At the same time the white light of an "Auer" lamp, the electric light, or acetylene light is to be preferred.

Electric lamps, as constructed so far, produce rather weak light, even Edison lamps of 32 or even 50 candle-power are not sufficiently powerful. Small incandescent lamps on a forehead band or similar contrivance are applicable, provided the light obtained in this way be reflected from a perforated mirror as in Kirstein's lamp. In using other lamps the light should be reflected by means of a concave perforated forehead-mirror.

If the opening of the nose be examined with good light, but without turning up the tip of the nose, one can see even under the most favorable conditions only the anterior extremity of both inferior turbinated bones, the atrium, and the anterior portion of the middle meatus of the nose. In order to look further in, and provided one wishes to inspect only the anterior portion of the septum and the entrance of the nose, the tip of the nose may simply be pressed up with the thumb. But it is only with the assistance of a speculum that a deeper view can be obtained. The funnel-shaped specula are only of use in protecting the sensitive entrance of the nose, particularly during galvanocaustic operations. For other purposes bivalve specula are preferable. In the Duplay model, which has been modified a number of times, the two leaves are attached to a complete ring and can be separated by screws or other contrivances. O account of this ring the passage of larger instruments and the removal ofrthe speculum after insertion of the instrument are rendered difficult. For this reason the model of B. Fränkel is better. In this instrument two plates or rings, uniting at an oblique angle to form a handle, are separated by a screw. It is light and does not occupy much space, but, so far as practical usefulness is concerned, it is decidedly inferior to the most ancient form of instrument, examples of which have even been excavated in Pompeii. In the latter model the two leaves are fastened at an oblique angle to long handles and are separated by pressure upon the latter. On being relieved of pressure they are closed by the force of a spring. For practical purposes the handles are made sufficiently long to be grasped by the whole hand. It is thus possible with one hand to lift up the tip of the nose and at the same time by pressure upon the handles to separate the valves. Locking devices are superfluous. The various models of this form vary according to the shape and size of the leaves and handles. Good work can be done with all of them. The author himself generally employs the so-called Cholewa speculum. The blades, when closed, should leave a small space between them; otherwise, in removing the speculum at the end of the examination, some of the stiff hairs situated at the entrance of the nose (vibrissæ) are easily torn out, which is not at all agreeable to the patient.

Upon looking into the nose, with the head of the patient held horizontally, the line of sight being in the same plane, the tip of the nose elevated and the examiner provided with good light, he can see the greater portion of the inferior meatus of the nose and a portion of the middle meatus. If one wishes to inspect the entire length of the inferior turbinated bone, the speculum as a whole must be pressed against the

septum, at the same time avoiding any rotation of the instrume
by so doing one is very liable to injure the delicate mucous mem
of the septum with the edge of the speculum and cause troubl
hemorrhage. If the patient throws his head back and directs t
of his nose upward, and the latter be then raised sufficiently, on
see only the anterior portion of the inferior turbinated bone; bi
the other hand, provided the inferior turbinated bone be not too
developed, one will be able to see more of the middle turbinated
and the middle meatus. Toward the side of the septum the v
more concealed by the projection of the anterior extremity of th
binated bone. By means of a speculum with long blades, suggest
Killian, the inferior and even the middle turbinated bones can be i
aside. But as this generally causes violent sneezing, if not severe
it is necessary to employ cocaine. As a matter of fact, the auth
seldom been able to accomplish more with these long specula than
the ordinary shorter ones after thorough cocainization. In or
obtain a better inspection of the middle meatus of the nose, one
as suggested by Cholewa, force the middle turbinated bone towar
septum with the help of a thin elevator. As the turbinated bone i
elastic, fracture is rarely caused in this way; but even by this m
one does not accomplish much more than by simple cocainization.

FIG. 327.

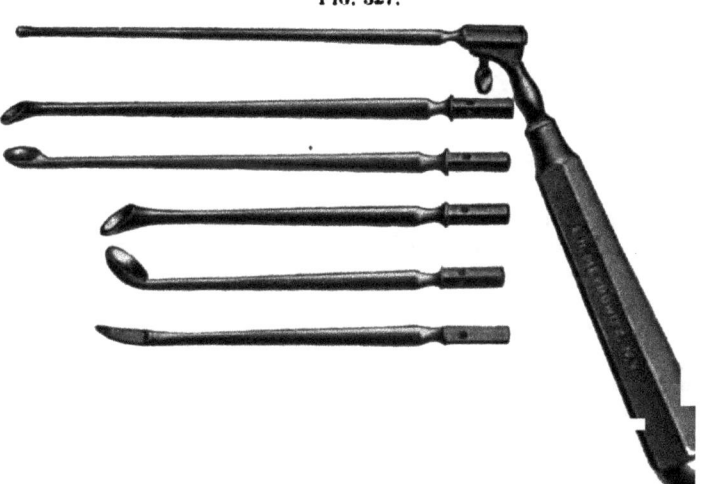

Grünwald set, consisting of a probe, four curettes, and a curved, sharp-pointed bistoury
each of which can be inserted into a common handle.

In general, cocaine has become absolutely indispensable for r
delicate examinations of the nose. By producing anæmia, the thick
of the mucous membrane of the nose is considerably diminished.
at the same time, after cocainization, even considerable hypertroph
the mucous membrane may escape notice entirely. Cocaine is

applied by means of cotton wrapped about a fine applicator. The cotton must project somewhat beyond the end of the carrier. In sensitive patients in whom contact with the cotton frequently causes violent reflex sneezing, it is advisable to apply a small quantity of a 1 to 5 per cent. cocaine solution with a spray apparatus. The spray alone, however, does not act sufficiently. More recently the ischæmic action of suprarenal extract (painted on) has been much employed for the same purpose.

The probe is another indispensable instrument in examining the nose. It should be united to the handle at an oblique angle, as in all other nasal instruments. It should not be more than 1.5 mm. thick, must have a well-rounded tip, and be easily bent. With a probe one can push aside swollen portions of the mucous membrane, examine tumors and other formations in regard to their mobility, but the probe is pre-eminently important in determining the position of the openings of the accessory sinuses.

In probing the maxillary sinus the probe usually employed is one bent to nearly a right angle a little less than 1 cm. from its tip; for the frontal

FIG. 328.   .   FIG. 329.

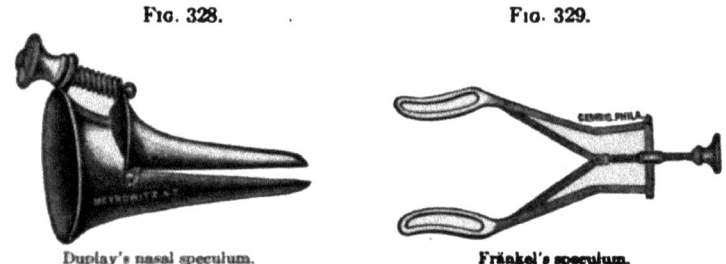

Duplay's nasal speculum.   Fränkel's speculum.

sinus, one which is bent in the form of a quadrant about 2 cm. from its tip. In locating the opening of the frontal and maxillary sinuses the anterior lip of the hiatus may serve as a guide, as it is visible from in front if the middle turbinated bone is poorly developed. In entering the *maxillary sinus* the probe is passed, with the convexity of the curve upward, to just behind the anterior lip of the hiatus, and an attempt made to direct the tip of the probe laterally by turning the instrument upon its axis. If this can be done without causing pain, the handle of the probe should be pressed against the septum, and with the latter be pushed toward the opposite side. If this meets with no resistance, it is safe to assume that the maxillary sinus has been entered. The only possible error is that the probe might have entered the ethmoidal bulla. The latter is, however, rarely deep enough to allow of the straight part of the probe being pressed against the septum without causing pain. The probe for the frontal sinus is best passed with the tip turned upward until the meatus is entered, attempting then at the same time to turn the tip of the probe slightly sideways, and to depress the handle so that the tip moves in the direction of the curve of the probe upward and side-

ways. If, with handle depressed, the tip of the probe is easily n
laterally and forward, the frontal sinus has been entered unless the
should have slipped into one of the anterior ethmoidal cells proje
from below into the frontal sinus. This error is, however, betr
generally by the fact that in markedly depressing the handle of the
it meets with resistance, and at the same time the patient feels pai
at least a sensation of pressure, in the depths of the eye instead of a
the eye, in the forehead.

If the middle turbinated bone be more developed, the hiatus ca
be directly inspected. Under these circumstances the probe mu
entered in the same direction as described above, between the m
turbinated bone and the lateral wall of the nose. If the tip of the
be turned slightly sideways and an attempt made to withdraw the p
one can feel the resistance of the anterior lip of the hiatus. The
manipulations should then be carried out as were described a'
Frequently it requires a great deal of patience, more on the part c
physician perhaps than on that of the patient, to probe these ca
successfully. Where the anterior extremity of the middle turbii
bone is much developed, it may be absolutely impossible, and the ren
of this portion of bone becomes necessary. The opening of the spheni
sinus can be safely entered with a probe, under guidance of inspec
only where the middle turbinated bone has been removed or is
small. It can, however, frequently be found if a straight probe be pe
close behind the anterior extremity of the middle turbinated lon
an angle of 45 degrees with the floor of the nose, as far as the ro
the nose, carefully feeling the way, and then, continuing to feel,
fully attempting to penetrate with the probe still further in the
direction. If the entrance into the sphenoidal sinus be discovered
probe will suddenly proceed without resistance for 1.5 cm. and s
against a firm wall of bone. At the same time the patient refer
sensation to the back of the neck, having hitherto localized it ii
nose itself. It is characteristic to feel an impact against a sm
hard, bony surface without being able to displace the probe as a v
upward or downward. If the probe be pressed against the bony
the head of the patient will be moved at the same time, which i:
the case as long as the probe impinges against the nasal mucous r
brane.

Probing the ethmoidal cells requires an accurate knowledge o!
normal anatomical relations and their very numerous variations
is rarely of any great surgical importance, and its description
therefore be left to text-books on rhinology.

A considerable portion of the nasopharynx can frequently be inspe
by anterior rhinoscopy if there is no swelling of the inferior turbin
bone and no marked projection of the septum. For this purpose, I
ever, the tip of the nose must be well raised with the speculum.
obtain a view of the deep relations in this region it is best to let
patient phonate the letter "e." This causes the levator veli pala
by its contraction, to produce a swelling of the floor of the nose, w

corresponds exactly to the edge of the posterior nares. In a broad nose this swelling can be seen prolonged in a vertical groove at the lateral wall of the nasopharynx, forming the mouth of the Eustachian tube. A better view of the nasopharynx is obtained by posterior rhinoscopy. In carrying out the latter the base of the tongue must, as a rule, be depressed. For this purpose the author prefers to employ a Turck tongue-depressor, the plate of which should, however, not be too large, and allow sufficient room between the teeth for those portions of the tongue that have been pushed aside. The author does not like the narrow depressors, like those, for example, recommended by B. Fränkel. More convenient to carry than the large Turck depressor, is a simple glass depressor, which generally serves the purpose, or a Czermak palate-hook, used as a depressor by Gottstein, Moritz Schmidt, and others. This is a pear-shaped wire ring bent upon its surface, attached to quite a long handle. This is placed with the convex surface upon the base of the tongue, and the latter forced forward by pressure downward and at the same time somewhat forward. The Turck tongue-depressor can be held by the patient in case an operation is to be performed.

Avoiding as much as possible any contact with the uvula or posterior pharyngeal wall, the mirror should be passed in such a way as to lie as high as possible, without being thrown into shadow behind the velum, within the curve between the uvula and the palatopharyngeal arch. By slightly turning the mirror in the vertical and horizontal plane the different portions of the nasopharynx and posterior nares come into view. In order to see the roof of the pharynx the mirror must be raised rather high and its surface made to approach a horizontal plane. It is difficult to interpret clearly the inverted image and the distortions of the picture in the mirror due to perspective. The landmarks are: the two openings of the tubes and the posterior border of the septum, which usually lies exactly in the median line. Very frequently formations, situated upon the posterior pharyngeal wall or the roof of the pharynx, are estimated to be much smaller than they really are, because in a certain sense one is looking beyond them from below and behind. The posterior nares are only obscured to any considerable degree by tumors situated above and behind if the latter are of some size. For one who is not skilful it is difficult to recognize what structures in the picture in the mirror are situated in front or further back. The location of the respective structures should be compared with that of the septum.

If for any reason the examination with the mirror is not possible, or if it is desirable to determine the consistence and manner of attachment of a structure situated in the epipharynx, palpation is to be recommended. It is best to stand behind the patient; the head being embraced and steadied with one arm, the index finger of the other hand, slightly bent, is passed to the posterior pharyngeal wall. At the same time the angle of the mouth of the same side is forced back, with the fold of skin between index and middle fingers. As soon as the posterior pharyngeal wall has been reached, the tip of the finger is made to glide rapidly upward, the

opening patent. Occasionally it has been necessary subsequently to bougies.

This malformation is not without danger during infancy on acc‹ of its interfering with suckling through obstruction of respira through the nose. Ronaldson's case actually died from this cause. on account of this danger, one should attempt operating upon suel obstruction during the first days of life, it must be borne in mind the opening of the posterior nares in the newborn is placed very obliqu almost horizontally. Perforation must therefore be directed backw and downward, otherwise there might be danger of injuring the v‹ bral column. As bony closure would hardly be expected at this it is best in such cases to employ a slightly curved trocar (as in p centesis of the bladder), using the finger in the nasopharynx as a g‹ in thrusting the instrument through. As a matter of fact, the au‹ is aware of no such cases in which operation was performed early. will probably be possible to postpone operating until a more advar age, and to provide nourishment with a spoon or by means of the stom‹ tube. There would only be danger, moreover, if closure existed on ‹ sides. This condition was observed in about one-half of the cases. the remaining cases, about one-third were affected upon the left s and two-thirds upon the right side.

Malformations of the nasopharynx possessing any surgical significa hardly ever occur. Abnormal band-like cords, with intervening pocl are frequently present, but they are of significance only in the treatn of chronic catarrhal pharyngitis.

CHAPTER XXIII.

INJURIES OF THE NOSE.

INJURIES of the external nose produced by sharp weapons possess nothing to distinguish them from injuries of the rest of the face. Many of the frequent injuries of the external portions of the nose produced by blunt objects are included among injuries of the face. Only those injuries will be discussed here that lead to changes within the cavity of the nose.

Such changes are always the result of violence with blunt objects, most frequently a blow or a fall upon the nose. Such acts of violence are not always severe; a slight blow with a cane, for example, may, if unfortunately directed, produce a serious lesion of the frame of the nose. Most frequently traumatism affects the nose from in front, as in the case of a blow or a fall. At the same time the nasal septum is compressed from before backward, shortened and bent. This may be followed by an injury of the bony bridge of the nose or a fissure of its root, the adjacent portions of the upper jaw, or the walls of the orbital cavity. This is particularly liable to happen when the root of the nose suffers severe trauma (blow with a fist, thrown stone). The bony septum is rarely injured by violence. As a rule the elastic cartilage takes up a certain amount of the force of a blow and is either broken or loosened from its attachment and laterally displaced. This dislocation (luxation) takes place almost exclusively along the sickle-shaped articulation of the quadrangular cartilage with the vomer. Very rarely dislocation takes place along the articulation with the perpendicular plate of the ethmoid, which is much thinner and very elastic. Partial or complete fracture of the cartilage of the septum occurs quite frequently, accompanying, or independent of, dislocations. According to Zuckerkandl's investigations, longitudinal fracture in a nearly horizontal direction is the most frequent. In every case in which the author was able to examine a recent fracture of the cartilaginous septum in the living subject, the line of fracture followed the above direction. But occasionally a fissure will run in any one of many directions. In the cadaver the author has found cartilaginous septa which showed on the crest of a bend an oblique ridge which extended from behind and below upward and forward. It cannot, however, be positively stated that this was caused by a previous fracture. It is only in exceptional cases that it is possible to determine exactly the character of the dislocation or change in form produced by violence shortly after injury, as there is almost always profuse hemorrhage into the nasal cavity. In fractures and dislocations the mucous membrane is generally stretched beyond its limits of elasticity and torn.

(745)

Usually, however, the edges of the wound do not gape, because in tl region of the cartilage the mucous membrane is quite firmly attache and cannot retract. Furthermore, the elastic cartilage usually sprin back after having been bent, so that the edges of the wound are aga closely approximated, and by the presence of coagulated blood in tl wound the latter may be rendered entirely invisible. Occasionall mucus covering the site of the tear is aspirated into the wound, so th coagulated blood at the bottom of the wound is infected from tl outset.

According to Zuckerkandl, the repair of such fractures regularly tak place by means of a connective-tissue callus. The development of ca tilage callus in general is still much disputed. Repair takes place an no permanent deformity results if the cartilage resumes its origin position or if it is artificially replaced immediately after injury. But a rule little attention is paid to such injuries, so that in many cas there remains a partial fracture or dislocation of the cartilage backwa and against the border of the vomer, which frequently leads to deformi of the outer nose. This deformity nearly always occurs at the time injury. Solution of the articulation between the vomer and the cartilag causes a deflection of the tip of the nose toward the side to which tl cartilage is dislocated. More serious deformity is caused as a rule k fracture of the cartilage, in consequence of which the line of the bridg of the nose frequently shows a very sharp and distinct deflection situate usually about the middle of its course. The tip of the nose may k displaced toward one side and also upward. This deformity is quit noticeable immediately after injury. In the course of a few days, how ever, it becomes less distinct as a result of a gradual extravasation blood into the subcutaneous tissues. The contours of the nose ar obscured as if by a cloak, and it is only after the original swelling ha subsided that the deformity again becomes more distinct. Occasionall and in the course of time the original dislocation is smoothed over t a certain degree, but complete obliteration rarely takes place subse quently. The deformity is permanent unless treated at the proper time In addition to the outward deformity there is in most cases interferenc with respiration through the nose on account of the projecting edge of th fractures or dislocated septum. This varies much in individual case and is followed by different unpleasant manifestations.

All these considerations render it important to examine carefully th interior of the nose, and to institute proper treatment whenever, followin an injury, any outward change in the form of the nose is noticeable Owing to the presence of coagulated blood, it will not as a rule b possible to obtain as much information by inspection as by palpatior For this purpose it is best to employ a stout probe or, even better stil a thin, straight elevator. In inserting the latter, however, one shoul be guided by the eye. It can best be accomplished if the mucous mem brane be previously cocainized. By pressing with the instrument a attempt should be made to displace the septum. In this way any existin mobility of any part of the septum can easily be determined. Occasion ally there may be a slight feeling of crepitation. Particularly the region where the cartilaginous septum and the vomer articulate should be carefully examined. The instrument should be passed in a horizontal direction and along the floor of the nose. If in this way a fracture or dislocation of the septum be discovered, treatment should be immediately applied. A short time after injury reposition can always be safely and completely accomplished by simply packing with strips of iodoform gauze, as v. Bergmann recently pointed out.

The displaced piece of cartilage should be first brought into proper position with an elevator or probe. Long, narrow woven strips of iodoform gauze are then inserted along the instrument. The first strip is passed in the inferior meatus on the side of the nose toward which the septum has been displaced, back of the site of fracture, into the space between the floor of the nose and the inferior turbinated. Here it readily obtains a firm hold. This having been accomplished, the middle meatus of the nose is filled with the continuation of the gauze strip, beginning again posteriorly in the same way, so that the first tampon comes to lie behind the displaced portion of the septum. Having made sure that the fragments have been reduced as well as is possible, or any improvement in their position having been effected, the middle and after this the inferior meatus are filled with iodoform gauze as far as the orifice of the nose. At the same time and in the same order that the packing is carried out the instrument used in effecting reposition is withdrawn. Finally, considerable pressure must be exerted in order to overcorrect the deformity. Unless the septum is fractured on one side and dislocated on the other, as occasionally happens, it will only be necessary to tampon loosely the other nasal passage. If, however, there is marked dislocation toward both sides, both nasal passages must be firmly tamponed. V. Bergmann recommends the employment of one single tampon, because, if several pieces are used, one of them is liable to be forgotten later. It is much more difficult, however, to insert a large single tampon, and still more difficult to remove it subsequently without causing pain and hemorrhage. The author would therefore recommend using two or three long narrow strips. Care must be taken, however, that the end of each strip extends forward as far as the nostril. The anterior end of the narrow strip that is used in packing the posterior portions, if pressed along the floor of the nose, will interfere very little with the view, so that reposition of the anterior portion of the septum, which is generally more seriously injured, can easily be controlled and the septum retained in its proper position by the anterior tampons. Obstruction of the nose by the tampons will cause some suffering, but the patient is more liable to be annoyed by the swelling, which is usually marked in the neighborhood of the alæ of the nose and the eyelids. One should, however, leave the tampons in place for several days whenever possible, in order not to interfere with the results of the treatment. By means of cold compresses soaked in a solution of aluminum acetate or lead wash the subjective symptoms can be materially relieved. A slight rise of temperature not infrequently follows tamponing. This is more liable to occur if some time has elapsed after injury before **tam**-poning is carried out, and can best be prevented by insufflating a little iodoform before inserting the tampon. If considerable rise of temperature should occur, it will, of course, be necessary to remove the tampon. It is better, however, to expose only the anterior portion of the septum and to ascertain whether perichondritis has not developed in this situation. If this is the case, the remaining tampons may remain in place after opening the abscess.

If it is only necessary to remove the tampons after three or four days, no further measures will be required. By this time the fragments will in most cases have become sufficiently united. Should it become necessary to remove the tampons sooner, they must be renewed. Should several weeks have elapsed since the injury, any attempt to repair the damage by these simple measures will be ineffectual. Under such circumstances it will be necessary to adopt the methods of treatment employed in case of crests and spurs (cristæ and spinæ) of the septum, which will be described later

The nasal bones, with the nasal processes of the frontal and superior maxillary bones and the cartilage of the septum, constitute a single system of arches; a little of the perpendicular plate of the ethmoid enters into its construction at the uppermost portion only. Thus it happens, according to Zuckerkandl, that whenever one of the above-mentioned bones is broken or dislocated, the cartilage of the septum is regularly injured. Most frequently there is a typical fracture of both nasal bones about at the junction of the middle and lower third. In most cases the lower fragment is displaced downward toward the cavity of the nose. Frequently both lower fragments are broken apart and occasionally separated to a considerable degree. This may be noticeable as a gutter-shaped depression after recovery has been completed. In such fractures the outward deformity is marked. But they can be reduced in recent cases without great difficulty by tamponing the nasal cavity, as described above.

Fissures and fractures of the frontal and superior maxillary bones may extend into the nasal cavity. Necrotic splinters from these bones may be evacuated through the nose and portions of the turbinated bones themselves become necrotic—the inferior turbinated bone in fractures of the upper jaw, the middle turbinated in fractures of the ethmoid. These injuries are generally the result of direct violence against the upper jaw or forehead. A blow of moderate force usually affects only the septum and the nasal bones. With this progressive destruction there is extensive extravasation of blood into the regions in the neighborhood of the nose, particularly into the tissues of the eyelids and the orbital connective tissue. If fissures extend through the ethmoid or superior maxillary sinus, the surrounding regions may be infected from these cavities and a phlegmon of the orbit or face be produced. The same thing occurs not infrequently if the anterior wall of the frontal sinus is broken by direct violence. A very alarming, but not very serious and rather infrequent manifestation in cases of fissure of the accessory sinus is emphysema. This originates in the sinus and extends over the entire face. It may remain present for a long time. In injuries of the nasal process of the frontal bone, which are rare and occur only as a result of extreme violence, the floor and even the roof of the frontal process may be fractured. In such cases it is always reasonable to suspect that other portions of the base of the skull are fractured. The latter condition is very liable to complicate all cases of extensive comminution of the nasal bones. Such an injury possesses an entirely different significance with respect to the organism as a whole than do isolated fractures of the frame of the nose. These complications have already been discussed.

The prognosis of uncomplicated fractures of the frame of the nose may on the whole be considered favorable. The only unpleasant consequences which result from inadequate treatment are, in the first place, the possibility of a subsequent outward deformity, and, in the second place, interference with breathing through the nose on account of a possible dislocation of the septum. Although all such fractures are really compound, infections processes rarely follow. The most frequent complication will be discussed in the following chapter.

CHAPTER XXIV.

HÆMATOMA AND ABSCESS OF THE SEPTUM.

EXTRAVASATIONS of blood beneath the mucous membrane after injury occur almost exclusively in the region of the cartilaginous septum, because it is here that fractures most frequently take place. Communications regarding this affection are still quite rarely published. Probably it is not of frequent occurrence. The author has seen about a dozen such cases, several of which were described by H. Theissing.

In recent cases there is found in front, upon the septum, a rounded swelling, limited to one side or occupying both sides symmetrically, bright red, yellowish, or orange in color, which in most cases completely fills the nostril. Upon being touched with a probe this swelling may be very painful. It is easily dented, tense, and elastic in consistency. The few who have seen such cases early found upon making exploratory puncture that these tumors contained a pale-red fluid or pure blood.

Such extravasations of blood are rarely absorbed without further disturbance or without special intervention. The author knows of only the one case which was cited by Ball; in all others suppuration followed. The general condition, which up to this time has been but little disturbed, suffers through lassitude, drowsiness, loss of appetite, and headache; the patients look pale and sick. The nose becomes still more obstructed, at times completely so. The rise of the body temperature may reach a considerable height, and thus lead to the erroneous diagnosis of a febrile general infection if the injury and the immediate effects of the latter are overlooked. For various reasons, children frequently remain silent in regard to having sustained such injuries, and, if the nose is not examined, the diagnosis may remain doubtful for a long time. Besides the swelling, which is visible within one or both nostrils, in most cases, when infection is rather severe, the parts adjacent to the nose are much puffed up. At times this puffiness is of such a character as to lead one to suspect erysipelas. The swelling itself, however, is as a rule pale.

The unpleasant disturbances caused by such an affection can be readily removed by incising the abscess. Incision should be free, as otherwise the lips of the wound become glued together, pus reaccumulates, and the former symptoms return. It is best to make a crucial incision and to pack loosely the cavity with iodoform gauze. Fresh accumulation of pus may occur after several weeks. At the same time that the incision is made the septum should be placed in the event of its having been dislocated.

(750)

As a matter of fact, there are cases clinically very similar which occur without injury as a result of acute infectious diseases (influenza, erysipelas). Occasionally they occur without apparent cause (perichondritis idiopathiea).

Incidentally may be mentioned here serous cysts, an accumulation of a purely serous or at times a slightly hemorrhagic fluid beneath the mucous membrane of the septum. These peculiar pathological products do not always occur in consequence of injury. In reference may be mentioned a case described by Lacoarret. There is no clear explanation for these cysts more than there is for analogous changes in the external ear.

Incision is the best method of treatment, though under some circumstances simple evacuation by puncture will suffice.

DEVIATIONS AND SPURS OF THE SEPTUM.

Deformities of the septum may be of significance owing to the fact that they interfere with respiration through the nose or because they produce outward deformity. These affections are frequently very difficult to remove. The following types may be distinguished:

Ridges and Spurs.—In ridges and spurs along the line of articulation between the vomer and triangular cartilage, which is probably the most common form, there is occasionally a congenital predisposition (frequently hereditary). But this form is usually found in later years, after the fifth, more frequently still after the tenth year, as has been proved by the anatomical investigations of Zuckerkandl. Irregularities of growth occurring during the time that the different parts of the septum approach each other might be the cause. In other cases there may be ecchondroses or exostoses similar to those occurring during the age of development, at other chondroosteal boundaries. Finally, traumatic solution of continuity between the vomer and the bony septum may produce similar deformity. In such cases the latter is usually combined with fracture of the cartilaginous septum. Deviation, as well as projection, of the cartilaginous septum is probably frequent in apparently congenital spurs also.

These spurs are, as a rule, pyramidal in shape, varying in height, usually situated little above the floor of the nose, and provided with sharp borders. They frequently bury themselves in the opposite-lying turbinated bone, and may become united with the latter. At times they extend posteriorly as far as the middle turbinated bone. The length of these projections is frequently underestimated, as from in front they are seen in transverse section. It is necessary therefore to examine these cases with a probe. The latter will also aid in determining the bony or cartilaginous character of these growths, and also whether there is union between the spur of the septum and the turbinated bone.

Deflection of the Cartilaginous Septum.—This frequently occurs in combination with the above-mentioned ridges and spurs, and varies in

direction and extent. It is almost always the result of trauma, a[
frequently recognizable by an external deformity, a deviation of t
bridge of the nose. In such cases there may be considerable bendin
frequently combined with deviation of the anterior border of the bo[
septum, which may be displaced close to the ala of the nose. The no
may be completely obstructed by these projections. It is frequently ve
difficult to determine regarding the location and extent of such deflectio
owing to the fact that the nose is closed immediately behind the nar[
One is successful, however, in many cases if the mucous membrane
thoroughly cocainized and a thin bivalved speculum inserted and sligh[
opened in order to determine whether there is narrowing of the no
behind the most prominent portion of the projection. If this precanti[
is not observed, it may be very annoying and surprising to find that aft
tedious surgical removal of the projections breathing through the no
is in no respect improved.

Deviation of the anterior extremity of the cartilaginous septu
from the middle line occasionally occurs without other bending. It cau
considerable difficulty in breathing through the nose, as during forcib
inspiration the ala of the nose is applied to the displaced septum, p
ducing closure. If the nose be inspected during quiet respiration, pa
ticularly after inserting a speculum, it is possible that quite a wi
opening may be present. But even in such cases one must be prepar[
to find that respiration is interfered with by an obstruction situated mo
posteriorly.

In most cases of deformity of the septum obstruction of the nose
the principal symptom. The latter naturally varies in degree. In son
cases there occur so-called reflex neuroses, especially asthmatic distur[
ances of varying degree. The same law applies here as in other refl[
neuroses of the nose, that the removal of the assumed cause does n
always make the resulting disturbance disappear. The external d
formity very rarely causes the patient to consult a physician, and the
only if there is marked deviation resulting from trauma, but not if the[
is only lateral displacement of the tip of the nose. It is generally easi[
to remove the cause of obstruction of the nose than to correct the extern[
deformity. The latter usually can be improved only if the patient h[
not attained his full growth, and the nasal bones can still adapt then
selves to any changes in the position of the cartilage of the septum. B[
in these growing patients it is extremely difficult to retain the septu[
in its proper position after it has been reduced. This requires a gre[
deal of patience on the part of the surgeon and the patient.

In order to remove the obstruction which interferes with respiratio[
it is sufficient in many cases simply to remove the bony or cartilagino[
projection, without making any attempt to correct the position of th
septum. This simple excision is applicable, however, only in the cas
of the ridges and spurs described above. Excision may be accomplishe
by means of a chisel, saw, or trephine.

Removal by means of the chisel presupposes that the extent of th
projection, and particularly its length, have been accurately ascertained

The straight chisel used for this purpose should not be too narrow. It ought to be about 1 cm. wide. The tip of the nose being elevated, the chisel should be passed in a horizontal plane, following the direction of the floor of the nose. This direction is important, as otherwise the chisel is certain to slip above or below the spur before the latter has been entirely removed, and the resulting hemorrhage, which may be profuse, renders further operation impossible If, however, the chisel is passed in a horizontal direction, even if it does slip, the crest is removed as far as that portion encroaching on the inferior meatus of the nose is concerned, and any small remaining projections can be pinched off. This portion of the nose is almost the only one concerned in respiration. After recovery from the first operation minor secondary ones are frequently necessary in order to remove remaining projections. It is absolutely necessary before inserting the chisel to determine exactly in what direction, as compared with the median line, and how far it is necessary to proceed, for as soon as the chisel penetrates hemorrhage will prevent all further inspection, and unless the conditions have been previously ascertained there is danger of going through the septum to the other side, or of glancing from the septum on the side of the projection. In either case the posterior part of the projection, which is the most prominent part, will be allowed to remain. A great deal depends upon firmly inserting the chisel in the

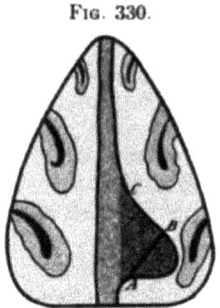

Fig. 330.

Diagrammatic representation of a spur on the left side of a septum. *A.* Point at which sawing should begin. *C.* Point at which saw should emerge. *A B.* Line along which the saw will travel unless care be taken. (Coakley.)

right direction from the beginning and completing the operation as quickly as possible. General anæsthesia cannot be employed unless the ·nose be tamponed behind, on account of the severe hemorrhage. This would cause more annoyance than the whole operation as conducted after careful cocainization, provided it is completed fairly rapidly.

Ridges of considerable size can be easily removed with the saw. For this purpose pointed saws, with thin and narrow blades, are employed. The handle should be bent at the angle usually found in nasal instruments. The best instrument of this kind is Beckmann's saw. The latter is very thin and only cuts on the out-stroke. The danger of deviating from the intended direction is greater when using the saw guided by the hand than with the chisel. This danger is much less, and almost certain to be avoided, if the saw is combined with an electromotor or dentist's drilling engine by means of a handle, which transforms the rotary motion into reciprocating motion by means of an eccentric. With such saws, which work very rapidly, these small operations can, as a rule, be so quickly completed that hemorrhage causes very little interference. If only very little osseous tissue is contained in the projection of the septum, a cartilage-saw is employed, instead of the usual toothed saw-blade. This is a sharply ground, thin knife with an undulating edge. In bony

tissues this saw is not practicable, and is very liable to slip. If
is used by hand, the head should be carefully fixed, as otherw
employing considerable force, as is sometimes necessary, a sudde
may cause the head to change its position and the proper bearin
be lost.

Trephines driven by electromotors or dentists' drilling machine
been used a great deal, particularly on the strength of Spiess'
mendation. A cylindrical piece is drilled out of the spur, the op
lying turbinated bone being protected by a bivalved speculum, pr
with a long lateral and a short median plate. This method i
simple and effective, but the trephine is very liable to slip.

Fig. 331.

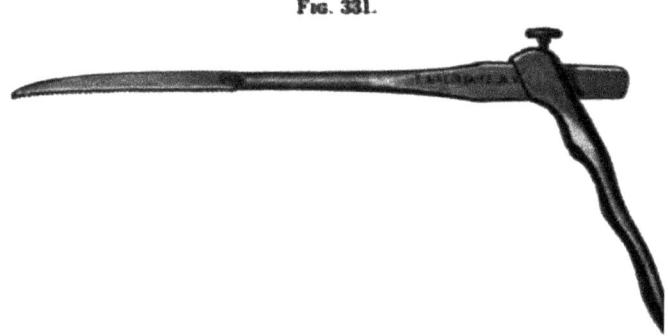

Mial's saw.

Electrolytic and galvanocaustic destruction for the removal o
jections of the septum are of more interest to the specialist than
surgeon. By means of the galvanocautery only cartilaginous proje
can be removed, and, as is true of other galvanocaustic operations,
follows a marked reaction, necessitating long after-treatment.
method is of advantage, therefore, only in timid and anæmic pa
By means of electrolysis, which is usually employed by the h
method, even bony projections of considerable extent can be ren
A large number of sittings are frequently necessary for this pu
But the patient suffers no annoyance either during or after the oper
In case of individuals who do not wish to interrupt their occupatic
method is useful. There is hardly space here to enter upon a full de
tion of its technic. The same is true of subperiosteal or subperi
drial resections, in connection with which there are many methods
by rhinologists.

Correcting the position of the septum, instead of excising the
must be considered in those rare cases of simple fracture without
ening at the site of the injury. If in these cases the projecting p
is excised, perforation may result. At the site of such perforation e:
tion is liable to take place. This is very annoying to the patien
should be carefully avoided. Besides, after excision in such cases
ticularly in growing individuals, but also in those who have att

full growth, deformity frequently occurs. On the other hand, if the projection is not excised, but the position of the septum simply corrected, the latter can be maintained in its proper position, even in growing individuals, by passing bougies. This correction is more easily effected the more anteriorly the deformity is situated and the more vertically it is directed. The best way of performing this operation is to cocainize thoroughly, and if the projection is situated well anteriorly, by submucous injection of cocaine, using Schleich's solution.

An incision is made with a narrow, pointed scalpel on the concave side of septum. This incision should almost completely divide the cartilage. With a pair of forceps, each blade of which is inserted into a nostril, the portion of the septum situated in front of the incision is firmly grasped and sharply bent in the direction of the convexity. The forceps should then be passed further posteriorly and the part behind the incision bent toward the side of the previous concavity. Owing to the fact that hemorrhage is usually considerable in amount, it is generally necessary to tampon the side of the previous concavity. It is better in that case to pack first the side of previous convexity, thus pressing the septum toward the opposite side. After several days the tampons are removed and replaced by suitable drainage-tubes, or, better still, by celluloid catheters of suitable diameter which have been softened by being exposed to steam and then pressed flat. The insertion of these bougies may be discontinued during the daytime after two or three weeks, but for some time, at least several months, the patients should insert them at night, as otherwise displacement is liable to recur. In cases of marked deformity it is better, after the position of the septum has been corrected, to remove the marginal portions of the cartilage along the line of fracture on the side of the incision in order to reduce the length and breadth of the septum, where these dimensions are too large. Occasionally rather large portions must be removed.

In simple deviation of the anterior border of the cartilage of the septum the latter can be simply trimmed off with a scalpel, but in order to prevent perforation the mucous membrane on the concave side should first be freed. This is accomplished in cases with marked deformity, according to Escat's suggestion, by submucous injection of Schleich's solution.

FOREIGN BODIES AND RHINOLITHS.

The majority of foreign bodies found in the nose occur in children, who are themselves usually instrumental in placing them there. Beans, peas, cherry-stones, buttons, and a very miscellaneous variety of objects have been found. During the acts of coughing or vomiting certain substances may also find their way from the nasopharynx. These may remain in the nose for a long time and lead to strange mistakes in diagnosis, such as an empyema of the accessory sinuses. A condition of this kind may also be brought about by bits of sponge or gauze introduced for checking nose-bleed, and organic products introduced during play. Substances employed for therapeutic purposes, such as pi tin-foil placed between cauterized turbinates and septum to p adhesions, may be forgotten and then set up an inflammatory p In exceptional instances bullets or fragments of exploded pro may find their way into the nose. Finally, it is to be noted i certain industries—cement-mills, paint-mills, and chemical wo large amount of pulverized material is inspired by the workmen, in the course of time becomes agglutinated and forms hard ma, considerable size. In this manner the rhinoliths are formed. masses of agglutinated cement particles often furnish curious calculi. Several cases have been described in which the irritatio duced by such foreign bodies along the anterior part of the septu resulted in ulceration and perforation, with the opening occupi the smaller part of the calculus. Rhinoliths, however, are u formed by incrustation around some foreign body, such as a fruit. a clot of blood, or inspissated mucus. The method in which this i tation takes place has not been explained. Gerber, Moure, and contend that the lime-secreting properties of various micro-orga is an essential factor in the process, but this view is energetically hated by Lantin.

Analysis of these concretions discloses great variation in their position. Usually they are made up of the phosphates and the carbe of calcium and magnesium. In one instance a calculus, whicl formed around a particle of iron, consisted of ferric sulphide.

Nasal calculi are found as a rule on one side only. A few ca which they could be detected on both sides may be explained h projection of a large concretion through a previously perforated se Isolated calculi in each nostril are rarely found. A moderate ar of calcareous matter may incrust a foreign body in a comparatively time, but the large calculi undoubtedly require a long period for development. The largest stones examined have weighed from 4 grams.

Symptoms.—The principal symptoms of calculi and foreign b are nasal obstruction and purulent secretion, with their attendant nomena, mainly headaches and facial neuralgia. Occasionall inflammatory œdema of the affected side of the face is seen (recu erysipelas?), and acute meningitis and encephalitis have been ol s when the foreign body has been forced into the nose and has penet the lateral masses of the ethmoid or the sphenoid bone. Substi which have remained for some time may cause marked inflamm swelling and tumor-like masses of granulations. In one case a malig growth was suspected, but when a rhinolith hidden away in a ma granulation-tissue was removed, the entire process rapidly subs Palpation of a hard, rough, movable body may make one think bone sequestrum and so lead to the idea of a specific lesion. erroneous impression of an empyema of the accessory sinuses is readily gained, though this condition may be rendered possible b' presence of a nasal calculus.

Treatment.—The removal of most foreign bodies from the nose may be accomplished with little difficulty. The restlessness of children, in whom the majority of these are found, often necessitates general narcosis. Thorough cocainization of the nose may suffice, however, as the swelling of the mucosa is thus diminished and extraction simplified. The forceps is the instrument commonly used, but really least suitable. More can be accomplished with a flexible probe having one end bent at right aagles, a blunt book or similar device. There is almost always room enough to pass beside or over the object, and getting behind to pull it out with the instrument. It is not advisable to pass under the object, as the latter, if small, may be easily pushed out of view into the space between the middle turbinate and the lateral wall. If the foreign body is large or if one of those enormous rhinoliths is present, it ought first to be crushed with strong forceps, a lithotrite, or similar instrument. For the removal of large bone sequestra it may be necessary to free the alæ by previous incisions. In most cases preliminary operations are unnecessary, as it is usually possible to make most foreign bodies accessible after thorough cocainization and cleansing irrigations. It is not advisable to flush out the object by directing the stream into the free nostril, for if the other is totally occluded by the foreign body, the pressure of the accumulating fluid may force some of the latter into the Eustachian tube and set up an otitis media.

In difficult cases it has often been recommended to push the foreign body back into the nasopharynx. This is not advisable, as the difficulties of extraction are increased in this locality. Especial care must be taken during narcosis, and if this method is employed, it is well to pass the finger into the nasopharynx to catch the object as it emerges from the posterior nares.

The occurrence of animal parasites should be noted, as they may produce severe inflammatory symptoms. Foreeps or irrigations may be employed in their removal, this being preceded by killing them with inhalations of chloroform or turpentine vapors.

NASAL HEMORRHAGE.

Although widely differing etiological factors may contribute to the production of nasal hemorrhage, the subject as a whole may be appropriately considered as a separate topic at this point. Clinically speaking they may be of considerable importance. In the majority of cases, at least in 80 per cent., the source of the bleeding may be traced to ulcerations or granulations along the anterior part of the cartilaginous septum.

This subject deserves greater attention than is usually accorded to it. Frequently cases are seen in which a comparatively slight hemorrhage is not checked by tamponade of the nares, for, as this is ordinarily applied, it includes everything except the crucial point, and that is the extreme anterior part of the nasal passage. If the bleeding continues, the other nostril may likewise be plugged. The hemorrhage may cease,

but usually does so of its own accord. Tamponade of the nasoph
moreover, especially if long continued, is very liable to be follow
an otitis media, and should not be practised unless absolutely nec
It is often difficult to recognize the bleeding point, as the entire
mucosa may be covered with blood, and even if a speculum is em
one of the blades may cover the ulcer.

As the hemorrhage usually comes from the locality already
(sometimes called "Kieselbach's point"), it is always best to tamp
nasal opening tightly to the very outer tip of the nostril. If the bl
does not stop, then the Belloc method should be used. When l
rhage proceeds from a granuloma, the so-called bleeding polypus
septum, its removal is called for.

Other causes for nasal hemorrhage frequently found are di
indirect injuries to the nasal mucosa accompanying fractures
nasal bones. This rarely assumes serious proportions. Bleeding
from malignant growths, particularly the sarcomata, is usually
Benign mucous polypi, if incompletely extirpated, may cause free
ing. Tuberculous ulcerations and glanders may occasion mo
hemorrhages. Operative injuries to any part of the nasal muco
attended by considerable loss of blood.

Tamponade is preferred in all these cases, but before doing it i
other measures should first be tried. Very often the bleeding ma
when the patient is put into the reclining position with the head
constricting articles of clothing removed, and absolute mental
insisted on. Much good often follows the injection into the nos
2 per cent. solution of gelatin in physiological salt solution, or satu
tampons with the same. Subcutaneous injections of gelatin oft
well. Tetanus following this procedure has been reported, but the
sterilization ought to obviate this danger.

THE INFLAMMATORY DISEASES OF THE NOSE

The simple catarrhs of the nasal mucosa are without surgical im
Most of the acute cases, independent of their cause, respond to m
measures or recover without treatment.

The chronic inflammatory processes may be designated as si
hypertrophic, and atrophic forms of rhinitis.

Hypertrophic rhinitis may lead to marked nasal obstruction
necessitate removal of the enlarged parts. As a rule the anterio
posterior ends of the middle turbinates are most involved and may
sionally be confused with mucous polypi. They are to be differen
by the vascularity, by shrinking under the influence of cocaine
more particularly by their situation on the inferior turbinate. S
hemorrhage may come on several hours after removal, due no doubt
paralytic action of the cocaine employed for anæsthesia. This com
tion may be avoided by using the Schleich solution, which has the
vantage, however, of not reducing the swelling of the mucous mem

For the extirpation of this hypertrophied tissue, the ordinary cold snare, the galvanocaustic wire snare, or the lately devised scissors of Beckmann may be employed. Some methods formerly in vogue depended on the formation of scar-tissue which followed scarification with chemicals or the galvanocautery. The unreliable character of such procedure has led to their abandonment.

Atrophic Rhinitis.—In atrophic rhinitis, which in many cases is attended by the formation of crusts and characterized by a very foul discharge (ozæna), Volkmann recommended a thorough curettage of the mucous membrane with the sharp spoon. This heroic procedure has not met with success in cases of genuine ozæna, and is now rejected. Treatment has been relegated to the specialist, but is still far from satisfactory, and the disease retains some surgical interest because of the possibility of confusion with empyemas of the accessory sinuses, which may present the same conditions of incrustation and foul discharge. Grünwald's claim, that all cases of ozæna depend primarily on diseases of the accessory sinuses, has not been substantiated.

The extension of an acute rhinitis into the accessory sinuses is of considerable surgical importance. It occurs quite frequently with the severer acute catarrhs, but is usually without evident manifestations and generally of short duration. At times the inflammatory process may extend into the sinuses after it has apparently ceased in the nose.

INFLAMMATIONS OF THE ACCESSORY NASAL SINUSES.

General Remarks.—Inflammatory processes in the accessory sinuses may be due to general infection or an extension from the nasal mucosa or neighboring organ.

When a general infection is present, it is often impossible to decide whether the infection is direct or has reached the accessory sinuses through the medium of a nasal catarrh. Influenzal coryzas are very often followed by this complication. The other infectious diseases, with the exception of diphtheria, where it occurs in a relatively large number of cases, do not present as great a liability. Acute inflammatory lesions are often found at autopsy in cases which have succumbed to an infectious disease (Harke, Dmochowski), but such processes were probably unimportant, and would have resolved spontaneously if the primary disease had not ended fatally.

There are certain localized nasal conditions which may bring on disturbances in the accessory sinuses; for example, the acute rhinitis which follows operations, some chronic catarrhs, and malignant new growths which have become disintegrated and foul. Benign tumors (polypi) may produce a mechanical occlusion of the orifices, leading to the accumulation of secretion and increasing the chances for infection.

The antrum seems to furnish the chief danger outside of the immediate boundaries of the nose. The molar teeth are overlaid by a plate of bone which in some cases is very thin and therefore readily penetrated

by an inflammatory process starting around one of these teeth,
of the lining mucosa of the antrum follows. Dentists believe
instances of maxillary sinusitis occur in this manner. Milit
however, claim to see more cases following influenza. Seventh
general prevalence of carious teeth confirms the possibility, th
eased teeth may be at fault in most cases. The author has
2 cases of antrum disease in individuals with absolutely perf
that had never been treated by dentists.

Trauma must also be considered at this point. The antrum
exposed through the cheek, the nose, or the mouth by blo
missiles or an animal's horn. Projectiles may penetrate in t
way, and in all cases infection is liable. The frontal sinus
injured by similar agencies. Foreign bodies, such as hair, bits
tips of foils, are often carried into the sinuses and produce
purulent processes. The ethmoid cells and the sphenoidal sin
less often involved in these accidents, though occasionally t
harbor projectiles.

Clinically the acute and chronic inflammations of the accessor
must be sharply differentiated.

Acute Inflammations.—The most prominent features of
accessory sinusitis which complicates a general infection are
the signs of septic intoxication unless these are obscured by th
toms of the systemic disease.

The pain may be severe, involving, for example, in a m
sinusitis, the corresponding side of the face. Pressure over the
cavity elicits pain. In frontal sinus inflammations the pain is k
in the supraorbital region, and is especially marked after pel
eye-strain or mental activity. By determining the outlines of
which is sensitive to pressure, the extent of a frontal sinusitis
quite accurately mapped out. Inflammation of the ethmoidal
usually accompanied by severe pains and intense injection of th
junctival vessels. Thus far the author has not been able to diagn
acute inflammations of the sphenoidal sinuses. The statements
in the literature of the subject regarding the localization of pai
likely refer to chronic conditions. It is a common experience
that blowing the nose increases pain in all cases of sinusitis. A
may complicate some of these conditions, the supraorbital and infra
nerves being distributed in the walls of the frontal and maxillary s

Inflammatory œdema of the immediately overlying skin or
membrane is occasionally observed. The swelling from a ma
sinusitis is usually soft and pale, seldom congested in appearan
presents local heat and tenderness, and sometimes pits on pr
Its soft and pale character serves to distinguish it from an a
periostitis; but if the pus from an empyema should break throu
bony wall, a similar firm, red, and fluctuating swelling would
With most accessory sinus inflammations there is an œdema of th
mucous membrane in the vicinity of the middle turbinate, wl
especially well marked in sinusitis of the ethmoid cells.

The effects of the septic infection vary greatly in intensity, and are sometimes obscured by the primary systemic disease or even the local rhinitis. As a rule there are irregular rises of temperature, occasionally with evening exacerbations—the temperature curve being influenced in many cases by the incompletely resolved primary disease. The temperature usually returns to normal with cessation of the pain, but a slight evening rise and general malaise may persist for some time after.

Symptoms.—The clinical course of these diseases cannot, as a rule, be followed because the patients do not often apply for treatment; and if they do, the condition is very apt to be treated as neuralgia following a cold, as malaria or similar affection, or possibly not treated at all. A cure usually results after a few days or weeks. If such patients are examined during the acute stage, the symptoms mentioned above may be readily elicited, at first increasing, then decreasing in intensity. In the second week, while the attacks of pain become less frequent and severe, a very profuse, mucous, amber-colored discharge pours from the nose, which gradually ceases. In some of the cases the discharge continues, but changes its character, becoming white, cloudy, and, after a time purulent, also more scanty and intermittent. In this manner a chronic empyema has resulted.

Disinclination for mental effort and general torpor have sometimes been noted in these patients; even marked psychic disturbances and acute maniacal attacks, as observed in a case by Ziem. But little attention has thus far been directed to such complications.

Diagnosis.—The diagnosis of acute accessory sinusitis depends mainly on the effects of the inflammations on the walls of the respective cavities, especially as regards the frontal and maxillary sinuses.

Pain on pressure elicited at the points of exit of the supraorbital and infraorbital nerves is a point of great diagnostic value. A valuable, but not always reliable, sign of involvement of the ethmoid cells is localized pain at the inner canthus of the eye. For this, as for all other cavities, the swelling of the mucous membrane around the middle turbinate may be considered an important symptom. Severe and continued pains of a neuralgic character in the head and face, following a coryza or any infectious disease should always lead to a careful examination of the accessory sinuses, especially if a profuse nasal secretion is present. Localization of the inflammation is difficult during the acute stage on account of the swollen mucosa in the middle turbinal region, which obstructs the view and prevents the introduction of instruments. If severe septic disturbances call for more detailed knowledge of the particular sinus involved, careful cocainization of this area should precede any attempts to locate the pus by irrigation. Even then, if severe pain is caused, it is advisable to forego this method of diagnosis. A convenient, although at times unsatisfactory, diagnostic aid is the method of transillumination. Having placed the patient in a darkened room, a small incandescent lamp, appropriately mounted, is introduced into the mouth and the lips closed. The normal maxillæ can be distinguished by a pink color, which is most clearly marked around the lower lid and the eyeball. The pupil is brightly illuminated and the patient experiences a subjective sensation of light. These signs are absent the antrum contains pus or its mucosa is thickened by an inflammatory swelling. The intensity of the illumination varies with individual case and an empyema of the antrum is not always marked by a shadow The frontal sinuses may be transilluminated in a similar fashion from their inferior aspects. The employment of the x-rays also gives evidence of shadows if any of the cavities contain pus.

Treatment.—In the treatment of acute inflammations of the accessor sinuses, antipyrin, phenacetin, and to a lesser degree quinine are c more value for the relief of the pain than the narcotics proper. Th application of cold seems to be the best remedy, especially for maxillar and frontal sinusitis. The continued application cannot be endured b many patients, and it then becomes necessary to employ the ice-bag o compress intermittently for, say, an hour at a time. The evacuatio of secretions by irrigation through a cannula introduced into a foramer is, as already noted, very painful; if demanded, the nose should b thoroughly cocainized and the irrigation done with very little pressure As many of these inflammatory processes subside spontaneously, it i better to omit any procedure which might aggravate the condition. I very severe pains are present, however, which are not relieved by othe means, it may become necessary to remove the secretions in the manne noted above. In some cases evacuation results after complete anæs thetization of the neighborhood of the foramen without further step being taken.

An acute inflammatory process of the accessory sinuses rarely break through into the surrounding tissues; this is more apt to occur witl exacerbations of a chronic process.

The common anatomical lesions associated with acute sinusitis an swelling and brawny œdema of the mucous membrane. These may become very extensive, filling up the lumen of the cavity and displacing the opening. Ulcerations or hemorrhages rarely occur; if a slight bleed-ing takes place, the secretion of the sinus assumes an amber color.

Chronic Inflammations.—Accessory sinus inflammations, which have taken on a chronic character from their beginning, are sometimes found with certain dyscrasias (tuberculosis, malignant neoplasms), but it is more likely that most chronic empyemas result from the continuation of an acute inflammation. The history reveals an influenza or acute coryza, followed by painful sensations in the face; after these have subsided a purulent nasal discharge appears, together with the other evidences of an empyema. In the case of a maxillary sinusitis the process is usually ushered in by some acute dental trouble. As patients apply for treatment ordinarily a long time after suppuration has begun, it is difficult to obtain details of early symptoms.

Symptoms.—Clinically the empyemas of the various sinuses differ markedly, yet a number of signs common to all may be considered together. The most constant symptom, although many patients give it scant attention, is the purulent nasal discharge. A characteristic feature is the intermittent flow, which depends on the relative position of the level of the fluid in the sinus to the natural opening, and therefore varies with the position of the head. The total quantity of the discharge during the day is considerable, especially if the larger sinuses are involved. The secretion is usually mucous and viscid in character, of a white, yellow, or green color, and sometimes brown or amber if mixed with blood. It may contain small brittle lumps or tough yellow flakes. Cheesy masses, sometimes of considerable size, are found, accompanied by a scant secretion. They are brown or gray in color and have a most disagreeable odor. Some accidental cause or an irrigation may cause their release, and the author believes that these cases form the basis of the condition described as rhinitis caseosa. The discharge of such masses presupposes, of course, a larger communication between the lumen of the nose and the cavity of the sinus than exists normally. With a scanty secretion present, thick brown crusts are apt to form on the mucous membrane of the nose and pharynx, producing a condition similar to ozæna. A profuse secretion is distributed both anteriorly and posteriorly; in the nose it leads to the formation of hyperplastic processes, exuberant granulations, and sometimes typical polypi, and in the pharynx the irritation is more apt to produce a chronic catarrhal condition, accompanied by the deposit of tough, glossy laminæ. The secretion may even find its way into the lyranx and produce a chronic laryngitis, accompanied by induration and thickening in the interarytenoid space and along both false and true vocal cords. The symptoms of these secondary affections, as manifested by the interference with nasal respiration, by the irritation felt in the throat, by difficulty experienced in swallowing, by occasional or constant hoarseness, finally lead the patient to apply for treatment.

One of the most disagreeable accompaniments of these empyemas is the decomposing secretion with its foul odor. It usually occurs with maxillary sinusitis, but is also found in the other varieties. Very old cases of empyema, however, often lack this symptom. The cheesy masses already described also possess a very foul odor. At times the odor is only evident to the patient, when changing the position of the head causes a sudden gush of pus.

Prognosis.—The prognosis of the chronic accessory sinus empyemas without operation is, according to most authorities, unfavorable for final cure and somewhat doubtful for life. This view, however, is probably too radical—some cases of long standing certainly get well and the diseased mucosa returns to its normal secreting function. Severe complications of ordinary empyemas are also comparatively rare, even those of the ethmoid cells; frontal or maxillary sinnses lead to the dreaded intracranial invasions less often than similar processes in the middle ear. Dreyfuss has collected from all sources only a very limited number of cases. Acute exacerbations of chronic inflammations often perforate into adjoining regions, *e. g.*, from the antrum into the cheek, sometimes into the orbit, the alveolar process or the canine fossa, from the frontal sinus through its inferior wall into the orbital fat, and from the ethmoid

cells into the inner canthus of the eye. In such cases marked
and septic symptoms may appear, and orbital cellulitis may
cranial complications. As a general rule, however, these infec
a milder course. Aside from the danger of intracranial compl
perforations into the orbit are worthy of attention, as they ma
lowed by an optic neuritis which does not always disappear a
the purulent process has been eradicated, and may eventually
blindness.

Treatment.—The cure of chronic accessory sinus empyema
brought about in two ways, either by a restitution of the diseased
or a replacement of the latter by a layer of scar-tissue. Resolu
tion aims to accomplish the latter result by complete eradication
affected mucous membrane. This is followed by the formation
lation-tissue on the exposed bony surfaces, and the lumen of t
is gradually obliterated. "A simple abscess with walls of gran
tissue is substituted for the suppurating mucous membrane." I
tion does not cause a complete obliteration of the cavity, a re
of the previously diseased mucosa may result or proliferation of
mucous membrane may take place from the edges of the o
wound. As the mucosa is restored with so much difficulty, it h
been proposed by Jansen to transplant epidermis on the expo
surface. The author has had no personal experience with this
but fears that the constant saturation to which the tissue is
would result in disintegration.

The aim of most operative procedures is to provide free drai
the secretions or unobstructed means of access for irrigati
medicinal applications. In theory the latter ought to answer
same purpose if given through the natural ostia of the sinus
opening, however, of an accessory sinus cannot be compared
of an abscess in the cellular tissues. A simple abscess heals af
ough incision, granulation-tissue forming in all parts, but a fistul
accessory sinus retains part of its mucosa or becomes lined wi
epithelium, which continues to give off a mucopurulent s
Cicatrization results only when the cavity is completely emptie
prevalent misunderstanding regarding this subject seems to ju
above explanatory remarks.

Medicinal applications require a thorough removal of all se
which is often difficult by way of the natural orifices of the
Irrigation may be done with an indifferent or mildly antisep
The excess of fluid must be gotten rid of by forcing a curre
through the cannula if the opening is narrow, or drying it out wi
gets of cotton or gauze if the opening is sufficiently large. Dis
can then be applied, preferably iodoform glycerin, astringents,
silver nitrate in from 2 to 20 per cent. solutions, or dry powde
ing boric acid and the newer antiseptic powders. The dry m
treatment cannot be commended to the same extent as in oth

Occasionally medicinal treatment is of no avail. In such ca
seated changes in the mucosa are usually present, and cystic d

tion, ulcerations, and true polypi are often found. When necrosis of the bone has resulted, extraction of the sequestrum is indicated. The author desires to note, however, that in all the operations done in severe cases he has never observed the condition, which has been described as "caries and necrosis," similar to that found in the ear. He cannot take for granted the view entertained by Hajek and others, that these osseous changes are present in many cases, and believes that probing has often conveyed false impressions. Even the numerous post-mortem examinations which have been done rarely afford illustration of this condition.

The other deep-seated changes, such as cysts and polypoid proliferations of the mucosa, are encountered more frequently. They can be removed by means of the snare or the sharp spoon—if merely curettage of the mucosa is done, they are apt to escape the instrument.

When medicinal treatment has not met with success or the inaccessible situation has rendered it impracticable, an obliteration of the lumen of the sinus must be sought for. The attainment of this end depends upon a thorough operation, followed by cicatrization and approximation of the walls of the cavity. All traces of mucous membrane must have been eradicated. This is hardly possible when the sharp spoon alone is used, as small remnants are likely to escape in inaccessible corners, and the scraping in some cases may induce a necrosis, which would further prolong the healing process. As a rule, if the sinus is well exposed, the mucous membrane may be peeled out *in toto* with a dull periosteal elevator. When this is done, the necessity of maintaining a communication with the nose is only of value for permanent drainage, in order to hasten closure of the artificial opening.

EMPYEMAS OF THE INDIVIDUAL SINUSES.

Empyema of the Maxillary Sinus.—Statistical evidence shows that empyema of the antrum of Highmore is more frequent than that of any of the other accessory sinuses. This does not mean, however, that the condition is readily diagnosticated by the general practitioner, and it is probable that the relative frequency of the disease is greater than is ordinarily supposed.

Etiology.—Diseased teeth as an etiological factor in this condition have already been discussed. Dentists are prone to ascribe too much importance to this cause, whereas the patients usually refer their trouble to a previous rhinitis or influenza than to a diseased tooth. The infection as a rule results from an alveolar periostitis, the pus perforating or infecting the wall of the sinus by contact. Although the cause is removed, the inflammatory process often continues. Occasionally a communication exists between the cavity and the affected tooth sufficient to admit a fine probe. When a tooth is extracted in order to gain access to the cavity, it is common to find the root tipped with a bit of granulation-tissue, which is separated from the sinus by only a thin layer of tissue.

If this thin membrane is torn away in the process of extractior antrum is exposed. The empyemas of dental origin apparently pi a better prognosis than those which arise from the nose.

Symptoms.—Subjective sensations of smell are often present. pus is marked by a disagreeable, foul odor, and considering the si the cavity is very abundant. It may be discharged with a sudden when the head is tilted forward. The formation of crusts is rare ii disease.

In many of these cases severe pains are present, usually diffuse l ache and pressure-sensations. Neuralgia, especially in the doma the superior maxillary nerve, may also occur. Patients afflicted uncomplicated antrum disease often complain of sharp pain on one of the forehead, and their condition may readily be erroneously sidered a frontal sinusitis. Toothache is frequent, and is describe the patient as being aggravated by cold, a draught, or even by blo the nose.

In some cases proliferation of the mucous membrane may take] in the region of the hiatus semilunaris, or the process may begin ii antrum itself and extend through an enlarged ostium into the i chambers.

Diagnosis.—If antrum disease is suspected, the confirmatory diag is in most cases quite easy. An empyema of the sphenoidal sinus o posterior ethmoid cells may be ruled out if the pus, after the nasal c is thoroughly swabbed out, reappears in the region between the mi turbinate and the lateral wall of the nose, and not in the olfactory fis The rather small anterior ethmoid cells, which are rarely involved a can be left out of consideration if the secretion is very abundant only remains, therefore, to distinguish between frontal and maxi sinusitis. This can often be accomplished by introducing a fine can into the normal or an accessory ostium, if present, and flushing ou cavity. The point at which the pus reappears after wiping out the can then usually be determined. If this procedure is unproducti result, an exploratory puncture may be made in the middle or inf meatus.

Exploratory puncture through the inferior meatus is best done a strong, straight needle, introduced about 5 cm. along the floor o nose. The needle is then directed upward and to one side and pre against the lateral wall close to the origin of the middle turbinate cartilaginous septum being held to one side. A quick, short push f the needle-point into the cavity; the absence of further resistance sl that the latter has been entered. Aspiration is often negative; if : is advisable to inject some sterile fluid and wait for it to emerge the ostium, carrying with it any pus which the cavity may have tained.

Puncture through the middle meatus is somewhat easier, as antrum-wall back of the hiatus and just over the inferior turbina made up of mucous membrane only. The most suitable needle i: bent in the form of an ear-catheter. The puncture should be r about 1 cm. back of the hiatus, and no force is to be used if marked resistance is felt. Carelessness may result in pushing the needle through the very thin-walled ethmoid cells, and so entering the orbit. The contents of the latter are then liable to infection by the irrigating fluid.

An erroneous impression may, however, be created by the appearance of pus in the irrigating fluid, for it is possible that this pus may have found its way into the maxillary ostium from the frontal sinus or ethmoidal cells. If this is the case, pus will reappear in the middle meatus in a comparatively short time after the antrum has been evaenated, for the simple reason that it comes from one of the sinuses which had not been disturbed by the irrigation.

Treatment.—Although the diagnosis of maxillary sinusitis is a comparatively simple matter, treatment is usually tiresome and unsatisfactory. Even after the most radical operative procedures a cure fails to result or the healing process is protracted. Yet at times chronic empyemas get well after ordinary irrigations through the natural or an artificial opening. As the prognosis in any given case is so uncertain, it is well to employ for a time simple irrigations through the natural ostium in all cases. If no benefit results, it may be necessary to make a supplementary opening in order to simplify the process of irrigation. The simplest, but by no means the best, procedure is to provide an opening through the alveolar process. The affected tooth is first extracted, or if several are involved, the second molar is selected. Should examination with a probe fail to disclose free communication with the antrum, the latter can be opened with a bone-awl or bone-gouge. A close-fitting wedge of soft rubber can be used to close the opening, which is removed for purposes of irrigation. If the patient wears a dental plate, the wedge must be accommodated to it, but should never be firmly attached. In case a sufficiently large drainage-opening is present, iodoform-gauze strips or drainage-tubes may be employed; but they must be properly secured, for if they should slip back into the cavity their extraction, especially when the opening is small, would be attended with considerable difficulty. Their retention greatly prolongs the suppurative process, and they give rise to a very foul odor.

A relatively larger opening than the one just described can be made through the canine fossa. An incision is carried down to the bone, about 1 cm. above the free edge of the gum, from the canine tooth to the molars. The mucous membrane and periosteum are pushed upward, and an opening as large as desirable readily made in the thin wall of the antrum by means of a chisel or trephine. The operation can be done under cocaine anæsthesia, and the opening secured is sufficiently large to permit the introduction of an aural speculum and the inspection of the entire cavity. It is prone to close very quickly, however, and the author has always found it necessary to prevent contraction by cannulæ or obturators. A much more complete exposure is secured by resection of the entire facial wall of the antrum, which should preferably be done under general anæsthesia. Even after such a complete operation, the author has seen the opening contract to such an extent that irrigations

could only be done after dilatation of the narrow sinus by mean:
bougie.

An almost complete obliteration of the antrum is possible if the
as well as the facial, wall is removed. The creation of an openin
the nasal passage, in addition to resection of the facial wall acco
to the method of Luc, merely provides drainage for parts of the
not previously reached. If, on the contrary, the nasal wall is en
removed, as lately recommended by Bönninghaus the nasal mucos
then grow into the cavity and unite perhaps with that from the che

With the exception of the last, the procedures mentioned provid
drainage and also ready access to the cavity, but have the disadva
of affording a communication with the month, which may lead to
sequent recurrent infections. As a rule, this does not apply whe
canine fossa has been opened, for in this case the mucous meml
of the cheek usually forms a valve-like fold, which prevents to
extent the entrance of infectious particles.

To avoid this complication Mikulicz has suggested an approa
the cavity through the nose. A strong stilet, the end bent at a
angle, is introduced along the inferior meatus (similar to the explo
puncture) and forced into the sinus. The opening thus made m;
enlarged by rocking the instrument to and fro. The cut edges o
mucous membrane, however, are apt to proliferate, and constant a
tion is necessary in most cases to prevent contraction of the wc
margins. These objections also apply to the method of opening by
of a trocar, as recommended by Krause. The methods outlined a
a general thing successful only in simple uncomplicated cases, and t
moreover, often get well without such radical procedures by the a
irrigations and medicinal applications through the natural open
A method for the severe cases, ideal and not too radical, has not
far been devised.

The most satisfactory procedure would consist in a complete rese
of the nasal plate of the antrum, but this would entail sacrifice o
inferior turbinate bone and the liability of injury to the nasolachr
duct. Before undertaking such an operation, however, a thor
knowledge of all the landmarks is essential, for the operative field lie
back and to one side, rendering access to the same a matter of cons
able difficulty. The author has operated on a few cases in this ma
but within the limits of the middle meatus, securing a fairly good e
ure and an improvement of the purulent process, sufficient at lea
satisfy the patients. Siebenmann has proposed breaking througl
nasal wall of the sinus with the finger introduced into the middle m
after cocainization. The author has not been able to accomplish
feat. Incising the ala and turning up the flap might make the open
easier, but would certainly make it too extensive. For the comb
empyemas of the frontal and maxillary sinuses attention is called t
method of Killian, which is discussed more fully later.

Empyema of the Frontal Sinus.—Chronic suppurations in the fr
sinus are less common than those of the antrum. By far the gr

number is caused by infection from the nose or systemic disease, especially influenza. Occasionally traumatic empyemas result from a compound fracture of the anterior wall or from a penetrating projectile or knife, part of which may remain as a foreign body.

In connection with a frontal sinusitis there is often present disease of the anterior ethmoidal cells or the maxillary antrum, for the secretion from the frontal sinus can readily find its way into the others. In such cases the inflammation in the frontal sinus occupies the foreground in the clinical picture, and as it subsides the trouble in the sinuses becomes evident.

Symptoms.—The frequent involvement of other sinuses causes an empyema of the frontal sinus to present a varied clinical picture. The main symptom of this condition is pain. Generally it is characterized by a sense of cerebral pressure or a feeling of fulness in the frontal region, and then the anterior wall is extremely sensitive to pressure. Quite often the pains are localized along the distribution of the supraorbital nerve, the point of exit being particularly sensitive. The intermittent character of the pain in some instances may lead to an erroneous diagnosis of malarial neuralgia.

The excretion of pus is particularly troublesome in the morning after awakening and when the erect posture is assumed. Inspissation of the secretion and the formation of cheesy masses is often found in this condition.

Eye disturbances are not uncommon, but probably on account of the involvement of the ethmoid cells. Patients are tired readily by occupations which require continued accommodation, and complain of pain similar to that observed with insufficiency of the internal recti. It is impossible to say whether these muscles are the site of inflammatory changes such are found, after a laryngitis, in the muscles controlling the vocal cords. The vertigo which is sometimes present seems to point to such a condition, but in one of the author's patients, in whom the sensations of dizziness entirely subsided after flushing out the sinus, the most careful search failed to reveal any disorder of the eye muscles. Visual disturbances have been observed by Kuhnt, but are quite rare. Scintillating scotoma are most frequently seen; optic neuritis, iritis, and similar lesions only come on after perforation into the orbit has occurred. Aside from the danger to the eye, such an infection may indirectly cause a meningitis, and therefore requires prompt and energetic treatment.

Intracranial complications may also be the result of a direct transmission of the infection through the upper wall of the frontal sinus by a phlebitic process, without destruction of the bone itself (Hinsberg).

Treatment.—If no complications are present, it is well to treat the inflammation by irrigations through the natural ostium. The frontal is the most readily accessible of all sinuses for this method of treatment, and usually responds to its effects in a very satisfactory manner. If irrigation is impossible or does not effect a cure, or finally signs of a perforation are present, it becomes necessary to open the sinus either

in front or below. The usual trephine-openings in the anter
which have been employed by surgeons for a long time past
permit flushing out of the cavity in a superficial manner. If a c
to take place a persistent fistula results, accompanied by cons
discomfort and deformity. After subperiosteal resection of th
anterior wall, however, a method which has been recommended
time past and revived lately by Kuhnt, the cavity becomes alm
erated and healing takes place, though with much disfigurement
the cavity is large, the lateral recess, which often extends into th
bone, cannot be reached by this method, and may prolong the s
tive process indefinitely.

A more or less complete exposure of the large cavities is
according to Jansen, by the resection of the entire inferior (orbit
The lumen of the sinus is then occupied by the orbital contents,
lateral recess, already mentioned, with its dense lower wall, is
with difficulty and does not readily become obliterated.

According to several authorities, healing may be delayed by s
tion in the ethmoid cells. To meet this complication several o
procedures have been suggested by which these cells are expo
nasal drainage provided. They will be described later. If th
boring soft parts, however, sink into and fill the cavity (really the
of the operation), the lateral recess may become shut off from th
age-opening and a discharging fistular tract remains. In a front
of this form operative openings, made both in front and below,
lead to better results.

The formation of a flap consisting of skin, periosteum, and bo
the anterior wall of the frontal sinus, was recommended about th
time by Czerny and Brieger. Taken alone the method is of littl
as the lumen of the cavity remains. In cases with prolonged supp
it is necessary, therefore, to delay the union of the flap, and whe
does take place the cosmetic result is by no means brilliant. Th
bination of this procedure with a wide opening into the nose
practicable, however. An incision is made along the lower b
the eyebrow, a second one perpendicular to its middle point
periosteum is pushed back from the inferior wall, and the latter
forated, can best be removed with a light and slightly bent Luer
Otherwise the anterior and inferior walls of the sinus are cut
in the lines of the skin-incision, with a chisel or circular saw, to th
of the cavity, as determined by the probe. The bone-flaps a
appropriately notched along the upper and lateral borders, fre
the chisel and lifted up. Care must be taken not to tear the
thickened lining membrane of the cavity, so that it can be pee
of all the corners in its entirety. Finally, if the bone-flap is p
trimmed so as to permit its approximation to the posterior wal
frontal sinus, and a communication with the nose is secured by
of the neighboring ethmoid cells, the conditions are favorable fo
eration of the lateral recesses of the cavity. The vertical incision
closed by suture, the horizontal one being left open for tampona

disfiguration is not prominent and the results in cases which the author has treated in this manner most satisfactory. A prolonged and careful after-treatment, however, is essential. This operation may be advantageously combined with the one proposed by Killian for opening the ethmoid cells, and the entire skin-wound sutured. Killian has also suggested another even more radical and extensive operation for opening the frontal and ethmoidal sinuses (see *Archiv f. Laryng. und Rhinol.*, vol. xiii. pp. 28 and 59).

Suppurations in the Ethmoid Labyrinth.—Isolated suppurative processes in the ethmoid cells are extremely rare. They are usually combined with empyemas of the other sinuses, and the majority of recent authors claim that suppurative inflammations of the frontal sinus and ethmoids should be regularly associated. The author cannot quite agree with this view. Not only has he seen a series of cases of frontal sinusitis heal under treatment by simple irrigation without subsequent signs of suppuration being found in the ethmoid cells, but he has also seen the ethmoid cells perfectly intact when they were opened for drainage in operations for empyema of the frontal sinus.

Diagnosis.—The diagnosis of ethmoiditis can be determined by the reappearance of pus in the hiatus or in the olfactory fissure after the nose has been thoroughly cleaned and after empyemas of the other sinuses have been excluded. Any one or all the ethmoid cells can be emptied by irrigation after the middle turbinate is removed, or when it is atrophied. The former procedure also makes the cells accessible for operative interference. If these requirements are carried out in making a diagnosis, the number of cases of ethmoiditis is very much diminished. According to Grünwald and others, the condition is very frequent. The author agrees rather with the views of Zuckerkandl and Hajek. Nevertheless in cases in which, after opening a suppurating accessory sinus, no pus appears in the wound, although it continues to discharge from the nose, it is always well to examine the ethmoid cells for traces of a hidden empyema.

Symptoms.—The symptoms are seldom characteristic. The purulent secretion, on account of the small size of the cells, is not very copious. The inflammatory thickening of the surrounding mucous membrane is usually quite marked. Very often the pus, of which part flows back into the nasopharynx, dries and forms thick crusts. Among other symptoms, pain may be entirely absent or it manifests itself as a ciliary neuralgia, follows periods of mental exertion, and may be especially marked in occupations which tax accommodation.

It is not definitely known whether this condition is due to inflammatory processes involving the internal recti or the nervous mechanism of the eye. The author is not prepared to say whether true functional disturbances of sight occur.

In disease of the anterior cells a swelling may become manifest, which is sometimes difficult to differentiate from abscess of the lachrymal sac. As a rule, however, the former is situated somewhat higher and extends further into the orbit. Perforations into the orbit are occasionally seen,

but the author has observed this complication occurring much
with frontal or maxillary empyemas.

Treatment.—An isolated ethmoiditis, when it does occur, can i
cases be treated through the nasal passages. If the posterior c
involved, a total, if the anterior cells are concerned, only a partia
tion of the middle turbinate is necessary. A number of the cells a
opened; the remainder can be exposed by breaking down the bon;
Care must be taken in flushing out the ethmoid cells to introdu
cannula very carefully, for by harsh treatment the orbital plate i
broken and the orbit invaded. The author has also seen severa
in which a subcutaneous emphysema of the lower lid followed the f
introduction of air into the ethmoid cells.

It should be noted that the complicated structure of the ei
labyrinth renders the suppurative processes very obstinate in cha
As the condition is usually simultaneous with one in the frontal
operative interference may be made to include both. The anterio
may be easily reached from the floor of the widely opened frontal
and removal of the inferior wall permits ready access to the po
cells. It is well to exercise great care at this point to avoid dam
the optic nerve. The deep-seated hemorrhage from the anterie
posterior ethmoidal arteries is also very troublesome. Operati
this region may endanger the trochlear nerve, and injuries to the su
oblique ocular muscle are not infrequent. If the trochlear nerve
turbed at the point where it lies in contact with the frontal bon
its articulation with the ethmoid, it will adjust itself again aft
periosteum grows fast; but the author doubts whether the traces o
injuries to either muscle or nerve ever disappear entirely. Dij
especially marked on looking downward, gives the patient very dis
able sensations, often remaining for a considerable period, but to
he gradually becomes accustomed.

Killian and, in similar fashion, A. Barth employ for the expos
the labyrinth a temporary resection of the nasal bone. The skin
nose is incised in the median line from the glabella downward
middle of the bridge, the periosteum over the frontal sinus is p
back and the cavity opened. The nasal bone is then disarticulate
together with the overlying skin, reflected to one side. A probe is
into the sinus and through the canal of exit. The nasal process
frontal is then cut away with a chisel down to the probe and ren
Winckler follows the old method of Langenbeck, with the except
turning the osteoplastic downward instead of upward.

For the exposure of both ethmoid labyrinths Winckler recom
the later procedure of Gussenbauer, which includes the temporary
tion of the upper part of the bony framework of the nose.

The author desires to reiterate that for the cure of ethmoid suj
tions the ordinary intranasal methods are usually sufficient. The
nosis is relatively good for these cases. Unless free drainage is pre
for, however, there is danger of perforation into the orbit, injury
optic nerve, and eventually septic infection of the meninges or the

organism. Perforations directly through the cribriform plate, followed by extradural or cerebral abscess, have also been observed.

Empyema of the Sphenoidal Sinus.—Suppurations in this sinus seldom occur alone, but are found quite frequently associated with other empyemas.

Diagnosis.—The diagnosis is simplified when the turbinates, especially the middle, are atrophied, as with an ozæna, or are reduced in size by the expulsion of bone sequestra, as in syphilis. The ostium, which is ordinarily covered by the middle turbinate, can then be seen and a probe or fine cannula introduced to determine the presence of pus. Under other conditions diagnosis is difficult and the empyema may easily be overlooked.

Symptoms.—The most prominent sign of sphenoidal sinusitis is the presence of very foul-smelling crusts, sometimes found only in the upper part, but frequently in the cutire nose. The clinical picture may lead to an erroneous impression of a genuine ozæna, but experience makes it possible to detect a difference in the odor of these conditions. At times an empyema of the sphenoidal sinus may really be a complication of an ozæna, and the crusts may be gathered around the ostium so that the latter cannot be identified. As soon as they are removed, the pus is usually seen issuing from the opening.

Granulations and inflammatory hypertrophies of the mucosa rarely occur, but an atrophic pharyngeal catarrh is often present, and the dryness and burning in the throat, the accompanying laryngitis and hoarseness are most annoying. The subjective symptoms have been studied by Berger and Tyrman, and also more lately by Schäffer and Grünwald. They all agree on the prevalence of functional eye disturbances, scintillating scotoma and amblyopia particularly having been observed.

Treatment.—The diagnosis being usually made in cases in which the floor of the sinus is rendered accessible through atrophy of the turbinates or their diminution in size by operative measures, the cavity can readily be reached through the nose by removing the inferior wall below the ostium with the aid of a sharp spoon, cutting plyers or, as lately suggested, by a motor-driven trephine. The cavity can then be packed with iodoform gauze. The external operative procedures, by which the ethmoid is exposed, as a rule also permit a good view of the ostium and the sphenoidal sinus if done with proper illumination and the hemorrhage is thoroughly controlled.

ULCERATIONS AND INFECTIOUS GRANULOMATA.

The nasal mucosa is affected perhaps oftener than any other organ by distinctive infectious processes and neoplasms, the entrances to the nasal passages being particularly exposed.

Ulcers.—The most common condition is the simple non-perforating ulcer. These ulcers are found as a rule in connection with some chronic inflammatory process, and are kept up by picking with the finger-nails and the forcible removal of adherent crusts. The trouble occur often during childhood, and then results from the introduction of tious material by the fingers. In adults the cause is usually more d and workmen in arsenic, color, and cement works are particula tacked. The finely divided, irritating dust is the main etiological in this class of cases.

As a result of hemorrhage into the tissues resorption of the clc lead to degeneration of the cartilage, with pigment-deposits, a ₱ called by Zuckerkandl xanthosis. Perforations of the septum then expulsion of the bits of necrosed cartilage. So long as there is no in the cartilage the ulcers are quite flat, and covered with brown or crusts which are tightly adherent. The edges are irregular, not sl marked, but never undermined, and are crossed by the tortuous in capillaries. The base of the ulcer usually presents a small mou granulation-tissue. Severe bleeding and the crust formation con: the only troublesome symptoms, and in many cases therefore the is observed only by accident, sometimes not until perforation has place and the mucous membrane has grown over the edges of the w When the latter takes place, the disease process practically comes to a

Tuberculosis is the most frequent specific infection leading to u tions and the formation of granulation-tissue. It may be present nose with a well-advanced pulmonary phthisis or in its early stag even without demonstrable general infection. In the latter ca: lesion is generally found on the cartilaginous part of the septum ι part of the inferior turbinate lying directly opposite and the floor nose. At times the anterior end of the middle turbinate is affecter the disease seldom extends backward further.

Ulcerations similar to those of lupus may be present, with partly undermined edges, and a necrosed bleeding base. These ar rounded by small disseminated fresh foci. The condition differs the tuberculous process in the skin in the extensive growth of gra tion-tissue, which often forms tumors as large as peas or cherries. ′ are not particularly characteristic except for the tendency to ulcer In color they are pale red, usually covered by squamous epithelium the surface is coarsely granular. Histological examination often to reveal their tuberculous character; the bacilli are only rarely ι after a prolonged search. The diagnosis, even with this aid, is the difficult, and especially in individuals who are apparently well othe·

With advanced tubercular disease typical ulcers may be fou various parts of the nose and nasopharynx, which break down rɛ and may often be entirely overshadowed by the severity of the sys infection.

Tuberculous lesions of a mild form can often be completely eradi by prompt and thorough surgical procedures. Recurrences take ι however, in many instances, and a view of the new foci may be obstr by the contractile scars at the nostrils. Nevertheless, the progno most cases is not unfavorable; a final cure may result even afte disease has been present for years.

Syphilis frequently causes ulceration, but rarely results in the formation of tumors or granulation-tissue. Gummata which involve the cartilaginous or bony framework of the nose and manifest a marked tendency to destructive processes, are frequent. Their favorite site is in the septum, near the nasal floor. It is also claimed, and perhaps with truth, that most syphilitic perforations of the palate have resulted from gummata of the vomer which have broken through into the oral cavity. These lesions present all the characters found in syphilitic ulcers elsewhere and do not require special description. In the septum, however, the usual appearance is often modified by the early perforation and the extensive destruction of the septum itself. The clinical picture may also be complicated by the ulcerative processes which accompany sequestration and the signs of infection of the accessory sinuses. The condition may continue for years and add to the misery of these patients, who are already rendered hypochondriacal by their disease. The administration of mercury and potassium iodide is not always effective in such cases. A most careful and systematic rhinoscopic examination and treatment are called for, and even then a cure is only effected with difficulty. Volkmann in his day recommended the complete removal with the sharp spoon of all involved parts of the mucous membrane and the framework of the nose. At present, however, the procedure is more properly limited to the parts of the bony framework in which necrosis is demonstrated by rhinoscopic examination. Diseases of the accessory sinuses should be treated according to the usual rules. These procedures it must be noted, should not be instituted until the systemic disease has been brought under proper control by the rational administration of mercury and the iodides.

Granulomata occurring in the course of nasal syphilis have only lately been brought into notice by the observations of Kuhn, Manasse, and Kuttner. They are uncommon and are present usually as flat structures, pale, smooth, and quite transparent, and bearing a strong resemblance to ordinary mucous polypi. They are commonly found on the turbinates, but the author has also seen them in the maxillary antrum. Tumor-like masses of granulation-tissue may occur, accompanied by ulceration and the formation of crusts, sometimes resulting in marked displacement of the alæ. These tumors are often multiple, but in other cases may extend *en masse* over a considerable area. If antisyphilitic treatment has not been inaugurated, they display a marked tendency to recurrence, and often lead to the diagnosis of a malignant growth on account of the extensive destruction, especially of bone, which is commonly present.

A histological diagnosis is also difficult. These tumors are made up of a mass of granulation-tissue, which is often œdematous and encloses solitary, or sometimes numerous, giant cells and occasional patches of fatty degeneration. The well-known arterial changes are as a rule the only specific signs, and these are not often well marked.

Treatment of the general disease is the main therapeutic indication. Oftentimes the administration of potassium iodide is not sufficient, and

mercury should be given simultaneously, as diagnostic errors are
made. On the other hand, this method must not be continued
nitely, especially if there is suspicion of a malignant growth, for
case the best opportunities for operative interference might be fo

It should be noted in conclusion that the entrance to the nose
sionally the seat of a primary specific lesion. The infection
instance probably results from an abrasion produced by an i
finger-nail, and the diagnosis is rarely made before general syn
have appeared. The condition may be suspected if a marked s
of the lymphatic glands accompanies a rapidly growing and infil
tumor at the entrance to the nose. Surgical interference, which
be suggested by the suspicion of a malignant growth, is naturally u
for, but thorough and energetic systemic treatment is indicated to
possibility of resulting destruction and deformity.

Glanders.—Among the other infectious processes which are
rarely seen is glanders. This disease is not localized in the nose
usually distributed over the skin of the face and in a few other loc
The ulcers of glanders bear a marked resemblance to those of
culosis, but frequently show an even more distinct undermining
edges. Aside from these punched-out ulcers, small disseminate
tular foci, each surrounded by an area of redness, are also found.
picture is quite characteristic, but the diagnosis should always be
to depend on the typical skin lesion and on the finding of the baci
one of the author's cases granulomata of a considerable size were
on the middle turbinate, the upper surface of which was occupie
large, sharply defined ulcer with a yellow necrotic base.

Leprosy.—Increasing attention has lately been directed to the
of leprosy. Infiltration is the most prominent symptom of this d
The process is usually localized at the entrance to the nose, ext
later on to the septum, where it forms pale, flat, granular masse
adherent crusts. There is little tendency to ulceration—as a ru
amounts merely to defects in the epithelial covering. This infil
usually results in the formation of crescentic cicatricial bands
extend from the septum to the lateral wall and reach their greatest
opment at the posterior border of the vestibule. Perforations
anterior part of the septum also occur, but these are rarely exte
The crusts, which often interfere with the proper inspection of the
can only be removed after thorough soaking, which in some case
take days.

Rhinoscleroma is one of the rare affections met with in the nose
characteristic feature is also infiltration, and the flat, slightly el
masses show a tendency to the formation of cicatricial bands and
from their centres. These masses are covered by thick crusts, v
however, can be readily removed. The process of infiltration
become so extensive as to displace completely the nose, and the c
mation may cause stenosis. This sclerotic condition usually beg
the anterior part of the nose and rapidly involves the entire
extending backward even into the nasopharynx.

According to the generally accepted view, local treatment in leprosy, glanders, and rhinoscleroma can only be of value as a palliative measure. Radical surgical procedures are inexpedient, and can only be thought of in rhinoscleroma, although even here the results reported are not very encouraging. One of the author's cases, in which he hoped for a complete cure, developed a recurrence after six years.

Aside from these specific infectious granulomata, there are others of a non-specific character, which the author believes should be made to include the so-called bleeding polypi of the septum. They are represented by nodular tumors, sometimes of considerable size, pediculated and freely movable, which spring from the anterior part of the septum. As they are very vascular, the hemorrhage from them may assume considerable proportions. Numerous vessels and granulation-tissue make up the greater part of their bulk. Their histological structure often causes them to be mistaken for sarcoma, angioma, angiosarcoma, or

FIG. 332.   FIG. 333.

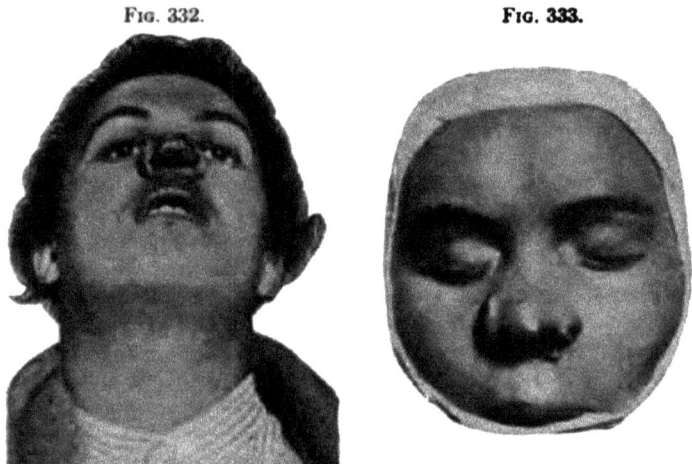

Rhinoscleroma.

similar growths. The narrow pedicle permits of ready extirpation; but as they are particularly liable to recur, malignancy is often suspected. If the attachment of the pedicle is completely eradicated, however, they do not as a rule recur quite so readily.

The treatment of granulomata and the analogous forms of ulcers is about the same. The simple ulcers of the septum heal quite rapidly if a sufficient quantity of a mild ointment is applied regularly every evening. At intervals a thorough cauterization of the base of the ulcer is indicated. The main consideration, however, is the removal of the cause, whether a traumatic or chemical irritant.

The presence of other specific inflammatory products calls for more active interference. The diseased tissues must be removed by means of a sharp spoon, curette, or snare, and in many cases injuries to the cartilaginous and bony framework of the nose cannot be avoided. these measures do not always protect against a recurrence. In culons cases the treatment may be supplemented by tamponad gauze strips impregnated with a 50 per cent. solution of lactic aci 2 to 5 per cent. ointment of pyrogallic acid. If the ulcerative prc from any of these causes have destroyed the larger part of the bony 1 work of the nose, especially the turbinates, the progress of the d may be stayed, but the lining mucosa of the enlarged nasal pa often becomes covered with thick crusts, which in time becom foul and a source of great annoyance to the patient. This con closely stimulates an ozæna, and the treatment is limited to pal measures, frequent irrigations, dry tamponade (Gottstein's me massage, etc.

THE INFLAMMATORY DISEASES OF THE NASOPHARYNI

Catarrhs of the nasopharynx result largely from previous inflamm conditions in the nose or follow diseases which have caused a contra of the lumen of the nasal passages. Aside from these, systemic tions, such as syphilis, may also prove etiological factors. Of the ch inflammations, the greater number are localized in certain folds c nasopharyngeal space, and also in the sinuses between the indiv lobules of the pharyngeal tonsil.

The acute catarrhs of the nasopharynx usually receive scant atter the patients complain merely of an ordinary coryza. A careful examin of the nasal passages, however, shows that the anterior part of the n not involved, but there is an acute inflammation of the pharyngeal 1 and its immediate neighborhood. Certain acute coryzas, characte by scanty secretion and marked interference with respiration, may be accounted for in this way. Other forms of nasopharyngitis are and are of no surgical importance. If the catarrh becomes chronic a tonsillar hypertrophy or a chronic suppuration of the crypts en removal of the pharyngeal tonsil is indicated. Attention should be called to the fact that ozæna and diseases of the accessory sinuses may also enter into the question of differential diagnosis. accumulation of secretions constitutes the main symptom of catarrhs, part of which flow into the nasopharynx and part inte nasal chambers. A not inconsiderable part remains *in situ* and f large dry crusts. The flow of the secretions into the nose furn the symptoms of a chronic coryza. The flow into the oropharynx rise to atrophic changes in the mucosa, to a swelling of the lymp follicles on the posterior pharyngeal wall, and finally, if the secre find their way into the larynx, to chronic laryngitis and atrophic cha especially marked along the posterior wall. For this reason the s toms of such chronic catarrhs are of a most varied nature, and the sc of the trouble is often difficult to find, as the irritability of the chroni inflamed pharynx renders a posterior rhinoscopic examination difficult in many cases. The greater number of these catarrhs depend either on a localization of the inflammatory process in one of the folds of the palatal tonsil or on a chronic pharyngeal tonsillitis; therefore the treatment should include the removal of the pharyngeal tonsil even if it is only moderately hypertrophied, and also the application of caustics or the galvanocautery to the suppurating crypts and sinuses of the palatal tonsil.

The secretion is sometimes very profuse, and in certain cases may be characterized by a foul odor which often leads to the suspicion of a purulent accessory sinusitis, or if crusts are formed to a true ozæna. To avoid this mistake, it is necessary to determine at which point the pus reappears after the nasal passage has been thoroughly cleaned. This class of diseases is rarely treated in a sufficiently careful or a satisfactory manner. Swabbing out the nasopharynx with weak astringents (iodin-glycerin and similar preparations) does not bring about favorable results; still the procedure is continued with the utmost faith and confidence by both patient and physician.

HYPERTROPHY OF THE PHARYNGEAL TONSIL.

The distinction of assigning the proper place to hypertrophied pharyngeal tonsil in the pathology of the ear and its effect on the entire organism, must be accredited without prejudice to W. Meyer, of Copenhagen. The far-reaching influences of these hypertrophies on the diseases of the upper respiratory passages has since been more thoroughly investigated, and still furnishes material for numerous publications, some of which carry too far, perhaps, the campaign against this organ. The enlargement of the pharyngeal tonsil in children and up to the twentieth year of life affords by far the most frequent reason for obstructed nasal breathing with its various consequences, and likewise the most common cause for acute and chronic inflammations of the middle ear.

Whether the hypertrophied tonsil also serves as a point of entrance for pathogenic micro-organisms has not been definitely proved. Recent investigations have shown tuberculous changes in certain cases. These statements cannot, however, be unequivocally accepted: the demonstration of the tubercle bacilli has rarely been successful, and when present they were few in number. A further discussion of this still undecided question does not properly belong here.

Symptoms.—Obstructed nasal respiration is the principal symptom of hypertrophy of the pharyngeal tonsil. This cannot be distinguished from interference due to other causes, and the degree varies with the size of the enlarged tonsil. In most cases seen, month-breathing is the principal symptom, and it is followed by serious results in the upper air-passages which may extend to the bronchi. It is out of place to discuss here the complications, which belong more properly to the domain of the specialist. Attention should be called, however, to the charac-

teristic deformity observed in the superior maxilla during ado
In many of these cases, if the hypertrophy has not been removε
the permanent teeth appear, the upper jaw becomes narrowec
consequence the hard palate is abnormally arched. The t
not properly accommodated and the canines are pushed forwaı
alignment. It still remains a matter of doubt, however, whetl
changes are really the result of an enlargement of the ph
tonsil or whether such an hypertrophy merely causes a disturl
those particular individuals who happen to possess a small maː
a contracted nasopharyngeal space. The condition just desε
observed very often; in many cases the face is likewise narrov
in connection with such abnormalities frequently are found dε
of the nasal septum. More extensive bodily deformities, iι
torticollis, scoliosis, thoracic changes similar to the rhachitic "ι
breast," have been ascribed by some to this hypertrophy, but t
of the statement seems questionable.

The most prominent external deformity associated with thiː
tion is undoubtedly the constantly open mouth and the dull,
facial expression.

Diagnosis.—The lesion can be demonstrated by both anteı
posterior rhinoscopy; or, if this fails, by palpation. The latter
reveals a firm irregular tumor or sometimes a number of soft
folds, giving the impression of grasping a mass of earth-worms.
nasal opening is sufficiently wide, anterior rhinoscopy reveals
posterior part of the nose a flat irregular mass of a yellowish·
if acutely inflamed, a bright-red color, and presenting a sharply
lower border. When the patient phonates, the contraction of the
veli muscle causes an elevation of the entire tumor mass. In the n
of cases this method of examination is amply sufficient for all p
purposes, and at the same time more agreeable to the patient tl
pation. Posterior rhinoscopy reveals usually on the upper wall
pharynx a vivid red tumor, divided in some cases by a series of l
into folds, and in other cases presenting a number of dependent,
tite-like villi. Care must be taken in this method of examinati
to underestimate the size of the growth—anterior rhinoscopy ;
mented by palpation affords a much more reliable estimate
degree of the hypertrophy.

Prognosis.—In giving a prognosis it should be remembered
moderate degree of inflammatory swelling of this as well as
palatal tonsil may subside spontaneously. It has been state
these growths have a tendency to recede at the approach of pι
but this has never been definitely proved. Many observers
the opinion that obstruction to the passage is diminished merely
expansion in the nasopharynx which ordinarily takes place abo
time. At any rate, there are many adult patients who still ι
marked adenoid enlargement. It is not advisable therefore to ν
this condition, for any retrograde change to take place in the coι
advancing years.   .

Treatment.—In treating adenoid hypertrophy the value of the application of caustics and the galvanocautery, and sometimes even general treatment—*e. g.*, brine baths, cod-liver oil, change of climate—is not to be denied. All these measures are not, however, followed by lasting benefits. The only reliable form of treatment includes the complete removal of the growth. Many methods have been devised for this purpose, each having its enthusiastic adherents; so that for the beginner the choice is usually a difficult matter. Ablation of the pharyngeal tonsil with the galvanocaustic or the cold snare possesses the advantage of affording an operation with little or no hemorrhage. This method is therefore to be preferred in individuals who are anæmic or are liable to bleeding. It requires, however, a considerable amount

FIG. 334.

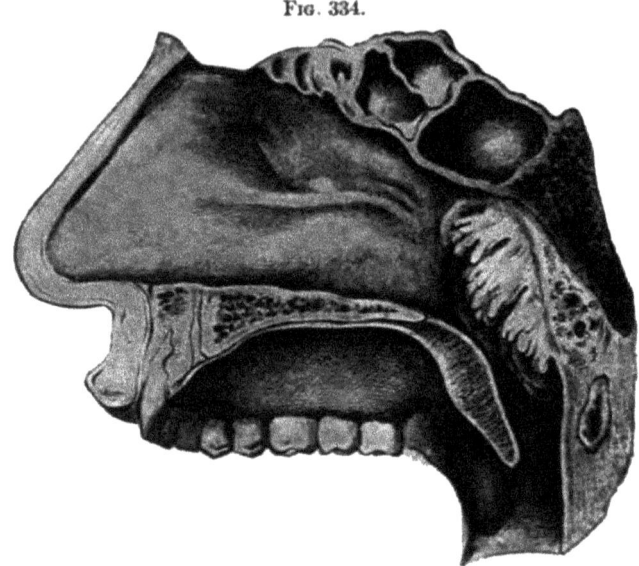

Anteroposterior section of the head of an adult, showing the situation and gross structure of hypertrophy of the lymphoid tissue of the nasopharynx. (Zuckerkandl.)

of skill in the use of the proper instruments, and its successful employment is restricted to specialists. The surgeon need only consider one of the methods about to be described.

The numerous instruments which have been devised for the removal of these growths can be grouped in three general classes, the oldest and most favored being the ring-curettes. That devised by W. Meyer, which was introduced through the nose and applied to the growth under the guidance of the finger, has gone out of use, and in its place that suggested by Gottstein, which is applied through the mouth, is now largely employed. The original Gottstein model has been modified in many ways, most successfully perhaps by Beckmann. In this instru-

ment the blade is directed backward, and forms with three c}
rods a square frame with rounded corners. The handle is in:
an acute angle into the frame opposite the blade. The instru:
closely into the nasopharyngeal space, and when in use it sl
carried back of the soft palate and along the septum to the ro:
pharynx. When closely approximated to the latter, the blade is
posteriorly. The knife is rotated around an axis correspo:
that part of the frame to which the handle is attached, a
pushed backward and downward. The knife cuts the ton:
to its base, and it comes away with the instrument or remain
nasopharynx. A strong nasal inspiration then causes the mas
into the pharynx, whence it can be readily expectorated. It se:
the tonsil is rarely swallowed; where this is assumed, it is mc
likely that the ablation has not been successfully accomplishe:
Beckmann instrument usually permits removal of the tonsil *in* :
on its cut surface there may be attached fragments of the basil:
cartilage. Subsequent palpation, in order to determine the comp
of the operation, is not necessary, as all the information requi
be gained from an inspection of the excised tonsil.

The hemorrhage accompanying this operation varies consic
The more profuse bleeding is usually seen in those cases whi:
been previously operated upon, and also in individuals between :
of ten and eighteen years. Cases of fatal hemorrhage have p
ported, but the author is of the opinion that in these instance
complications were the cause. Although he has seen a number
severe cases of post-operative hemorrhage, they all ceased spontar
and in only one instance did he find tamponade necessary. The e
feature is to calm the more or less excited young patients, to keep tl
high, and to instruct them to avoid unnecessary coughing or sn
If blood finds its way into the stomach, severe vomiting is apt to
and may cause recurrence of the hemorrhage. When this ass:
dangerous aspect, tamponade of the nasopharyngeal space is ind
packing the nose alone merely masks the bleeding.

When no hemorrhage takes place, after-treatment is unnec
The wound heals in from eight to fourteen days, and during this i
severe coryza may arise, which may be treated with insufflati:
iodoform or astringent applications. Nasal irrigations are oft:
ployed after the operation, but as a general thing are not to be
mended, except in those instances in which there has been a
hemorrhage and the nose and the upper part of the pharynx ar
with numerous blood-clots. In the latter case infection of the :
grating clot may otherwise take place and lead to subsequent i:
ment of the middle ear. Fortunately these are rare complicatio
seldom lead to severe suppurative processes.

The so-called "cutting forceps" have found a number of adh
and a number of models have been devised. The least effec
these forms appear to the author to be that modelled after th:
bone-forceps, or the double curette, as it is necessary to appl}

successively a number of times to the growth, and even then its complete removal is apt to remain a matter of doubt. More practical is the forceps suggested by Kuhn, which consists of two hollow ground rings fitted one into the other—it is about the form and size of the epipharynx and permits the entire tonsil to be seized at once and removed. The instrument is quite effective and the resulting hemorrhage moderate; yet the most severe hemorrhage the author has ever encountered followed its use in one case. The entire procedure is more disagreeable perhaps than the use of the ring curette, and probably less complete, but the instrument is particularly applicable for seizing and removing small fragments of tonsils.

The question of narcosis for these operations has long remained a matter for discussion. Cocaine is of little value, it readily excites nervous children in a most disagreeable fashion. With general narcosis there is always danger of aspiration of blood or bits of tissue, which at times has produced asphyxia and caused a fatal result. It would seem advisable therefore to employ an anæsthetic from which recovery is rapid, such as nitrous oxide or ethyl bromide. An operation conducted without an anæsthetic is, however, to be preferred. Patients who cannot be relied on to keep quiet must have the head and arms firmly held by an assistant. Children can be held in the lap and the body and extremities firmly fixed by the nurse. The index finger of the left hand, protected by a Langenbeck metal shield, is then introduced between the molar teeth and the tongue depressed. In place of this, a thin, narrow spatula may be used, and when the tongue is firmly depressed the mouth is necessarily kept wide open. The operation should then be done as quickly as possible, the instrument employed being carried well back to the posterior wall before it is pushed downward. The bleeding, which is usually severe at the beginning, soon ceases. Fragments of tissue hanging down into the pharynx are prone to excite a very disagreeable cough and retching, and should at once be removed. This can be readily done by grasping the fragment with a long curved hooked forceps and tearing it off, care being taken not to pull in a downward direction, as this merely strips off a section of mucous membrane. The mistake is also made at times of grasping the uvula. Cooper's scissors or the wire snare are convenient instruments for seizing and removing these fragments. In certain cases, when the operation has been incomplete, a posterior rhinoscopic examination may be necessary, and eventually the fragments should be removed with a snare introduced through the nose. After complete and thorough extirpation recurrences are extremely rare. Small remnants may remain without causing trouble, but larger ones increase in size and cause the previous disturbances.

TUMORS OF THE NOSE AND NASOPHARYNX.

Benign Tumors of the Nose and Nasopharynx.

Tumors of the Nasal Connective Tissues.—The rarest ti the nose of connective-tissue origin are probably the *lipoma* only authentic case on record is that of Gomperz, in which th sprang from the mucous membrane at the junction of the bony with the fibrocartilage. True fibromata are also quite rare, for th does not include here the so-called mucous polypi. The fibroi scribed in the literature are all apparently derived from the pe: or the perichondrium of the septum. They are usually hard composed of densely matted connective-tissue fibres containing f

Enchondromata are also uncommon. According to Macken: favorite site is the cartilaginous part of the septum. They are fou frequently during adolescence, but usually persist after the comp this period. In spite of their slow growth they may attain an ei size; in some cases the bones of the face were forced apart, i in a horrible disfigurement.

The operation for the removal of these growths is attended wit difficulties and sometimes calls for extensive sacrifices of the facis The smaller fibroma and chondroma can be removed through by means of the snare. In some cases, however, a knife or sciss be used; or if the tumor is very hard, the chisel may be ne Although these tumors may be considered benign, recurrences place, and in some instances are apparently metastases.

Osteomata are uncommon, but still more frequently encounter the growths above mentioned. Those of the accessory sinus already been described, and those of the nasal cavity proper n them in every respect.

Polypoid Growths of the Nose and Accessory Sinuses.— number of nasal tumors manifest a tendency to pedunculatio assume, in other words, the form of a polypus. This term, h is erroneously applied to a large number of tumors which properly should be looked upon as inflammatory new growths.

The pathological status of these polypi has not been difinitely mined. Although they are frequently associated with inflam disturbances in the nasal mucosa, their process of growth is no itely understood. It is probable that the first stage in the forms a polypus is a chronic inflammatory œdema of a circumscribe of mucous membrane. The exuded fluids collect in the most dep part and a club-shaped swelling results, which in time assum characteristic pedunculated form. The influence of the respirato rent is often alluded to as an etiological factor in the production o polypi; it seems to the author, however, that this theory is of little Structurally these tumors closely resemble certain œdematous g mata, being made up of a spongy, coarse-meshed tissue, enclosing leucocytes and containing large numbers of glandular acini wit gated ducts. They usually contain but few vessels and are deficient in cellular elements.

Clinically these polypi also resemble granulomata. Recurrences are apt to occur, and the author has noted this fact in 2 cases. Greenwald and some of the earlier writers believe that most polypi were caused by a "focus of suppuration," such as an accessory sinus empyema. The author has never seen any traces, in numerous cases which have come under his observation, of a macroscopically accessory sinus or bone disease. He inclines rather to the view of Hajek, who assumes that a chronic ostitis is present in the interior of the turbinate bones.

Fig. 335.

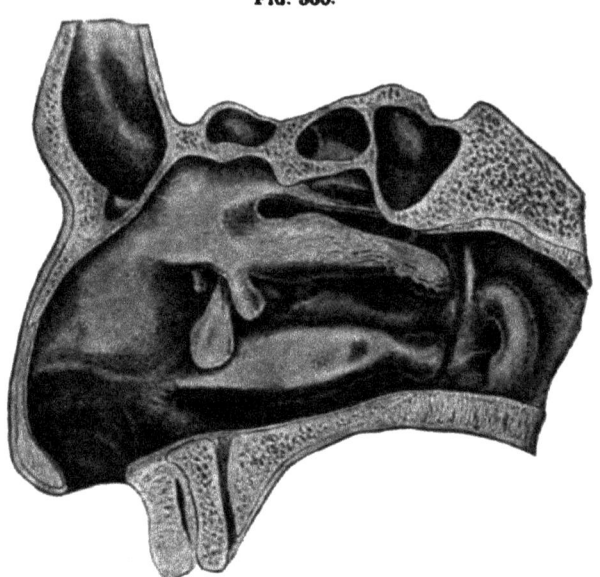

Outer wall of the right nasal cavity, exhibiting three polypi. (Zuckerkandl.)

Most rhinologists seem to be in accord with the latter theory. The point of view is not a matter of indifference, for, if the theory of Greenwald is correct, it would be necessary in the case of all, and especially recurring polypi, to search for such a focus of disease regardless of consequences.

Whatever the origin of these polypi, they may be considered benign growths, which, however, are a source of annoyance to scores of patients. The opinion is prevalent that nasal polypi invariably recur. The latter is only true when the operation has been incompletely done, and this happens quite frequently, for, as the polypi are often multiple, the larger masses are easily removed, but the remainder, becoming covered with blood, are readily overlooked. As the patients do not as a rule apply for treatment again until the nose is once more occluded, the entire symptom-complex is repeated. Even if the growth has been completely extii there may be a liability to recurrence, but this only takes place : prolonged period.

Diagnosis.—The majority of the larger polypi situated in the at part of the middle meatus can be readily recognized as such. Tt ditions which may lead to a mistaken diagnosis are: polypoid sw surrounding malignant new growths, bone sequestra, etc., or gr mata due to certain dyscrasias, of which syphilis need only be cons here. Otherwise the characteristics of the tumors in question at known: the peculiar transparent, gelatinous appearance, the yell gray color, the rounded form, the softness and ready mobility. S polypi are often difficult to find. Their favorite site is in the between the middle turbinate and the lateral wall, and the onl visible is that which p into the middle meatus. impossible to recognize which originate in one i accessory sinuses until the secondarily invaded the cavity. In these cases the c of the sinus involved is markedly enlarged, and a companying suppurative p also affords a clue to the i

Fig. 336.

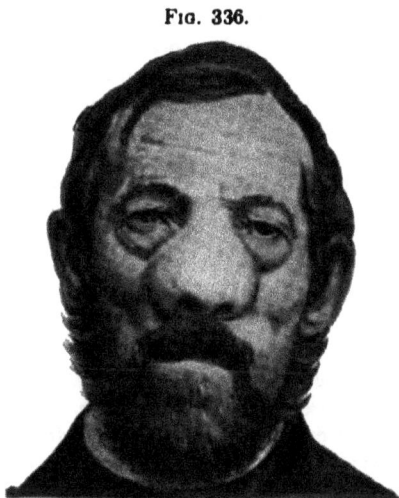

Broadening of bones by nasal polypus.

Nasal occlusion is the characteristic symptom in ing the presence of a pol In addition there is usu: profuse discharge, either w or mucous in the simple i and purulent in those co cated by an accessory emp} Anosmia is quite comn present; also headache ii form of a dull pressure-pain, and various conditions designati reflex neuroses, which include asthma, migraine, hay fever, etc.

Treatment.—The intranasal method is practically the only one ployed at the present day in the treatment of polypi and other pe lated growths. Formerly the sovereign instrument for the ablati nasal polypi was the so-called "polypus-forceps," a small-bladed to forceps, slightly curved on the flat. In order to obtain a firm gra the growth the blades were corrugated or sometimes furnished small hooks. In doing the operation the site of the pedicle was d mined by a probe with the aid of reflected light. The pedicle was grasped by the forceps near its insertion and the entire mass for torn away from its attachments to the mucous membrane. This cedure was usually successful in the case of a small polypus with a na pedicle. Extensive lacerations often resulted. The author has se number of patients with several recurrences who had been operated on in this manner years ago, and in whom almost the entire turbinated bones were sacrificed to this heroic procedure. Such an attack is uncalled for, because the parts from which the polypi usually spring, namely, the region of the hiatus semilunaris and the lateral surface of the middle turbinate, lie quite well protected and are therefore rarely reached; whereas other parts on which polypi rarely occur and which are of great importance in the functions of the nose, such as the mucous membrane of the inferior turbinate, are often entirely destroyed.

The necessarily cumbersome forceps interfered with manipulation and the proper illumination of the parts so that it was often a matter of difficulty to reach the base of the polypus. It was soon superseded by the method of ligation, and numerous instruments have been on this principle. The first to be generally adopted was the wire snare, the introduction of which was largely due to the efforts of Zaufal. There are many useful instruments of this type. The author prefers the Wilde snare, as modified by Zaufal, because it is light, easily handled, and yet sufficiently strong for all purposes. The tube forms an acute angle with the handle, so that the closure of the snare may be readily followed with the eye. The majority of the numerous modifications of these snares depend on variations in the curvature of the tube and on the attachment of the wires. Others are constructed with a transverse partition at the free end of the tube, which permits of firmer adjustment of the snare and of complete separation of the tumor without tearing. In some snares—e. g., that recommended by Jarvis—there are appliances for drawing the wire taut, consisting of screws or ratchets. This construction is unnecessary and even inconvenient for the removal of ordinary polypi. Steel wire of the thickness usually employed will readily cut through the growth if the hand alone is used to tighten the snare. Piano or zither wire is the most suitable and is commonly used, some preferring the soft, others the tempered variety. The flexibility of these snares renders their introduction into the nose an easy matter.

In doing the operation, the loop of the snare is held vertically, parallel to the septum, and is then carried back of the polypus. An effort is then made to pass the loop over the dependent portion of the polypus and along the pedicle to the point of insertion of the latter. The loop is then gradually tightened until the pedicle is severed. As a rule only a moderate amount of bleeding follows the operation. More severe hemorrhage occurs when a considerable section of mucous membrane has been cut away with the pedicle. It may also take place when the club-shaped anterior end of the middle turbinate bone has been cut away by mistake for a part of the polypus. If no extensive laceration of the mucous membrane has taken place, the bleeding usually stops of its own accord; if it does not cease, tamponade of the nose may be required.

Some difficulty usually arises when numerous and partially pediculated polypi are present. It is necessary in these cases to remove partially the anterior growths in order to secure a proper exposure of the nose. The resulting hemorrhage is apt to interfere greatly with the determination of the nature of the remaining polypi; and if there immediate reason for ending the operation at once, it is advisa complete it after an interval of several days. Pain, even without application of cocaine, is slight. Wounds of the mucosa itself, how cause intense pain, and for that reason the operation for pa pediculated polypi is usually more painful than for those with a formed pedicle. With the aid of cocaine it is possible to excise the anterior end of the middle turbinate quite painlessly.

The application of the snare may be rendered more **difficult t** projection of the polypus into the nasopharyngeal space. This por apt to be more extensive than that in the nose itself, and will not r the largest snare which it is possible to introduce into the nose to be r around it. Such polypi are also quite movable and readily escape the grasp of the snare. It is well to fix them with a long hooked fo, which is carried through the loop of the snare, but care must be not to tear through the friable tissues of the polypus. The blunt devised by Lange may be advantageously employed for polypi w long pedicle, the hook being forced into the latter near its origin when a good hold has been secured the entire mass may be torn with a quick jerk.

If marked bleeding follows the operation, the nose may be lightly poned with iodoform gauze. If the hemorrhage is slight, a little iode powder may be insufflated to maintain asepsis, but as a rule this i necessary. The site of operation becomes covered with a crust of blood, which is cast off after a short time without further disturba Irrigations have apparently no influence on the healing process and therefore be omitted.

Benign Connective-tissue Tumors in the Nasopharyngeal Spa, Enchondromata and osteomata are exceedingly rare growths, and i nate usually from the basilar process of the occipital or its sym droses, or less frequently from the posterior edge of the septum addition there are certain neoplasms arising from the edge of the sep which resemble nasal polypi in every respect; they are furnished w well-developed pedicle, they are firm and dense, and hanging down even reach into the pharynx. They cause disturbances similar to of the true nasal polypi, and are to be treated in the same fashion.

The typical connective-tissue neoplasms of the nasopharyngeal s are the fibrous ploypi.

Pathology.—Pathologically these tumors have been described as fibroma, occasionally also as fibrosarcoma. The former point of is probably the correct one, although it is not to be denied that, i like sarcomata, they break through and invade the surrounding of bone. True metastases, however, do not occur. As a rule t tumors consist of a dense network of connective-tissue fibres enck a few cells. The fibres are in long bundles, which interlace and en in their meshes small round nodules. This results in a structur dense consistency, but which may be readily dissected in the dire of its fibres. Large numbers of leucocytes may be enclosed in meshes of the network, sometimes so plentiful in certain localities as to obscure the fibrous structure. This appearance usually indicates the presence of an inflammation; but it is evident that it may readily lead to the mistaken diagnosis of a sarcoma, instead of a mere fibroma.

The vascularity of these tumors varies, but is usually quite marked, and single vessels may assume the dimensions of the radial artery. The vessels are mostly of a venous character and often form a spongy, cavernous mass. Strange as it may seem, these polypi were formerly described as containing but few vessels (Billroth), due to the fact that they were examined in an exsanguinated condition and the demonstration of the vascular structure was not possible by the older histological methods.

The tumors in question originate from the base of the skull or from its bony prominences. They are developed from the basilar fibrocar-

FIG. 337.

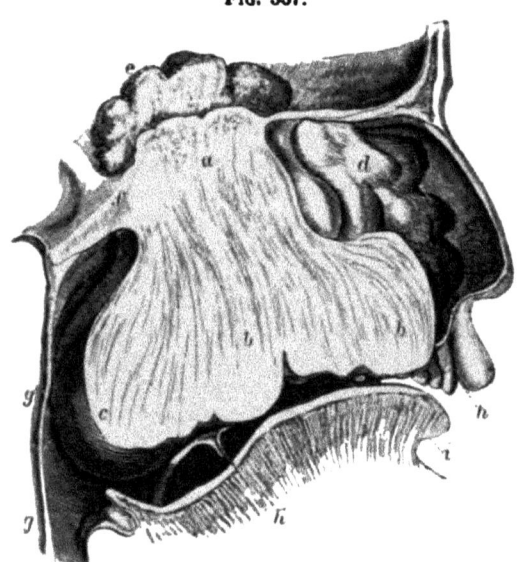

Fibrous nasopharyngeal polypus, with invasion of skull cavity. (O. Weber.)

tilage, which, firmly united with the periosteum, extends from the under surface of the basilar process at the posterior border of the septum and along both wings of the sphenoid bone into the pterygopalatine fossa. The mucosa of the nasopharynx forms a covering for these tumors, and if subjected to irritation or injury it breaks down very quickly, and ulcerations result. The latter usually remain superficial and do not cause destruction of the deeper tissues, although the larger vessels may sometimes be laid bare, and severe and even dangerous hemorrhages result in consequence. The bleeding frequently follows bodily exertion, sneezing, blowing the nose, coughing, etc.; but it often comes on during perfect quiet. A marked influence seems to be exerted by one those parts of the tumor which are tightly enclosed and the infection of the ulcerated areas.

Symptoms.—Nasal occlusion is usually the first symptom by the patient; at the same time there may be a condition present is looked upon as a coryza and is characterized by a profuse or more rarely by a mucous or a purulent discharge. The int with nasal respiration is usually limited to one side. The pat ordinarily not seen until the entire nasopharyngeal space is fill

The most disturbing attribute of these tumors is their ten rapid growth. Usually they grow at first into the free cavities

Fig. 338.

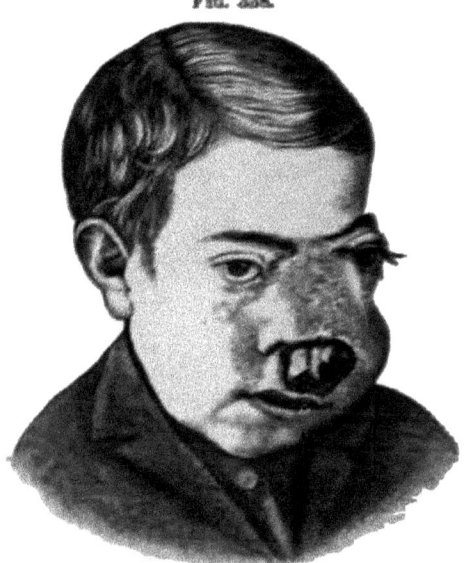

Nasopharyngeal fibroma in a boy aged fifteen years. Duration five years.

on the nasopharynx, invading in succession the nasal cavities. cases, especially if the tumor springs from the sphenopalatine soon begins to press against the temporal fossa. From the nasa the tumor may extend into the ostia of the sphenoid, maxill frontal sinuses, or into the ethmoid cells; prolongations may e cavities and more or less fill them, the continued pressure pr in time atrophy of the bony walls and finally perforation. may thus penetrate the base of the skull by breaking through t of the sphenoidal sinus, or, more rarely, through the ethmoi From the latter they may also perforate the orbital walls and p eyeball forward and to one side; this is more often seen in the malignant growths. Perforation of the base of the skull in the just detailed is quite common, and is seldom accompanied b which are at all severe or easily recognizable. The tumor may also perforate the maxillary antrum through its relatively thin posterior wall. Among others it may penetrate the sphenomaxillary fissure, and from this eventually reach the cranial cavity through the sphenoidal fissure. If the growth has originated near the foramen ovale, it may find its way through the latter into the cranial cavity. Perforations through the foramen lacerum, or other ostia for vessels and nerves, have rarely been observed.

An interesting clinical feature of these growths is their association with certain definite periods of life. They are almost invariably found in young individuals, usually between the ages of fifteen and twenty-

FIG. 339.

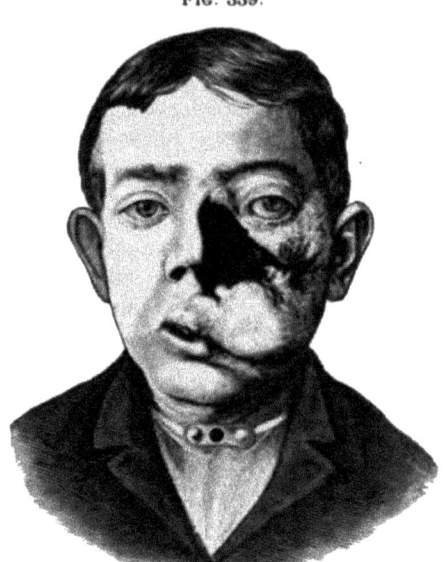

Same patient after the removal of the growth. The defect was closed by plastic operation.
(K. Rosin.)

five. The greater number of cases are found in the male sex; when observed in girls, they usually occur before the fifteenth year. Although true and undoubted cases in females of more advanced years have rarely been reported, it does not seem advisable to accept the assertion of Bensch, that they do not exist at all.

Another remarkable fact which has often been observed in connection with these tumors is their disappearance after the completion of the period of adolescence. This disappearance may be spontaneous or it may follow even incomplete efforts at extirpation. For this reason the attempt has been made to associate the development of these neoplasms with the growth of the skull, with puberty, and with various other etiological factors, but no one has gone beyond the formation of hypo-

theses. The retrograde development of these tumors is no doub
great clinical significance; for recurrences are frequent even
thorough extirpation, during the period of adolescence, but fortun
they are not any more malignant than the original tumor.

The results of the clinical examination in patients who present
form of nasal polypus show little variation. As a rule the entire n
pharyngeal space is occupied by the mass of the tumor, with the exp
surfaces in the nose and pharynx extensively ulcerated. The c
varies from a bright pink to a dark red, the ulcerations being cov
with yellowish-brown crusts. Very frequently the tumor and
remaining structures in the nasal cavity on the same side are co
with a white or yellow slimy secretion, which is occasionally so abunc
as to interfere with the proper view of the shape and size of the tur
The accumulation of secretions is by no means so marked in the n
pharynx. The tumor itself is of the consistency of dense cicatri
tissue and is quite elastic. It bleeds readily when touched with a pr
or subjected to slight injuries. This applies particularly to the n
part of the tumor, for the main mass in the nasopharynx can often
handled quite roughly without producing hemorrhage. The tur
possesses only slight mobility, as a proper pedicle is rarely form
The growth, however, may be moved slightly *en masse* from side to si
the prolongations taking part in the movements of the body of
tumor. The point of attachment of the growth cannot as a rule
readily determined, as it is usually covered on all sides by the mass of
tumor. The probe affords little assistance, and unless very carefu
used, it may give rise to severe bleeding. It is well to bear in mi
when doing an operation that the insertion is ordinarily to be found
the inferior surface of the body of the sphenoid or of the basilar proc
of the occipital.

The external disfigurement caused by these tumors is often rema
able. The nasal prolongations may lift up the ala on the affected s
and force apart the nasal bones. An orbital prolongation may cau
an exophthalmos. An extension into the maxillary antrum produ
a swelling of the cheek similar to an abscess from a tooth. A ret
maxillary prolongation produces a swelling, often of considerable si
in the temporal region. The occlusion of the nasal passages causes
patient to keep the mouth constantly open, and this, together with c
or more of the features just mentioned, affords a typical picture of
severer forms of this affliction.

Diagnosis.—The differential diagnosis must be made from an ordin
nasal polypus, the body of which projects into the nasopharynx.
the mirror the latter appear of a blnish-gray color; the fibroma, pi
or dark red. Polypi are rarely ulcerated except perhaps at the na
entrance; fibromata are frequently ulcerated in the nasopharynx. Bo
involvement is an extremely rare occurrence with ordinary polypi,
is the rule with fibroma. The hemorrhage and the results of perforati
are the unfortunate complications of the fibroma. The latter conditi
are also associated with the presence of malignant tumors of the n

and nasopharynx, and the differentiation from sarcoma is not always possible. The finding of a greater or lesser number of cells in a histological examination does not afford conclusive evidence. Clinical signs such as the restriction of the fibromata to the male sex and the period of adolescence, the tendency to a retrograde development, etc., may help to simplify the diagnosis. In addition, the fact should be noted that even a firmly enclosed nasal polypus, with numerous prolongations, possesses a certain degree of mobility, which may be elicited with one finger pressed against the tumor in the pharynx and the other in the nasal opening. This mobility is wanting in the case of an infiltrating malignant growth. Evidences of cerebral pressure, such as choked disk and optic neuritis, when they appear relatively early, indicate a malignant tumor. With fibroids they do not appear until quite late. Simple atrophy of the optic nerve, however, is more apt to be associated with the fibromata.

Tumors of the superior maxilla, usually of a malignant nature, may give rise to similar appearances. These are more frequently accompanied in the early stages by dental neuralgia and swelling at the canine fossa. Such symptoms are generally the last to appear in the case of a nasopharyngeal polypus. Complicating antrum empyemas frequently occur with tumors of the upper jaw, but rarely with those of the nasopharynx. When a fibroid polypus has perforated the superior maxilla, an orbital prolongation is usually present, which displaces the eyeball forward and outward, whereas maxillary tumors which have penetrated the orbit displace the eyeball upward.

Finally the diagnosis of retropharyngeal growths must be considered. These tumors arise in the retropharyngeal connective tissue in front of the upper cervical vertebræ and are usually fibromata, rarely sarcomata. They are freely movable on the deeper structures and the overlying mucous membrane is unattached. In all cases they displace the pharyngeal mucosa and eventually the soft palate, and no trace can be detected of fissure between the tumor and the posterior pharyngeal wall. Such a fissure is always present even with the largest fibroma of the nasopharynx. As these growths in other respects imitate the clinical picture of a typical nasopharyngeal fibroma, proper value should be given to the foregoing points in the differential diagnosis, as the operative procedures indicated in retropharyngeal tumors must be essentially different from those for fibroma of the nasopharynx.

The differential diagnosis from chondromata and teratomata of the nasopharynx, on account of the great rarity of these growths, need only be considered in exceptional instances. Palpation usually reveals the cartilaginous character of the chondroma, or the presence of hard nodules in a soft network of tissue in the case of a teratoma.

Prognosis.—The prognosis of fibroid polypi is not favorable. This is largely influenced by the possibilities of a fatal hemorrhage. Moreover, unless removed by operative means, they may cause extensive destruction and cause death by perforation into the skull. If there is present a complicating inflammation of the accessory sinuses or one

has been brought on by reaction after an incomplete operati
dangers of a meningitis are considerable. These dangers are mii
if the patient has reached or passed the period of adolescenc
certain degree of retrograde development may be safely coun
Tumors which reach down into the pharynx and sometimes co
larynx may cause serious obstruction to the act of swallowii
interfere with respiration.

Treatment.—The treatment of the smaller growths and tl
patients who have almost reached adolescence may be directed
mere destruction of the tumor. At the present day galvanocaus
electrolytic methods are alone employed for this purpose. Eith
be applied under cocaine, without pain, hemorrhage, or other d;
When the scabs which result from cauterization are cast off, es
if septic infection has taken place, severe bleeding may occur. Fol
electrolysis, the risk of hemorrhage is much less, but infection
place more readily. Electrolysis is most effective when the n
pole, consisting of one or more needles of steel or platinum-i
thickly covered with shellac to within a short distance of their
is plunged deeply into the tumor, while the positive pole in th
of a broad plate is placed on or near the sternum. A rheostat
be employed and the current gradually increased from 0 to
milliampères, this being the extreme amount which can be er
without anæsthesia. In from five to fifteen minutes considerab
integration takes place in the interior of the tumor, the needles b
loosened, and when the current is gradually turned off they c
removed without causing bleeding.

For excision of the tumors more direct methods may be emp
By means of a wire snare analogous to that used for nasal wor
having the tube curved upward, the tumor, or at any rate its phar
part, may be seized through the month and torn from its attachi
The strength of the latter often interferes with this procedure,
severe hemorrhage is likely to result. The same applies to the
forceps or to digital manipulations, although these methods are
satisfactorily employed. Through the nose a snare can usua
applied only to the nasal process of the growth; in order to cut th
the same an incandescent wire is necessary on account of the tong
sistency of the tumor. It is possible therefore to remove these g
piecemeal, partly through the nose and partly through the ph
but the application of the snare is ordinarily a difficult procedui

One who is not skilled in rhinological methods can perhaps a
plish better results with electrolysis. If this cannot be done or imm
relief is required, it may become necessary to perform a prelin
operation, such as will be described later, in order to expose the t
Only the most urgent conditions should call for this procedure, a;
bloody operations are too dangerous for the removal of a growth
may resolve spontaneously. If intracranial complications are susp
however, it may be possible by means of such an operation to p
a meningitis.

PLATE XIII.

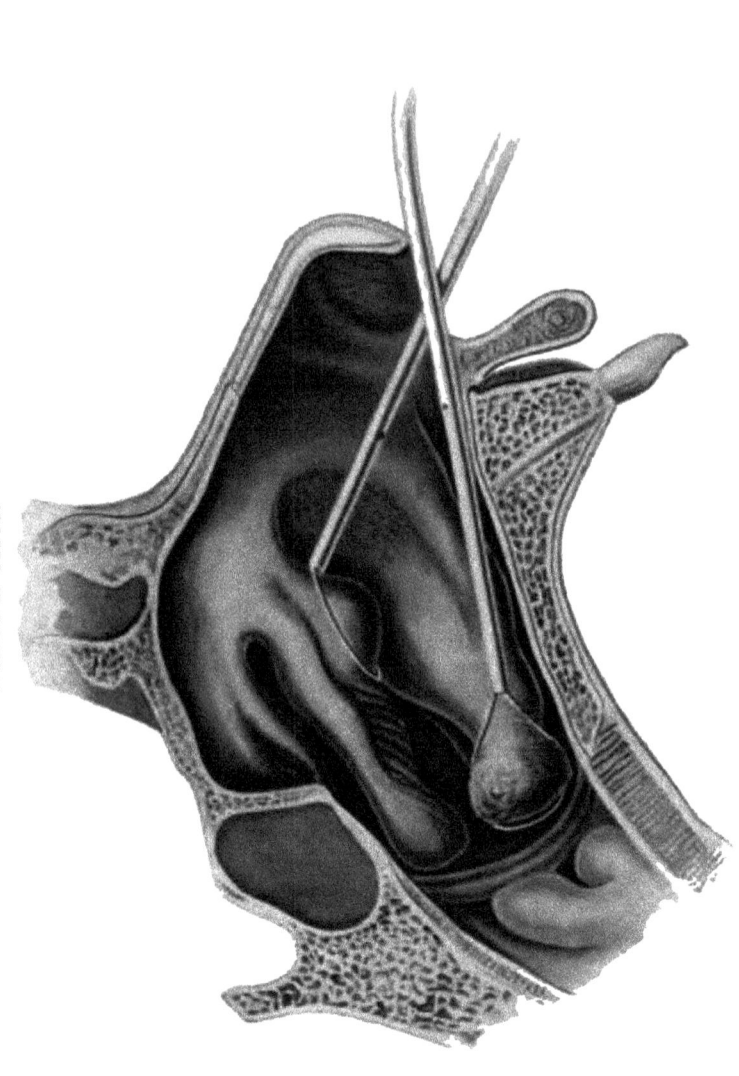

Hypertrophy of the Posterior End of the Inferior Turbinate and of the Anterior End of the Middle Turbinate. The Vertical and Horizontal Adjustment of the Wire Loop for removing such Hypertrophied Mucous Membrane is shown. (Coakley.)

When the tumor presents a large temporal prolongation which cannot of course be reached directly, P. v. Bruns has suggested that the nasal and pharyngeal part be removed directly; then after temporary resection of the malar bone, and, if necessary, permanent resection of the coronoid process of the mandible, the temporal prolongation may be excised down to the sphenopalatine foramen without opening the upper air-passages.

If bleeding results, nasal tamponade with iodoform gauze is usually sufficient to check it. To prevent recurrence of hemorrhage, irrigations with aseptic solutions and insufflations of iodoform powder may prove of value.

Teratoma and *dermoids* of this region are extremely rare.

Attention must also be called to tumors derived from displaced parts of the embryonic gill-arches and the external gill-clefts. The completed processes which occur in this region and result in the development of the nose, palate, floor of the month, and lateral pharyngeal wall, are predisposing factors in the formation of these growths.

Benign Growths of Epithelial Origin.—Certain tumors, found more particularly on the lower turbinate, which clinically and histologically resemble the ordinary nasal polypi, quite frequently assume the character of a superficial papilloma. They cannot, however, be considered in a separate class. Growths in which the epithelium forms the important element, as in dermal warts, are rarely encountered. In them the epithelium may become horny or remain soft. In both varieties epithelial columns and tubules may extend into the underlying tissue, so that the growth may perhaps be spoken of as an epithelioma (adenoma)

None of these tumors can with certainty be called benign; they recur readily, they manifest a tendency to infiltrate the surrounding tissues, and may become encapsulated. Kiesselbach, and later Hellmann, observed such a case, which finally became carcinomatous. In some instances extirpation seems to have resulted in a permanent cure. If they are sharply defined, they may be treated as ordinary polypi; if the histological examination discloses traces of malignancy, recurrences should be more radically dealt with; if they again return, one is justified in regarding them as true malignant growths, and in extirpating them together with the surrounding tissues, especially the underlying bone.

Tumors of this character are apparently never found in the naso-pharynx.

The Malignant Tumors.

The malignant tumors of the exterior of the nose have been considered elsewhere. The various types of malignant growths in the interior of the nose rarely come under observation. Comparatively speaking, they occur more frequently in the accessory sinuses than in the nasal cavities. Some of the tumors of the accessory sinuses clinically resemble those of the interior of the nose in every respect, and may properly be discussed at this point, whereas others—*e. g.*, certain sarcomata of the antrum—cannot be separated from those of the body of the superior maxilla, and must be considered in connection with the diseases maxilla.

Sarcoma.—Sarcoma is the most frequently occurring tumor interior of the nose. The author is familiar with but one case, t Duplay, in which a sarcoma was found to have originated directly the mucous membrane of the nose. The majority are appa derived from the cartilaginous or the bony framework of the nose, the perichondrium or the periosteum.

The round-cell and spindle-cell sarcomata preponderate over all varieties. The former most frequently spring from the walls antrum or the ethmoid cells, less often from those of the frontal the latter usually originate from the septum. Giant-cell sarcomata in rare instances been observed in different parts of the nose. rare, but interesting from the standpoint of general pathology, lymphosarcoma. This is found exclusively in the nasopharyngeal originating from the lymphoid tissue of the roof of the pharyn: pharyngeal tonsil, but may invade the rim of the posterior nares. tumors are often associated with similar ones on the palatal tonsil are usually accompanied by marked swelling of the lymph-gl They can only be differentiated with difficulty from the clinical p of a pseudoleukæmia. The melanosarcomata are also quite rare are probably derived from the oftentimes richly pigmented mu Those cases which have been diagnosticated as myxosarcomata usually indefinitely or incompletely described, and some of them better be classed among the granulomata—the bleeding septum p The author has never heard of an undoubted case. A unique ins of a rhabdomyosarcoma has been reported by Richardson, which ably originated from the superior maxilla or the epipharynx.

Endothelial Growths.—The tumors which are derived from endothelium can only be considered malignant under certain ci: stances, as many of them grow very slowly and only gradually le destruction of the neighboring tissues. It is possible, however, after a long period of comparative quiet they may begin to grow rapidly and then assume the clinical as well as the histological aeters of a malignant type of sarcoma. These endothelial tumo difficult to differentiate from the sarcomata on the one hand an carcinomata on the other, and this is explained by the extreme vari in their histological structure. The favorite site for these tumors accessory sinuses, and they are apparently found more often i antrum than in the frontal sinus. In both cases they are prone to a in the anterior part of the middle meatus, and form at this point tu resembling the ordinary mucous polypi. After a time they cause a bt of the walls of the cavities and may perforate into the cheek, the or the cranial cavity. As long as they remain within the sinus or appear at the ostium they may readily be mistaken for benign tu: If, on the other hand, they do not become evident until they pene the bony wall of the sinus, it is practically impossible to differe them from sarcomata.

Carcinoma.—The carcinomata of the interior of the nose, although derived from a mucous membrane which is covered with ciliated epithelium, are, strange to say, usually made up of typical, horny, squamous cells. Probably in many cases the appearance of the carcinoma was preceded by an ozæna or a fetid accessory sinus empyema, and it may be assumed that the conversion of the ciliated epithelium into squamous, which is a constant accompaniment of an ozæna, prepares the way for the production of an epidermoid growth. These carcinomata usually originate from the ethmoid region—that is, from the roof of the nose. Transformations of the so-called mucous polypi into sarcomata or carcinomata have often been described; but these statements should be accepted with doubt. It is well known, however, that polypoid growths may coexist with carcinoma, as well as sarcoma and endothelioma. In some cases both varieties may be brought about by the same cause—*e. g.*, an accessory sinus empyema or other form of chronic irritation affecting the mucous membrane. In other cases the irritation due to the growth of the tumor itself, or that due to its disintegration or an accompanying accessory sinus empyema, may lead to the formation of polypi on the mucous membrane.

In the accessory sinuses, on the contrary, carcinomata made up of cylindrical epithelium are apparently more frequent than those composed of the squamous variety. They occur in the antrum more often than in the frontal sinus, and occasionally they may be derived from the ethmoid cells. The cylindrical carcinomata all show a structure similar to that of an adenoma; they usually present a surface covered with papillæ and contain a number of glands, part of which have undergone cystic degeneration. It is very probable that many of these carcinomata are derived from tumors of an adenomatous nature.

Symptoms.—The symptomatology shows great variations, depending on the site of the tumor, but yet does not differ in essential respects from the various kinds of malignant growths.

A symptom common to all is nasal occlusion, and this is often of a very severe grade. In carcinomata which are undergoing rapid disintegration it may not be a prominent symptom, and in tumors of the accessory sinuses it may not appear until comparatively late. The rapidly growing malignant tumors, more often than the benign, cause a marked displacement of the nasal skeleton, which is accompanied by horrible disfigurement. Moreover, the malignant growths not only produce atrophy, but also replace the neighboring bony walls and soft parts, and in this way readily invade the cavities bordering on the lumen of the nose—the mouth, accessory sinuses, orbit, and cranial cavity. The evidences of perforation are usually very prominent with sarcomata, but less so with the rapidly disintegrating carcinomata. The process of disintegration in sarcomata ordinarily takes the form of a central softening, and for this reason superficial ulcerations and fetid, necrotic masses are less liable to be found than with carcinomata. This condition is particularly marked in carcinomata of the accessory sinuses, or in those which have penetrated the latter or have caused their infection. Very fetid empyemas, however, are also found wi comata.

The local symptoms, which vary with the point of origin of the may be considered in the following groups:

In the case of tumors of the septum the signs of nasal oc occupy the foreground of the clinical picture; more charac symptoms only appear after the neighboring regions have been ir

Tumors of the upper and anterior region of the nose first m themselves by a swelling at the root of the nose, by perforation i orbit, and an infiltration of the cheek, and eventually by invol of the tear-ducts.

The tumors of the roof of the nose become evident by their ir of the orbit and the base of the skull. They behave somewhat diffe depending on whether they originate in front in the region of the e or further back in the region of the sphenoid.

In the presence of tumors of the anterior ethmoid region the n of the eye and their nerves, especially the internal rectus and the sı oblique, are the first structures to be involved. With further the movements of the eyeball become more restricted, and fina optic nerve becomes injured by pressure. The tumors of the pc ethmoid and the sphenoid region cause an earlier involvement optic nerve, the abducens, and the oculomotor nerves in the cavity. Those in the domain of the sphenoidal sinus may in rar produce lesions of the chiasma with their peculiar symptoms. variety of tumor may perforate into the anterior fossa of the sku may introduce infection, which is followed by meningitis and c abscess. Such a perforation may not become evident for a long for it is well known that injuries of the frontal lobes may give few symptoms, particularly those of a focal character. In the stages indefinite headaches, a feeling of pressure and like sens are usually complained of. The appearance of more severe sym indicates the beginning of the terminal stage, and they are ord not observed until just before the fatal ending.

Perforation in the sphenoid region is more commonly follow meningitis than by cerebral abscess; but the reverse happens perforation has occurred in the anterior part of the ethmoid Generally, the injury to the nerves which usually accompanies tumo ated quite far back, long precedes the appearance of symptoms rel to the interior of the skull. The optic nerve is especially prone t atrophy, with or without the preliminary appearance of choked d

In many cases in which these tumors are located in the region posterior ethmoid cells or the sphenoidal sinus, symptoms refere the trigeminus nerve are prominent. This is usually due to perfo of the growth through the posterior part of the lateral wall of the noidal sinus, and causes an involvement of the second branch foramen ovale and later of the other branches. The optic ne ordinarily affected about the same time. When the condition from the posterior ethmoid cells, an early involvement of the first l of the trigeminus in the sphenomaxillary fissure is observed, combined later with optic nerve atrophy. Exophthalmos is rarely absent in the case of these tumors, and the simultaneous paralysis of certain muscles of the eye makes the clinical picture conspicuous.

Involvement of the trigeminus first manifests itself by severe neuralgic pains in the affected region. Anæsthesia in these cases is not well marked. In rare instances in which the tumor reaches the nerve far back a keratitis neuroparalytica may be present.

Diagnosis.—Tumors of the lateral nasal wall, in the stage in which they are usually first seen, can scarcely be distinguished from those of the body or the cavity of the superior maxilla. Their differential diagnosis also presents great difficulties. Almost all tumors of this region are accompanied by an empyema of the antrum which is often the cause of more annoyance than the tumor itself. A circumstance which often renders the diagnosis very difficult is the fact that the pressure of these growths against the healthy mucous membrane causes the production of swellings and polypoid thickenings. These are very apt to be considered, together with the evidences of an antrum empyema, as forming the symptom-complex of a single lesion. In these cases the extensive destruction of the nasal-wall of the antrum readily permits the introduction of an irrigating cannula and the presence of pus can be easily demonstrated. The method of transillumination reveals a shadow which is just as dense as that due to an empyema. The cardinal symptom which usually distinguishes a malignant growth from an empyema is the severe pain, which ordinarily does not disappear even after thorough irrigation and the evacuation of the pus. Nevertheless, this continuous pain is often observed in severe acute empyema.

Even if external perforation of a tumor has taken place, the idea of a simple perforating empyema is still possible. If successive perforations have occurred at different places, the case should always be viewed with suspicion. Moreover, the unhealthy appearance of the granulations, their large extent, the continuation of the suppurative process although free drainage has been provided, should always arouse suspicion. Perforations usually take place in the malar region. Rapidly growing sarcomata, however, may break through into the month and also into the nose. An ordinary phlegmonous inflammation of the surrounding soft parts may sometimes precede the act of perforation. Unusual perforations are those into the lateral part of the floor of the orbit, and also those into the inner canthus of the eye, which probably result from involvement of the ethmoid cells.

Clinically these malignant tumors reveal little that is characteristic unless a considerable displacement of the facial and maxillary bones has occurred. The symptoms of many carcinomata are disguised by the accumulation of inspissated masses of secretions, of which the removal is often difficult and may be attended by profuse hemorrhage. The complete displacement of the nose which is sometimes caused by a large sarcoma may be accompanied by an enormous accumulation of mucus, which is usually gotten rid of with difficulty. The carcinomata

are, as a rule, covered with ulcerations and are of a gray or g
brown color, while the sarcomata are only ulcerated where expe
the nasopharynx or at the nares; otherwise, they present a i
surface. Fibrosarcomata and spindle-cell sarcomata are of a pa
color, of a firm consistence, and bleed readily. Round-cell sarc
on the other hand, are of a bright-red or bluish-red color; they
down readily and the hemorrhage is often alarming. Melanosare
are of a dark-red or brownish-gray, rather than of a black color.

The differential diagnosis of malignant growths in the nose fr
histologically benign nasopharyngeal polypi, from the benign tun
the accessory sinuses, from ordinary nasal polypi, especially i.
nection with empyemas, finally from granulomata, particularly
of a tubercular or a syphilitic nature, is always a difficult matter.
latter conditions may only be diagnosticated with certainty after i
careful examination of the entire growth. So-called bleeding po
the septum, even after a thorough microscopical examination, ha
quently been taken for sarcomata, as they are made up entirely of
lation-tissue and are freely supplied with vessels. Their delicate p
however, is characteristic. The displacement of the nasal sk
which is prevalent with malignant growths, is usually the most ei
means of avoiding confusion in the diagnosis between benig
malignant tumors. The presence of pain, unless an empyema is p
may be considered as indicating in most cases a malignant g
A fetid odor, if there is no complicating empyema, is rarely foun
benign tumors. The characteristics which are usually associate
benign growths, especially the slow increase in size, must alwa
most carefully considered in all cases.

Typical nasopharyngeal polypi are often difficult to distinguish
malignant growths. Tumors which occur in young men are mo
to be mistaken for fibromata. The nasal prolongation which is
narily present in these cases is sharply marked off from the m
membrane for the greater part of its length, and the entire mas
be readily moved forward and backward. Severe and partic
spontaneous hemorrhages likewise point to a typical nasophar
polypus.

It is impossible to formulate definitely signs for the differentia'
malignant tumors of the superior maxilla, the antrum, and the
nasal wall. The symptoms which point to a lesion in the uppe
are an early swelling of the face particularly near the canine fc
thickening of the alveolar process accompanied by a loosening
teeth, all combined with severe pains along the upper row of teet
none in the distribution of the infraorbital nerve.

Prognosis.—The prognosis of the various malignant tumors
universally unfavorable. It seems to be worse with the carcinom
the round-cell sarcomata, especially, if these extend into the et
cells. As in other localities, the compact sarcomata need not b
sidered so very unfavorable, and the myelogenous sarcomata m
looked upon as relatively benign. It is a remarkable fact that m

sarcomata present varying clinical properties; some may be benign, others of a most malignant character.

Localization has an important bearing on prognosis. Tumors confined to the septum may be removed with comparative ease and without much damage to the surrounding parts. Those on the anterior part of the roof of the nose and the frontal sinus are readily reached, but require a greater sacrifice of tissue, and some part is liable to remain. Malignant tumors of the antrum, and even more so those of the ethmoid cells, afford the gravest prognosis, and can rarely be operated on with good results. If an operation is decided on, no hesitancy must be felt in attempting the most radical procedures. These operations will be more fully discussed in the following chapters.

CHAPTER XXV.

PRELIMINARY OPERATIONS FOR THE EXPOSURE OF T INTERIOR OF THE NOSE.

THE view of the interior of the nose afforded by inspectio the speculum and artificial light is often insufficient, and for thes various preliminary operations have been devised. The perfec the technic of rhinoscopic examination and operations has diminished the necessity for these procedures, but they still mee approval for the removal of recurring nasal polypi and also at for the correction of deformities of the septum. However, no the simplest of these operations are justified by the mere fact tl operator may not have acquired the necessary skill in rhino technic. The question assumes a different aspect, however, wh removal of tumors is concerned, which are extensive or difficult of in which leaving behind even small remnants might cause consequences, and which it would be impossible or impractice extirpate piecemeal. In the nose itself this would include among growths the larger cartilaginous and bony tumors, especially tl the ethmoid region, and also with few exceptions all malignan plasms. In the nasopharyngeal space all malignant growths, i suitable for operation, call for one of these preliminary operatio fibrous polypi, however, only when the growth cannot be re *en masse* with the wire snare or when its removal piece by piece gradual destruction is prevented by the suspicion that the base skull may be very much thinned or possibly perforated. In the case the danger of producing an infectious meningitis must alw considered.

Of the many operations which have been and are still being d a number have been abandoned; either the exposure secure insufficient, or the bleeding was too severe, or because they in too great a disfigurement after healing was completed. Th permanent resection of the upper jaw for the removal of nasophar polypi was formerly performed very frequently, but is now aban although an excellent exposure was secured, the operation itself p so many dangerous features that it does not appear warrant tumors which only in a very restricted sense can be considered mal To a lesser degree this also applies to the temporary resection upper jaw.

The operations just noted and a few others are more fully dis elsewhere. It is only necessary to mention that for the expos the posterior part of the nose and the nasopharyngeal space a me opening may be secured by the permanent or temporary resection of the upper jaw, an intermaxillary passage by separating and forcing apart the two superior maxillæ, and finally a palatal opening by dividing the soft and eventually resecting the hard palate. In this connection attention should be called to the method of reseeting the malar bone for reaching the retromaxillary prolongations of nasopharyngeal polypi, which has already been mentioned. This procedure also affords a favorable access to malignant tumors on the lateral wall of the nasopharynx which have invaded the neighboring soft parts and the posterior wall of the maxillary antrum.

OPERATIONS WHICH INCLUDE THE SPLITTING OR THE FORMATION OF FLAPS OF THE NASAL SOFT PARTS.

The simple procedure of splitting the nose along or near the median line has been employed since the time of Hippocrates. Quite as simple is the separation of the alæ at their line of insertion, as recommended by Garengeot and Wutzer; the exposure is equally good and the resulting scar less noticeable than in the Hippocratic method; but neither affords a better view of the interior of the nose than that which may be secured with the skilled use of the speculum.

The operation of Rouge provides a somewhat readier access and avoids outward scars. The upper lip is separated from the jaw by an incision carried through the mucous membrane where the latter is reflected from the alveolar process. The incision is then carried subcutaneously through the septum and the line of insertion of the alæ up to the bridge of the nose. The entire soft parts of the nose together with the lip may then be reflected upward. This procedure is accompanied by considerable hemorrhage, and, moreover, provides a communication between the seat of operation in the nose and the oral cavity which may have an unfavorable influence on the process of healing.

The same objection applies to the method of Furneaux Jordan, which has been specially recommended by v. Baracz. The upper lip and the cartilaginous skeleton are divided near the median line and the entire flap of tissue dissected free and reflected to one side. The same procedure is then carried out on the other side. If the median incision is continued upward to the root of the nose this method may be combined with that of Linhart, which is about to be described.

If the method of Castex is employed it does not become necessary to open the oral cavity. The alæ are separated at the boundaries of the apertura pyriformis, the septum cut through in the same plane, and then the entire cartilaginous part of the nose reflected upward.

All these methods, however, afford a restricted view of the depths of the nose. A much better exposure is secured by a resection of the bony framework.

**OPERATIONS WHICH INCLUDE THE SPLITTING AND RI
TION OF THE ENTIRE NOSE.**

Splitting the hard and soft parts of the external nose along the 1
line is merely a further elaboration of the method of Hippc
There are many variations in the technic of this operation, an
often combined with other preliminary procedures. König recom
the method of Linhart. Here, after dividing the skin and the
aginous part of the nose close to the median line, the nasal bo1
separated from their attachments to the frontal bones, and the
process of the superior maxilla is resected with a chisel or a saw
outer coverings are left in place. A periosteal elevator is then
duced into the split, and by causing a fracture in the region
lachrymal bone the entire half of the nose may be reflected ou
If necessary, the same procedure may be carried out on the othe
In many of these operations the Kuzy-Gigli wire saw may be em
with advantage.

Of the methods for the reflection of the entire nose, that devii
Chassaignac, and more completely described by P. v. Bruns,
most favorably known. The incision is carried from the inner c
of the eye across the bridge of the nose, and then encircling the
nose at its line of insertion ends at the ala of the side where it s
The skeletal parts of the nose and the septum are divided i
saw or chisel, and the resected nose may then be reflected to the o1
side. As this osteoplastic flap is very well nourished, it may 1
reflected for a period sufficiently long to allow for a more or le:
tinued observation of the seat of operation, and may then be s
secondarily.

In the method of Ollier the nose remains fixed at its lower
insertion, the incision encircling the nose from one ala to the
The nasal processes of both superior maxillæ and the septum ar
cut through in the plane of this incision with a wire saw. As ,
further separation of the cartilaginous parts is not necessary, t
nose may now be readily reflected downward. One of the disag1
features of the method is that the flap is very much in the way,
feres with narcosis, and is apt to become infected from the 1
The cosmetic result, moreover, is not very favorable as a rule.

Of the methods which are concerned with the exposure of the
and posterior parts of the nasal cavity, the most important one c
of the temporary resection of the nasal bones and the nasal pr
of the maxillæ. In doing this operation v. Langenbeck cart
incision from the middle of the glabella to the end of the nasal
and from this point along the apertura pyriformis to the ala.
resulting skin-flap is separated without injury to the periosteu
nasal bones are freed from each other, and the nasal process cut t1
along its base down to the orbit by means of a wire saw intr<
through the apertura pyriformis. The nasal process and the nasa

which are still connected with the periosteum and the mucous membrane, may then be reflected outward and later replaced.

Closely related to this method are those recommended by Killian and A. Barth for the purpose of opening the frontal sinus and the ethmoid cells, which have been discussed elsewhere. A better exposure of the upper part of the nose may be secured if, in addition to this procedure, an osteoplastic flap is made of the anterior wall of the frontal sinus and reflected upward together with the nasal bones.

The method of Gussenbauer permits an exposure of both sides of the nose. The incision extends from the middle of the eyebrow along the edge of the orbit to the nasal process of the superior maxilla, then across the nose on a line with the origin of the nasal bones, and is continued to a corresponding point on the other side. Both nasal processes are chiselled through to the orbital margin and separated together with the lachrymal bones, the orbital plate of the ethmoid, and the nasal process of the frontal bone, and finally the perpendicular plate of the ethmoid to its line of junction with the vomer. The entire wedge-shaped flap of bone may then be reflected upward, affording an exposure of the upper precincts of the nose of a varied degree which depends largely on the anatomical relations. For the purpose of also exposing the frontal sinus, Winkler proposes a continuation of the incision upward at each end of the wound, which readily permits a resection of the anterior wall.

A result similar to that secured by the method of Gussenbauer is gained by a modification of the temporary resection devised by Chassaignac-Bruns, which is described by Kuster. In this the cartilaginous part of the nose is severed from the bony part by a transverse incision. The former remains in situ, the latter is separated by the same incisions as in the previous method, and reflected to one side.

The numerous combinations which it is possible to make aside from those already mentioned cannot all be described here. Neither is it in place to discuss the indications and contraindications for each method. The choice must be left to the surgeon, who is to be governed entirely by the extent and the locality of the disease. In general it may be said that only those methods are of value in which the bony framework of the nose is included; but they are coupled with the disadvantage of being attended with more bleeding than those which involve the soft parts only. The hemorrhage is especially profuse in the resection of the ethmoid cells, and must be checked by tamponade before the removal of the tumor itself can be proceeded with. Moistening the tampons with hydrogen peroxide may be of value in this case. If, as in the case of very vascular tumors, much bleeding is expected, it is well to pack the nasopharyngeal space in order to prevent the influx of blood into the pharynx and trachea.

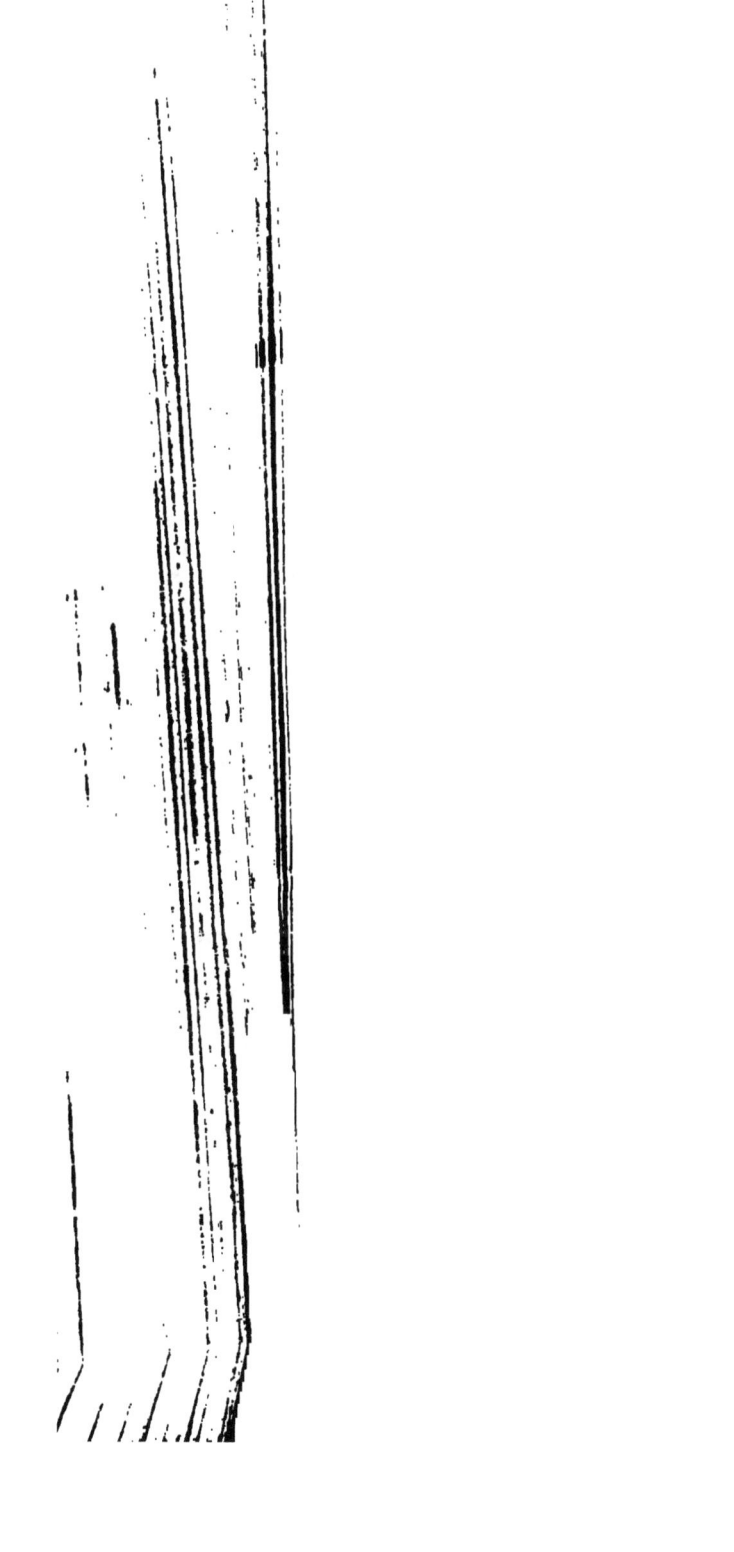

MALFORMATIONS, INJURIES, AND DISEASES OF THE MOUTH.

CHAPTER XXVI.

MALFORMATIONS AND CONGENITAL DISEASES OF THE MOUTH AND TONGUE.

THE formation of branchial clefts has been discussed in preceding chapters. Mention was also made of synchylia and microstoma, and of the double lip. The congenital tumors of the blood- and lymph-vessels, the cysts, and several other tumors of a teratoid and sarcomatous nature, will be considered when treating of neoplasms of the mouth. The following conditions may be appropriately discussed at this point: absence of the entire tongue, the cleft tongue, the adherent tongue, ankyloglosson, the abnormally long tongue, and certain cases of epignathy.

Jussieu (1618) observed a case of total absence of the tongue in a girl of fifteen years, the locality being occupied by a small flat wart-like papilla. Spiller (1816) saw a similar condition in a newborn infant, in which there was also a cleft palate.

Griffith has seen a case in which in connection with other defects in the oral cavity the greater part of the tongue was missing. The gums were confluent with the checks, the hard palate was cleft, and only the posterior section of the tongue remained as a stump.

These observations seem plausible enough if it is assumed that the defects are produced by the formation of amniotic bands and adhesions which restrain and interfere with the development of the embryonal fissures. In a case reported by Welde, and figured in Ahlfeld's atlas, the fetal membranes are shown adhering not only to the edges of the facial cleft, but also to the tongue. The malformations of the upper half of the face do not affect the tongue, the latter being more often involved in the rare condition known as "agnathy" (Ahlfeld).

A preparation in Ahlfeld's collection shows the face apparently made up of two halves which have failed to come together below the level of the nose. The tongue and both the upper and the lower jaw are divided in the median line.

As a rule the bifid tongue is always seen in cases of agnathy. An exception to this is reported by Parise, who saw a case in which the lower jaw was divided and the tongue split down the median line. Pooley records a similar case.

The congenital bifid tongue can be readily distinguished from that which is the seat of a sclerotic syphilitic glossitis, although deep furrows

may be present in the latter case. The bifid tongue is soft and is
where covered, including the edges and the furrows, with pe
normal epithelium. The fissures in a syphilitic tongue may a
found in the median line, but in addition there are others runr
various directions, some of which are cicatrized, and others are st
rounded by indurated areas and ulcerations. When there is any n
membrane present, it is red and glistening in appearance, for the ι
are absent.

Another congenital condition is that known as "lingua plica
"dissecata." The tongue is always moderately enlarged, but the u
and smooth surface has disappeared, and instead there are pre
number of longitudinal and transverse folds. The mucous men
is unchanged and the parenchyma retains its soft character.

The term "adherent tongue" refers to a coalescence betwee
inferior surface of the tongue and the floor of the mouth, or to a
tion in which there are bands present which bind it to the inner ε
of the mandible. Such bands may be attached merely to the edge
tongue. In extremely rare cases a band of tissue may extend frε
tongue across the alveolar border to the cheek.

A union between the epithelium of the tongue and the floor of the
is often found; it is very delicate in most cases, and similar to the
sions which occur between the labia of newly born girl babies. Iι
cases the adhesion may be readily broken up with the finger or a sμ
Tougher bands and adhesions may be cut with scissors. The cο
movements of the tongue usually prevent the formation of fresh
sions; but in case they threaten, it is well to break them up daily w
finger.

Bands between the cheek and the gums, as described by Volk
occur but rarely.

The most widely known form of lingual deformity is that prο
by a large and anteriorly displaced frenum (ankyloglosson). Ι
the protrusion of the tongue the point is turned downward, and t
of suckling cannot be successfully accomplished by a nursing child.
importance of this condition is often overestimated by motheι
nurses. If the finger can be introduced beneath the tongue aι
latter pulled forward over the alveolar border, an incision of the f,
is unnecessary. If required, the frenum can be cut with a Coope
sors. The bleeding is slight and readily controlled with a gauze ta
A history of hæmophilia in the family naturally excludes any opι
procedure.

In 1742 Petit reported in the memoirs of the newly found sι
academy 3 cases in which an abnormally long tongue served as ,
stant menace from the danger of swallowing the same. Two οι
children were actually suffocated. The possibility of suicide by ι
tion of the tongue has often been discussed in forensic medicine. Aι
always fails to reveal the condition, as the tongue sinks into placι
death, and most of these cases can be explained on other grounds.

The presence of a pure muscular macroglossia in the newboι

been asserted, but it is difficult to substantiate this statement, as only small isolated pieces of the tongue can be examined. Bundles of hypertrophied muscle-fibres are also found in a typical macroglossia which is dependent on a lymphatic hyperplasia.

Girod describes a case in which the tongue was so long that it could be extended about 7 cm. beyond the line of the incisor teeth. No changes were evident in either the mucous membrane or the parenchyma.

In the few cases in which an attempt has been made to remove a projecting epignathus which interfered to some extent with the respiration of the newborn infant, very complex accessory structures were found, so that the excision was attended with difficulty and was usually unsuccessful. The only case reported as ending successfully is that of Sonnenburg.

CHAPTER XXVII.

INJURIES OF THE MOUTH.

WOUNDS, BURNS, AND SCALDS OF THE MUCOUS MEMB OF THE MOUTH.

In considering wounds of the oral mucosa, only those are x of attention which are connected with wounds of the lips, cheeks, maxillæ, and nasal cavity, it being immaterial whether the obje flicting the same proceeded from the face or from the oral cavity. I wounds in the mouth cause the most extensive lacerations of the m membrane of the tongue, cheeks, and gums. Of force applied exte1 blows dealt with the fist occur very frequently, and may, without I ing the skin, knock out the teeth and cause a fracture of the al processes. In such a case the gums are also lacerated.

Wounds limited to the mucous membrane are frequently se children who have fallen while holding in the mouth some p object which has been forced into the cheeks, the floor of the n or the soft palate. These small wounds heal rapidly after the re of the foreign body. In spite of the numerous saprophytic and | genic organisms which inhabit the oral cavity, the repair of these wounds, erosions, and deficiencies in the epithelial coverings takes rapidly. The same applies to wounds of the gums, even the irr ones resulting from the extraction of teeth, healing without f disturbances. For this reason but little attention need be paid accidental wounds inflicted during the act of eating by bits of bon\(in the food or to the slight contusions and lacerations caused t teeth in mastication.

Yet severe and even fatal infections following wounds of the m membrane are seen, especially if these are complicated by injui the bones. As long as the mucosa is intact the presence of pa_{th} organisms in the mouth does not do harm, but the slightest injur; afford a point of entrance for these germs. It has often been ob\(that the extraction of a tooth may be followed by traumatic myelitis of the maxilla, and the pus may creep along the bone : base of the skull and even enter the cranial cavity. Miller has tab\(60 cases of this character, but in almost all the bone was either in or exposed. Superficial abrasions of the gums are rarely succeed such consequences, and this seems the more remarkable, as small w on the fingers of dentists inflicted by the ragged edge of a tool often followed by a rapidly spreading phlegmonous inflammation. is undoubtedly caused by the streptococci present on the tooth. In

(810)

of the tongue are frequently caused by these ragged teeth, but they are seldom followed by serious results. Rosenthal has shown that from two drops of 10 c.c. of water used to flush out the mouth, at least one hundred, and often twelve hundred colonies of bacteria developed on a proper culture-medium. Black in 10 cases found *Staphylococcus pyogenes aureus* present in 7 and the albus and the streptococcus in 3. It is evident therefore that the smallest wounds of the mucosa are constantly brought in contact with a large number of pyogenic germs, and yet inflammation rarely occurs. For this reason a relative immunity of the oral mucous membrane has often been spoken of and accounted for on various grounds. It has been assumed that there is present an antagonistic condition between the numerous saprophytes and the more sparsely represented pathogenic bacteria; that the stream of saliva is constantly flushing away whatever may be adherent to the epithelium; that the oral secretion possesses bactericidal properties (which have never been conclusively proved however); that certain leucocytes are endowed with specific influences; that the virulence of bacteria varies greatly. These are among the numerous theories proposed in explanation of this condition, but all are more or less unsatisfactory, and the fact remains that the enormous numbers of micro-organisms found on the oral mucosa only cause infection in exceptional cases; whereas if they gain access even in the slightest degree to an operative wound, the aseptic condition of the latter is at once brought to an end.

As wounds of the oral cavity are well protected against infection, it is questionable whether the attempt to disinfect the mouth thoroughly before operation has any practical value. Undoubtedly the mechanical cleansing of the mouth by washes and gargles, and the brushing of the teeth, are of the first importance. It may be assumed, moreover, that the daily cleansing of the mouth has a certain prophylactic value in regard to wounds of the tongue and cheeks.

The author's method for disinfecting the mouth before operation or in the presence of an accidental wound, in order to prevent infection, is as follows: The mechanical cleansing of the field includes a thorough wiping of the mucous membrane covering the gums and checks, and also the surface of the tongue, with a cotton swab dipped in normal salt solution. This is followed by a thorough rinsing of the mouth, for which the most suitable fluid is a solution of mercuric chloride in the strength of 0.5:5000 to 1:5000. The author believes it is harmful to do more; too much friction and the application of alcohol, ether, or tincture of iodine produces an irritation which is very apt to lead to a stomatitis.

The presence of an inflammation of the mucous membrane always increases the virulence of the bacteria inhabiting the mouth. After operations, and the author refers particularly to those on the tongue, and excepts those of the teeth and maxillæ, it is therefore advisable to do even less. He is contented with irrigations of normal salt solution, to which may be added as a deodorant a quantity of hydrogen peroxide. The latter seems preferable to the formerly much vaunted potassium permanganate. The author has never seen any advantage i chloride of lime, the various odorous and non-odorous antise the ethereal oils, but has always feared a harmful effect on wound. For the large cavities which result from operations tongue or the floor of the mouth he prefers the firm and care ponade with iodoform gauze.

As previously noted, a pointed tool, pin, or similar object hel mouth may accidentally penetrate the tongue. A fish-bone mi lacerations, and usually becomes embedded near the base of the Foreign bodies in certain instances pass beyond the tongue. mentions a case in which the mouth-piece of a pipe was forced b; into the internal carotid and in which the resulting hemorrhi fatal. -

Incised wounds of the tongue are sometimes caused by a tak improperly used. Children often inflict deep cuts on the tong lips with a blade of grass drawn back and forth between the play.

Blunt objects which wound the tongue are either projectiles ments of the fractured inferior maxilla, or the teeth. Wounds by the teeth are the most frequent.

In every institution for epileptics recent and healed wound: tongue are commonly seen, having been inflicted during the spasms. The edge of the tongue is usually involved, and the r white scars are often plentiful in old cases and serve as an in of the severity and duration of the disease. More extensive lac are sometimes found in tetanus, large sections of the tongue re: attached only by a small band of tissue. In other instances a struck on the lower jaw at a moment when the tongue is exten teeth may penetrate the substance of the tongue to a greater extent, and some may occasionally be broken off and remain em A case is reported by Vilches in which the free edge of the maxilla almost amputated the anterior section of the tongue in a that had fallen and struck on its chin.

The most serious consequence of extensive and deep wound: tongue is hemorrhage. The danger may be due to the actual blood, to the influx of blood into the respiratory passages, or extensive infiltration of the soft, distensible tongue parenchyn blood. It is essential therefore to stop immediately all bleeding wounds. The tongue should be drawn forward, the wound tho dried out, and the spurting vessel seized and ligated. Superficial rhage may be stopped by suture; that deeper and less accessibl times calls for tamponade. Infiltrations or true hæmatomata tongue are only recognized in from one to three days after the is inflicted, by a considerable swelling which steadily increases It then becomes necessary to reopen the wound, turn out the c and to tampon.

In two cases of attempted suicide by shooting in which the entered the submental region and caused extreme laceration tongue, the author found it necessary to perform a preliminary tracheotomy, and then sutured the wounds in the tongue. The author desires to recommend this procedure in all cases of serious hemorrhage from the posterior part of the tongue before any reparative measures are attempted. While the operation is being conducted in the mouth the tampon-cannula may be inserted, which may be replaced by an ordinary double tube. In a few days after the inflammation and the œdema have subsided the latter may be removed.

Recent hemorrhage may ordinarily be controlled in the wound itself. This does not apply, however, to the secondary hemorrhages. Here the forceps and clamps cannot secure a hold in the friable inflammatory tissue. It then becomes necessary to tie off the lingual artery. Bullet-wounds have even necessitated ligation of the carotid.

Wounds of the tongue may be complicated by the retention of foreign bodies. Fish-bones and needles constitute the larger number of these. Teeth and projectiles have been known to remain embedded in the tongue for a considerable time without having caused pain or noticeable swelling. Usually they lead to the formation of abscesses or produce ulcerations, and may at times be confused with a benign tumor, as they simply present a hard nodule in the tongue which may remain in evidence for years. Foreign bodies, whether diagnosticated early or late, should always be extracted, an incision being made for their exposure if necessary.

All recent wounds of the tongue, even if they are extensively lacerated, should be sutured, for, as already noted, most wounds of the mouth usually heal quite rapidly and without suppuration. The author has given up the use of mouth-washes in these cases during the period of healing. The tongue may at first be coated with a thick white fur, but this disappears in a short time and interferes in no way with the process of repair. The presence of a tenacious mucous secretion on the lips may call for a cleansing of the mouth, but in no case should irritating antiseptics be employed; it is better to use normal salt solution with the addition of hydrogen peroxide in the proportion of about 4:1.

Brief mention may be made here of the stings of bees and wasps, which may be accidentally introduced into the mouth on articles of food. The tongue may swell rapidly and attain such a large size that tracheotomy need sometimes be considered. In rare instances in which snake-charmers have been bitten by vipers introduced into the mouth the immediate danger to life was proportionately greater. The enlargement due to the stings of wasps usually resolves quite rapidly.

The traumatic but not necessarily acute lesions of the tongue also include the ulceration which accompanies dentition and pertussis in children and the decubital ulcers of adults.

In infants in whom the lower incisors appear early or in whom they are already present at birth, there is usually present at the point where the frenum is inserted into the tongue an elongated ulcer with a dirty yellow base. This is caused by the rubbing of the frenum against the teeth, and does not occur otherwise. The application of a 25 per cent.

solution of silver nitrate, which is quickly neutralized by the n
a drop of tincture of myrrh, is ordinarily sufficient to cause th
to heal. This also results spontaneously when the teeth in the
of two weeks rise further above the level of the gums.

The ulcer found in children with pertussis is due to a similar
the tongue during the coughing-spell being constantly rubbed
the lower teeth. It is found along the frenum or sometimes on th
side of the tongue.

Long-continued pressure combined with friction is apt to aff
edge of the tongue where it comes in contact with a broken tootl
improperly fitted dental plate. If any swelling occurs, the teetl
an impression in the form of transverse furrows. As the swellii
sides these furrows disappear; but if the increase in size is a c
one, they are prone to remain. Inward displacement of a tc
excessive deposits of tartar may produce a pit-like depression ꞇ
a normal tongue. These regions are often the seat of sensitive e
tions. Ragged and sharp teeth cause even more irritation and
to the edge of the tongue, producing a chronic inflammatory ind·
or the so-called decubital ulcer. Very often the history of thes
discloses a previous transitory superficial inflammation of the ꞇ
and probably during this time the swollen organ was brought int
intimate contact with the ragged, carious teeth. The induration
condition is circumscribed, quite hard, and becomes painful
mastication, swallowing, and speaking. It is at first superficiꞇ
later becomes deeper and seldom attains a larger size than thꞇ
pea or hazelnut. At the summit there appears a flat or a craꞇ
ulcer with a foul base. Its site on the free edge of the tongꞇ
sensitiveness, the induration, and the funnel-shaped character
ulcer readily leads to a suspicion of a beginning carcinoma. Tl
that an indurated ulcer is found opposite a bad tooth, and that it r
as soon as the irritating cause is removed, must always be givꞇ
weight and consideration.

A discussion of the effects of exploding gases may be admitteꞇ
as the preponderating symptoms are those of the lacerated and c
wounds.

Burns of the mouth result from contact with heated objects, ꞇ
hot fluids or steam. The elastic character of steam streaming ·
boiler, or freed from it by an explosion, forces it into the moutl
and pharynx, from which it may be inspired into the deeper air-pa
Therefore we usually find after boiler explosions, in addition to the
sive burns of the skin, severe scalding of the mouth and pharynx,
may also extend back of the epiglottis into the larynx. The anaꞇ
changes in the mucosa are similar to those which result from th
lowing of hot fluids. The general use of the samovar in Russia ꞇ
the report of numerous cases of burns of the mouth in children wl
applied the lips to the spout of this utensil. Of objects which causꞇ
the most frequent are hot food substances or the lighted end of
thrust into the mouth by mistake. Pitts (St. Thomas' Hospita

don) reports that of 77 cases of burns in children, 67 resulted from the inhalation of hot steam or the drinking of boiling water from the spout of a tea-kettle, and in only 10 were they caused by the ingestion of other hot foods or drinks. Even severe burns of the mouth would be far less dangerous if they did not extend deeper and involve the œsophagus and stomach, and more particularly the larynx. The latter is really more often affected than the digestive tract. This is explained by the fact that the ingestion of hot fluids induces an immediate retching, and the substance is expelled before it has entered the œsophagus, but has nevertheless remained sufficiently long in contact with the entrance of the larynx to leave its traces. In the cases reported by Pitts this complication was always present, the epiglottis, the arytenoid folds, and the mucous membrane being scalded. Instances are not uncommon in which no traces of a burn can be detected on the tongue or any part of the mouth, but yet after the ingestion of very hot liquids patients may suffer from œdema of the epiglottis. The laryngeal lesion is usually the most prominent symptom, and on it the degree of the danger depends; in Pitts' series of cases tracheotomy was found necessary in 23.

The first symptom of scalding is the severe pain, which in children may often produce convulsions. The pain soon disappears, however, but swallowing remains a matter of difficulty for some time. Cold water and bits of ice afford the greatest relief. In the more severe cases blisters form which soon rupture. The epithelium is separated in grayish-white strands. In the severest cases sloughing may result. The sloughs which result from the application of the Paquelin cautery for the purpose of destroying ulcers and neoplasms separate quite readily, and leave a smooth white scar. Burns confined to the mouth have only a transitory and very little penetrating effect, and the mucosa soon returns to its normal condition. They only become of moment by involvement of the epiglottis and the larynx. If the œdema has produced an obstructive dyspnœa, tracheotomy is indicated.

Ulcerations of the mucosa which remain after burns can be treated as are burns and ulcers elsewhere.

Lesions of the oral mucosa are produced by corrosive poisons, concentrated acids, and alkalies, swallowed accidentally or with suicidal intent. Medicinal substances prescribed as mouth-washes, such as potassium permanganate, etc., are often used in the undiluted state. Superficial but extensive sloughs may result surrounded by swelling and œdema, all of which disappears in a few days. These grayish-white sloughs, if situated on the palatoglossal folds, may readily be confounded with a diphtheritic membrane. The treatment consists in all cases of demulcent mouth-washes, decoction of althæa, and gruels.

The ingestion of corrosive poisons taken with suicidal intent is followed by much more serious effects. These include caustic soda, spirit of ammonia, and sulphuric acid. Their corrosive action involves not only the mouth, but the œsophagus, stomach, and air-passages as well. The extent of the destruction in the latter localities entirely governs the prognosis; the lesions in the mouth are of secondary consequence. The

color of the corroded areas may give some indication of the sul
taken.   The sloughs caused by sulphuric acid are a dark-red
almost black; those of nitric and nitromuriatic acids, a distinct
color.   Most of these caustic sloughs are white or gray, with ir
outlines, but circumscribed, and are more numerous on the lips, t
soft palate, pharynx, and epiglottis.   If the patient survives the
diate effects of the poison, there is the liability of the formation of
sions between opposing granulating surfaces at a later period.   ]
then become necessary to break up these adhesions at various tim
sometimes a plastic operation is called for in order to prevent the g
together of opposing raw surfaces.

CHAPTER XXVIII.

DISEASES OF THE MOUTH.

Of the numerous circumscribed or diffuse inflammatory diseases of oral mucosa and the tongue, only those will be here considered which partly from their bearing on purely surgical affections, partly from their mode of origin or treatment, merit the interest and attention of the surgeon. The various superficial affections of the mucous membrane need not be discussed in this connection. Of the numerous occupation diseases which affect the mucous membrane of the oral cavity, the periostitis due to phosphorus-poisoning and the lesions of the maxillæ seen in workers in mother-of-pearl have been spoken of. The discoloration seen along the gums as a result of poisoning from lead, silver, or bismuth, is not so well known as that produced by mercury. Of the affections of the mucous membrane in acute and chronic infectious diseases, syphilis and tuberculosis alone are mentioned. The mycotic diseases are considered with actinomycosis of the mouth and the tongue. Affections of the mucous membrane which are part of a general exanthema (herpes, lichen, pemphigus, urticaria, etc.) do not properly belong here. The same applies to those which are derived from certain constitutional diseases, including diabetes, Barlow's disease, purpura hæmorrhagica, and scurvy. It is a matter of importance to give proper attention to the so-called idiopathic leucoplakia as a distinct disease with especial reference to its bearing on cancer of the tongue.

STOMATITIS ULCEROSA.

A proper definition of this disease has not been agreed upon. Numerous authorities, particularly the French, consider it to be an infectious disease of an epidemic nature; others deny its contagious character and believe that its appearance in epidemics in orphan asylums and hospitals is due entirely to unsanitary conditions.

Etiology.—The presence of teeth is apparently the only absolutely constant etiological factor, for the disease is not known to have occurred in their absence. The immediate cause has not been determined, although a priori it may be either a variety of bacterium or leptothrix.

Symptoms.—The clinical aspects of the disease are well marked. A swelling and intense redness are developed along the portion of the gums next the teeth, the process being accompanied by severe pain. This condition is never seen in infants who have not developed teeth, nor is

it found on those parts of the jaw where teeth are wanting. Du
process of dentition it only appears where the teeth are presen
disease therefore, as far as its first appearance is concerned, is de
on the presence of teeth, and only later does the mucous memb
the cheeks, lips, and tongue become involved, and the process
usually confined to one side.

The gums in the neighborhood of the teeth are puffy and of a
red color, and are noticeably thickened in the interstices. Slight
readily causes bleeding, and blood even appears between the lips
attempts at drinking and swallowing. The saliva is increased
breath becomes fetid. The temperature is never high, but the
of depression and fatigue is always marked. After from two to fo
the free edge of the gum assumes a dirty-yellow color and beco
and pulpy. The ulceration usually begins at one of the cani
extends around to the incisors and the molars, gradually includi
the posterior alveolar borders. Finally all the teeth become surr
by a flat ulcerated area, the base of which is covered by a diph
like exudate. After the process has involved the entire gum, it
extends to the inner aspect of the cheek, the lips, and the edge
tongue, invading those sections which come in contact with the ul
surfaces when the mouth is closed. The same changes take plac
mucous membrane, and the lips and tongue become swollen, t
with the lymph-glands in the retromaxillary and submaxillary a
submental regions. The ulceration rarely appears on the hard or
palate, and the faucial isthmus ordinarily marks the limits of the
In very severe cases the alveolar processes may be exposed, the te
out, and parts of the jaw even become necrotic. Up to this p
general condition of the patient is merely affected by the inability
sufficient nourishment. Later a septic temperature and pulmona
plications may develop, and may endanger life. The transition
process into noma has also been observed in cases in which gang
the cheek occurred as a result of the ulceration on its internal su

Ulcerative stomatitis is primarily a disease of childhood. It ma
on soon after the appearance of the lower incisors. It is rarely e
tered after the tenth year. Affected children usually include the
are poorly nourished, pale, and weakly, and present the pietu
scrofulous diathesis. Living in small, overcrowded, and poorl
lated dwellings is also a contributing factor. Most cases are fo
occur during the first and second periods of dentition. The di
seen in adults sporadically and even epidemically, in barracks
and other crowded quarters. Gerhard calls attention to the fact
spite of its great frequency the contagiousness of the disease has nev
demonstrated. In epidemics which have occurred in the Frenc
gian, and Portuguese armies the officers were apparently never a
but only the more unfavorably quartered privates. In adults the
also begins in the gums, usually along the incisors and canines.
lary injection appears early in different parts of the mucosa of the
and a marked redness and swelling extend along the inner

usually of one cheek, opposite the line of contact of the upper and lower teeth. Kraus has called attention to the appearance in three or four days of a slough which covers the flat, rapidly spreading ulcers. It separates in five or six days and the underlying pulpy mass becomes covered with small red granulations over which the mucous membrane grows rapidly. Similar ulcerations are produced along the edges of the tongue corresponding to the depressions caused by the teeth.

The disease may run its course in a few days, but may extend over a period of two or more weeks. The separation of the slough is ordinarily followed soon after by the complete healing of the ulcers.

Diagnosis.—The differential diagnosis in the early days is concerned principally with noma in its initial stages, the consideration of which follows. If the disease is present in adults in epidemic form, it may be confused with certain scorbutic affections of the mouth which also show a predisposition for attacking the gums. In scurvy, however, aside from other manifestations, there is an immediate involvement of the mucous membrane of the cheeks and lips situated in the proximity, and the presence of ecchymosis in the mucosa and the red nodes in the spaces between the teeth should afford ready aids in the differentiation.

Treatment.—The treatment of this disease is usually followed by favorable results. It is important to keep children in the open air. The author has often placed the cradle or the bed out-of-doors when the weather permitted. There is scarcely a disease in which a sojourn in the open meets with such beneficial results. The pain which accompanies the act of swallowing often interferes with the proper nourishment of the patient, as the children are loath to place the food in their sore and bleeding mouths. Applications of a 2 per cent. solution of eucaine have been employed before feeding in order to diminish the sensibility of the oral mucosa. Great benefit results from the internal administration of potassium chlorate in the form of a 5 per cent. solution given every two hours, in the early stages of the disease. This drug should not, however, be continued for longer than three days. Locally brushing the ulcers at least once daily with spirit of camphor is of value. Children who have learned to rinse their mouths may be given a 10 per cent. solution of hydrogen peroxide for this purpose.

STOMATITIS GANGRÆNOSA, OR NOMA.

Noma, from the Greek *νομή*, *νέμεσθαι*, meaning to destroy, is a gangrenous, sloughing, destructive process of the oral cavity, involving by preference the cheeks, less often the gums, the hard and soft palate, and the lips. Other gangrenous processes of a similar nature, and bearing a close resemblance in their etiology and clinical histories, are encountered on the mucosa of the anal and vulvar orifices, and to them the same term is applied.

Etiology.—Noma is usually limited in its occurrence to weak individuals with an impaired nutrition, and more particularly to children

from two to twelve years of age. In adults noma has only been o
in a few cases, and then appears to have begun as an ulcerative sto

The diseases which are apt to be followed by noma are measles,
and the mercurialism of syphilitic infants. The noma of adi
usually appeared after severe cases of typhus, especially among
diers in a campaign. In the 75 cases collected by Perthes o
occurring in children, measles antedated the disease in 20, typh
cases. In the remainder the health and strength of the child were
mined by either syphilis, mercurial stomatitis, diphtheria, dy
tuberculosis, or unfavorable surroundings and improper or insi
food, before the disease actually appeared. The occurrence of i
epidemics, as maintained in former years, can probably be traced
demics of measles, which were complicated by noma in numei
stances. Thus Blumer and McFarlane report an epidemic of
in an orphanage, in which of 173 cases, noma followed in 16.

Symptoms.—The well-marked signs of the disease are usua
ceded by inflammatory disturbances of the oral mucosa in the
an ulcerating or a mercurial stomatitis. General symptoms
absent at this time or even later. On the contrary, it is often no
the children do not complain, remain playful, and are troubl
slightly in eating. The characteristic disturbance is first noted
mucous membrane of the cheek, less often on the mucoperiostea
ing of the alveolar process or the hard palate. A small vesi
cloudy contents is first seen, or a macerating yellowish spot
spreads rapidly over the surface. This is succeeded by a slou
gray color, which is surrounded by an infiltrated area. The cheel
but is neither red nor œdematous, only somewhat pale. Pi
reveals a hard mass in the substance of the cheek. The skin c
latter then assumes a bluish color, which fades off into that of the
skin. This appearance, together with the rapid increase in size
black spot, is characteristic of noma. After a time the cheek t
indurated and is surrounded by an extensive area of œdema wl
cludes the nose, eyelids, ears, and the temporal regions, and finally
the neck. A remarkable fact is the slight degree of pain which tl
feels—the cheek may be pinched and squeezed without resistanc
part. The sloughing process then rapidly advances in the mo
volves the mucous membrane of both upper and lower jaws and
forms it into a pasty, foul mass, which fills up the cavity of the
The odor is very penetrating and is manifest at some distance fi
patient. The loosened teeth drop out; the bones are exposed i
come black and soft. Finally the outer skin covering the cheek
away. The more rapid the process of destruction, the sooner des
be expected to end the miseries of the patient.

This gangrenous process runs a similar course if the gums or t
palate is the starting point. The foul-smelling breath of the
then an early symptom. The dark-brown lips are covered witl
and the deep-red gums present a number of dirty ulcers and bla
spots which soon become transformed into a soft, stinking, pulp

The teeth fall out and the inferior and superior maxillary bones are completely exposed. The cheeks swell, grow tense, and assume a waxy, grayish-yellow color.

If the process starts on the hard palate, a black spot appears in this locality, after the child has been troubled for several days with a more or less severe grade of stomatitis.

It is rare that the disease becomes limited spontaneously. In such cases the necrotic area is surrounded by a deep circular slough, which penetrates the entire thickness of the cheek and marks off the gangrenous patch from the healthy tissue. An early perforation of this kind can always be considered a favorable sign. A similar process of demarcation may also take place if the area of necrosis begins on the gums, the hard palate, or even if it involves the bones. In the latter case, however, it consumes more time, especially if fragments of the jaw are cast off. During the course of this procedure gangrene may begin in some other part of the oral mucosa not previously affected. In one case such recurrences were noted three times. After the sloughs all disappear large defects remain, resulting later in malformations within the cavity of the mouth and in contractures of the jaws, which, if the child recovers, may necessitate extensive plastic operations. If the process of demarcation is effective in the early stages of the disease, only a stellate-shaped scar may result, which displaces the corresponding angle of the mouth and the ala of the nose and causes no further deformity.

Diagnosis.—The diagnosis of noma is not attended with difficulty. The gangrenous fragments of mucous membrane may readily be seen on inspection of the mouth. During the first few days the condition may be mistaken for an ulcerative stomatitis, but the rapidly spreading gangrenous process in the mouth and cheek soon leaves little doubt of its true nature.

The sudden appearance in an apparently healthy tissue and the marked similarity in the clinical pictures of the cases have led to the supposition that noma is a microparasitic disease. Schimmelbusch and others have made attempts to transmit the disease to animals by inoculation of bits of the sloughs, but without success. Symptoms of sepsis appeared in all of these animals, as well as in those in which sloughs from other sources had been introduced simultaneously. Microscopical examination of the gangrenous tissue discloses the presence of all the species associated with the floor of the mouth, none of which can, however, be considered an etiological factor. The slough forms a good culture-medium for numerous saprophytes present in or carried into the mouth. An important discovery is that of Perthes, who isolated from the diseased tissue a fungus, the streptothrix of noma, with numerous long hyphæ, forming a mycelium which is particularly dense at the junction of the healthy and the gangrenous tissue. It is assumed that the fine terminal filaments invade the living tissue, surround the cells, and cause their death. Observations made by Krahn, Ferie, Blumer, and McFarlane agree in some respects with the assertions of Perthes. A pure culture of this fungus has not thus far been secured, nor has animal inoculation with infected bits of tissue been successfully accomplished. In the latter inoculated material produced neither suppuration nor gangr leptothrix has also been found in the sloughs from the mucous me of the cheek in the ulcerative form of stomatitis, by Netter and Fr in addition to spirilli, bacilli, and cocci.

Prognosis.—The fatal ending which usually takes place resu one of three causes. The most frequent is a complicating inflar of the lung, which is due to the aspiration of infectious material t month and is of the lobular and peribronchial type. The foci in are apt to suppurate or become gangrenous. Severe diarrhœas r bring on a fatal issue, and are undoubtedly due to the ingestion of Finally the heart may be paralyzed by the septic infection. A the latter may not be present in the early stages, and the genera tion of a child even with extensive sloughing of the mucous me may be comparatively good, it becomes a most formidable comp at the end, especially if any involvement of the respiratory o added. Fever is present—104° F. and over; the patient becon thetic, and sinks from hour to hour.

Treatment.—The treatment of noma is based on the observat early perforation of the cheek is usually followed by a favorable o The author therefore recommends the destruction of the black the mucosa, passing the point of the Paquelin cautery through th thickness of the cheek and including a considerable area of the su ing mucous membrane. Two cases in his clinic were treated manner by converting a soft gangrenous into a firm, dry slon life saved. It is advisable to maintain this hard character b cations of pyroligneous acid or alcohol until a line of inflan demarcation results. The mouth itself may be kept clean by th strong solutions of hydrogen peroxide.

The author would not advise a substitution of the knife for the cautery for the following reasons: There is sure to be more hem with the former, and it opens up tissue-spaces which would ot remain closed. The heat radiating from the cautery probably beyond the actual limits of the destructive process and ex influence on toxic substances which have penetrated beyon boundaries.

If this local treatment is to meet with success, it must be doi in the disease. V. v. Bruns has collected 413 cases from the lit in which a cure was reported in 123. This figure is probably to however, as the cures are almost invariably reported, the deaths Nevertheless the figures show that the prognosis is not invariab and that prompt and energetic measures should always be institu

The author has never had any success with the methods of ir carbolic and other solutions, which were recommended for a tir desires to protest at this point against their employment.

It is necessary to exert every means to improve the nutrition r weakly young patients, a task to which particular attention must during the periods of demarcation and repair.

If the noma does not begin in the cheek, the application of the cautery may be difficult. In such cases solutions of zinc chloride may be used, or, what is probably better, absolute alcohol.

SYPHILIS OF THE MOUTH.

Syphilis can by no means be considered an exclusively venereal disease, as proved by the numerous cases of extragenital infection. Münchheimer has shown that of every 100 cases of extragenital infections, 39 occur in the mouth, in the following order of frequency: lips, tongue, palate, cheeks, and gums. The infection results from direct contact with a syphilitic lesion on the body of another person; from knives, forks, and other eating utensils previously used by a syphilitic person; from pipes, cigars, and cigarettes passed from one individual to another; from the mouth-pieces of musical instruments exchanged by musicians; from glass-blowers' pipes; from the tongue-depressor of the physician; from dental instruments, and numberless other causes.

The initial form of the disease is the hard chancre or the papule, similar to those found on other mucous membranes. On the lips the eroded papule is seen more often than the chancre, or the lesion may take the form of a superficial ulcer covered by a crust, resembling a localized eczema, an ecthyma pustule, or a herpes erosion. The ulcer grows to the size of a twenty-five-cent piece and palpation reveals an indurated base. The lip swells in proportion to the rapidity with which the ulcer grows. An enlargement of the lymphatic glands in the submaxillary and submental regions takes place much more rapidly than involvement of the corresponding glands with a chancre of the genitals. They are not particularly sensitive, however, and manifest no tendency to coalesce. If the diagnosis of any given case is doubtful, the induration and the lymphatic involvement aid in deciding the question even before the characteristic secondary rash appears. In the few cases in which the primary sore occurs on the gums or the hard palate the lesion runs the same course as that just described on the lips and cheeks.

The initial lesion commonly found on the tongue is the hard chancre. Its site is usually the upper surface or the edge of the anterior part, and consists of a bright-red indurated area the size of a bean, with edges sharply marked, elevated, and smooth. There is a slight central depression, and in the course of five weeks the sore is covered with a scab. In a short time the submaxillary and submental lymph-glands become involved, and can be felt as distinct hard nodes. The differential diagnosis from the gumma of late syphilis, even from cancer, is therefore not a difficult matter. In place of this typical beginning and the later change of the induration into a flat ulcer with bleeding base, the primary sore, especially if situated on the edge or the tip of the tongue, may be lacerated by the teeth during mastication, although little pain is felt by the patient. The fact that the neighboring lymph-glands are enlarged to a marked degree at an early stage, and, moreover, the site of the lesion, help to

differentiate this condition from other inflammatory processes.   I
the stage of erosion it is, of course, almost impossible to distingui
epithelial exfoliation from that seen in a superficial glossitis, or that
succeeds mechanical or thermic irritation.   In such cases it is nec
to wait for the development of the induration.

The further course of a syphilis which is the result of an extraç
infection does not vary from that acquired through the channels
genitals.   The prognosis is neither better nor worse.

During the secondary stage of any case of syphilis the mouth
site of both varieties of lesions which usually attack the mucous
branes, erythema and papules.   A diffuse redness appears in th
pharynx at the same time or shortly after the breaking out of the g
roseola.   This is of a catarrhal nature, and involves by preferen
soft palate and the pharynx, leaving the rest of the mucous mem
practically exempt.   There is nothing in the color or the disposit
this condition of the soft palate to distinguish it from the reduess
other causes; the only characteristic points are the time of its aj
ance, its protracted presence, and its rapid disappearance under
curial treatment.

The papular syphilide of the oropharynx spreads very quickly
sharply marked clinically.   It is the usual manifestation of this
on the mucous membranes.   The size of the papules varies from t
a small pea to that of a bean.   Over the cellular infiltration of th
epithelial layer there is always a layer of hypertrophied epith
which becomes macerated by the moisture in the mouth and gi'
the lesions its characteristic pale-gray color.   In this condition th
thelial covering may remain for some time, or a greater degree of d
cration may take place and a superficial loss of substance occur
ducing an erosion which may extend still deeper and result in an
A more marked development of the papule and a thickening of th
thelium afford a picture similar to the broad flat condylomata se
the genitals.   During the first two years after infection the pa
syphilide is usually found on the lips, the tongue, or the palatal tc
it then gradually disappears, and is not seen after the eighth year. '
is no difficulty in finding and distinguishing the peculiar grayish-
spots on certain parts of the tongue.   Their differentiation from aj
ances found in the leucoplakia of the tongue and cheeks will be disc
elsewhere.

The appearance of the papules at the commissure of the lips ai
the back of the tongue is quite characteristic.   On each lip nea
angle of the mouth is a grayish crescentic papule; they lie in appo
when the mouth is closed.   In the angle of the lips is a narro
sure, which is very sensitive and bleeds readily.   Where the infilti
extends beyond the vermilion border of the lips the skin is copper-cc
and covered with an adherent crust.   On the back of the tougu
affected area is a little darker than normal, but the attention is attr
to its mirror-like smoothness and the circumscribing elevation, the
coated with a dirty-white fur.   Fournier designates this condition k

term, "plaque lisse." Although these mucous plaques disappear rapidly under appropriate treatment, they are very apt to return during the first few years after infection, a recurrence which, on account of the extremely contagious nature of the eroded papule, favors transmission of the disease.

Surgical interest attaches more to the later lesions of syphilis. The circumscribed gumma and the gummatous infiltration are both represented in the oral cavity. They usually appear between the tenth and fifteenth years after inoculation, rarely before the fifth or after the fifteenth. The male sex is more often affected than the female, in the proportion of 6 to 1. This relation is explained by habits commonly found in men—smoking, chewing, and the daily use of alcohol. Both forms of gumma take their origin either superficially in the submucous connective tissue, or more deeply between the muscle-fibres, and for this reason the clinical picture varies greatly. The tongue and the floor of the mouth are most frequently involved, very often at the same time or in connection with the lower lip or the lower jaw.

The gummatous infiltration of the lip usually begins at the angle of the mouth as a hard induration, at first circumscribed, but later involving the entire lip. In the check it is characteristic that when disintegration occurs perforation always takes place externally, and the serpiginous ulcers are formed followed by the deformities described in a preceding chapter. The extensive involvement of the lips, cheeks, and their surroundings is usually associated with localized syphilis in other parts, especially the skull and the testicle.

The superficial as well as the deeper circumscribed gummata of the tongue form distinct protuberances, limited usually to the anterior part. Very often the gummata are multiple and appear simultaneously in different parts of the tongue, in contradistinction to the nodes of carcinomata and actinomycosis, which are usually single and remain so. In some instances they occupy only one-half of the tongue. In the submucous tissue the nodes are numerous and also small. Those in the depths of the muscle are less in number and develop more slowly, and may attain the size of a walnut. The surface is covered with a smooth mucosa, smooth because the papillæ have disappeared. The centre of the mass then begins to break down, the mucous membrane is perforated, and from the opening is discharged a tenacious fluid containing yellowish lumps. The thin and undermined edges of the fistulous opening slough away and the crater-like ulcer becomes larger. The base of the latter is of a dirty-yellow color, and the process of granulation goes forward very slowly, with constant remissions and further necrosis at the expense of the surrounding tissue.

While the circumscribed gumma at the height of its development, unless influenced by antisyphilitic measures, breaks down, owing to disintegration of its cellular elements, the infiltrating lesion pursues a different course. As a rule even during its growth it stimulates the formation of new connective tissue around its periphery. In the course of time this goes on to the production of cicatricial bands which manifest a ten-

deney to contract, and finally there results the typical syphilitic inc
tion with characteristic deformities. The gummatous infiltration us
affects the tongue in its longitudinal planes, and this, together witl
deep furrows which are brought about by the process of contrac
especially if one of the latter is in the median line, causes the to
to be divided in the middle, and forms the so-called double to
of syphilitics. The mucous membrane which remains between
furrows is thickened and tender and shows a tendency to super
ulcerations.

A superficially situated gumma, especially if ulcerated, can be di
guished from the initial lesion by the fact that along with one gu
a second or a third is likely to be found, while the primary sore is al
single. The primary lesion, moreover, is soon followed by well-ma
swelling of the adjacent lymphatics, these being absent in the later s
of syphilis.

Fig. 340.

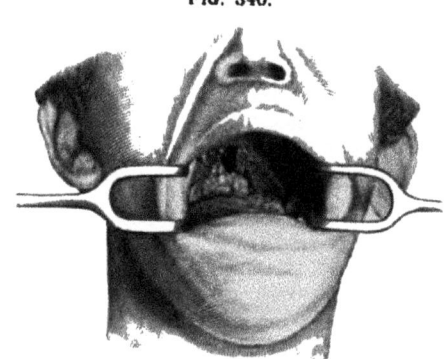

Hereditary syphilis of the soft palate in a boy aged sixteen years.

The differentiation of the ulcerating gumma from actinomyc
tuberculous lesions, and carcinoma will be discussed more fully
where.

As already noted at another point, the hard palate is perhaps ı
often the seat of the later lesions of syphilis than either the lips
cheeks, or the tongue, and was there described as an accompanime:
a continuation of nasal syphilis. As a matter of fact, the gumma iı
middle line of the hard palate is due more commonly to the perfori
of the palatine process of the superior maxilla. This perforation anc
separation of the sequestrum leave a small ovoid tumor in the me
raphe, covered with mucous membrane, which either breaks dow
disappears if it has been possible to extract the sequestrum throngl
nose.

The so-called "smooth atrophy of the root of the tongue" has ‹
been looked upon as a specific syphilitic phenomenon. In this cond
the follicles disappear, the epithelium becomes very much thinned

PLATE XIV.

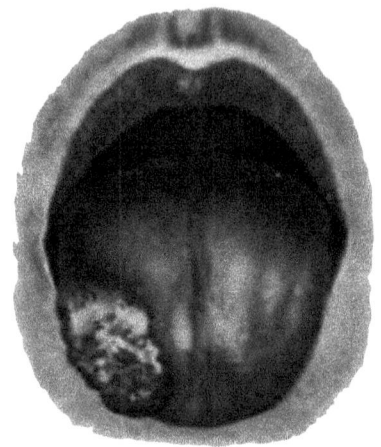

pithelioma of the Tongue. (Grünwald.)

and later muscular atrophy and occlusion of the mucous glands result. Goldschmidt's researches have shown, however, that these disturbances are also found in other diseases which are accompanied by degeneration of the tongue, including tuberculosis and other debilitating conditions, and old age.

Prognosis.—The prognosis of gummatous processes in the oral cavity is not unfavorable if prompt treatment is instituted, consisting of the use of large doses of potassium iodide and mercurial inunctions.

Treatment.—The constitutional treatment of the disease is of the first importance, as is evidenced by the favorable effect produced on the gummatous processes of the tongue. The combination of inunctions with the internal use of potassium iodide has been particularly favored, and forms the main points in the treatment at Aix-la-Chapelle. As the potassium iodide is frequently not well tolerated by a delicate stomach, Nobl has substituted injections of iodipin subcutaneously.

Although many cases of late syphilis are cured by these methods, recurrences are nevertheless numerous. Many patients are sufferers for years, and are only free from the disease during the periods of actual treatment.

Local treatment is appropriate in all cases. The softened gummatous nodules may be scraped out with a sharp spoon. In the same manner the deep furrows in the tongue may be cleaned out. This procedure is to be followed by cauterization, preferably with a 10 to 20 per cent. solution of chromic acid, applied with a brush or a cotton swab. The application of the silver nitrate stick is also serviceable. Particular attention must be given to cleanliness of the mouth. Finally, as the indurated and painful tongue interferes greatly with the taking of food, the nutrition, especially of the weaker patients, must be carefully attended to.

TUBERCULOSIS OF THE ORAL CAVITY.

Although the oral cavity is so frequently exposed to the effects of pathogenic agencies, it is a remarkable fact that up to the present time it has rarely been demonstrated as affording a point of entrance to tuberculons infection. It is apparent therefore that the epithelium which covers the mucous membrane of the mouth affords ample protection against the inroads of infectious materials as long as it remains intact. An instance is known in which a physician, otherwise in perfect health, accidentally inoculated himself with a cigarette which had been allowed to come in contact with freshly grown tubercle bacilli. At the angle of the mouth where he had been accustomed to hold the cigarette an ulcer developed, which soon extended over the cheek and was accompanied by swelling of the neighboring lymphatics. Tubercle bacilli in great numbers were demonstrated in the ulcer. The entire diseased area was removed, including the glands, which had meanwhile undergone cheesy degeneration. Microscopical examination and animal inoculation confirmed the diagnosis. A series of cases has been collected by Frank and Hildebrand in which the development of a general tuberculosis has been traced initial lesion in the oral cavity. A primary tuberculosis of the tongu also be thought of in those cases reported by Chrostek, in which at showed a chronic ulceration of the tongue and a recent miliary tul losis of the lungs, kidneys, pleura, and meninges.

A secondary involvement is much more common than the pri The mouth may become infected in one of three ways. In th place, by extension of a lupus from the lips and nose to the m membrane of the mouth, which as a rule is most marked on the lip. The small nodules creep from the outer skin over the ver border and the mucosa, where they become converted into eh ulcers. As the process extends there results a surface covered granulations, marked by a number of deep furrows, which gra involve the gums and in time the hard and soft palate. The meanwhile drop out. If the disease is present in the nose, the soft becomes involved by direct extension, or in some cases it may be i sible to trace any line of continuity between it and the original fo the nose. In any one individual the various stages of develop comprising nodules, ulcers, and scars, can usually be seen at the time.

From the velum pendulum the process extends along the p arches to the posterior wall of the pharynx and the base of the tc and gradually encroaches upon the entrance to the larynx.

The diagnosis depends on the presence of a florid lupus (outer skin or at least one that has run its course, and without means it is impossible to make it. Other forms of tuben ulcerations of the mouth are characterized by pain, while lupus (little pain and always runs a chronic course. Periods in whic process is at a standstill alternate with those in which advance is an apparent cure is followed by quickly growing recurrences, and fore the white scars of the healed and the fresh ulcers of the lesions are found in proximity. Swelling of the adjacent lymph- is an early accompaniment of other forms of oral tuberculosis, usually absent in lupus. The demonstration of tubercle bacilli i difficult in the products from lupous ulcerations, but is readily a plished in other tuberculous lesions.

Another manner in which the mucous membrane of the mout become secondarily infected is by the transmission of tuberculous s from a diseased lung. It is a difficult matter, however, to demor this satisfactorily, as in most instances the surgeon is dealing severe and extended general infection, and the disease may have transmitted through the medium of the circulation. The findir Strassmann and Schlenker show that an infection of the ton readily possible, as in these cases there is almost always prese advanced pulmonary phthisis, and inoculation by sputum is accomplished. Dmochowski reports 15 cases of phthisis in whi involvement of the lingual tonsil was found in 10. It seems remar considering the large amount of infectious material which con contact with the numerous small abrasions and wounds of the mucous membrane of the mouth, that specific infection does not develop oftener. As the affection of the tongue represents only a part of the general disease, it seems more reasonable to consider its origin in connection with the third method of dissemination, the circulatory system.

Tuberculosis of the mouth usually manifests itself in the form of a large node at the edge of the tongue, or numerous small scattered excoriations which are derived from superficial ulcerating vesicles. The nodes are usually solitary, but the excoriations are always multiple and form groups which are most marked on the oral surface of the soft palate and along the arcus palatoglossus.

The tuberculous lesion is invariably found on the edge of the tongue and cannot be distinguished from an actinomycotic nodule, a gumma, or an induration which is due to pressure or contact with the teeth. In the latter case the immediate presence of a decaying tooth may furnish an explanation. Although it would be a very desirable matter to distinguish these lesions at an early stage, the inability to do so is not of great consequence, as the treatment is the same for all cases, namely, complete extirpation. In comparing tuberculous with carcinomatous nodules, it is found that the former are most always multiple, the primary lesion being supplemented by others on the back or the under surface of the tongue, while an initial carcinomatous induration is invariably solitary. The same may be said of actinomycosis. The mucous membrane over a tuberculous nodule is characterized by a marked red color. The further course of these lesions differs greatly. A rapidly growing nodule breaks down and forms an ulcer which shows its tuberculous character by its thin, undermined edges, which gape slightly and disclose a base dotted with red and grayish-yellow points, the "tuberculous rhagade." These slit-like ulcers may be distinguished from the furrows of a syphilitic glossitis by the absence of the hard circumscribed edges, the extensive induration, and the swelling between the deep furrows which run at right angles to each other. The tuberculous "rhagade" is a simple slit; the syphilitic fissure is branching and crossed by others. The sensitiveness of tuberculous ulcers is marked when compared with the comparatively painless syphilitic lesions. As the tuberculous ulcer enlarges by the breaking down of its edges, it still remains superficial and resembles closely the ulceration which results from disseminated nodules. The latter is another way in which the process may begin, and usually accompanies a severe pulmonary or laryngeal tuberculosis. Numerous small grayish-yellow nodules appear almost simultaneously at the angle of the mouth, on the tongue, and the soft palate. They project but slightly above the surface of the mucous membrane, occur in groups or scattered, and gradually extend around the edge of the tongue. From these miliary tubercles are derived round or irregular ulcers, with sharply marked edges, a yellowish-red base, and surrounded by an area of intense redness. By confluence of several of these, large ulcers are produced of varied forms. Around them appears a fresh miliary eruption, and underneath is a well-marked infiltration. \\

opportunity is afforded to make an examination of the latter, it w
found to be made up of numerous characteristic grayish nodules. '
tuberculous ulcers are extremely painful, and especially those de
from the disseminated tubercles, so that swallowing and attemp
speaking become very painful. Nutrition is interfered with, an
patient's strength declines more rapidly than is warranted by the s
extension of the disease. The diagnosis depends on the extreme
bility, and furthermore the association with a tuberculosis of the pha
larynx, or lungs. The determining factor is the demonstration o
tubercle bacilli in the débris scraped from the ulcer. Finally, in dou
cases it may even be advisable to employ the subcutaneous injecti
tuberculin, care being taken to use only a very small dose, as the
pulmonary infiltration which often follows is apt to prove fatal t
patient.

Prognosis.—A comparatively favorable prognosis attends those
of tuberculous affections of the mucous membrane which are orig
derived from a lupus on the external skin. The ulcerations whic
the result of disseminated tubercles run a protracted course, recur n
after healing has apparently taken place, and as they are usually ac
panied by a more severe form of laryngeal or pulmonary tuberei
final dissolution may be looked for at an early date.

Treatment.—The treatment is both general and local. The ge
treatment is directed against the constitutional disease. The
measures fulfil two indications: first, to lessen the sensitiveness c
lesions; and second, to convert the advancing ulceration into a
granulating surface, which is thus given an opportunity to heal.
first indication is met by brushing the seat of the disease with a sol
of cocaine or eucaine, or applying the lately devised anæsthesin.
the treatment of the nodular form the author recommends extirp
of the nodule or ablation of the entire tip of the tongue. Whe
distribution of the smaller ulcers is not too extensive, they ma
curetted after thorough cocainization. This may be followed,
.bleeding has ceased, by application of the thermocautery or a sol
of iodoform in ether. The former belief in the specific action of
acid in these cases has given way to the present employment of iodo

ACTINOMYCOSIS OF THE MOUTH.

In the greater number of instances actinomycosis of the mouth o
in connection with the same process in the cheeks, jaws, or the

The mucous membrane of the mouth and pharynx is the ord
point of entry of the actinomyces fungus, and also probably of
varieties of the streptothrix. Illich has shown that in 392 cases in v
the point of entrance could be determined with certainty, it was t
to be in the mouth in 234 instances. Of the latter, the tongue
involved in 16. The method of inoculation has been determine
many cases to be the result of the introduction of the fungus on g

of cereals or a splinter of wood which had been taken into the mouth. The sharp point of these objects penetrated the mucous membrane, and the fungus on reaching the submucosa proliferated rapidly. An opera- tion done for the resulting disturbance always showed the foreign body in the centre of the focus of the disease. These cases have been collected by Hummel, and Jurinka has also added a number of interesting obser- vations made at the clinic in Gratz. In one instance a nodule extirpated from the tongue contained parts of a kernel, the intracellular spaces of which were filled with the fungus. The latter had entirely enveloped the grain and undoubtedly reached the parenchyma of the tongue in this manner.

In most cases the wound is minute and, as it rapidly undergoes cica- trization, cannot be recognized. In any given case it may be a difficult matter to trace the path of the infection, as the immediate disturbances

Fig. 341.

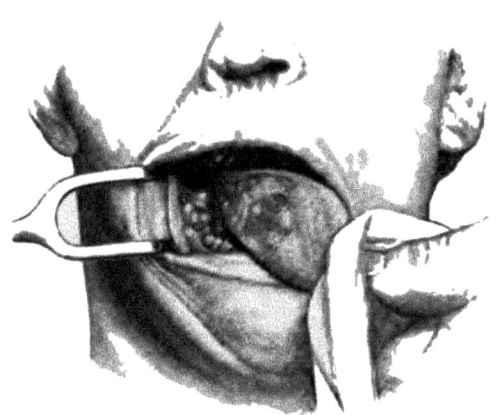

Actinomycosis of the tongue.

at the point of entrance may have entirely subsided, and later and more marked lesions appear at another site. In cases in which the jaw is affected, the point of inoculation has rarely been found.

The swelling of the cheek, which is at first doughy, later becomes indurated, and soon leads to trismus; it is also accompanied by a second- ary involvement of the oral mucous membrane. The induration of the latter extends upward along the posterior section of the cheek or con- tinues along the palatopharyngeal fold. Small abscesses are discharged into the mouth or outwardly through the skin of the cheek or the tem- poral region. Sinuses are formed leading down into the masseter muscles, and the markedly swollen cheek may become tunnelled in all directions. In the mouth these sinuses appear as small round funnel- shaped openings filled with soft yellowish-red granulations.

The infiltration starting from the under surface of the tongue extends over the floor of the mouth and gradually involves the musculature in

the submental region, and even spreads down over the neck.
time when abscesses are discovered on the neck the swelling
tongue may have subsided, and all that remains is a certain deg
stiffness and impaired mobility, or in certain cases there may
cicatricial bands in the floor of the mouth. The inflammatory nec
due to the fungus is rarely found on the mucous membrane of the
Partsch in one case observed a solitary nodule near Stenson's duc
the tongue, on the contrary, these nodules are the most frequent
The nodule is embedded in the substance of the anterior half
tongue, and the overlying mucous membrane may be unchanged
bright-red color, but is not freely movable. It is of slow growth
firm consistence. After some months, or perhaps years, it reach
size of a hazelnut or even that of a walnut, and softens in the
If it ruptures or is incised, the contained pus will be found to c
the typical actinomycotic granules. The process may remain qui
or, what is more usual, new foci and sinuses may arise arou
periphery, but it ordinarily subsides under appropriate treatment

Diagnosis.—The diagnosis of actinomycosis can always be mad
certainty by the finding of the characteristic yellowish-brown gr
either in the pus or the tissues of the lesions. The induration is co
to both syphilitic and actinomycotic processes, and may lead to
confusion. It is well to note that the base of the syphilitic ulce
a dirty-yellow color and ragged, whereas in actinomycosis the
pockets and undermined ulcers filled with flabby granulation
surrounded by small and large abscesses or bands. Those c:
actinomycosis which originate from the gums or are brought
carious teeth have been considered in connection with the diseases
jaws.

Treatment.—The treatment follows the lines already laid
Nodes in the tongue should be excised, hemorrhage checked, at
wound sutured. Healing invariably takes place without suppu
Ulcers should be thoroughly curetted, and if a cure does not follo
operation should be repeated. The soft tissue surrounding them.
also be removed. The smaller abscesses are evacuated and their
and the fistulæ curetted. The latter method has been successfu
number of instances in which the cheek was extensively involve
trismus was present. Energetic and timely treatment is the only
of protecting the patient against extension of the process alo
sphenomaxillary fossa to the base of the skull and into the cranial
The success of this procedure is shown in the author's clinic,
Schlange first demonstrated in a series of cases the value of su
treatment, and altered the previous conception of actinomycosis
incurable disease. About five-sixths of these cases were traced
with the exception of a few instances, all remained cured. The :
does not close the wounds, but keeps them open with iodoform
packing. If the granulations become pale and break down, they :
be removed and the opening of a hidden sinus looked for. The
must be slit open and thoroughly cleaned. The internal use of pot

iodide, as formerly recommended to prevent the spread of the infection, has not met with favorable results in the author's hands.

LEUCOPLAKIA OF THE MOUTH.

This term, as first used by Schwimmer, is applied to an idiopathic disease characterized by the gradual development and extension of opaque, milk-white patches on the mucous membrane of the cheeks, lips, and palate, but most frequently on the upper surface of the tongue, where they may extend as far back as the circumvallate papillæ. On the mucous membrane of the cheek they are arranged in mosaic fashion, are small, and scarcely project above the surrounding level. A similar condition is found on the lips, the gums, and the palate. On the tongue, however, they give the impression of a thin rind only a few millimetres in thickness, applied to the upper surface, at first smooth, but later wrinkled and furrowed. Some of these furrows are ulcerated and penetrate more or less deeply into the mucous membrane.

These patches, whatever their site, are sharply marked but of irregular contour, and are often compared in appearance to a map. The edges may become closely approximated, and in certain places the patches are confluent. In this manner the entire upper surface of the tongue may be covered with white flakes of varying thickness. Palpation shows that these patches are hard, and in advanced cases they feel like roughened horny plates. The furrows and the ulcerated areas are very apt to bleed at times.

Mauriac claims to have observed small circumscribed red points as the initial stage in the formation of these plaques. Undoubtedly these white patches appear as if the mucous membrane had been swabbed with a dilute solution of silver nitrate, and the underlying red color of the parts was simply veiled. As the disease is a progressive one, the various stages in the development of the process can usually be observed at the same time.

The favorite site of this disease is the upper surface of the anterior section of the tongue. The edges and the under surface are less likely to be involved, or at least not until the process has extended over the entire upper surface.

In the beginning the process causes but little disturbance; but as it extends and the patches become larger and eroded, the tongue becomes very painful, and speech, chewing, and swallowing are interfered with. This sensitiveness may reach an extreme degree, affecting the nutrition of the patient, and before each meal recourse must be had to cocaine. Even more importance must be attached to the possibility of this process degenerating into a carcinoma. In the author's clinic a history of leucoplakia preceded the appearance of carcinoma of the tongue in 53 per cent. of the cases.

To the researches of Nedopil and Schuchardt surgeons owe the knowledge of the anatomical relations of these lesions to carcinoma.

In the larger number of cases the white patch consists merely of mu
thickened squamous epithelium deposited in many layers and al
a tendency to cornification. The author has often observed, in
ining the white patches in the neighborhood of a carcinoma excise
the tongue, the same sort of proliferation of the epithelium,
cornification of the superficial layers. The papillæ lying directly
neath were unchanged, but the vascularity both here and over the
area of the plaque had largely disappeared, and the layer of epit
was capable of removal without causing much bleeding. Schu
was able to show that the substance called "eleidin," which a
during the process of cornification in the cells of the Malpighiar
could be demonstrated regularly in the leucoplacic patches as a
granular zone stained red by carmine and situated directly und
horny layer.

Although in the author's examinations the majority of the
examined disclosed the changes just described, without involven
the underlying tissues of the tongue, a certain number showed a d
state of affairs. In these, and in fact in a large number of the p
tions made by Nedopil and Schuchardt, were found an hypertrop
hyperplasia of the papillæ, and more frequently formation of new
and an infiltration of leucocytes in the subepithelial layers. The
also covered the bottom of the deeper furrows. Finally Schuchar
after him all other investigators, demonstrated mitosis in the
layers of the proliferating epithelium. But the most important fa
the development of carcinoma from leucoplakia is the atypical i
of epithelium, which in the form of flattened bands extends b
the papillæ into the deeper layers.

Etiology.—The etiology of this disease has by no means been
itely established. It is a well-known fact, however, that it occur
often in smokers and is rarely seen in women. In 596 cases co
by Schongarth, only 28 were females. One patient whom he
saw presented a typical picture of the disease, but on the next c
patches had almost disappeared. The man had often observe
phenomenon, and declared that the condition always subsided a
as he stopped smoking, only to reappear when he smoked even on
The fact that men present this disease more often than women
seems, be most readily explained by the almost universal use of t
by the former. Among the few cases the author has treated in the
sex, was one Russian woman, who according to her own statement s
at least eighty cigarettes daily. As Ludwig has demonstrated th
ence of carbolic acid in tobacco-smoke, it is not unlikely that the
of the latter on the mucous membrane is similar to the action c
paraffin, and carbolic acid on the outer skin, and in the long-con
irritation produced by the products of dry distillation the explana
the epithelial proliferations may be sought.

The similarity which exists between these lesions and the plac
secondary syphilis may have led to combating the claims of Schwi
who considered the disease entirely idiopathic. This was mos

getically done by Kaposi, and the idea seems to be upheld by the frequency which leucoplakia is found in individuals at some time infected with syphilis. Schongarth calculated that syphilis was present in 65 per cent. of the cases, and these figures confirmed the earlier claims of Erb. If this fact has any relation to the disease, it can only be looked upon as a remote one, in the sense that syphilis may have afforded a predisposing cause for the later appearance of a leucoplakia. But even this theory is not tenable, when it is remembered that although women are not less frequently infected with syphilis than men, they are rarely afflicted with leucoplakia. A notable case is cited by Schwimmer, who observed a fresh syphilitic lesion in a man with a well-developed leucoplakia. Finally, the employment of mercurial treatment undertaken in many cases has never caused the disappearance of a patch of leucoplakia, but, on the contrary, has made it worse, whereas the secondary symptoms of syphilis in the mouth readily subside under the same treatment.

It has also been claimed that there is a connection between leucoplakia and psoriasis of the skin. Lissauer in 50 cases of general psoriasis observed a leucoplakia of the oral cavity in 10.

Diagnosis.—The diagnosis and the differential diagnosis of this disease are not difficult. The plaques are commonly confused, however, with the mucous patches of syphilis. A point to be remembered in this connection is that the lesions of secondary syphilis in the mouth are usually found during the first two years after infection has taken place. At the same time similar spots are found on the palatal tonsils, a situation in which a patch of leucoplakia has never been observed. Syphilitic papules are usually situated on the edge of the tongue, leucoplakia on the back of the tongue. The former remain soft, the latter in time become hard. The papular syphilide of the mucosa is never so widely distributed as the leucoplakia, which may gradually occupy the entire tongue. The most marked differences are found, however, in the manner in which these affections develop. Syphilis begins acutely or subacutely; leucoplakia is chronic from the first, increases slowly, but is continually spreading. In the former an enlargement of the cervical lymphatic glands is regularly present, but is never found accompanying a leucoplakia. Finally, syphilitic lesions of the mouth are usually only a part of other manifestations of the secondary period on the skin or other mucous membranes. The differentiation from a beginning carcinoma is much more difficult, especially if a thick white patch is present and there is the possibility of a newly forming neoplasm underneath. Severe pain accompanying a leucoplakia may be attributed to a simultaneous neuralgia of the lingual nerve.

Treatment.—The treatment of this condition should begin as soon as the diagnosis is made, for experience has warned surgeons of the possibility of the white patches forming the starting point of future carcinomatous growths. Fournier has stated that this takes place in 30 per cent. of the cases. This affords, however, a pretty favorable outlook, and the author has seen instances in which leucoplakia has been present for twenty-seven years or longer without signs of malignant degeneration

having taken place. Smoking must be absolutely prohibited, and
early stages this may be sufficient to check the further progress
disease. A bland mouth-wash may also be prescribed, such as ɪ
cent. solution of borax in water and aqua menthæ in equal parts.
the disease is more advanced, cauterization is recommended witʰ
mate, papayotin, or a solution of chromic acid in water in the proɪ
of 1:10. The author has never seen any permanent results foɪ
the employment of these methods, but desires to recommend the ɪ
lin cautery as first advised by Volkmann. The tongue may be
anæsthetized, particularly with the recently introduced anæsthesi
means of a sharp spoon the thickened epithelium is scraped awɪ
bleeding arrested with a gauze tampon, and the cautery applieɪ
ciently long to produce a superficial slough. The pain followiɪ
procedure is severe, but may be relieved by holding a piece of ice
mouth. After the slough has separated, it is well to use a moutʰ
to promote healing of the underlying raw surface. If there ar
furrows running through the patch, or ulcers are present which
heal kindly, the application of the cautery is indispensable, as the
of malignant degeneration is imminent, and this is only the way in
the diseased tissues can be reached and destroyed.

PHLEGMONOUS GLOSSITIS.

Although a number of the diseases already described are not
by the border-line between the mouth and the oropharynx, knɪ
Waldeyer's lymphatic ring, this is especially noticeable in regard
phlegmonous processes of the tongue and the pharynx. At any
is usually considered a difficult matter to distinguish a deep glossit
a phlegmonous process in the region of the palatal tonsils. The exɪ
of any inflammatory swelling of the palatal tonsils to the so-called
tonsil is readily possible, and probably always occurs in every ɪ
acute pharyngitis and tonsillitis. The clinical picture of a sup
glossitis as regards the redness, swelling of the papillæ, and coat
different types, is part of that of a general disease, more particul
one of an infectious nature. (The strawberry tongue of scarlet ɪ
a good example of what has been claimed by numerous special
the mouth, nose, or throat, as an affection *per se* and belonging
of their particular fields of endeavor.) There are various otheɪ
tions of the tongue which need not be considered here; these inch
feline and the geographical tongue, the papillary glossitis of Micʰ
and the exfoliative glossitis of Möller. Consideration, howeveɪ
be given to the surgically important phlegmonous glossitis.

The tongue manifests a marked tendency to diffuse inflammatic
swelling. If during the asphyxia produced by a general anæsthɪ
tongue is seized with a forceps or is tightly grasped by the fingers,
enlarges and turns a bluish-red color. This swelling disappears
ever, just about as rapidly as it comes on, and in twelve hours' tɪ

organ usually returns to its normal condition. Pronounced irritation, even if transitory and superficial, is liable to cause a similar swelling. Chewing the bark of the spurge laurel is said to produce the same effect. The swellings which follow scalds, wounds, insect-bites, mercurial and other forms of stomatitis, and their consequences, especially the extension to the entrance to the larynx, have already been discussed. The most serious swelling is that due to erysipelas of the oral mucosa, on account of the danger of an œdema of the glottis. Although this erysipelatous process usually affects only the mucosa and the uppermost layers of the submucosa, it induces a very pronounced swelling of the entire tongue. It rarely happens that any phlegmonous process results from this cause, and the swelling ordinarily subsides without leaving any traces.

Fig. 342.

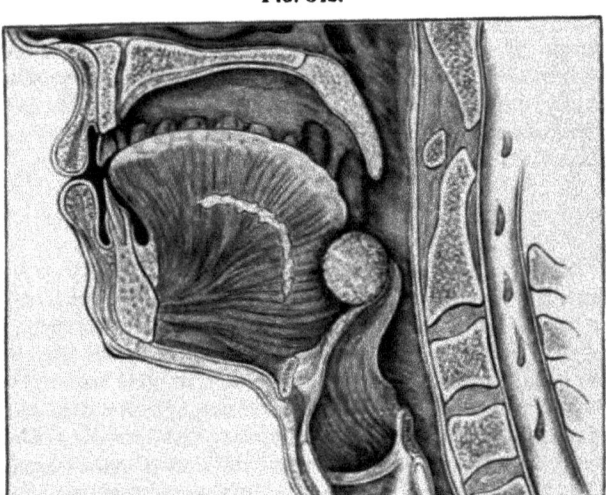

Showing accessory thyroid gland at base of the tongue. Tumor is nearly spherical, 2.5 x 3 cm. Color, grayish-red. Microscopical examination shows structure like thyroid.

A peculiar form of this transitory swelling of the tongue is known as hemiglossitis, which is described as a very acute and painful enlargement of one-half of the tongue, accompanied by high fever. The latter lasts but one day and the swelling subsides in about three days. Güterbock, who has written a monograph on this disease, believes that it depends on nervous influences, and is analogous to herpes zoster, the distribution following the branches of the lingual nerves.

Mention may also be made at this point of the swelling of the tongue which is found in man infected with the mouth-and-hoof disease of cattle. Siegel has closely observed this condition during one epidemic, and describes it as dominating the clinical picture. Of 6 patients, 2 died of sepsis. In 3 of the 4 who recovered the swelling subsided without further complications, but in the fourth the larger part of the tongue became gangrenous, probably from the pressure of the teeth, for it pro; about 2 cm. beyond the latter.

The diagnosis of this infectious inflammation of the tongue mu based on the other symptoms of the disease present. A feverish dromal stage is followed by the development of a vesicular erupti the lips, and especially on the mucous membrane of the mouth, ir ing the tongue, similar to an aphthous stomatitis. The same eru appears on the prepuce or the vulva and on the breasts of nursing wo while the entire outer skin is covered with an erythema and pete spots. Other complications follow, such as scorbutic-like hemorr from the oral mucous membrane and also the skin, chronic exhau gastrointestinal catarrhs, or finally chest symptoms. The vesicl the mucous surfaces become ulcerated and the invasion of strepto results in mixed infection. The fatal Ludwig's angina observed by ! in some of his cases is attributed by him to the latter cause. Siege found in the liver and kidneys of the victims of this disease ba which produced, when inoculated in calves, the typical hoof-and-n disease usually found in these animals.

Lymphangiomata of the tongue, especially those of the diffuse are often accompanied by an inflammatory process. This ordi subsides in a few days, but may lead to deeper abscesses and exte sloughing.

Considering the numerous injuries which the tongue sustains an number of foreign bodies which enter it, such as fish-bones and splinters, phlegmonous glossitis is a comparatively rare disease. . inflammation is limited to the pre-epiglottic region, which is ofte region where foreign bodies are liable to be caught, it resembles an angina, especially in the difficulty experienced in swallowing. Shou abscess form, a rise of temperature, swelling of the lymph-glands dyspnœa are the symptoms which quickly appear, so that immediate t eotomy may even be necessary. It may be that in these cases ther swelling of the tongue only when there has been a previous peritor phlegmon of the palatal tonsil which has spread down over the to The more acutely the swelling develops, the greater the dang asphyxia. In some cases the disease runs a very chronic course, i may be weeks before the abscess develops. The milder cases are us limited to the movable parts of the tongue; those of a severer for vade the root. The latter type is apt to attack one side only, and n bles very often a tonsillar angina. The tongue swells to such an e that there seems hardly room for it in the mouth. It forces its between the teeth, presses down on the floor of the mouth, pushe gullet backward and the palate upward. In this manner respirati interfered with mechanically and without the presence of an œdei the glottis. The patient therefore bends his head back as far as pos in order to be able to draw the air through the nose over the back (tongue. This is a very characteristic position, and as a result the appears extremely congested. The movements of the tongue are gi interfered with; it can no longer be projected, speaking becomes ir sible, and the acts of chewing and swallowing are extremely limited. The saliva is constantly dribbling and the edges of the tongue become sore from the pressure of the teeth. The swelling at the root of the tongue is evident as a board-like hardness in the submental and the hyoid regions. The temperature nevertheless is not high, and in the milder cases there may be no rise at all.

Among the dangers attending this condition, aside from the mechanical interference with respiration produced by the swelling of the root of the tongue, is an œdema of the glottis. The phlegmonous process may also extend through the floor of the mouth and down along the neck. The origin of the acute condition, well known as Ludwig's angina, which invades the deep connective-tissue planes of the neck, may usually be looked for in a suppurative peri-odontitis. The focal point of the resulting inflammation is in the floor of the mouth and to one side along the capsule of the submaxillary salivary gland. An inflammatory process may extend from the tongue in a similar manner into the loose connective tissue between the genioglossus and the mylohyoid muscles, and may also invade the neck like a Ludwig's angina.

To the dangers of asphyxia and of an extension of the phlegmon must be added the possibility of an inspiration pneumonia, for the stagnating saliva which constantly bathes the diseased tongue swarms with pathogenic organisms. As the patient is unable to swallow, this is continually flowing into the respiratory passages and induces peribronchial infiltrations and pneumonic processes. For this reason the treatment of a phlegmonous glossitis must be energetically conducted. The finger should be passed backward as far as possible over the root of the tongue, and under it, as a guard, a scalpel or, better, a curved bistoury is introduced until its point reaches beyond the circumvallate papillæ. The point of the instrument is plunged deeply into the substance of the tongue and then drawn forward so as to cut to one side or the other of the median line, for the process is usually unilateral. Very often only blood and a cloudy serum issue from the wound, at other times there may also be pus. This procedure is ordinarily followed by an immediate reduction in size of the swelling, and is accompanied by very little hemorrhage. The wound is allowed to remain open, and although it appears quite deep when first made, it gives the impression of a mere superficial scarification after the swelling of the tongue has subsided. If marked hemorrhage takes place, the wound may be temporarily packed with iodoform gauze, and later closed by suture. Mouth-washes may now be prescribed, but should always be of a bland character. If the swelling develops rapidly from the very beginning, causing marked interference with respiration, accompanied by stridor and lividity of the face, an immediate tracheotomy should be done before incisions are made in the tongue.

Finally, in cases in which there was a marked induration in the submental region, and the skin red and œdematous, the author has made a deep incision extending between the genioglossi muscles and enlarged the wound in the substance of the tongue by blunt dissection. The evacuation of the foul-smelling pus always produced an immediate

amelioration of the pain and the dyspnœa. This incision has the ɛ
tage, moreover, of a complete evacuation, without the danger of pɩ
blood finding their way into the air-passages.

Sloughing of the tongue as a result of compression of the vess
the tension of the inflamed tissues has rarely been observed. It iɛ
likely that gangrene is produced by the pressure of the teeth on a sᵗ
tongue projecting beyond their borders, as in the case reported by ɩ

The author has already noted the more or less circumscribed gaɩ
of the tongue which may take place as the result of wounds or I
tions of the organ, with insufficient vascular connection to mainta
nutrition, or those which are due to hemorrhage which dissects ɩ
parenchyma of the tongue sufficient to produce a degree of tensio
may obstruct the vascular supply. A deep inflammatory glossiti
in a similar manner. Severe burns, as well as cauterization with
alkalies, or the actual cautery, also produce a gangrene of the m
membrane. Sloughing may be due to sutures introduced too
together or tied too tightly. Brindelle and Lafarelle claim that ɩ
tial gangrene of the tongue may result from pressure on the necɩ
cite an instance in which a man of seventy was seized by the
and partially strangled. This brought on an extensive hæmatomɪ
the hyoid bone, and from this locality the blood found its way in
root of the tongue and produced a swelling. A non-traumatic gaɩ
may also result from extension of a noma from the floor of the n
Gangrene of the tongue has finally been observed as a complicat
typhoid and puerperal fever, and Partsch reports having seen it ɛ
spontaneously in a case of diabetes.

The chronic abscesses of the tongue are quite rare. They are ɩ
a swelling which has been circumscribed from the beginning.
number of instances where reported they have undoubtedly been coɩ
with suppurating actinomycotic nodules.

TUMORS OF THE MOUTH.

Hæmangioma.—The simple angioma—telangiectasis—is u
present on the tongue as an elevated patch the size of a pea, ɛ
a deeper bluish-red color than its surroundings. On the m
membrane of the check it is apt to be larger. Its make-up of
lacing vessels is evident by the small dilated venules plainly visɪ
the periphery. At times the highly colored nævi usually found ɩ
external skin may extend over the lips into the mouth and ɩ
gums. Angiomata may appear, either single or multiple, on the tɩ
the cheek, or the soft palate, and exist alone or combined with ph
tasias. They may also cover or adjoin the second form of angiom
cavernous, which projects above the mucous membrane in the fo
dark-blue ridges and bunches, and also sinks deeply into the suhm
tissues. The size and elevation of these growths vary with the aɩ
of blood they may contain, increasing in diameter and tension ɩ

the act of stooping, and collapsing when the head is again held erect. They afford a soft impression to the palpating finger, and may be squeezed out like a sponge. As soon as the pressure is released they return to their original form.

These growths assume a clinical importance on account of the tendency which many of them show of extensive invasion of the surrounding tissues. It has already been noted that the cavernous tumors of the lips and cheeks may steadily increase in size and extend through the intervening soft parts until the mucous membrane is reached. In this way the entire cheek may be converted into a soft compressible tumor of a

Fig. 343.

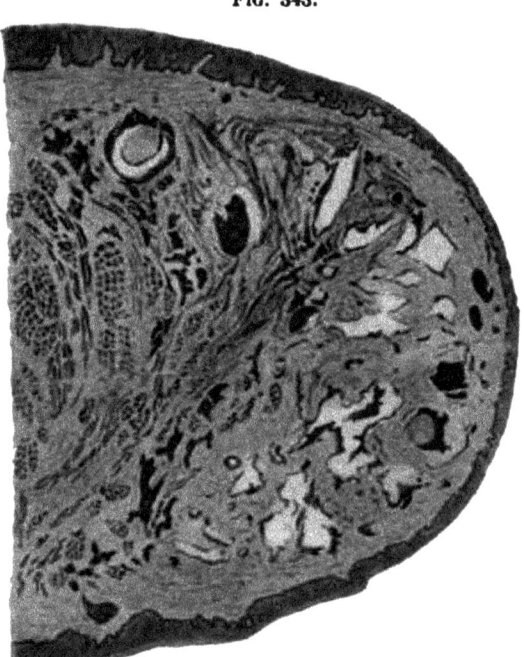

Cavernous angioma at end of the tongue.

bluish tint, with knob-like projections on the mucous surface and nowhere sharply marked off from the surrounding tissues. In other cases they may extend over the floor of the mouth and the soft palate, and may even involve the tongue, so that the entire side of the mouth is taken up by this enormous cavernous tumor. The snout-like protrusion of the lips is a very characteristic sign when these have become the site of such tumors. The atlases of v. Bruns, v. Mikulicz, and Michelson illustrate instances of this condition, and the author has also known cases in which the upper lip, the nose, the cheek, the eyelids, and the mucous membrane of the mouth back to the velum have all been verted into one large, soft, dark-blue tumor mass.

The tumors confined to the mucous membrane of the cheek for puffy elevations of a bluish color, over which the mucosa is thinne often excoriated. They are very liable to be caught between the and injured. Isolated cavernous tumors are rarely found on the of the mouth; when present, they are likely to have extended fro lower lip.

On the tongue these tumors are found as solitary growths of various sizes. Landerer describes one which involved the anterior half tongue and attained the dimensions of a fist. At times there m present simultaneously isolated cavernous tumors on the lips and to or on the lips and soft palate, and in other combinations.

The development of the smaller as well as the larger growths u proceeds from a telangiectatic patch, which may have been presen birth, but to which little or no attention was given. In this sen cavernous tumors may be looked upon as congenital, although main growth does not take place until a later period of life.

In considering the effects produced by these tumors, the res deformities are found to be of less importance than the sudde frequent hemorrhages or the inflammations to which these growt liable. Hemorrhages are very liable to occur from the large cavernous tumors, from progressive thinning and rupture of the lying mucous membrane, or traumatism. An inflammatory pro brought on by the entrance of an infection through a wound or ex tion. It may lead to suppuration, thrombosis, embolus, and g sepsis. Although this presents a very unfavorable course for one larger angioma, it may produce healing of the smaller varieties by cration of the dilated vessels. Such a process, however, has neve observed in the angiomata of the cheeks and tongue.

V. Mikulicz reports having seen a case of racemose aneurysm external maxillary artery which was particularly well developed the gums, and bled profusely on several occasions when teeth extracted.

Treatment.—The treatment of these angiomata depends on th of the growth. The small, blue, circular spots on the tongue : be left alone. In certain cases, in which patients were worri the fear of their being cancerous, the author has removed the cauterization.

The small circumscribed cavernous tumors may be extirpated. hemorrhage from these cases is not so severe as one would e especially, if the incision is made quickly and outside of the limits enlarged vessels. In the case of an extended flat angioma on the t or the inner surface of the lip, temporary compression may be s by the fingers of an assistant or the ring-shaped instrument recomm by v. Mikulicz for the tonsils. After local anaesthesia has been s a longitudinal incision is made through the growth and the spong scraped out with a sharp spoon down to healthy tissue. Wh pressure is released, the few small spurting arteries may be readily seized and ligated. The attempt has also been made to apply a provisional ligature around the base of the tongue.

The larger cavernous tumors call for operation when spontaneous hemorrhage has occurred several times. In these cases the patient's head must be kept low, and a preventive tamponade of the trachea may be necessary. The excision should be done as rapidly as possible.

The principal procedure directed against the diffuse and extensive cavernous tumors when they have become an element of danger by reason of frequent hemorrhages or continuous growth, is the method of ignipuncture introduced by Thiersch. If the tumor is especially soft and vascular, it is well to precede the operation by ligation of one or both lingual and external maxillary arteries. With the fine point of the Paquelin cautery at a dull glow a series of punctures are made into the substance of the growth quite close together. The inflammatory reaction and its consequences cause an obliteration of the growth, although it may be necessary to repeat the operation a number of times. Hemorrhage is liable to occur when the sloughs separate, and then a Péan's forceps may be applied to the bleeding point and allowed to remain in place for from twenty-four to forty-eight hours. The author has also had some success with a bit of sterilized sponge applied directly to the wound, which adheres by suction and may be left in place for several days. He has had good results with the injection of absolute alcohol into the depths of the tumor; an injection directly under the surface is very apt to cause sloughing of the mucous membrane.

Lymphangioma.—The lymphangiomata of the oral cavity are either cystic or cavernous. The cystic lymphangiectases occur in two forms: In the first place, as simple cysts, which are only recognized as being derived from a lymphatic origin by the detection of the endothelial lining in a microscopical section. They are situated on the end of the tongue or in the cheek, and Ratimow reports one case in which they occurred in the soft palate. They attain a considerable size and present an irregular outline. Along the base may sometimes be felt a ridge made up of smaller cysts or of cavernous tissue filled with lymph. The latter condition may point to the development of a single-celled cyst from what was originally cavernous lymphangioma, or at any rate it shows the close relationship between these two structures. Although their serous contents differed from the viscid fluid in the smaller cysts of the cheek, they were not considered as distinct until Ranke proved that the one was an enormous lymphatic varix and the other merely a retention-cyst.

The nodular type is another form of lymphangioma. This consists of small, isolated, hemispherical elevations scattered over the edge and the back of the tongue singly or in groups. Closer inspection with a hand lens shows the roughened surface covered with minute vesicles containing a watery, turbid, or a bloody fluid. In a few instances Dollinger has shown that the fungiform papillæ were the seat of the cystic degeneration. The firm base upon which these lesions are found

is an inflammatory product, and it is characteristic of these g1
that at irregular intervals they may become inflamed, and durir
period increase in size, which, together with a greater degree of
ration, remains as a permanent feature. A marked swelling
tongue may accompany this process, but it rapidly disappears
inflammation subsides.

The large simple cysts are also congenital tumors, but are not per
until some time after birth. They manifest themselves by their gra
increasing size or by an inflammatory process. If examined at ar
stage, groups of small vesicles in the vicinity of the nodular elev

Fig. 344.

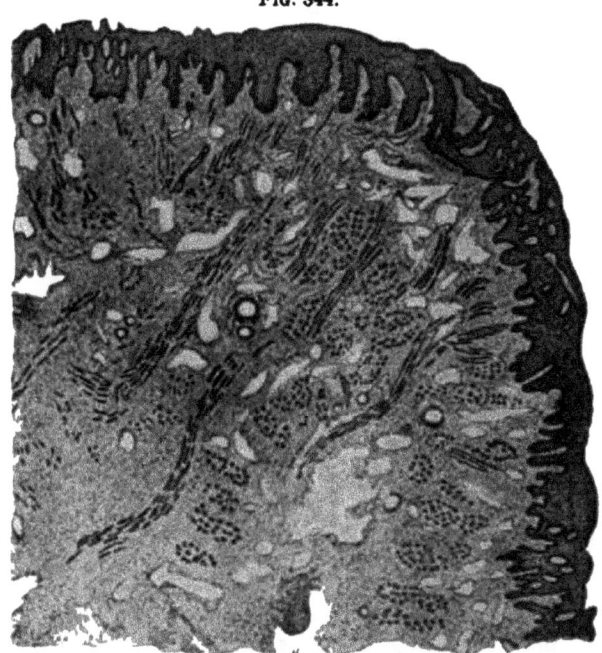

Section through a lymphangioma of the tongue (macroglossia). a, Lymphanode

may be seen on the part of the tongue that is yet perfectly n
This gives an impression as if the small cystic spaces under the el
epithelium constituted the original change, and the indurated base,
gives them the appearance of nodules, is the result of intercurrent i
mations. The latter are undoubtedly due to an infection which :
takes place through one of the numerous cysts which are present
surface of the tongue. This may also result in exceptional ex
abscesses, which appear after the swelling subsides, or in a phlegn
process which extends down the neck.

Treatment.—Treatment of these cases should be instituted a:
as possible. The lately introduced preparation known commerci

anæsthesin (a para-amidòbenzoic acid-ester) manifests its effects more rapidly than cocaine or eucaine, and the same is more lasting. By this means the tongue may be thoroughly anæsthetized and with the aid of the Paquelin cautery the growths thoroughly destroyed. The applications may need to be repeated, and months elapse before the lesion entirely disappears and the tongue is restored to its normal condition.

Macroglossia.—The cavernous lymphangiomata of the tongue may finally lead to that condition known as macroglossia. Formerly this was looked upon as a general hypertrophy of the tongue, until the researches of O. Weber, Virchow, Maas, and especially Wegner, showed conclusively that it was a true cavernous lymphangioma.

A macroglossia exists at birth, but usually does not become noticeable until the tongue has attained such a size that it projects beyond the teeth and lips. From this is derived the old name of the condition,

FIG. 345.

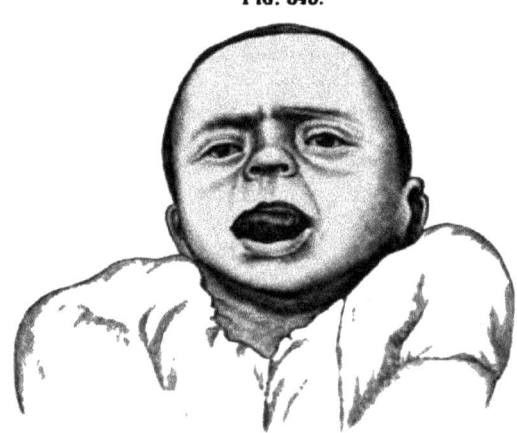

Macroglossia.

prolapsus linguæ. A good representation of the condition is seen in the appended illustration (Fig. 345) of a child one and a half years of age. That part of the tongue projecting beyond the teeth is of a dark-red color, excoriated, fissured, and ulcerated, and here and there presents a number of adherent brown crusts. A deep furrow caused by the teeth or the free edge of the alveolar process surrounds the tongue and divides it into two parts. That lying within the line of the teeth may entirely fill the cavity of the month, which accounts for the disturbances in speech and swallowing, and the interference with respiration, all of which may gradually assume a dangerous aspect. If it is possible in an early case to obtain a view of the back of the tongue, the entire surface of the latter is seen to be covered with vesicles of about the size of the head of a pin. The constant pressure of the protruding tongue gradually produces an eversion of the lips and also results in changes in the lower jaw. If teeth are present they are forced to assume a horizontal position, and

the middle section is bent outward and downward. This interfere
the development of the bone, and in consequence it remains narro
thin.

As long as the diseased tongue remains within the limits of th
cavity it may not annoy the patient very much for some years, bu
painful inflammations are apt to come on at more and more fr
intervals. During such an attack the tongue becomes very large
held between the teeth. In the interval it sinks into the mouth, a
mains in a quiescent state until a fresh swelling again causes it to p

A histological examination of one of these enlarged tongues
that it is traversed by a large number of irregular hollow sinuses.
clefts extend down to the upper surface of the papillæ or further,
rating the muscle-fibres. The connective tissue contains many cell
does not form compact masses, but merely extends as a loose ne
between the sinuses. At various points are large collections of lyn
cells resembling the lymph-follicles. A distinct endothelial linir
be demonstrated in all the sinuses. The relations between the enc
connective tissue and the sinuses depends on the dimensions
latter. If these are large and dilated, the connective tissue is
represented, and *vice versa*. The marked development of con
tissue and the cellular infiltration may properly be considered as
quences of an inflammatory proc es. Blood has also been repe
found in these sinuses, pointing to a mixed growth—a hæmatol
angioma.

A congenital macroglossia may in rare instances involve the
tongue. In the case illustrated, only the anterior half of the
was altered, the part on the distal side of the circumvallate papillæ
apparently unchanged. Aside from the large diffuse lymphangi
which involve such extensive sections of the tongue, a circums
form is also known. The latter may afford the impression of a fi
or a sarcoma, as they appear in the form of a sharply marked-off
in the anterior part of the tongue. They are moderately hard,
little in size, and are only slightly compressible. Their surface
guishes them from the other forms of tumors. The mucous men
is tightly adherent and cannot be separated from the growth,
covered to a greater or lesser degree with the small vesicles pre
described. When the diagnosis is doubtful, it is always well to e
the lesion with the hand lens.

Treatment.—The treatment of the smaller tumors, in order to
hemorrhage and infection, should consist in their destruction wi
thermocautery. The site of operation may first be anæsthetized
suitable constricting clamp applied before cauterization.

The large diffuse tumors, the macroglossia, may be diminis
size and finally removed by a series of wedge-shaped incisions. Fe
has observed that a diminution in size followed ligation of both lir
and it may be advisable to do this before the operation. A wedge-
section of tissue is then excised from the tongue on each side
median line, with the base corresponding to the upper surface

tongue, and the point directed downward into its substance. It may be necessary to repeat this operation several times, and finally a similar piece may also be excised from the tip, with its base consisting of the latter itself. The wounds should be closed with deep sutures placed close together. The operation is not without danger to a young child, both on account of the time necessary for its execution and the possibility of infection from the ulcerated surface.

Cystic Tumors of the Mouth.

Cysts of the Mucous Glands.—These cystic tumors must be distinguished from the lymphatic cysts discussed in the preceding section. Like them, they are situated on the inner surface of the lips and cheeks, but more rarely on the edge or the under surface of the tongue. They are, properly speaking, retention cysts, and consist of small, transparent, spherical tumors of a bluish color. The contents consist of a fluid, viscid, mucoid or colloid material. Their derivation is from the mucous glands, and examination of their thinned-out walls often shows the presence of small islands of epithelium on the inner surface.

The peculiar bluish gloss and the thinned-out mucous membrane may lead to mistaking it for hæmangioma. The latter, however, is not so well localized, and usually appears in more than one part of this region as irregular elevations of a darker blue color. The characteristic differences between these mucous cysts and the lymphocysts have been discussed, consisting chiefly of the larger size and irregular form of the latter together with the presence of palpable ridges in their bases.

As a rule these small retention-cysts cause very slight disturbances and are only discovered when situated on the lips or on the cheek near the line of contact between the teeth. During the act of mastication they may be caught between the latter and crushed or torn open.

Their removal may readily be accomplished by shelling them out, or they may be incised and the walls scraped away with a sharp spoon.

A larger interest, on account of their origin, is shared by the cysts in the posterior part of the tongue near the foramen cæcum, the third tonsil, and the valleculæ. They may arise from the mucous glands of the tongue, which often have a comparatively long excretory duct, or from one of the larger mucous glands which open into the furrows between the circumvallate papillæ, or finally from the remnants of the pars lingualis of the thyroglossal duct. The latter forms a number of freely branching tubules lined with ciliated epithelium. These structures do not possess any particular clinical interest, and are usually overlooked or only discovered by accident. Any symptoms which they may cause are similar to those due to an hypertrophy of the lingual tonsil. Contact with the epiglottis may cause a reflex cough or afford the sensation of a foreign body, such as a hair, deep down in the throat. Inspection with the laryngeal mirror, or better, with the autoscope of Kirstein, readily reveals the source of these disturbances, and their removal may be accomplished by means of a small bistoury or cauterization.

A peculiar and rare form of cyst is sometimes found on the tip tongue. It is quite transparent, reaches the size of a walnut, projects one side, and is covered with the pale-red mucous. This is a ... of retention-cyst, and is derived from one of the glands of Nuhn under the mucous membrane and a single layer of longitudinal fibres.

Echinococcus cysts are found in rare instances in the tongue floor of the mouth, where they may be confused with ranula. The ... of the cysticercus have been observed a number of times on the floor of the mouth, and on the tongue. They are often like the mucous cysts, but are much harder, less transparent, and can be about with the fingers. Finally they are always multiple, never less three have been seen on the tongue, and are found in ...
body at the same time.

Fig. 246.

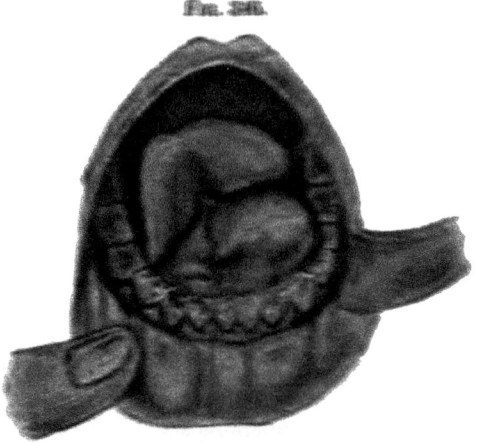

Ranula.

Ranula.—The term ranula is applied to a cyst situated under tongue, which occupies the space between the frenum and the ... the jaw and displaces the tongue upward (Fig. 246). They ... on one side, but with advancing growth, extend across the mid ... and are then notched by the frenum. The larger cysts may ... dent under the chin and may invade the tongue to a considerable ... Very rarely a ranula may begin in the median line and remain attached near the line of the teeth.

These cysts are present in the form of a rounded tumor in the ... the mouth, of a grayish-red color and quite transparent. The ... the overlying mucous are plainly visible, and the latter appears ... but is readily movable over the mass. A probe can easily be ... Wharton's duct. The entire appearance may be compared to a ... filled with water lying under the tongue, and this resemblance ... throat of a frog has probably led to the application of the term ...

The cyst, which is almost always unicellular, and only in rare cases multilocular, contains a viscid fluid of the consistency of egg albumin, and is ordinarily colorless, though at times it may assume a greenish, red, or brown tint.

A ranula may occur at any time of life and also congenitally. Its growth is slow but progressive. Little attention may be paid to the growth at first, but as it increases in size it causes mechanical interference with speech and nutrition, and in very large tumors respiration may be affected, especially if infection and sloughing of the floor of the mouth are added. The latter fortunately is a rare occurrence. The more frequent course which the affection may take is known as acute ranula. This refers to the acute enlargement of a previously unnoticed small cyst, in which, owing to some irritation, there is a sudden and pronounced transudation from the capillaries of the cyst-wall. In these cases the symptoms are apt to be much more pronounced than in the other form.

Fig. 347.

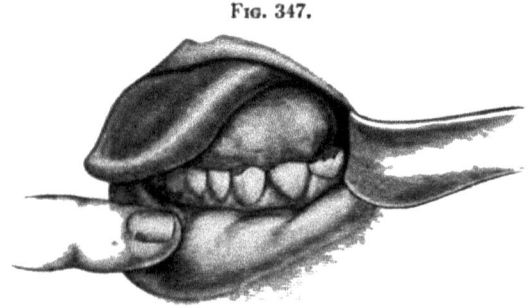

Ranula.

If a ranula attains a considerable size during the years of early childhood it may produce marked disturbances of growth in the inferior maxillary bone. The lower jaw may then·project beyond the upper to the extent of several centimetres, rendering approximation of the teeth impossible when the mouth is closed. The teeth, moreover, do not develop to their full size, are separated by a considerable interval, and are directed outwardly.

According to the modern conceptions, this growth may be one of three things: either an epithelial cyst derived from the tubule of one of Bochdalek's glands (Neumann), or a cyst of the gland at the end of the tongue, known as Blandin-Nuhn's gland (v. Recklinghausen), or a retention-cyst of the sublingual and in rare cases the glandula incisiva (v. Hippel).

Regarding the first, it may be said that the frequent finding of ciliated epithelium on the inner wall of the cyst serves to demonstrate the truth of Neumann's theory. This cannot be considered abnormal, as claimed by v. Recklinghausen, but must be ascribed to a derivation from ciliated epithelium found in the tongue in only one locality, namely, the ducts of Bochdalek's glands. The latter, according to present embryological knowledge, are derived from the lingual duct, which is a branch . upper part of the thyroglossal duct.

The theory advanced by v. Recklinghausen, that the typical ran derived from the gland of Blandin-Nuhn, does not appear to be s substantiated. Undoubtedly a cyst may result from occlusion and tation of the excretory duct of the gland at the end of the tongu the clinical picture differs greatly from what has been accepted f well-known ranula. The point of the tongue itself is the seat of the in this instance, and it seems improbable that in the further grow latter should by any possibility appear under the chin.

All the symptoms are more easily understood if the subli salivary gland is looked upon as the point of origin of the n According to v. Hippel, the cyst begins in one of the smaller exc ducts of this gland. The first step is a chronic interstitial inflamn of the sublingual gland, and the new connective tissue which forms compresses the smaller ducts. This results in retention of the sec and dilatation of the passages. By pressure, atrophy of the walls cysts follows and a number of the cavities become confluent. The f growth results from a profuse transudation from the numerous cap vessels in the cyst-walls and from a mucous degeneration of the c epithelial cells in the cavity. This accounts for the viscid character contents, which originally consisted merely of saliva.

The researches of v. Hippel are of particular value because they carried out on completely extirpated ranules, and not merely on a the excised wall of the cyst. The sublingual salivary gland pro serves as the point of origin of the majority of these ranules, an accounts for the fact that in the extended growth of these tumor invade the substance of the mylohyoid muscle. Morestin has d strated in addition that the sublingual gland may normally send prol tions between the fibres of the mylohyoid muscle, which explair presence of a swelling in the submental region after the ranula has been excised. The rare instances of median ranula, which directly behind the teeth, are traced by the same authority to the dula incisiva of Suzanne and Merkel, a group of glands found di under the mucous membrane in the middle line close to the inner s of the inferior maxilla.

There are a number of affections which may closely simulate the cal picture of a ranula, so that it may be a matter of difficulty to whether a ranula in the restricted sense as just defined is present. distinction has ordinarily little influence on the therapeutic me employed, and need only be considered in case an angioma migh been mistaken for a ranula and treatment instituted consisting of excision or the injection of tincture of iodine. In such a case unpl consequences would be likely to follow.

Diagnosis.—The differential diagnosis is concerned rather wi cysts of the floor of the mouth than with solid tumors. Of tumor be mentioned those of the sublingual salivary gland and the lipo the floor of the mouth, both of which are extremely rare. The

abandoned since their anatomical construction has been determined. These growths can only arise from abnormal invaginations of the outer germinal layer during embryonic life, in one of several localities. The most common is the embryonal cleft between the second and third gill-arches, next the region of the junction of the first and second gill-arches and the incompletely developed parts of the inferior maxilla. As a matter of fact, the majority of these dermoids are found in the hyoid or submental regions between the skin and the floor of the mouth, in some cases attached to the hyoid bone, in others to the inferior maxilla. A few are directly under the skin and outside of the mylohyoid muscle, which forms the diaphragm of the floor of the mouth. The larger number are

FIG. 348.

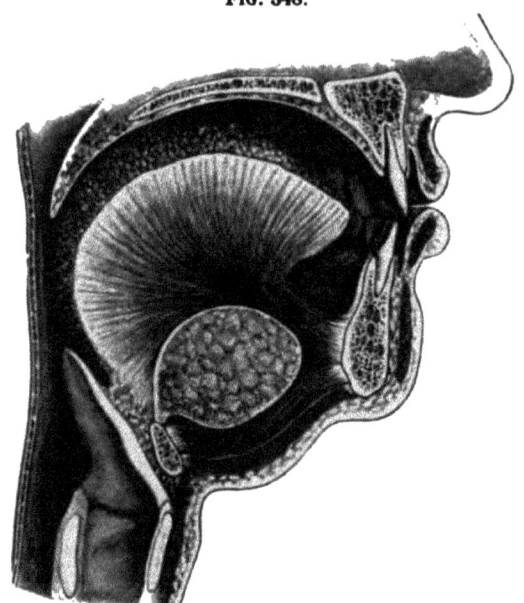

Dermoid cyst at base of tongue. (Marchant.)

situated more deeply between the geniohyoids, and some may extend between the genioglossi even further into the substance of the tongue. In the latter case they form a cavity in the tongue, change its shape, and cause a projection of the surface in the posterior section. It is possible that the presence of a dermoid in the epiglottic region may be due to a growth which has penetrated further than usual into the deep muscles of the tongue.

The dermoids of practical importance are the submental forms, which are separated from the cavity of the mouth by the mylohyoid muscle, and the sublingual varieties, which are situated between the geniohyoid and genioglossi muscles and therefore close to the floor of the mouth.

The former can be included in the upper region of the neck, the mental region; the latter belong more properly to the cavity of the n

The submental dermoids first become evident as a projection the chin directly in the middle line, and readily afford the impress what is commonly known as a double chin. The tumor is of a hemi ical shape and varies in size from that of a hazelnut to that of an o The overlying skin is unchanged and easily thrown into folds, the s of the tumor is smooth and elastic, and fluctuation is indistinct. can sometimes be produced by firm pressure, or the latter affor impression of a doughy mass. If the examination is conducted th the mouth, the tumor can be made more evident by pressure a under the chin; but if the growth has reached any considerable siz at once brought into view as soon as the mouth is opened. The

Fig. 349.

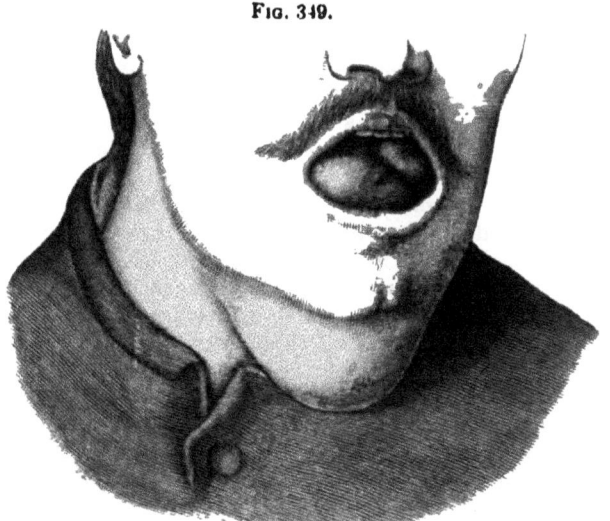

Dermoid of the floor of the mouth.

stages in the development of both varieties are practically alik when a tumor has reached the size of an orange it is impossible to mine from what source it may have originated.

A sublingual dermoid of moderate size can only be palpated th the mouth. As it enlarges it may also become evident in the subr region, but never to that degree caused by a tumor which origina this locality. When pressure is applied from within the mouth, i be felt in the space over the hyoid bone. The mucous membr freely movable over the smooth and ordinarily fluctuating tumo it increases in size it produces the same symptoms as those of a r disturbances of speech, displacement upward of the tongue, diffici swallowing, interference with movements of the tongue and respii

Dermoids are sometimes found to one side of the median line, and may be mistaken for ranulæ; the manner of differentiating these two conditions has already been discussed. The submental variety of dermoid may also resemble a lipoma. The latter, however, is not limited to the median line and discloses to the palpating finger its lobular character and softer consistency.

Diagnosis.—Although these dermoids are congenital structures, they are rarely recognized during infancy and only in cases in which continued difficulty in nursing may lead to examination of the mouth. Roland has published a tabulated statement of the time of life at which dermoids are found; in 50 cases, it was seen 4 times in children under five years, 4 times in those under fifteen, 27 times between the fifteenth and twenty-fifth year, and twice at the age of fifty. The growth of these tumors is extremely slow and gradual, but a more rapid increase may take place during the time of puberty, which accounts for the larger number of cases seen between the fifteenth and the twenty-fifth year. Occasionally suppuration has resulted from a puncture or an exploratory incision; the tumor then becomes tender and enlarges rapidly, the overlying skin or mucous membrane takes on a red tinge, and perforation or a spreading phlegmonous inflammation in the connective tissue of the neck may threaten the patient.

The walls and the contents of these cysts are characterized by the same features as found in other dermoid tumors. Rosenberg reports having seen in a dermoid of the lingual tonsil a tooth which was attached to a connective-tissue pedicle growing out from the inner wall.

Treatment.—Treatment consists in extirpation of the tumor. At one time this was always conducted through the mouth, probably because this and ranula were thought to be one and the same condition. The best way to reach the growth is through the suprahyoid region in a manner similar to that recommended by v. Hippel for the operation for ranula. The incision starts at the chin in the middle line, and extends over the growth down to the hyoid bone. The geniohyoid muscles are then pulled apart at their middle point and held to one side with the aid of blunt retractors. The surface of the cyst is then exposed, and the tumor may be readily freed by blunt dissection, the only adhesions which need cutting are those on the hyoid and the jaw. If there has been any surrounding inflammation, the removal of the cyst is rendered more difficult, and may lead to injuries of the mucous membrane. In the latter case the wound should be lightly packed with iodoform gauze, otherwise it may be closed by suture and a short drainage-tube inserted between the muscles. If no infection has resulted in the open wound during the first four days, the packing may be removed and the opening closed by secondary suture.

In the same class with the dermoids of the oral cavity, the author also includes the extremely rare teratoid tumors in the region of the tongue and palate. The discussion as to whether they are fetal inclusions or fetal derivatives, heterochthonous or autochthonous, is not appropriate at this point. The known cases of the tumors in question have been

collected by Niemczyk and are 20 in number. They are charactei
by a covering of hairy skin and assume a polypoid, club- or pear-shi
form. They are attached to the posterior wall of the pharynx neai
orifices of the Eustachian tubes, to the posterior aspect of the soft pa
the areus palatoglossus and pharyngeus, the tonsils, or even to the
palate. They ordinarily cause but little annoyance, and are only casi
discovered on inspection of the month or pharynx. In cases in w
they come in contact with the epiglottis they may bring about a r
cough, or if with the posterior pharyngeal wall, a tendency to retc
may be caused. More serious symptoms have occasionally appeari
infants from the interference with nursing or the production of asph;
In such cases their removal was readily accomplished with a knife
pair of scissors or the galvanocaustic snare.

These tumors are as a rule quite small and made up principally oi
so that they might be easily mistaken for pedunculated lipomata wi
not for the presence of the epidermoid covering. In certain insta
there were found in addition near the pedicle small cartilaginous pl
with a perichondrium and a few points of ossification, and stri
muscle-fibres. The resemblance between these tumors and the
called open dermoids of the rectum is plainly evident. In the l
the outer surface is also found made up of a hairy skin which covi
mass of fat and enclosing cartilage and bone, often teeth and nervi

The Solid, Non-carcinomatous Tumors of the Tongue.

Lipoma.—Lipoma of the tongue has been observed in a comj
tively small number of cases which have been collected from the
tered literature of the subject by Knoche and Krausnick. Knoche
that in 29 cases of lipoma of the oral cavity, the tumor was preser
times on the tongue, 9 times on the floor of the mouth, 7 times oi
lips, and once on the gums and soft palate.

These growths are usually discovered directly under the mu
membrane of the floor of the month, although they do not all arise ;
the submucosa, and many probably originate deep down between
muscular layers. The thinned-out overlying mucous membrane is
adherent and may be picked up in small folds. The loss of the pai
deprives it of the velvety appearance by which it is normally character;
and its thinness permits the light-yellow color of the lipoma to be ii
tinctly seen. In the majority of the cases reported the lipoma
situated on the tip of the tongue somewhat to one side, as show
Fig. 350. In the latter instance, when the tongue was withdraw
swelling appeared in the right cheek, giving one the impression
tumor of the upper jaw. When the tongue was protruded the wi
of the growth dragged it downward and to the right. The movem
of the tongue did not seem to be interfered with in the least, and
same fact has been noticed in the presence of other large lipomata.
lipomata in the floor of the month are distinctly lobulated, which rea
distinguishes them from ranulas and dermoids, aside from their n

lateral position. The lipomata of the cheeks are situated exclusively in the submucous layer, a position which distinguishes them from the large lipomata of the outer skin. They are easily recognized, as they present all the characteristics of a fatty tumor. Their treatment by extirpation does not present unusual difficulties.

A not inconsiderable part of these growths are apparently congenital. In one instance, reported by Poncet, connective tissue was present to such a degree that the growth might have been described as a transitional form of fibroma. A preponderance of adipose tissue is not only found in certain teratoid tumors, but also in other neoplasms of a mixed nature which may have cartilage and bone embedded in them. Such

Fig. 350.

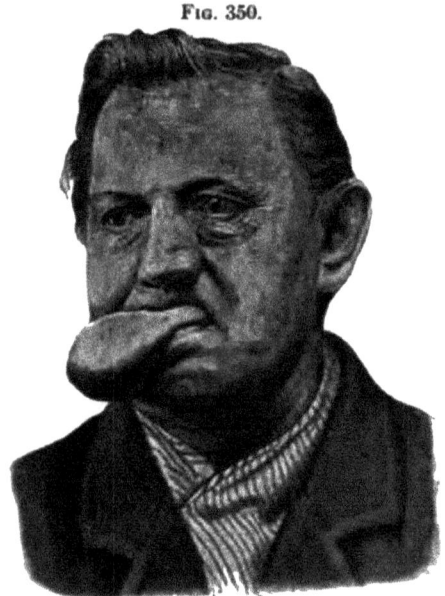

Lipoma of tongue.

cases have been collected by Lannelongue, and are also commented on by v. Mikulicz and Kümmel.

Papilloma and Fibroma.—Connective-tissue growths in a more restricted sense comprise both papillomata and hard fibromata. The papillomata are peculiar growths, usually found on the uvula, the palatal arches, or the dorsal surface of the tongue. They are often pediculated, and vary in size from that of the head of a pin to that of a hazelnut. The surface is nodular and their consistence varies from comparative hardness to extreme softness. As they are painless and cause but little trouble, no attention is ordinarily given them, and they are only casually discovered during an examination for some other purpose. If these growths cause annoyance, they may be easily snipped off with a pair

of scissors. When situated at the tip of the tongue a papilloma
sometimes be confused with a small cavernous angioma.

M. Kahn has seen 83 cases of papillomata of the mouth and phi
and compares them with others described in the literature of the su
A noteworthy point in his account is the frequent appearance of
growths after chronic inflammations in the mouth and pharynx.
calls attention to the coincidence which seems to exist between pi
mata on the posterior section of the tongue and similar multiple gr
of the larynx.

Hard fibromata are rare occurrences, even if there is included he
cicatricial-like connective tissue, which contains few cells but pr
a distinct form and outline. Most likely a number of inflamn
indurations have also been included in this group. Silbermann des
a swelling of the tongue which had been present for a period of
years and was about the size of a hazelnut. It was made up er
of broad bands of connective tissue enclosing scattered giant cell
considered by the author to be a reactionary hyperplasia, due t
irritation set up by a few wool-fibres which had penetrated the subs
of the tongue. The fibromata proper have been described as sn
hard tumors in the parenchyma of the tongue, which may reael
size of a pigeon's egg. These are usually only felt in the substan
the tongue, and rarely project above the surface. A marked chara
istic is their extremely slow growth, no change taking place in
cases in ten or more years, and their complete separation fron
surrounding tissues. Their differential diagnosis will be consider
connection with the sarcomata. The treatment consists in extirpa

Endothelioma.—But very few growths have been described t
the designation of an endothelioma of the oral cavity. Before I
defined the clinical characteristics of this group of neoplasms they
included with the sarcomata, adenomata, myxomata, and other I
of mixed tumors. The case described by Santesson as a "sar
plexiforme hyalinum linguale," and also that of Barth were und
edly of this character. The researches of Volkmann first helped to
up this obscurity. The plexiform disposition of the rows of cell:
a hyaline degeneration, seen on microscopical examination, establis
true status of these endotheliomata. Their clinical aspects pi
greater variations. As a rule the diagnosis can be based on the
growth, which may extend over many years, the soft consistence, a
degree of lobulation or furrowing, a freely movable mucous memb
and well-marked encapsulation. The size varies within conside
limits. Their favorite site in the oral cavity, of which the antho
seen four examples, is at the angle which the soft palate makes
the arcus palatoglossus, the region near the ascending ramus o
lower jaw. One of these tumors which he removed was the size
small apple, but elongated, and extended into the cellular tissue o
side of the pharynx. Considering its size, this growth caused com
tively little disturbance until it began to interfere with speech, pro
by coming in contact with the tongue. In all four cases remova

readily accomplished through an incision in the mucous membrane by blunt dissection.

Ulceration of these tumors may be the result of external trauma. Both the clinical and the histological diagnosis may be surrounded with difficulties in certain cases, for in several instances plates of bone and cartilage have been found in the connective-tissue stroma besides the hyaline, colloid, and other products of a retrograde metamorphosis.

Adenoma.—Tumors consisting of tissue derived from the thyroid gland are sometimes found at the base of the tongue near the foramen cæcum, and have until recently been described as adenomata. Attention was first directed to them by R. Wolf at the Surgical Congress in 1882. He found in an eighteen-year-old girl a firm, hard tumor, the size of a walnut, in the tongue near the epiglottis, which gradually enlarged and caused interference with the act of swallowing. On removal it was found to be made up of thyroid tissue. Since then a number of cases of such accessory strumous growths at the base of the tongue have been reported. Chamisso de Boncourt has collected about 18 examples, and later instances have been added by Benjamins, Watson, Teweles, and others. All of these were discovered in young women. The growths are invariably situated in the median line, their surface is smooth or slightly notched, they are elastic, and their vascularity is well marked. Dilated vessels are seen coursing over their upper surface, which is usually of a pinkish color. (Fig. 342.)

The thyroglossal duct empties at the foramen cæcum, and at this point are found embedded in the substance of the tongue the suprahyoid glands as remnants of the embryonic middle lobe of the thyroid gland. The further growth of these produces one of the neoplasms in question. Other fetal remnants are found in the neighborhood of the duct further down near the hyoid bone, the so-called accessory thyroids, which are also apparently only observed in the female sex. Bernays reports a case of this kind in which the growth penetrated deeply into the root of the tongue, and was removed through an incision in the suprahyoid region.

The extirpation of these tumors is usually possible through the mouth, but a preliminary tracheotomy, together with tamponade of the trachea, is indispensable. The tongue must be drawn forward by temporary ligatures passed through the anterior part, one on each side of the median line. If this procedure causes too pronounced narrowing of the isthmus the palatoglossal folds may be divided. When the growth is large and vascular, Wolf recommends temporary resection of the inferior maxilla near the angle.

An interesting observation is reported by Seldowitsch, who saw a myxœdema develop after the extirpation of an accessory thyroid tumor at the base of the tongue.

Sarcoma.—The rarely encountered sarcomata of the mouth are, as in the case of the other tumors just mentioned, usually found in the tongue, and more often during the period of childhood than otherwise. They do not seem to favor any particular part of the tongue, and vary greatly in size, from examples scarcely as large as a hazelnut to weighing 13 ounces, removed by Poncet.

The growth of the sarcomata is very characteristic. Small tu may remain stationary for a long time, then suddenly take rapid growth, or the increase in size may be rapid from the b ning. In this case they disintegrate very quickly, ulceration sloughing being in direct proportion to the rapidity of growth. is an accompaniment of even the smaller tumors, and becomes severe when the growth breaks down. The pain resembles that ca by carcinoma, is not constant, and radiates usually toward the ear. they are ordinarily of the round-cell type of sarcoma, they are a be quite soft, are not well differentiated from the surrounding tis and are closely united to the mucous membrane. After they reached a certain size ulceration of the surface is rarely absent. growth does not remain flat, but assumes a funnel or crater-like sh

Fig. 351.

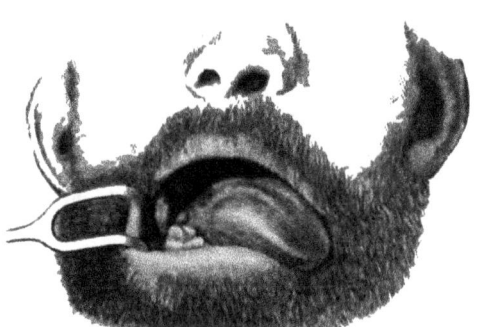

Interstitial sarcoma of tongue.

and at the bottom of this the presence of necrotic tissue may lea the diagnosis of a broken-down gumma or a carcinoma. This re blance may become even more marked when the sarcoma at its appearance is the seat of an ulcerative process. Korte reports a in which there was little evidence of any tumor, but there was pr a deep, irregular, discolored ulcer on the upper surface of the ton which caused intense pain and interfered with swallowing. Antis ilitic treatment did not meet with response, the tuberculin reaction absent, the examination of bits of excised tissue did not afford t worthy information. The rapid increase in size of the ulcer prom the cutting out and examination of a larger segment of tissue, w was finally proved to be round-cell sarcoma. An extensive oper was immediately done, but the patient soon succumbed to the ra appearing recurrences.

The rare melanotic tumors found on the soft palate can be recogn as sarcoma without difficulty. The only error may consist in mista their black pigmentation for the glistening appearance produced by a cavernous angioma.

Prognosis.—The sarcomata are attended by a good prognosis if they can be removed in the very early stages. Local recurrences, moreover, do not take place when the tumor has been present for a considerable time but has grown very slowly. The neighboring lymph-glands are ordinarily not involved. The outlook in the case of a pediculated sarcoma is also a favorable one. A bad prognosis, however, is afforded by the rapidly growing and ulcerating forms. Local recurrences quickly follow their apparently complete extirpation, the lymph-glands become involved, and metastatic deposits in the internal organs and in other remote parts of the body are common.

Nägele has collected 30 cases of sarcoma of the tongue (although 3 of these seemed to have been endotheliomata and 1 a decubital ulcer), of which 15 were located on the back, 7 at the base, 4 on the edge, and 4 on the inferior surface of the tongue. In 5 instances the tumor was pediculated. Three cases were congenital and rapidly assumed dangerous proportions. Aside from these there were 4 other cases found in children under ten years of age. Of 28 cases in which the course was influenced by extirpation, 14 were definitely cured.

Treatment.—The only method of treatment is the thorough extirpation of the involved sections of the tongue by the methods about to be described under Cancer of the Tongue.

Differential Diagnosis.—In every case of nodular tumor of the tongue the surgeon is placed in the position of not only distinguishing them from other tumors, but also from circumscribed inflammatory processes. These include the tumor-like syphilitic and tuberculous neoplasms, the nodules of actinomycosis, the decubital induration, carcinoma, cysts, lipoma, fibroma, endothelioma, and the accessory thyroid. The papilloma and the polypoid teratomatous growths are not included here, as their characteristic form establishes the diagnosis at once. Exceptionally a papilloma on the upper surface of the tongue may be mistaken for a pediculated sarcoma or a small cavernous angioma which projects above the surface of the mucous membrane. The wart-like surface, the slight degree of ulceration, and the absence of the peculiar color, serve as the means of distinguishing the papillomata.

The characteristic point about the cavernous lymphoma is the presence of the small vesicles on their upper surface, which may require a hand lens for their recognition. The angiomata are compressible, usually of a dark-blue color, diffuse or in patches, and combined· at times with telangiectases or phlebectasias. A decubital induration presupposes an irritating tooth in the vicinity, without which it may be impossible to make a diagnosis, and no doubt it has often been mistaken for a fibroma, a sarcoma, or a carcinoma.

The diagnosis of a strumous growth is simple. It is always found in the middle of the posterior part of the tongue, dilated veins run over it, the growth is slow, and up to the present it has been observed only in young girls and women.

There are many instances in which it may be impossible to d:
entiate a fibroma, endothelioma, sarcoma, or even a small lipoma
a tuberculous conglomerate in nodular form, a syphilitic induratio
hard gumma, or an actinomycosis nodule. The idea of a tuberci
neoplasm would be supported by the presence at the same time
tuberculous process in the lungs or the larynx. The initial sclero:
syphilitic infection is always accompanied by a swelling of the adjo
lymph-glands, and a gumma is usually multiple and associated w
characteristic history. The latter is also found almost invariably ii
centre of the movable part of the tongue and near its tip.

The transparency and the fluctuation of the smaller cysts and
of the larger cyst from Nuhn's gland have already been noted. A:
sarcoma is not the only tumor which is subject to ulceration, the l
characteristic is insufficient for making a diagnosis—ulceration
occurs in fibroma, endothelioma, and even in lipoma, as the resu
irritation or trauma. The nodule of actinomycosis often shows the s
yellow color through the thinned-out overlying mucous membrane
found in a lipoma. It may be distinguished from the latter, how
by its more rapid growth, its adhesion to the mucosa, and the palp
central softening. A gumma before breaking down may give the s
impression. There is one stage in the development of both in w
it is practically impossible to differentiate them from fibroma, end
lioma, or sarcoma. The lipoma may be recognized by their soft
sistence, their lobular form, and the fact that the overlying mucosa
be thrown into folds.

A hard sarcoma of slow growth may be readily mistaken for a fibr
and an endothelioma can only be differentiated from either by a m
scopical examination. The site at which one of these tumors is f
may somewhat influence the opinion as to their character.

As a matter of fact the diagnosis is of little benefit to the patient
in all cases extirpation at an early stage in their growth is indic:
Even a gumma is most readily gotten rid of by an operation, in add
to the necessary constitutional treatment. If an actinomycosis no
has broken down, the presence of the peculiar little yellow grains ii
discharge confirms the diagnosis. A broken-down gumma, how
will still be difficult to differentiate from an ulcerating sarcom
carcinoma. The latter topic will be treated in connection witl
diagnosis of cancer.

Cancer of the Tongue.—Adherents of the parasitic theory of
origin of cancer, who believe that the specific germ of the disease e
the body through the medium of the food, will hardly be prepare
explain that among 1000 women, only 13 are affected with carcin
of the lips, oral cavity, and tongue, while 243 suffer from carcinon
the mammæ. Of these 13 cases, 8 were found on the lips, 3 on
tongue, and 2 in other parts of the mouth. Of 1000 cases of canc
the male sex, 111 occurred in the oral cavity, of which 77 were ol
lips, 21 on the tongue, and 13 on other parts of the oral mucosa. Si
tics collected by Stützer from various hospitals showed that in 100 o

of carcinoma of the tongue the percentage of males affected is 83.55 and of females 16.45. This relationship is explained by the habits of smoking and the use of alcohol, which are more prevalent in men. Barker has aroused considerable interest by his claim that there has been a relative increase in the number of cases of cancer of the tongue during the last few decades. In England, during the years from 1872–1881, the number of cases increased from 26 per 1000 to 115 per 1000. In the author's clinic 178 cases were seen during the period from 1884 to 1891, of which 142 were males and 36 females. Operation was done on 159; the remainder were inoperable or refused treatment.

Oral cancer begins in one of three localities: the tongue, the mucous membrane of the cheeks, or that of the floor of the mouth. Proof of the development of carcinoma from a chronic irritation or a previous non-malignant tissue hyperplasia may be found in any of these situations. There seems to be a well-marked dependence of cancer on a leucoplakia; in the author's list of 159 cases, the growth was preceded by a leucoplakia in 34.6 per cent. of the cases, and in 19.2 per cent. the white patches were few in number and not prominent. In more than 50 per cent. therefore the two conditions were present at one time or another. This is not an accidental association, but a further proof of the claims made by Nedopil and Schuchardt, that a proliferation of the surface epithelium is followed by a penetration of these cells into the deeper layers, a transformation of a pachydermatitis of the oral mucosa into an epithelioma.

The larger number of cases of leuco-plakia are not followed by cancerous de-generation. This corresponds with the fact that unchanged papillæ and mucous glands are found under white plaques. The deviations from the normal described by Schuchardt are associated with the large and thick patches, where columns of epithelial cells extend down between the papillæ. The mitotic figures in these in-stances are easily recognized, indicating

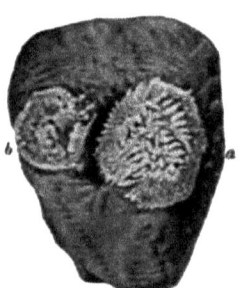

Fig. 352.

Carcinoma of the tongue.

active growth. In other cases the papillæ are merely elongated and thickened, and probably infiltrated with leucocytes. In one case which came under the author's observation a papillary excrescence and an epithelial invagination were seen on the tongue at the same time (Fig. 352); *b* referring to ulcerating carcinomatous nodule with raised edges, *a* to a papilloma adjacent to the latter and made up of papillomata cornified at their tips. Both of these lesions were covered by a leuco-plakic patch. In 21.6 per cent. of the author's cases, in which no traces of leucoplakia could be discovered, opposite to the growth was found either a ragged or a carious tooth. In these instances a decubital in-duration undoubtedly antedated, and its constant irritation formed the basis of a later cancerous growth.

The relation of cancer to syphilis has often been discussed.
longer believed that syphilis itself predisposes to the developı
cancer, and the only question not yet decided is whether a gumı
not become transformed into a carcinoma, or whether the late
ulcerations and their resulting scars may not undergo cancerous
cration.

Alfred Cooper, in his work on *Syphilis* (London, 1895, p. 1
scribes a case in which a nodule in the tongue was diagnosticat
gumma, which five months later was found to have been trans
into a carcinoma. It may be possible, however, that the first
was already cancerous. A diagnosis based on the microscopica!
ination of a bit of excised tissue is very uncertain, and yet iı
instances it is the only way in which a decision can be arrived
priori it may also be assumed that a cancer may develop from

Fig. 353

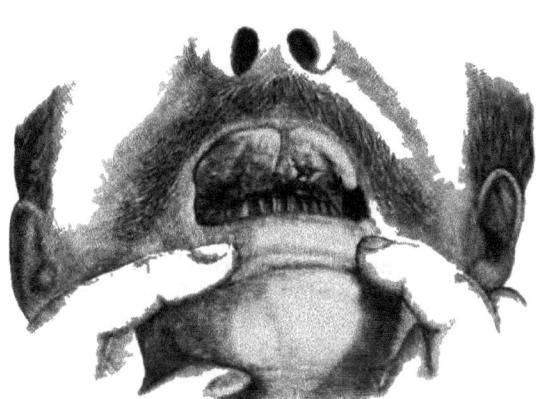

Carcinoma on under surface of the tongue.

lupus or a lupus scar, and in fact such cases have been reported b
Fournier, Gaston, Warren, and others. Ozenne even ascribes
tumors a growth which is very slow at the beginning, but this is a
apparently common to nearly all carcinomata.

In 24.38 per cent. of the author's cases no local factor of eti
moment was in evidence. Such cases are usually traced to the
irritation of a chronic superficial glossitis brought on by the use
alcohol or tobacco.

Age seems to exert a marked influence on the appearance of a
of the tongue as well as in other parts of the body. The perioı
during which most of the cases appear is between the ages of fı
and sixty-five. The author's statistics correspond very closely wiı
of other observers; 2.25 per cent. were found in patients between
of twenty-five and thirty, 7.91 per cent. between thirty and for
per cent. between forty and forty-five, 13.48 per cent. between fı

and fifty, 19.92 per cent. between fifty and fifty-five, 20.83 per cent. between fifty-five and sixty, 17.41 per cent. between sixty and sixty-five, 5.63 per cent. between sixty-five and seventy, and 5.05 per cent. in those over seventy. Wölfler reports 1 patient of twenty-five, and Weber 1 of 100, these including the two extremes.

The lingual cancers are almost always made up of squamous epithelium. The occurrence of a cylindrical-cell tumor, such as the one reported by Steiner, is an exception. Clinically surgeons may differentiate the cancers of the tongue into the superficial and the deep seated. The latter arise, with the exception noted, from the superficial epithelium, the latter from the glands in the mucous membrane. For this reason the deep varieties present at the beginning the picture of a growth covered over with mucous membrane, while the superficial variety becomes ulcerated at an early stage. It is possible therefore to distinguish a nodular and an ulcerative stage in these lingual cancers.

The nodular form invades the mucous membrane from below, the mobility of the latter is lost and an ulcer soon results. At no time is the nodule sharply marked off from the surrounding tissues. The ulcer which follows the breaking down of the nodule is characterized by elevated edges and a dirty, yellowish-brown base. The latter is not smooth, but extends into the parenchyma to a varying degree and present a number of furrows. The ulcer may also assume a crater-like form, the surrounding tissues appearing gray and necrotic. The tumor which starts on the surface of the tongue, after ulceration has fully developed, cannot be distinguished from that which began as a hard nodule. In many cases it is present as an elevated ulcer, with a number of small projections on the surface and clefts and furrows in between them, and resembles in a way the labial cancer. By pressure small hard white bodies may be squeezed out of the furrows, in which the typical epithelial pearls may be readily demonstrated. Papillary excrescences and cauliflower growths are rarely found on the tongue. There are two other characteristic symptoms usually present in a case of lingual cancer, hemorrhage and pain. These are apt to be quite severe, just as in the tuberculous ulcers on the edge of the tongue, and are often neuralgic in character. They radiate toward the ear and cause much suffering. During the later stages of the disease the carcinoma invades the surrounding structures by continuity, ordinarily in the following order: floor of the mouth, the inferior maxilla, the palatoglossal folds, the tonsils, the cheeks, and finally the parotid gland.

An involvement of the adjacent lymph-glands regularly occurs at an early date through the medium of the lymphatics, and invariably indicates an unfavorable prognosis. As a matter of fact, the recurrences, at least about 70 per cent., are not found in the operative scar, but in the neighboring lymph-nodes. This has been fully confirmed by the researches of Küttner on the lymphatic system of the tongue. The results of these observations have an important bearing on the diagnosis as well as the treatment of lingual cancer. The wealth of lymphatic channels in the tongue readily accounts for the early involvement of the

glands. The lymph-vessels from the mucous membrane and fi
depths of the tongue possess a single outlet, which also takes
lymphatic stream from the floor and the walls of the oral cavit
far as the latter would be concerned in the distribution of a car
On injection of one-half or even a small section of the tongue the n
is carried to all glands within the lymphatic system of the entire
which explains in a unilateral lesion of the latter the involvemen
glands on both sides. The lymphatic glands which drain the ton
the submaxillary, the deep cervical on the jugular vein, the sm
lingual, and those in the tongue between the genioglossi muscle
principal lymph-gland lies on the jugular vein at the level of the
of the carotids. From this point the infection may travel along th
cal glands to the base of the skull. There is also a direct path f
tongue to the supraclavicular glands. In every suspicious' tu
the tongue it is well therefore to palpate carefully the lymph
enumerated, in order to determine whether they are indurat
swollen.

In the list of 159 cases operated upon by the author the carcino
limited to the tongue in 29, almost all of which were preceded by s
plakia and were diagnosticated at an early stage. In 10 cases eitl
or both submaxillary glands were removed without being separate
the tumor in the tongue or through secondary incisions direct
them. Of the remaining 120 cases, an extensive extirpation of the
was done in 89. Furthermore, the floor of the mouth was excise
the lateral wall of the pharynx together with the palatal tonsil a
palatoglossal arch in 13, the ramus of the lower jaw up to the te
maxillary articulation in 6, the epiglottis in 1, the parotid in 2, tl
maxillary salivary gland in 80—the latter, in fact, in almost every ir
in which an operation included the resection of the lower jaw. T
tistical reports of Wölfler, Sachs, Meyer, Binder, and others
complete discussions regarding the frequency of extension of
cancers to the adjoining lymph-nodes, and the author's obser
fully agree with theirs.

Patients affected with a cancer which has invaded the surro
areas are in great misery, as the ulceration, tissue-necrosis, and slo
increase constantly both in extent and degree. To this are adc
profuse hemorrhage and the excruciating pain. The nutrition
patient declines rapidly, even if it is possible to feed through th
The adjoining diseased glands grow rapidly, even to the size of
soften, and break through the overlying skin. Where this occur
is found in the opening the red disintegrating and sloughing car
tissue. The duration of a cancer which is left to itself, is, on the a
about one year.

Diagnosis.—In the majority of instances the diagnosis is not a d
matter, especially if the characteristic ulcerations are present from
the small pearly-white nodules may be expressed. It is most con
confused with syphilis, less rarely with an ulcerating decubital
with tuberculosis, an ulcerating sarcoma, occasionally, perhaps, v

PLATE XV

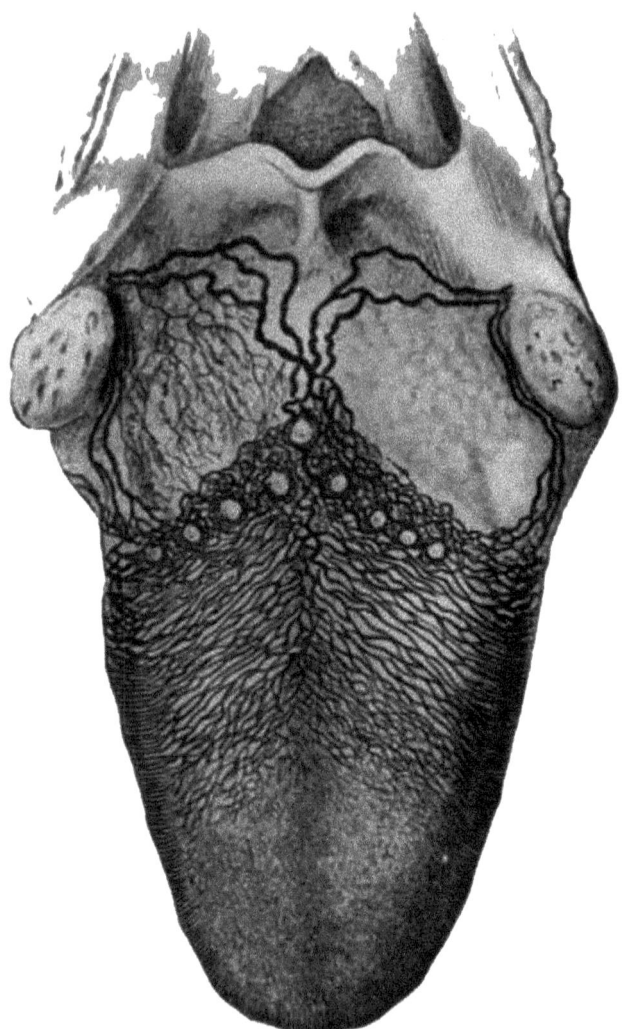

Lymph Vessels of the Mucous Membrane of the Back and Sides of the Tongue. On the right the lymphatics of the base of the tongue are shown.

ulcerating cavernous lymphoma, and finally with the nodules of actino-mycosis.

The provisional diagnosis of a decubital induration, a nodular benign growth, or actinomycosis, in place of a beginning carcinoma, is attended with considerable risk, as time may be wasted in waiting which had better be applied in considering the question of early operation. This question should be decided as soon as possible. The teeth adjacent to a doubtful indurated area must be extracted, and if the trouble has been due to a chronic irritation, resolution will usually take place in two or three days. In discussing the tumor-like tuberculous conglomerates the author has advised removal in all doubtful cases in which there might be any possibility of cancer. Even in the case of a gumma, an otherwise unnecessary operation would be justifiable when we consider the possibilities of over-looking a carcinoma.

It is also important to distinguish between the lesions of syphilis and a carcinoma. It is natural to hesitate before doing an extensive operation for a probable carcinoma of the tongue when there is a possibility of the condition being of a specific origin and likely to be favorably influenced by medical treatment. To eliminate any such possibilities the patient is subjected to a prolonged course of medication with mercury and the iodides, which further diminishes his strength. In case this method does meet with success and an operation is finally attempted, the latter must be done in tissues which are already more or less affected by a mercurial stomatitis. It is a well-known fact that the inflamed mucous membrane is not so resistant to infection as that which is in a normal, healthy condition, and the dangers attending an operation during this time are there-fore proportionately increased. The differential diagnosis between these two conditions is consequently a matter of great importance.

The author does not claim that the distinction between a carcinoma and the late lesion of syphilis may easily be made, but if based on very careful observations it is usually successful. Two factors common to both are the formation of new tissue and its early disintegration. This causes a marked similarity between them and accounts for the fact that up to the end of the eighteenth century every case of late syphilis of the tongue was considered cancer. The differences are to be found: First, in the multiplicity of the gummatous foci in contrast with the solitary lesion of a carcinoma. Second, in the site, which is almost exclu-sively, in the case of a carcinoma, on the edge of the tongue, somewhat back from the tip and opposite to the molar teeth. In a very small number of cases a cancer may be found on the tongue in the pre-epiglot-tic region; in three cases observed by the author, these were marked by an extraordinary hardness and were very nodular. This form is par-ticularly dangerous on account of the involvement of the epiglottis and the larynx, and may be confused with laryngeal tuberculosis. The fre-quent cough, which is never present in cancer of the larynx, and the find-ings in the sputum, usually afford sufficient evidence for making a diag-nosis. The majority of cancers at the base of the tongue are not primary in this locality, but have originated along the edge and extended forward.

The favorite site of the gumma, as well as of the sclerotic syp glossitis, is at the tip and the middle of the tongue. Third, fact that the base of a gummatous ulcer is covered with a laminated mass, bits of which may readily be picked off with a fe without causing much bleeding, while the base of the carcinom ulcer is soft, necrotic, and bleeds easily. Fourth, hemorrhages quite frequently in carcinoma and rarely in gumma. Fifth, p always present with cancer, but likely to be absent in gumma. Six adjacent lymph-glands very rarely enlarge in the presence of a gu but increase progressively in size with the advance of a cancer. A constant sign in connection with the latter is the swelling of the g over the bifurcation of the carotid and in the supraclavicular g Seventh, the presence of a patch of leucoplakia alongside of a susp nodule or ulcer on the edge of the tongue is indicative of carcinoma. combination makes possible an early recognition of the disease an mits of a successful operation.

It is evident from the foregoing that in most doubtful case preliminary constitutional treatment may be omitted and the diag made without the examination of a bit of tissue excised from the gr Personally, the author has seen more incorrect than correct diag from the results of these microscopical examinations.

Carcinomata are also found on the floor of the mouth, at the part of the angle which the mucous membrane of the cheek make the alveolar process, and on the hard palate near the molar teet

The cancer on the floor of the mouth first appears on the surf; the mucous membrane, or it may begin in its deeper layers. carcinomata made up of cylindrical-cell epithelium which are fou the floor of the mouth spring from the sublingual gland, and have discussed elsewhere. Cancers of the mucous membrane are seer the frenum and extend to the inner surface of the inferior m They appear as a flat uneven ulceration with an extremely hard and movements of the tongue cause intense pain. The progno these cases is unfavorable because the tumor soon extends into the or involves the under surface of the tongue.

Carcinomata of the inner aspect of the cheek and the hard grow slowly at first, and during this time present all the characte of a cancer of the mucous membrane. Later they grow more ra involving the entire thickness of the cheek and invading the retro lary fossa and the parotid gland. Both the upper and the lowe are easily invaded because the tumor is usually found in the angle the mucous membrane of the cheek is reflected to the alveolar p in close proximity to the ascending ramus. But even before this obstinate spasm of the jaws may result.

It has often been noted that a cancer of the cheek is preced leucoplakia, and sometimes a few spots could still be recognized vicinity. Its unfavorable prognosis is directly in proportion t distance which separates it from the labial commissure.

A carcinoma of the hard palate rapidly invades the superior m and in order to effect its removal, resection, partial or complete, of this bone is necessary.

Treatment.—Surgical operation is the only effective means of treatment in cancers of the mouth. A resection of that part of the tongue which is diseased may be accomplished in several ways, which will be considered in order.

1. In case the neoplasm is situated on the front part of the tongue, a resection may be done through the mouth itself. Of growths which lie on the back of the tongue beyond the circumvallate papillæ, only the smaller varieties, such as a papilloma, may be removed in this fashion. The procedure is only to be relied on in well-defined benign growths on the region in question or in the case of small sarcoma and carcinoma which have not invaded the posterior sections of the tongue. In all other instances the field of operation must be more effectually exposed than to the degree afforded by merely holding open the mouth.

The preliminary disinfection of the cavity of the mouth has been discussed on a preceding page. It is usually sufficient to brush the teeth thoroughly with potassium chlorate, followed by flushing with a solution of mercuric chloride (1 : 1000). The sloughing ulcers may be swabbed with a stronger solution of the same (1 : 250). If the mucous membrane is intact, such detail is not necessary, and anæsthesia may be immediately started. A 20 per cent. solution of eucaine or anæsthesin (recently introduced) is applied to the mucous membrane. The mouth may be kept widely open by a wedge of wood or hard rubber introduced between the molar teeth, and the angle of the mouth pulled to one side with a blunt retractor. An assistant seizes the tongue between his fingers and draws it forward as far as possible. The use of special tongue-forceps is not advised. In order to secure a firmer hold, and also to exert a transverse pull, it has been recommended to introduce two metallic (better than silk) threads through the tongue back of the diseased area, and employ these as retractors. Cauterization or extirpation may now be undertaken with the knife, the cold or the galvanocaustic snare, or the Paquelin thermocautery. There is considerable danger of uncontrollable hemorrhage from the tongue in all those cases in which the removal of a tumor is undertaken. If this threatens, or there is any subsequent bleeding which does not stop after proper tamponade, a preliminary or a later ligation should be done of the lingual artery according to Pirogoff's method.

In carrying out the latter procedure a curved incision is carried from the angle of the jaw to the hyoid bone, and ascending from this point to the neighborhood of the chin. Skin, platysma, and cervical fascia are divided, care being taken to avoid the fascial vein in the posterior angle of the wound. The submaxillary salivary gland is now freed from its capsule and reflected over the lower edge of the jaw. Under the thin posterior layer of the capsule is seen the edge of the anterior belly of the digastric muscle, and back of the latter the mylohyoid, from under the posterior edge of which the hyoglossus ascends to the tongue. The hyoglossal nerve crosses the angle made by the mylohyoid and the tendon of the digastric. In the small triangular space framed by the muscles and the nerve, the base of which consists of the hyogl muscle, lies, separated by only the muscular fibres of the hyogl the lingual artery. By dividing these fibres the artery is exposed

The attempts to render the field of operation bloodless by passi elastic ligature around the tongue have been abandoned, as well i temporary ligation or compression of the carotid artery.

2. In order to obtain a better exposure of the field of operation, i in 1831, proposed an incision through the cheek. If the new gro᙮ situated on one side or the edge of the tongue, it is only necessi cut through one cheek, otherwise both cheeks must be cut through. incision extends from the angle of the mouth to the anterior bor᙮ the masseter. Stenson's duct and the transverse artery lie abov line of incision. The circumflex and the external maxillary arteri᙮ ligated, and if the size of the growth and its vascularity warran᙮ lingual may also be tied off. By splitting both cheeks a very exposure is secured.

3. The tongue may also be reached through the submental hyoid), submaxillary, and retromaxillary regions. The author d᙮ to recommend this operation, done in the manner about to be desc᙮ for those cases in which the carcinoma is located on the anterior of the tongue and has invaded its lower aspect and the floor o᙮ mouth. For all the operations, but especially for this one, con᙮ narcosis by chloroform is necessary. He has never had cause to ᙮ its employment, and believes that by its aid the operations can be safely and completely executed. A preliminary tamponade of the tr᙮ is not necessary, unless the resection of the tongue also include removal of the epiglottis or a part of the lateral wall of the phary

In 1827 Cloquet attacked the tongue through the suprahyoid r᙮ His example was followed by Regnoli, who, in 1838, recommend᙮ extensive transverse incision, from the middle point of which an incision extended downward. Billroth (1873) also made a trans᙮ incision running along the lower edge of the maxilla, from the en᙮ which two others descended along the neck. Through the res᙮ wound the entire tongue was rendered accessible from the tip t epiglottis. It is necessary to divide the muscular attachments ᙮ middle point of the lower jaw, which becomes a serious matter, these cases an inspiration pneumonia is to be particularly feared. complication is not apt to result when a lateral incision is made i submaxillary fossa, as the elevators of the hyoid bone are spared. fact has been noted by Langenbeck and also by Kocher. The m᙮ in which the author carries out the operation for a cancer on the an᙮ part of the tongue is as follows:

The incision starts in the same way as that for the preliminary li᙮ of the lingual artery just described, and is continued further on ᙮ sternomastoid muscle to a point on a level with the bifurcation ᙮ carotid. After the cervical fascia is divided the facial vein is li᙮ and cut, and all the diseased lymph-glands and also the salivary g᙮

PLATE XVI.

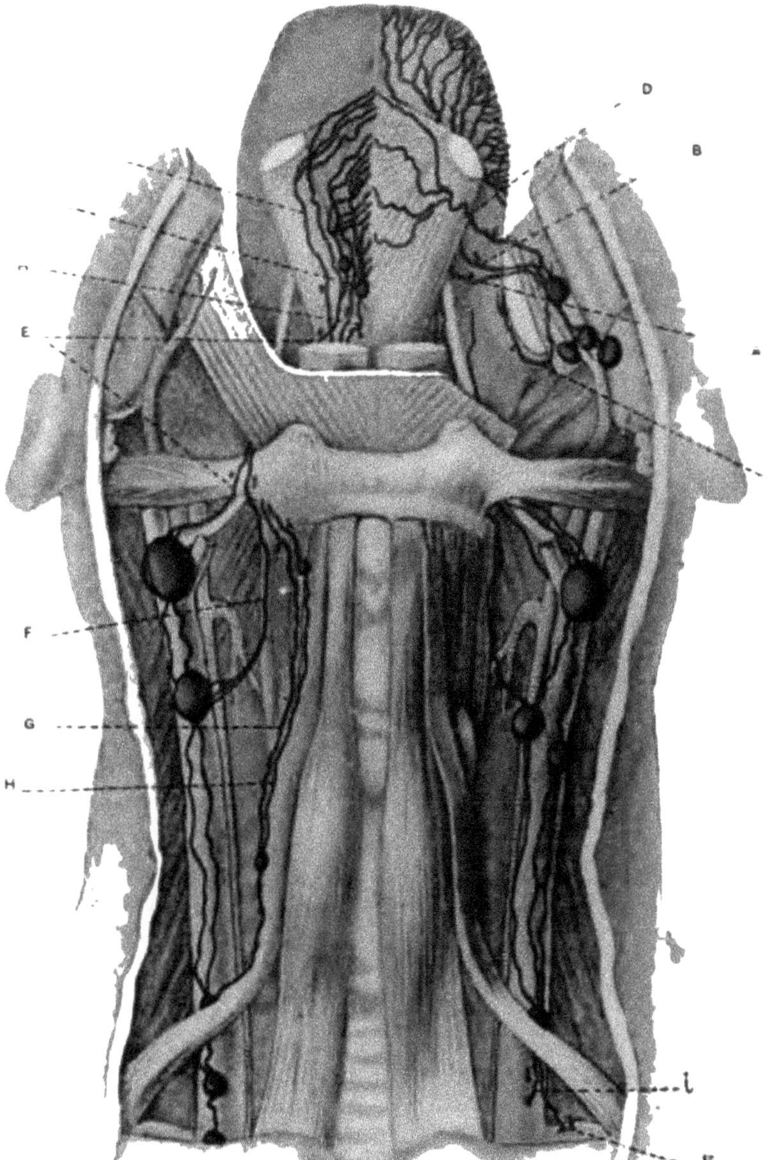

Anterior View of Lymphatics of Tongue.

The anterior portions of digastric and the geniohyoid muscles have been removed. A large window has been cut in the mylohyoid and the genioglossi muscles pulled apart. On the right side the lymphatic vessels which empty into the deep cervical glands and pass between the genioglossi are shown (G, F, H, K). On the left side the lymphatics of the tongue which empty into the sub-maxillary glands (A, B, C) are shown above. Below (at I and K) are seen the terminal lymph vessels of the deep cervical glands emptying into the large venous trunks.

PLATE XVII.

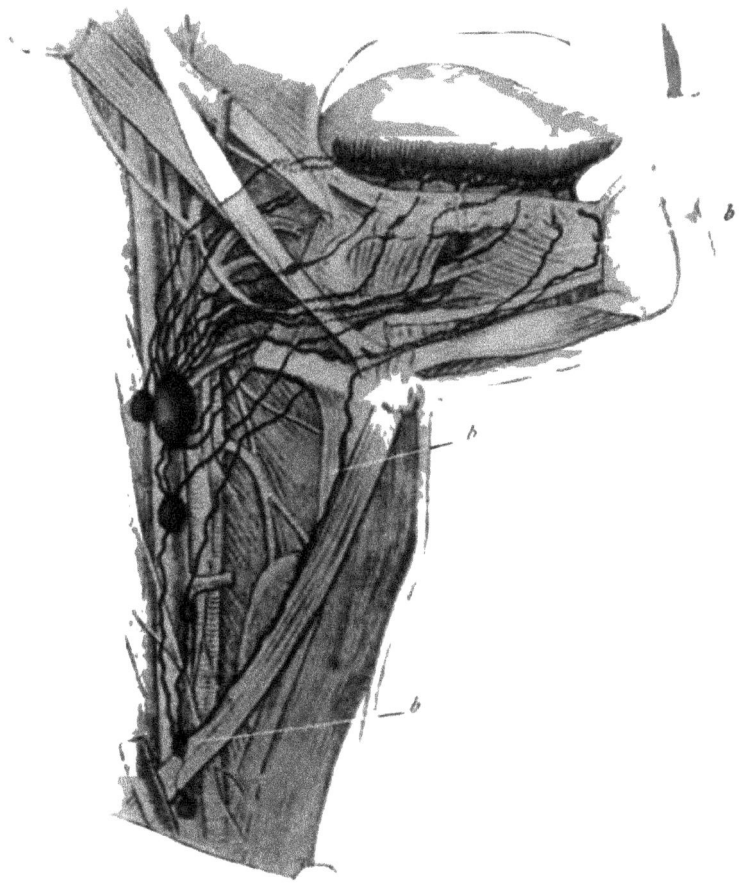

Lateral View of the Lymphatics of the Tongue Emptying into the Deep Cervical Lymph-nodes, some perforating and others passing between the Genioglossi.

in the capsule of which a number are always found, carefully removed. The mylohyoid and the hyoglossus, with the hypoglossal nerve, being now exposed, the lingual artery is tied off. The mucous membrane of the floor of the mouth is then cut through close to the lower jaw sufficient to expose completely the diseased parts of the tongue. It may also be necessary to divide transversely the anterior belly of the digastric, but in many cases it is sufficient to pull it to one side with a blunt hook. The only muscle which needs to be cut is the mylohyoid at its insertion, and this may be done through the same incision which separates the mucous membrane from the lower jaw. The operation is attended by the following advantages: (1) It is possible to extirpate completely the submaxillary and, if required, the lymphatic glands over the carotid. (2) A large exposure is afforded of the tongue and also of the floor of the mouth. (3) Free drainage is assured for the fluids from the mouth and for the discharges from the wound. When the diseased parts of the tongue have been excised and all hemorrhage checked, the wound in the tongue may be closed by deep sutures. The opening in the floor of the mouth may be packed with iodoform gauze, the end of which is allowed to project from the middle of the outer wound.

4. If the cancer is a very large one and has extended from the edges to the root of the tongue, or to the hard palate or the floor of the mouth, a resection of the inferior maxilla is imperative. Sédillot, in 1844, performed this operation in the middle line, and Langenbeck, in 1875, practised it on the side of the bone. The methods for operating in this condition are based on well-known facts and experiences. It is universally agreed that every bit of diseased tissue must be removed under all circumstances, and it is also a well-established fact that in no other form of cancer are the lymph-glands involved in such an early stage. If it be also remembered that metastatic deposits in internal organs are comparatively rare with a lingual carcinoma, it follows that the method which aims at the complete and successful removal of the primary growth and the adjacent lymph-nodes up to those over the carotid is the one which should receive due support and approval. Langenbeck's operation, which includes the lateral resection of the inferior maxilla, fulfils all these indications.

The author has employed this method in his clinic as follows: An incision is made from the angle of the mouth directly through the cheek to the edge of the masseter muscle. From this point it passes downward to the inner border of the sternomastoid, through the submaxillary and hyoid regions. The underlying tissues are dissected in layers, and if a number of enlarged glands are found at the lower end of the cut the latter may be extended still further down. The lymphatic and the salivary glands are removed and the facial and lingual arteries are ligated. The inferior maxilla is then sawn through with the Gigli saw in an oblique direction in the manner shown in Fig. 354, the cut beginning in the angle between the body and the ramus. The direction of the saw cut is downward, forward, and outward, and when near the end the saw may be turned still further forward so as to form a more

pronounced projection on the extremity of the posterior and lower
ment, on which the anterior and upper may rest.   Hooks are
inserted into the cut surfaces of the bone and the sections pulled a
The posterior belly of the digastric is then cut through, and als
mucous membrane in front of the palatoglossal arch and down t
pharyngolaryngeal sinus.   The wound now gapes to the width o
hand, and the entire diseased area of the tongue and its surroun
are in plain view and readily accessible.   Further operation or
tongue is then conducted in a similar way to that on the surface o
body.   If the bleeding has been properly attended to in every st
the operation, and the soft parts in the submaxillary region
free and left hanging from the floor of the mouth before the rese
of the jaw is done, there is no reason to fear an accumulation of

Fig. 354.

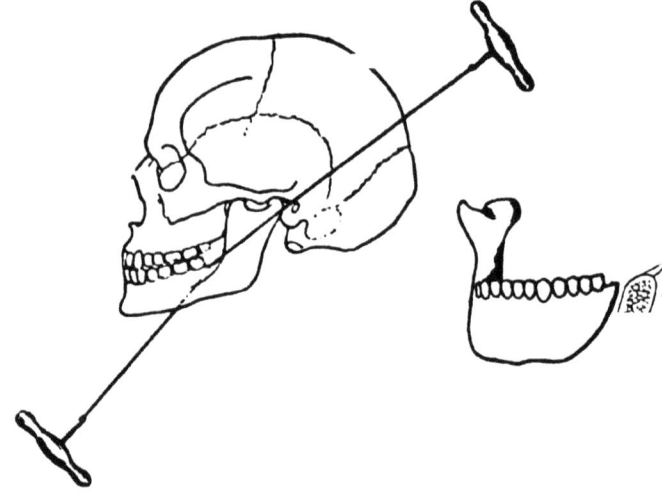

Method of dividing bone in resection of jaw.   Division of lower jaw in resect

in the pharynx at the entrance to the larynx.   If there is any uncerta
a small hook may be fixed on the epiglottis and the entire larynx
up and the operator assured that the walls of the pharynx down t
rima glottidis are free and clear.   During the remainder of the oper
an assistant provided with a sponge on a long handle can keep v
on the entrance to the respiratory passages and guard them agains
influx of blood.   The further steps in the operation, including the
patiou of the entire tongue or its greater part, are not difficult.   A
lingual is tied off, there is no interference caused by hemorrhage
limits of the diseased area are easy to recognize, and the incision
be carried well into healthy tissues.   The author always employ
knife; others prefer the thermocautery in the belief that the resu
slough acts as a barrier against infection of the wound.

PLATE XVIII.

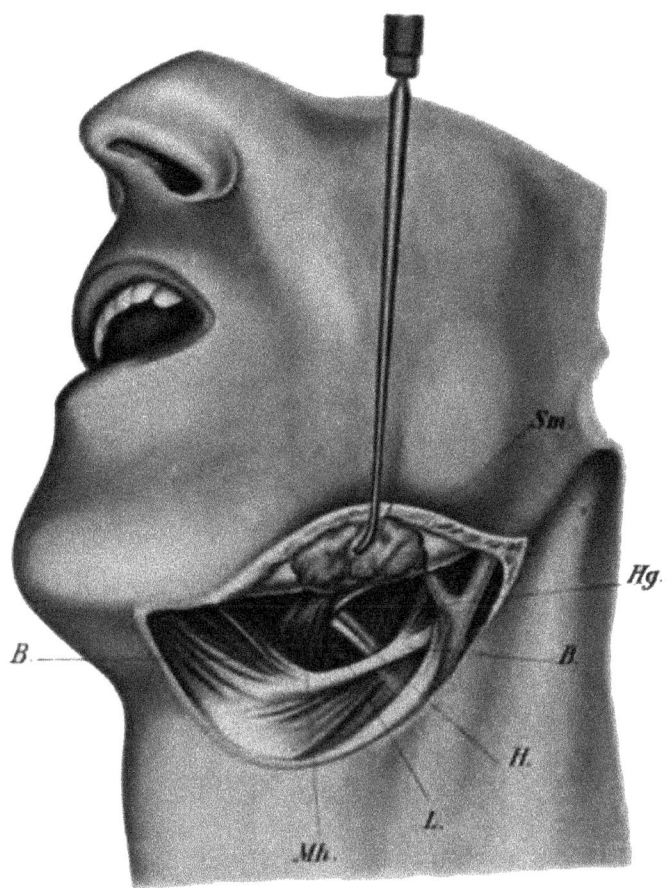

Exposure of the Lingual Artery.

Sm., Submaxillary gland.   *B.,* Digastric muscle.   *Mh.,* Mylohyoid.
H., Hypoglossal nerve accompanied by a vein.   *Hg.,* Hyoglossus
muscle.   *L.,* Lingual artery.

The main point in the closure of the wound and the after-treatment is the prevention of the accumulation of discharges. Proper drainage must be provided for the latter and also for the oral secretions which are apt to collect in various nooks and corners. The process is facilitated by suturing the mucous membrane of the pharynx near the larynx to the skin at the lower angle of the external wound, forming in this way a fistula which reaches to the deepest parts of the wound, and conducts the secretions from the mouth, nose, and pharynx away before there is opportunity for an accumulation to take place. Trendelenburg was the first to call attention to the importance of directly draining the space between the tongue and the epiglottis.

The above is accomplished by suturing both edges of the wound in the mucous membrane to the external skin near the lower angle of the incision. In this way the epiglottis and the entrance to the larynx are brought close to the outer skin of the neck which has been pulled inward by the sutures. This procedure is much more effective than the introduction of drainage-tubes, which in this locality are very liable to kink and become displaced, or they may irritate the epiglottis and bring on cough and retching.

One of the important points in this operation is the oblique direction of the saw-cut through the inferior maxilla. There is a constant tendency for the ramus to be pulled upward and for the horizontal part of the bone to sink downward. The obliquity of the cut overcomes this tendency, and the opposing forces equalize each other and keep the fragments well in place. Mikulicz for the same reason makes an angular cut in resecting the bone.

Two holes may be drilled through the ends of the divided bone, preferably with the electrical drill, because it can be done most rapidly, and sutures of aluminum-bronze wire introduced. To obviate infection of the raw surfaces, the periosteum and the mucous membrane should be carefully sutured. In none of the author's cases has he seen any inflammation of the bone or the separation of large sequestra. Occasionally small pieces may be cast off after a considerable period has elapsed, or one of the wire sutures may find its way into the oral cavity, and can then be extracted often with a small piece of bone. The operation is completed by sewing up the wound in the cheek and over the facial aspect of the lower jaw to the boundary of the previously mentioned fistula. The deep groove which is left in the mouth or the wall of the pharynx after the tumor is excised may be packed with strips of iodoform gauze which pass out through the fistula and are fixed to the outer skin with adhesive plaster, in order to prevent their aspiration into the pharynx.

Kocher has lately attempted to achieve the same ends by reviving and improving the old operation of Sédillot's, consisting of the resection of the inferior maxilla in the middle line, and believes that he has simplified the operation for excision of the tongue. As the author has had no experience with the method, he presents Kocher's description.

After cutting through the lip and the lower jaw in the middle line the geniohyoid and the genioglossus on the diseased side are separated ¦ the bone, and the halves of the jaw pulled apart. The tongue may be pulled outward and to the opposite side with the aid of a previc introduced suture. The mucous membrane on the floor of the mou then cut through along the edge of the tongue back to the anterior pa arch. The lingual vein is now brought into view, passing backward outward along the lateral surface of the hyoglossus, and also the lin nerve close under the mucous membrane at the edge of the tongue. hypoglossal nerve is seen at the anterior border of the hyoglossus mu Under it and between the hyoglossus and genioglossus appears the gual artery, which can be readily tied off. The hyoglossus is divided the thermocautery, and likewise the mucous membrane, which is pu the stretch by pulling on the tongue. If the new growth has reachec palate and pharynx, it becomes necessary to divide the styloglo Should the soft palate be involved the internal pterygoid muscle ma cut with the actual cautery, the latter muscle being exposed by cu through the mucous membrane in front of the tonsil and removing organ. Diseased parts of the soft palate are excised by the aid of cautery, and the same instrument is used on the tongue. Over ¦ cauterized surfaces Kocher applies xeroform and brings together the of the resected bone with wire sutures. The external wound is sut with the exception of a small opening at the lower end, into whi xeroform gauze drain is inserted. Kocher claims the following ad tages for his operation: a minimum degree of hemorrhage, abso drainage, and the preservation of the most essential muscles conne with the mechanism of swallowing. The only objection which the au can offer is that it does not afford an exposure of the important g of lymph-glands over the external carotid and the bifurcation of common carotid.

In addition to the median resection of the lower jaw Vallas also rec mends median division of the hyoid bone.

5. Removal of the tongue must be accompanied by resection of a la piece of bone if there is a simultaneous involvement of the inferior ¦ illa. In the majority of instances the ramus of the lower jaw is affec An incision is made similar to that required for the lateral resectic the bone. After cleaning out the submaxillary region and tying of external carotid artery the bone is cut through at right angles to its axis at a point anterior to the cancerous tissue. The ramus is then articulated at the temporomandibular joint, and the surgeon is now to remove the lymph-glands lying back of the parotid and parts of parotid itself.

These extensive procedures are attended by a high mortality rat the author's series of cases it amounted to 17.6 per cent. Accordir various other authors, the mortality varies from 8.3 to 25 per cent., c an average 16.2 per cent. The improved modern technic has undc edly improved the chances of recovery. The more extensive operat which include the methods mentioned for exposing the tongue, according to Loison, less apt to be followed by recurrences than t conducted through the mouth alone, the actual figures being 24.1 per cent. for the former, as against 34.2 per cent. for the latter. The mortality for the extensive operation is naturally greater, being 23 per cent. against 10.7 per cent.

The number of cases cured would be higher had it been possible to select them more carefully for operation. An operable case is one in which incision can be carried at least 1 cm. into sound tissue beyond the limits of the tumor. It must be possible also to remove all diseased glands. The latter may not be so firmly adherent to the surrounding tissues as to prevent their clean dissection.

Total removal of the tongue has been well borne in a number of cases. Thus a patient presented before the Twenty-third Congress of German Surgeons by Dombrowski could make himself understood and swallow without difficulty. The author can confirm these facts in a number of his own cases.

The treatment of inoperable carcinoma of the tongue is exceedingly unsatisfactory. Feeding the patient is extremely difficult, a feeding-cup with spout and the stomach-tube soon become useless. There remain only the passage through the nose, the use of rectal enemata, which soon fail, and gastrotomy. The pain constantly increases, preventing sleep and rendering continually larger doses of morphine necessary. Locally a solution of hydrogen peroxide may be employed as a mouth-wash, or suffering can be rendered less severe by wiping out the mouth with iodoform gauze and dusting with anæsthesin.

In operating for *carcinoma of the floor of the mouth* the same method is employed as in those cases in which carcinoma has extended to the floor of the mouth from the anterior portion of the tongue. If the bone is not involved by carcinoma, the operation is carried out from the suprahyoid region. Sufficient room can generally be obtained by a median incision, which should open up the space between the geniohyoid muscles, or if carcinoma has affected these muscles, a second incision can be made at right angles to the first along the lower border of the jaw. If the bone is involved, the middle portion of the jaw must be resected. The operation has already been described.

Carcinoma of the buccal mucous membrane can be readily surrounded by incision if situated in the region of the commissure of the lips, even if it should be necessary to cut through the entire thickness of the cheek. In the latter case a subsequent plastic operation would be necessary. A second incision is made in the submaxillary region in order to remove the glands. Where the tumor is situated further back, between the upper and lower jaw, it is very difficult to remove. If the growth is still small, it may be sufficient to split the cheek; but where it is larger, or if it involves the bone, a very extensive operation will be necessary. The tumor may be removed after lateral oblique resection of the lower jaw, as described above, or it may be necessary to resect the ramus of the lower jaw, possibly also to perform partial resection of the upper jaw.

MALFORMATIONS, INJURIES, AND DISEASES OF THE PHARYNX.

By Prof. Dr. W. KÜMMEL.

CHAPTER XXIX.

MALFORMATIONS OF THE PHARYNX.

MALFORMATIONS of the pharynx are rather rare. The only one that needs to be considered here is teratoma. On account of interference with respiration and nutrition true "epignathi" as a rule render it impossible for the bearer to live, even where the latter is otherwise well developed. But in several instances the tumor has been successfully removed during the first few days or months. In most of these cases the mass is attached by a broad base to the basilar portion of the occipital bone, and may extend through the latter into the cavity of the skull, to be attached to the region of the hypophysis or to some intracranial tumor-like formation. Externally the tumor usually presents a rounded mass, with a nodular or smooth surface. Its interior is traversed by hard particles, being rarely of a uniform density. On the surface there are occasionally found grotesque, deformed, or non-recognizable organs, such as the extremities, for example.

Diverticula which are due to errors in development of the branchial clefts always occur at a typical site. This is true also of cysts and fistulæ due to the same cause. The situation alone would therefore point to their branchiogenetic origin. Diverticula arising from non-closure of the first branchial cleft proceed from the wall of the Eustachian tube. They are very rare, and in most cases of little significance. Some of those originating in the second branchial cleft are associated with the posterior portion of the latter, which goes to form the fossa of Rosenmüller. They are usually simple dilatations of the above fossa, but may form true diverticula, extending as far as the outer skin. Diverticula arising from the ventral portion of the second branchial cleft, which goes to form the tonsillar fossa, are relatively the most frequent, though not so common as complete fistula. They proceed from the tonsillar fossa, have a wide mouth, and extend to some point in the anterior triangle of the neck, between the sternomastoid muscle and the trachea.

Diverticula due to non-closure of the third branchial cleft proceed from that portion of the pyriform sinus situated above the fold of the superior laryngeal nerve, between the cornu of the hyoid bone and the

thyroid cartilage, and may extend a considerable distance for\
downward. They must not be confused with diverticula of the \
of Morgagni, which are similarly situated. (See Vol. II., page 1

Diverticula of the lower portions of the pharynx are more \
They are not congenital malformations, and are discussed u
head of Diverticula of the Œsophagus.

Cysts and fistulæ can arise at all the places that congenital di
are found. It is extremely difficult, however, to determine theii
ital origin. In this group may be included certain cysts of the
sinus filled with tough, stringy mucus, and lined with ciliated c)
epithelium or with cuboidal epithelium. In the case of cysts si'
front of the epiglottis, in the vallecula, or in the glossopharyn₄
ment, it may be difficult to determine their branchiogenetic orig
question may arise in these cases whether they originated in th
branchial cleft or in the thyroglossal duct. Cysts which origina
latter are situated exactly in the median line, between the
cæcum and the root of the tongue. This is the same situation \
by the analogous accessory struma (thyroid gland). More rar
cysts extend downward as far as the middle lobe of the thyroi
Cysts of the second branchial cleft, on the other hand, would b
for in or behind the glossopharyngeal ligament. But where a c
considerable size it may be difficult to determine whether it
secondarily assumed a median or a lateral position.

These cysts produce a peculiar metallic tone of speech. Pati\
quently complain also of difficulty in swallowing. If the cyst 1
inflamed, as occasionally happens after the injection of chemi\
stances, or sometimes even after spontaneous rupture, severe inf
tory processes may be set up in the neighboring structures. Such
plete operations should therefore be avoided. If difficulty in swa
renders their removal necessary, a large portion of the wall of \
should be excised from the pharynx with knife or scissors, n\
Kirstein's direct laryngoscopy or of the laryngoscope, provid\
impossible to enucleate the cyst or to remove it completely wh\
pedunculated. Where a cyst extends to just beneath the outer
the neck, it is easier and preferable to remove it through an \
incision. Congenital fistulæ are discussed elsewhere.

CHAPTER XXX.

INJURIES OF AND FOREIGN BODIES IN THE PHARYNX.

ACTUAL injury of the pharynx is seen only as a result of burns or the action of caustics, as in attempts at suicide. In the former cases the resulting manifestations are situated in the mouth and œsophagus; in the latter, on the other hand, the coexisting injury of the larynx or trachea is so prominent that the symptoms of pharyngeal injury are hardly ever considered. At the same time it should be mentioned that in those cases which recover sloughing may be followed by adhesions or stenosis; that, moreover, after incised wounds there frequently remain annoying fistulæ, which secrete mucus and pus, and which require to be removed by dividing the integument from the mucous membrane and by carefully suturing the latter after its edges have been turned in. The outer wound should be allowed to remain open and be packed with iodoform gauze in order to avoid phlegmon of the neck, which might otherwise occur. Any remaining small fistulæ can usually be closed by cauterizing their edges.

Foreign bodies must still be mentioned. The latter are usually pieces of bone, fish-bones, and needles, which are swallowed with food, and which are apt to become lodged in the pyriform sinus or in the lowest portion of the pharynx. Such foreign bodies, situated in the sinus pyriformis, can be located with the laryngoscope, or, better still, by palpating with the finger. Those situated in the lowest parts of the pharynx can only be located by œsophagoscopical examination. What applies to them applies also to œsophageal foreign bodies. Those situated in the sinus pyriformis frequently are very difficult to diagnosticate and to treat; they usually produce marked œdema of the aryteno-epiglottidean folds and the mucous membrane of the arytenoid cartilages, which completely covers one side of the latter. This condition may cause dangerous asphyxia and, on account of the difficulty in swallowing, serious disturbance of nutrition. In addition there is the danger that septic manifestations, with the well-known danger of periœsophageal phlegmon, frequently follow. If such swelling has attained any considerable size, the diagnosis is absolutely impossible, and it is necessary to reach the foreign body from without by lateral pharyngotomy, or possibly also to expose the inflammatory focus by subhyoid œsophagotomy. If œdema is marked tracheotomy should not be postponed too long, as the danger of asphyxia may suddenly increase. It has frequently happened that in incising deep phlegmons of the neck a foreign body which had not been diagnosticated was unexpectedly found. For this reason it is extremely important to determine the presence of a foreign body either with the mirror, by Kirstein's direct laryngoscopy, or by palpation, before inflammatory œdema has set in.

INFLAMMATORY DISEASES OF THE TONSILS AND NASOPHAI

Acute Angina.—The term "angina" (sore throat) is generally a to all acute inflammatory diseases of the nasopharynx. They ge involve this entire region, but as a rule the affection of the tonsils nates the entire clinical picture. Nearly all the infections of this originate in the tonsils, and the latter are the seat of the pri symptoms. The terms "angina" and tonsillitis are therefore : synonymous.

General Remarks. Forms of Angina.—The various forms of litis are regularly ascribed to "catching cold" by the laity; but th hardly be considered an important factor unless pyogenic organisi present. A large number and various kinds of the latter exist in th sillar crypts of individuals who are entirely well: streptococci are th frequent; less frequent are *Staphylococcus pyogenes aureus* and *albi* pneumococcus, Friedländer's pneumobacillus, the bacillus of diphi and pseudodiphtheria bacilli, also many other bacteria. Actino (Lesin) occur only in the isolated cases. There is uncertainty as virulence of these different organisms constantly present in health; viduals and in those suffering from angina. There are few facts which to base any opinion regarding this question. It is known, ever, that most of the micro-organisms normally present in the ! possess a very low degree of virulence, but that the latter is at or creased to an extreme degree whenever the individual suffers fro slightest local infection, such as catarrh or sore throat ("ang Nearly all individuals who periodically suffer from angina have very large or very prominent tonsils, both conditions apparently ing accumulation of micro-organisms. At the same time removal tonsils does not always cause the tendency to disappear.

Different forms of non-specific tonsillitis are distinguished, b division into groups is obscured by the occurrence of various trans: forms.

1. In *catarrhal tonsillitis* there is usually marked involvement entire mucous membrane of the pharynx. The pillars of the f the posterior pharyngeal wall, frequently the region of the tongu the epiglottis, and not infrequently the entrance of the larynx as far vocal cords, present a bright scarlet-red or bluish appearance, gradually diminishes in intensity as the distance from the tonsils inc The swelling of the tonsils (usually both are involved), which is th

(880)

noticeable feature, may be due more to an old hypertrophy than to acute inflammation. In the beginning there is a sore feeling in the pharynx, especially during swallowing; the particles of food produce a rough or sharp sensation, and sometimes it is almost or quite impossible to swallow solid food. After three or four days, rarely later, the severe pain as a rule disappears; sometimes a sore feeling or sensation of roughness in the throat remains for a long time. This is usually limited in such cases to one or several points, and upon careful examination it is usually found that these correspond to the neighborhood of one or several crypts, showing marked redness and tenderness.

2. In *follicular tonsillitis* the inflammatory process is limited at first to the neighborhood of one or several crypts. There is a yellowish or whitish deposit, occasionally producing a spotted appearance of the tonsil. When only several crypts are involved the tonsils are frequently very little enlarged, and swelling may be limited to that portion of the tonsil concealed within the fossa between the pillars of the fauces. Follicular tonsillitis is more liable to affect only one tonsil than is catarrhal tonsillitis. The duration and severity of the clinical manifestations vary considerably. They frequently terminate within a few hours or a few days. At other times the course is protracted for several weeks, different groups of follicles becoming diseased in succession.

In these forms there is frequently pseudomembrane, of a whitish or dirty-yellow color, reminding one of a diphtheritic process. This occasionally leads to errors in diagnosis. As a rule this membrane can be readily wiped off, or if very firmly adherent can be torn off in small shreds without producing loss of substance or possibly only a slight loss of epithelium. At present the majority of physicians consider the most important point to be the presence or absence of diphtheria bacilli. The latter are, however, not infrequently found in cases of mild and harmless tonsillitis, and the discovery of these bacilli and their relation to prognosis must be carefully considered in each individual case. When the result of the examination is negative, it is advisable to make repeated examinations.

3. *Parenchymatous tonsillitis* occurs in combination with both the above forms as a result of more severe infection which invades the deeper tissues. It produces marked swelling of the tonsil, and as a rule causes more severe clinical manifestations than the above forms; pain on swallowing is very much more severe, and frequently the inability to take nourishment becomes quite serious. Speech is difficult and acquires a peculiar thick quality. Owing to the difficulty in swallowing there is much annoyance from the accumulation of saliva in the month, which renders speech difficult.

Swelling of the tonsils is characteristic of parenchymatous angina, but may be simulated by inflammatory swelling of the peritonsillar tissue. In the latter condition, however, the pillars of the fauces are pressed forward and tend to be stretched over the tonsils, while in parenchymatous tonsillitis the tonsil projects freely from its pocket; only where there are adhesions between the tonsils and the pillars of the fauces, caused by previous inflammation, do the pillars of the fauces project in the swollen tonsil. It is frequently impossible to distinguish peritonsillar abscess from parenchymatous tonsillitis.

Symptoms.—The clinical manifestations in the various forn sillitis are not essentially different, but are distinguished prin their severity and duration.

The onset of angina is always marked by general malaise, by decided chills, not infrequently the local symptoms are tran insignificant.

In fully developed angina *fever* is the most regular and most . symptom. A slight rise of temperature is rarely absent even in tive cases; in case of more severe infection the temperature ma than 41° C. (105° F.). The highest temperature usually acc peritonsillar abscess. In such cases the temperature may exc be intermittent in type, while in parenchymatous and **follicul** the temperature is almost always continuous, and in the catar it is generally only slight.

Hand in hand with fever there are usually *general malaise, lassitude, loss of appetite, muscular pain in the neck and shou* pain in the back. As in other general febrile conditions, there m swelling of the spleen, occasionally, also, swelling of the liver, alb and in rare cases actual nephritis. In young children headach less severe, but there may be more serious symptoms on the p central nervous system, such as convulsions, delirium, etc.

Locally the changes in the tonsils are always noticeable; in se there is also swelling of the neighboring structures, but as a involves only the uvula. The latter may form a pale-red, s parent club-shaped swelling which completely fills the space be enlarged tonsils. This swelling becomes most severe in case c cating peritonsillar abscess. In the latter cases there are more be inflammatory changes in the maxillary articulation and the muscles covering the latter on its inner side. This condition n in severe ankylosis of the jaw.

There is frequently a bad taste in the month. As on accot difficulty in swallowing, the month is not automatically cleansed normal conditions, the tongue is usually very much coated. T even be severe diffuse stomatitis. Saliva is swallowed with diffic accumulates in the month, so that apparently there is a conditio vation.

In all forms of acute tonsillitis, mild as well as severe, variou cations may occur on the part of neighboring structures, at some from the diseased organ and even in quite remote parts of t Frequently it is difficult to find any connection with the original particularly if they are associated with milder forms of **angim** for example, manifestations on the part of the nerves **following** attacks of diphtheria.

The commonest form of complication of angina is **peritonsi** below). The regional lymph-glands are regularly **affected,**

rarely leads to severe manifestations; at the same time suppuration of the nearest lymph-glands does take place occasionally. The glands most frequently affected are those situated between the angle of the jaw and the sternomastoid muscles; occasionally, however, those lower down between the latter muscle and the carotid artery are also affected. The lymph-glands situated in the floor of the month are occasionally enlarged; at times they are the only ones affected, but are difficult to palpate.

Slight torticollis occasionally occurs, associated with angina. Whether this is simply due to the painful glands of the cervical region, or whether it is caused by myositis of the sternomastoid, emanating from the angina or produced by the same cause, is difficult to decide. No observations in proof of one or the other theory have been made.

Swelling of the large salivary glands, the parotid, and the submaxillary, does occur, but may be due to enlargement of the lymph-glands embedded within the salivary glands.

The *larynx* is not infrequently affected, particularly on the lingual surface of the epiglottis. There is frequently inflammatory œdema; more rarely this involves the arytenoepiglottidean folds. In case of complicating peritonsillitis the above conditions frequently reach a very severe degree, and cause alarming or even dangerous dyspnœa. Moderate interference with respiration may be caused by enlargement of the tonsils.

General septic infection associated with tonsillitis is intensely interesting. Particularly its relation to articular rheumatism and acute infections osteomyelitis has recently attracted the attention of authors (see the comprehensive description by Suchannek). A number of conclusive cases were reported by A. Buschke. It is certainly true that angina frequently occurs during the onset of both diseases.

Severe septic infection is generally propagated by peritonsillar abscess and subsequently by thrombophlebitis of the pterygoid plexus, the veins of the neck, and septic endocarditis. The latter may be associated with myocarditis and pericarditis, also permanent valvular changes. Still more severe is pyæmic or septic general infection in connection with phlebitis. Occasionally there are seen in milder cases pleuritis, more rarely severe empyema, pneumonia, and affections of the kidneys. But more frequently, however, there is transitory albuminuria.

Disturbances on the part of the central nervous system, such as delirium, etc., are rather less frequent than in other acute febrile diseases. Through phlebitis of the pterygoid sinus and cavernous sinus meningitis may result, as observed recently in a case of the author's. Paralysis of the peripheral nerves is more frequent, but in these cases it has frequently been discovered that the diphtheria bacillus was the cause of the apparently simple angina; also the fact that paralysis most frequently affects the palatal muscles and the muscles of accommodation of the eye, would point to the diphtheria bacillus as the cause of the disease.

Diagnosis.—The diagnosis is generally easy; where the local changes are slight there is occasionally some uncertainty as to whether the existing difficulty of swallowing or the general febrile condition is due to the

slight angina or to some other disease. In the presence of otl
septic symptoms the possibility of a phlebitic process in the ve
neck or the cranial sinuses must be considered. As a rule the
the disease will soon decide the question. Occasionally it is fou
to one's surprise, that an apparently simple angina subsequent
to be syphilitic. This error is prevented by the fact that syphiliti
gitis as a rule exists for some time before the patient is presen
surgeon, while in the other forms of tonsillitis it is only durin
few days that the disease causes severe manifestations. Mo
syphilitic angina mucous patches are frequently found in othe
of the mouth. Of other forms of angina, diphtheritic infectio
liable to escape recognition. If every case in which Löffler's l
present is considered diphtheritis in its clinical sense, then, exce
positive or negative finding of the bacillus, there is no thoroug
nostic characteristic, and one is obliged to bear in mind that e
of angina may be diphtheritic until a microscopical examination
made. Follicular angina especially frequently causes confus
diphtheria. In recent cases of the former there is such a cl
deposit that there is no reason for suspecting diphtheria, as in
the deposit is more of a yellowish-white or dirty grayish-yell
But this quality must not be depended upon too positively, citl
against diphtheria.

Processes which produce vesicles on the skin and fibrinous de
the month are liable to be the sources of error; such, for exar
pemphigus, erythema multiforme, and other exudative dermatos
ring in the month. But in the latter affections the skin as well a
of the mouth is almost always involved. One of the process
occur only in the mouth and form vesicles, and which may be
with angina, herpes tonsillaris, will be discussed later. Aphthou
titis and similar efflorescences occurring in hoof-and-mouth disc
be localized in the tonsils and the mucous membrane of the mout
will always be prevented if the general disease be considered,
larly involvement of the mucous membrane of the rest of the mot
diagnosis of associated peritonsillitis is difficult, but very import
the point of view of treatment (see below).

Prognosis.—The prognosis of acute angina is generally favo
the occasional complications are so rare that their possibility nee
be considered. If, however, they do occur, they will determine t
nosis. Catarrhal and follicular angina usually terminate withii
days, but may continue for a week or even longer. The same a
parenchymatous angina; but in the latter, complications, such
tonsillitis, are more frequent. Follicular angina is extremely c
if accompanied by extensive deposits or with very deep follic
the openings into the latter are situated very high up. Un
circumstances a form of chronic tonsillitis may develop.

Treatment.—As in the majority of cases angina occurs in st
attacks, the surgeon is frequently asked to suggest some effectiv
of *prophylaxis.* When there actually is a tendency to "catchin

some hardening measures should be instituted. But in most cases it is more important to render it possible for the patient to breathe naturally through the nose. Particularly in cases of pathological mouth-breathing, inflammation of the tonsils is very liable to result from "catching cold." Removal of the tonsils may diminish very much such a tendency. The second principle in instituting prophylactic measures is to keep the surface and the interior of the nostrils as free from pathogenic organisms as possible. In this regard it is extremely important to incise tonsillar crypts that are very deep or which have narrow openings. By this means the latter can be regularly evacuated and the accumulation of plugs abounding in bacilli be prevented. As enlargement of the tonsils has some influence on the frequency of the attacks, the removal of hypertrophied tonsils may be advisable. But in some cases all prophylactic measures are unsuccessful, and many patients are not relieved of their constantly recurring attacks of tonsillitis.

An existing attack of tonsillitis may be treated by means of internal remedies and local applications. Of the former, sodium, salicylate, quinine, and tincture of guaiac are most frequently employed. They are not very successful as a rule. For local application, various astringent and antiseptic substances have been recommended. They are employed in solution to be painted on or gargled, or in solid form by insufflation. Solutions for gargling, which are still regularly prescribed for angina, are superfluous. Only in patients who have acquired a certain degree of dexterity does the solution reach the tonsils, and even then it acts for a few seconds only. In the presence of angina, moreover, gargling is very painful, or at least very unpleasant. A spray apparatus is more efficacious. With the latter, weak solutions of potassium permanganate, alum, etc., may be applied. Steam inhalation apparatuses are generally less pleasant to the patient, on account of the high temperature of the spray. Of the substances to be painted on, iodoform is the best in the author's opinion, particularly in follicular tonsillitis, in the form of a 10 per cent. emulsion of iodoform in glycerin or a thick iodoform paste. The small particles of iodoform lodge in the months and contents of the crypts, and thus produce a continuous disinfectant action. Astringents, especially alum, which is very generally employed, are of little use. Application of cold is more useful. Small particles of ice should be held in the mouth and the water swallowed, or if there is great difficulty in swallowing, the water can be expectorated. The external application of cold may be of service also in milder cases; the application of moist compresses to the throat according to Priessnitz's suggestion is to be recommended. These are frequently very grateful to the patient.

All these measures have very little influence in the various forms of tonsillitis; as the disease generally lasts only a few days, their usefulness is rather imaginary. When there is high fever, internal antipyretics or tepid or cold packs to the whole body may be of advantage.

Herpes Tonsillaris.—Herpes on the surface of the tonsil occurs primarily at the beginning of acute infectious diseases, in the same manner as herpes labialis, but is much less frequent. The herpetic vesicles are

... found in the vicinity of the tonsils as far as the ... the posterior palatine ... As in other parts of the ... they exist for a short time only, and may not be at all visible ... become transformed into flat erosions covered with a white membrane. These erosions may become confluent, and the picture of some other affection, such as diphtheria, for ... ... usually such confusion is obviated by accompanying ... other cases, however, the diagnosis may be extremely ... severe pain and the frequent occurrence of high fever with ... and redness of the surrounding structures may be of import ... ing a diagnosis. Treatment is hardly ever necessary in ... and it is of importance only on account of a possible com ... diphtheria.

Diphtheria of the Pharynx.—Diphtheria is most frequen ... the tonsils, and generally occurs there first. More rarely it ... down, in the upper air-passages. For the diagnosis of diphthe ... tion of the latter on the tonsils is very important; from the p ... of therapeutics, and especially surgical therapeutics, involve ... larynx and trachea is of greater significance. For this reaso ... important features in regard to the etiology, pathology, diagn ... diphtheria are discussed in Vol. II. It is only necessary to po ... that the first visible signs of diphtheritic inflammation occur i ... of the tonsils; that a typical diphtheritic membrane is for ... neighborhood of one or several crypts; that this membrane ... tends over a large portion of the tonsil, and, exceeding the l ... latter, extends over the pillars of the fauces and the vicinity o ... finally remaining stationary, and then disappears or advan ... larynx and trachea.

Treatment.—Little can be said in regard to the treatmen ... theria of the larynx. At present the serum treatment is indi ... cases in which the diagnosis has been positively confirmed. ... treatment of the membrane is so uncertain that there is ... method that has come into general use. Lime-water is ... employed for inhalation and local application. Iodoform wo ... useful, particularly in septic or gangrenous processes. Al ... numerous substances employed in its treatment are each fa ... by a few practitioners.

Phlegmonous Tonsillitis and Peritonsillitis.—Phlegmon ... mation of the tonsil and of the surrounding capsular tissues a ... together, as they furnish the same clinical picture, and i ... impossible to make a differential diagnosis between them. T ... of cases which at first are considered phlegmonous tonsilliti ... show themselves to be peritonsillitis in the course of their furth ... ment. Even if products of inflammation rupture at the su ... tonsil, it is no proof that the primary abscess occurred in ... itself. The so-called chronic abscesses of the tonsils, freque ... and stationary, encystered, phlegmonous tonsillitis, are pr ... abscesses lying free within the connective tissue of the ton ...

probably cystic dilated tonsillar crypts filled with purulent secretion and detritus.

In peritonsillar abscess the characteristic feature is the inflammatory swelling of the capsule of the tonsil, which forces both layers of the soft palate apart and causes marked bulging of the portions situated laterally from the pillars of the fauces. The swollen area is very painful, particularly on pressure; at first of firm consistence; later, after pus has formed, it is more soft. Sometimes swelling is more noticeable on palpation than on inspection. Infiltration of the peritonsillar tissues is usually most marked in those portions situated above and to one side of the tonsil. In this situation there is frequently circumscribed bulging. This is probably due to the fact that at this point the lymphatics of the tonsil unite to form a common trunk, or that here the lymphatics form follicles or glands. The lymphatics proceed from here through the wall of the pharynx to the region behind the maxillary articulation, and the glands situated in this region constitute a second stopping point. Accordingly swelling of these glands regularly accompanies peritonsillitis. Not infrequently these glands have been observed to suppurate.

The *starting point of infection* is regularly one of the tonsillar crypts, particularly one of those in the supratonsillar fossa. In the vicinity of this fossa the connective tissue of the capsule approaches nearest the inner surface of the crypts. Moreover, the crypts are more frequently situated here, whose openings are directed upward and filled with necrotic masses, so that they are very much exposed to infection.

The onset of peritonsillar abscess is usually ushered in by a chill and rapid rise of temperature, 40° C. (104° F.) or higher. Frequently peritonsillitis has been preceded by parenchymatous or follicular angina which has caused slight disturbance of swallowing. Under such circumstances involvement of the peritonsillar tissues is only betrayed by a marked increase in the symptoms. Swallowing of solids or even fluids becomes impossible, even if only slight objective changes are noticeable. Unless rupture occurs early, there will develop on the second or third day of the disease, in addition to the swelling of the lateral palatal region, inflammatory œdema of the nvula, causing the latter to be transformed into a transparent swelling the size of a finger or thumb. In a similar manner inflammation may extend to the epiglottis and to the arytenoepiglottidean folds. The mucous membrane of the floor of the pyriform sinus becomes much swollen, though this condition does not become distinctly noticeable to the eye. Under such circumstances swallowing of fluids becomes impossible and saliva flows out of the month. The condition becomes still more unbearable if there is dyspnœa. The latter frequently develops so rapidly that life can only be saved by means of tracheotomy. This danger should always be borne in mind in cases of severe tonsillitis.

It is difficult to determine the duration of the disease, as the symptoms are so severe attempts are always made to evacuate the pus, and the course of the disease is changed. In general, unless such attempts are made, the symptoms increase for three or four days in milder cases,

and for eight or even ten days in the severer cases. The disease
its highest point at the time of rupture, which almost always tak
into the supratonsillar fossa, being the point of the mucous me
situated nearest the capsule of the tonsil. Less frequently it tak
through the anterior pillar of the fauces. Occasionally perit
develops posteriorly, possibly as a result of congenital sacculatio
supratonsillar fossa behind the posterior pillar of the fauces.   A
edge of this occurrence is important particularly for therapeutic
as in the presence of this condition spontaneous rupture, as
artificial evacuation of the abscess, must take place through the p
pillar of the fauces. The latter forms a thick cord passing direc
the posterior pharyngeal wall, at a level with which rupture g
takes place posteriorly and near the entrance of the larynx.   F
through the inferior portion of the tonsil, formerly supposed to
hardly ever takes place spontaneously.

Spontaneous rupture of such an abscess during sleep is attend
certain dangers, as large quantities of pus may enter the lary
number of cases have been reported in which under such circum
death resulted from asphyxia. Furthermore, the carotid artery 1
eroded by an abscess and fatal hemorrhage result. It might be mer
also that pus may burrow in the deep tissues of the neck as far
aperture of the thorax or even into the mediastinum. In these
suppuration of glands or phlebitis of the jugular vein has app
prepared a bath. In cases of severe abscess severe septic general
tion may occur, particularly on account of the proximity of the
whether or not there is burrowing of pus. · The danger of phlel
the pterygoid plexus and also of the cavernous sinus, with subs
meningitis, has been previously mentioned.

All of which goes·to show that the prognosis of peritonsilliti
always be guarded, unless the abscess is emptied early. At the
time dangerous complications are rare.

Diagnosis.—The diagnosis of peritonsillitis is rarely difficu
palpation is carried out, it always shows dense infiltration of the
surrounding the tonsil; fluctuation is rarely felt. Malignant tumo
be mistaken for peritonsillitis, particularly if the former are the
inflammation. Such cases have repeatedly been reported, an
occasionally led to unpleasant consequences through the fact of a
having been incised, and serious hemorrhage produced. If such a
bility be suspected, it is advisable to make exploratory puncture
attempting incision, while otherwise it is better to make an in
immediately at the site of infiltration.

It is to be noted, moreover, that true peritonsillitis may occas
accompany other diseases, as, for example, primary syphilitic in
of the tonsil. Peritonsillar abscess is very easily simulated by s
induration accompanying such a primary lesion. Also when tl
phlegmonous inflammation of the gums in the vicinity of a wisdon
and in the intermaxillary fold, with formation of abscess, and t
advances toward the tonsil, the abscess assumes the same posi

in peritonsillitis. When there is marked immobility of the jaw, which may accompany either of these conditions, it is hardly possible to distinguish them. Incision should, however, be made in both affections in the same manner, and afterward it will be easier to determine the source of infection.

The vicinity of the wisdom tooth should be carefully inspected, as otherwise this source of infection might be overlooked.

Treatment.—The treatment of peritonsillitis requires incision unless rupture takes place very early. It is true that so-called spontaneous resolution of such abscesses does take place without evacuation of pus, but it is a question whether in such cases small abscesses have not ruptured into the supratonsillar fossa without being noticed by the patient or the surgeon, so that simple resolution was only apparent. Resolution cannot certainly be expected; and if severe manifestations set in, it will be necessary to incise even when the presence of an abscess has not been positively determined. Incision should be made at the most prominent point of the swelling or at the point of fluctuation. If such a point cannot be positively determined, it will be best to hold to the empirical fact that formation of pus first usually takes place at the above-mentioned site, in the prolongation of the supratonsillar fossa.

In order to locate the site of incision, Chiari's rule is without doubt very practicable. A line joining the base of the uvula and the last molar tooth is bisected, and the incision made at the point of bisection. At this site one may cut 1 to 2 cm. posteriorly without danger. A narrow double-edged knife should be used, with which it is possible to prolong the incision either upward or downward. Any other cutting instrument can be employed, but it must be extremely sharp as otherwise pain is much increased. It is very important, moreover, to incise sufficiently deep; not infrequently the abscess is only found at a depth of more than 1 cm. Even if pus issues from the incision the operation is not always completed. Following evacuation of pus the layers of tissue which were formerly separated come together and thus may easily prevent the further escape of pus. Or, if the incision is carried through sound tissues the edges of the latter may rapidly adhere, and pus again accumulates behind the wound. The incision should therefore be made as free as possible, but on account of the possibility of injuring the large vessels it should always be made in a strictly vertical direction. After the incision has been completed the opening may be enlarged by inserting a pair of blunt-pointed scissors and withdrawing them opened. This procedure is very painful, however. It is always advisable after incision to insert a bent probe and to determine whether the abscess extends further in one or the other direction, and to enlarge the incision accordingly. If the opening of the incision becomes closed, it is best to reopen it with a probe or scalpel. Inserting a strip of iodoform gauze may keep the opening free, but is unpleasant and painful for the patient.

It is very annoying if the incision fails to reach the abscess. This occurrence will be comparatively infrequent, provided the above rule is followed. It is more liable to happen when the attempt is made to incise

the point of greatest swelling, as ascertained by palpation, and this
is just missed.   In such cases pus will subsequently rupture int
wound, particularly if a blunt probe or closed scissors are in:
repeatedly.   If the first incision does not reach the abscess, an
parts have been well cocainized, incision may be repeated close 1
first, but this should not be carried too far, as the inflammation w
immediately increased, and the latter will quite properly be laid 1
operator.   It is better under such circumstances to wait a short
or possibly to insert a probe into the opening of the old incision
case incision at any other point has failed, it is always practical
incise again at the site of election.

Little need be said regarding the other methods recommended i
treatment of acute peritonsillitis.   König suggested the injection
per cent. or 3 per cent. solution of carbolic acid into the periton
tissue.   This method has found adherents.   The external applic
of poultices is a favorite remedy with patients and physicians.
certainly relieve pain.   External application of ice rarely affords 1
swallowing cracked ice may, however, be of great service.

Occasionally artificial means of feeding the patient are of the gr
importance.   As swallowing of even soft articles of food is quite un
able, it may be advisable to pass a small Nélaton catheter throug
nose, and introduce food to the upper portion of the pharynx thr
the latter.   From this point it can readily be swallowed without ca
pain.   It is certainly of the greatest importance to sustain the str
of patients suffering from this septic condition.   A number of physi
consider the administration of large quantities of alcohol useful.
pain is so severe that morphine acts only when given in large 1
The latter need not cause any apprehension, however, unless the
severe general sepsis.

Finally it may be noted that after the termination of the acute di:
particularly in cases in which such attacks frequently occur, incisin
tonsillar crypts may occasionally exert a good prophylactic influer

Retropharyngeal Abscess.—The formation of abscess behind
posterior pharyngeal wall may originate in the burrowing of
which results from disease of the vertebræ or the base of the 1
The loose connective tissue surrounding the pharynx laterally
behind is particularly adapted to such a process.   The diseas
be considered in this connection have been discussed in other 1
ters of this work, and a burrowing abscess possesses so few ch
teristic qualities to distinguish it from those suppurative proc
to be discussed immediately below, that a special description b
seems necessary.   The second group of such abscesses is cause
suppuration of the glands situated behind and at the side of
pharynx.   These lymph-glands are very numerous and form a
chain on both sides, close to the pharynx and in the median
along the cervical vertebræ.   There is a second chain parallel t
first, in the sheath of the cervical vessels.   Both chains probably
municate by anastomoses, knowledge in this regard being still impe

It is fairly certain, however, that these retropharyngeal glands receive the lymphatics from the posterior pharyngeal wall and the pharyngeal tonsil, possibly also the palatal tonsils. This chain of glands is frequently involved as a result of inflammatory processes in the tonsils occurring primarily or accompanying acute or chronic general infectious disease. In the majority of cases inflammation of these glands resolves spontaneously. In some of the cases, however, suppuration of the glands takes place. It may be difficult to decide whether suppuration is primary or due to a burrowing abscess, particularly in the case of tuberculous retropharyngeal abscesses.

Fig. 355.

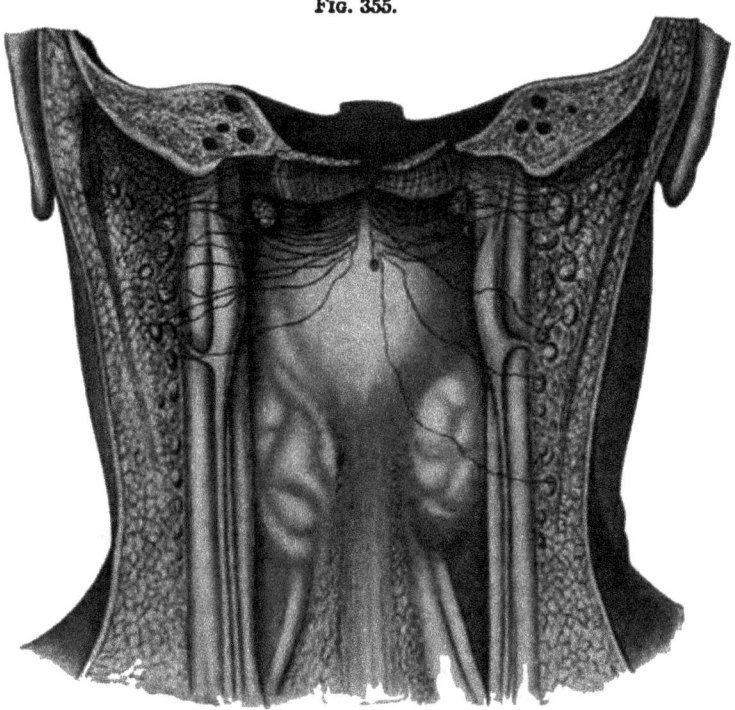

Posterior pharyngeal wall from in front, showing lymphatics.

A great number of diseases other than tuberculosis may cause such abscesses: erysipelas, scarlet fever, measles, and whooping-cough are the ones most frequently mentioned. Simple catarrh or traumatic infection of the nose, of the pharynx, or of more distant regions, as of the ear, superior maxilla, the orbits, base of the tongue, even the temporal region and the face, are regarded as causes. It must be borne in mind, however, that an infection of the ear may cause periphlebitis of the jugular vein, thus simulating the picture of a retropharyngeal abscess. Similar errors may occur under other circumstances.

Most cases of retropharyngeal abscess occur in childhood, more one-half during the first year, possibly on account of the frequen measles, scarlet fever, etc., during this time, and possibly also be in later years the retropharyngeal lymph-glands atrophy (Strübing

Inflammation of the retropharyngeal lymph-glands is not alway lowed by abscess. Even when there is considerable swelling accompa by severe symptoms complete resolution may take place. More quently, however, an abscess is formed. Naturally the abscess is siti a little to one side, but frequently it extends beyond the middle lir that it is apparently situated medially.

Examination is generally very difficult, especially so as most case met with in small children. The swelling produced by the absces: generally covered with normal mucous membrane; occasionally the l is reddened. In other cases again the yellow color of the pus can be through the mucous membrane.

Symptoms.—The clinical symptoms of retropharyngeal abscess sist principally of the manifestation of septic infection, which may considerably according to the virulence of the process and the raj of its development. In addition there are difficulty in swallowing disturbance of respiration. The latter is caused not only by the mec ical hindrance offered by the very sensitive abscess swelling, but al inflammatory œdema of the surrounding tissues. Both conditions develop to a considerable degree and threaten the life of the pa Danger to life may be caused also by rupture of the abscess as in tonsillitis. Unless such an occurrence takes place the chances of rec from "primary" abscess are good, provided it is recognized suffici soon and evacuated, and unless it was caused by tuberculous ly adenitis, or it occurs in a child suffering from hereditary syphilis. U the latter circumstances the power of resistance is so low that in sp an early diagnosis the patients die after evacuation of the abscess.

Diagnosis.—As far as the diagnosis is concerned, it is remarkable very frequently retropharyngeal abscess is overlooked. The severi the symptoms and the accessibility of the posterior pharyngeal wall (to prevent this occurrence. The existence of abscess, as distingu from tumor, may occasionally be readily determined by obtaining tuation or softening on palpation. Frequently, however, it rer doubtful whether there is only lymphadenitis or whether abscess formed. This condition will hardly be mistaken for malignant t if palpation is performed. Tumors are very rare in childhood. of these errors in diagnosis are due to the fact that palpation was om

Strumitis of retrovisceral struma would be difficult to distinguish retropharyngeal abscess. The situation of such struma is very si to that of the retropharyngeal glands.

Treatment.—The treatment requires first of all evacuation of th scess. This is usually easy, provided the diagnosis of abscess had act been made. Care should be taken, however, not to puncture too de as otherwise the scalpel may penetrate the vertebræ, which are so childhood. Care must also be taken in case of larger abscesses th

soon as pus escapes the patient is placed with the face directly downward, in order to prevent pus entering the larynx. Free incision is indicated only in case of acute abscess. In case of tuberculous process or burrowing abscess operation is indicated only when there is considerable difficulty in swallowing or disturbance of respiration. In these latter conditions the prognosis is grave, even after simple puncture followed by injection of iodoform, while under appropriate general treatment such processes sometimes do get well. At all events it is better when the abscess must be opened to perform an external operation in order to avoid secondary infection. For the same reason it may be better to make an external incision in case of simple abscess also when it occurs in very small children.

Chronic Tonsillitis.—It is hardly of sufficient importance to set up a distinct special clinical picture of chronic tonsillitis. After successive attacks of acute tonsillitis isolated portions of the tonsil continue to remain markedly reddened and moderately swollen. Freqnently such portions of the tonsil are divided from the rest of the tonsil by very deep clefts or by scars extending to the pillars of the fauces. In some cases the crypts occupying the cleft portion of the tonsil are surrounded by an area of redness while a deep-yellow plug projects from the opening of the crypt. In other cases no great change can be seen in the tonsils, only that a white deposit forms at the opening of one or several crypts which does not generally continue for any length of time, but causes an annoying sensation of pressure or burning. The tonsils are generally enlarged; in other cases again they are atrophic. In connection with the latter condition there are generally rather extensive adhesions with the pillars of the fauces, so that in a certain sense the tonsils are concealed by the latter.

In these various conditions the most noticeable feature is the great variation in the manifestations; there are periods during which the conditions are absolutely normal, alternating with periods during which there are mild manifestations of angina or more severe attacks of acute inflammation.

Diagnosis.—It may be impossible to make a diagnosis of chronic recurrent angina if the process is observed during a free interval. In those cases in which there are extensive adhesions with the pillars of the fauces the small inflammatory foci are only rendered visible by pushing aside or pulling forward the former.

Treatment during the free interval is directed to the hypertrophy and the cryptic condition of the tonsil.

Chronic Pharyngitis.—Those conditions which are included under the term chronic pharyngitis are of little surgical interest. Chronic catarrhs result from the action of various irritants upon the posterior pharyngeal wall (alcohol, tobacco) or are caused by infections or irritating secretions flowing from the nose, epipharynx, or the month, drying of the mouth as a result of mouth-breathing, and by many other conditions. This catarrhal condition causes enlargement of the lymphatic vessels of the posterior pharyngeal wall, producing so-called "granula," which is subsequently followed by atrophy of the mucous membrane.

In the former condition the follicles are conspicuous, of a yellowi:
color, and raised above the surface of the pharyngeal wall like fi
buds. Under the second condition the wall of the pharynx is su
glistening as if varnished, frequently also covered with tenacious (
mucopurulent secretion. In both conditions the patient complains
cipally of dryness, burning, or a sensation of pressure in the t]
Frequently there are reflex cough and intermittent or continuous h(
ness.

These conditions require special treatment, such as applicatic
astringents, cauterization, destruction of the "granula" with gal
cautery, and many other methods which need not be described he1
is important to seek the cause of this very annoying disease, partic
in the nose, epipharynx, and tonsils.

Hypertrophy of the Tonsils.—There is a great difference in op
as to the etiological significance of this very frequent abnormal (
tion. While formerly it was considered the expression of a scrofuk
lymphatic diathesis, it has been more recently maintained that in a
number of cases, at any rate, the surgeon has to deal with a latent 1
culous process. Tuberculous changes have actually been observ
cases with enlarged tonsils, but it must not be forgotten that in most
these changes were found on the cadaver of tuberculous subjects '
the tonsils were systematically examined. So far it has never been (
mined in a sufficiently large number of cases just how frequently 1
culous changes are found in the tonsils of individuals not suffering
phthisis. The same difficulties are present as in case of the phary
tonsil; the crypts of the tonsils very frequently contain necrotic m
dead horny epithelium, associated with numerous living and dead n
organisms, particularly leptothrix, but also many other kinds of bac
moulds, and fungi, deposits of lime, cholesterin, etc. At the bor(
the necrotic masses the epithelium of the tonsillar crypt is frequ
absent as a result of excessive infiltration with leucocytes, as has
described by Stöhr. Under these conditions a lymphoma-like stru
may develop about such necrotic masses in which giant-cells
sionally develop, similar to those occurring in granulation poly
the middle ear. Necrotic masses embedded in lymphomatous t
and giant cells have frequently, no doubt, led to the incorrect diag
of tuberculosis. For this reason such histological structures shou
carefully interpreted. There can be no doubt that in a large numl
cases the diagnosis of tuberculosis is correct, but to evolve theraj
indications from this fact, as several observers have done, seems 1
hazardous.

The conditions present in hypertrophy of the tonsils are well k1
Enlargement may be considerable, so marked that both tonsils touch
other. At the same time they project very much from their po
exposing their free surface, unless they have become adherent t
inner surface of the pillars of the fauces. In other cases only c(
portions of the tonsil are enlarged. Under certain circumstancei
difficult to determine this condition, particularly if the lowest porti

the tonsil nearest the tongue is involved. The surface may be smooth, but more frequently it is divided by clefts. The crypts are usually provided with a narrow entrance, frequently presenting yellowish-white plugs. Other crypts are very deep, having a slit-like or irregular-shaped opening. This condition is more frequently found in adults than in children. The enlarged tonsils are pale red or yellowish-red in color. If observed during the time of an acute onset, they may be vivid dark red in color, or in case of anæmic individuals very pale or almost white in appearance. The consistence of the tonsils varies considerably and within wide limits. In children hypertrophied tonsils are usually soft, particularly after repeated attacks. The tonsils of adults, on the other hand, may be extremely hard or occasionally entirely fibrous. Particular attention should be paid as to whether the tonsil is adherent to the pillars of the fauces. This cannot always be determined by inspection alone, but is easy with the assistance of a probe. As J. Killian has pointed out, it is not sufficient to examine the tonsil from in front only, as is usually done, but it is necessary to draw back the opposite angle of the mouth (mouth-retractor). The tongue should be drawn forward as in conducting laryngoscopy, in order to observe the tonsil and both pillars of the fauces from the opposite side. The posterior portion of the tonsils, particularly, can only be inspected in this way. The laryngoscope should also be employed in conducting the examination, particularly for the purpose of inspecting the lower portions of the tonsil.

Symptoms.—The clinical manifestations caused by hypertrophy of the tonsils vary considerably. Many of the disturbances which were in former times universally ascribed to the palatal tonsils (and such statements are still found in some text-books) have been referred to coexisting enlargements of the pharyngeal tonsil, whose importance was formerly not appreciated. Even considerable enlargement of the palatal tonsils frequently causes no clinical symptoms, while a very small pharyngeal tonsil may produce very unpleasant manifestations. It is necessary therefore to examine carefully the pharyngeal tonsil, even when the palatal tonsils are considerably enlarged. In the majority of cases both lymphatic organs are diseased at the same time, though to a very different degree. It may be difficult to determine sometimes which is the principal cause of the disease, and in doubtful cases it may be necessary to remove both.

The principal symptom actually produced by enlargement of the palatal tonsils alone is *disturbance of swallowing*. In some cases the latter is continuous; in others it is present only during the acute attack of inflammation. A sensation of difficulty of swallowing or of soreness, as if a bone were lodged in the throat, may frequently be present without the existence of any discoverable inflammatory condition. Occasionally patients swallow the wrong way. This is caused by a lack of mobility of the tonsil and consequent distortion of the soft palate, as a result of which the nasopharynx cannot be closed air-tight, or it is due to the fact that fluids when swallowed cannot pass over the entrance of the larynx in the normal way, but are deflected from their regular course by

the enlarged tonsil. Very considerable enlargement may occasio
especially in the case of young children, render the swallowing of
so difficult that the patients object to solid food.

Respiration may also be interfered with, but this is much les
quently observed than formerly, since the significance of the phary
tonsil has become generally recognized. Breathing through the
may be obstructed by large palatal tonsils alone, particularly at
when the patients lie on their backs and the enlarged tonsils fall
and close off the nasopharynx. There is frequently a snoring s
during respiration in this condition.

Hypertrophy of the palatal tonsil quite frequently causes refle:
turbances, particularly reflex cough. While speaking or during bal
respiration a peculiar sensation is suddenly produced in such
which has been described as a feeling as if a certain point in the t
had suddenly become dried up, or a feeling like that caused by the
of a pin, or as if a foreign body had lodged in the throat. This c
an irritable cough, and the patients cough a number of times, frequ
with such violence that tears come to their eyes. The attack pass
without any expectoration or possibly only a small quantity of mu
coughed up.

The most annoying consequence of hypertrophy of the tonsils i
common tendency to *acute attacks of tonsillitis.* And it is this which
frequently causes the patient to consult the physician. These at
frequently occur on the slightest provocation; most frequently the
ascribed to "catching cold."

A subject that has been little studied is *retrograde development*
tonsil. It is generally assumed that this takes place at the time of pul
this cannot be denied, but it is certain that tonsillar hypertroph
quently continues beyond the time of puberty. Undoubtedly retro
development may be associated with spontaneous or surgical art
evacuation of the crypts, or with suppuration of tonsillar tissue, or
peritonsillar abscess.

Treatment.—*Tonsillotomy* is only indicated in patients who
from repeated attacks of severe tonsillitis, and in whom there is co
crable enlargement of the palatal tonsils. But even in such cases it sl
be noted whether at the same time breathing through the nose i
structed, and in this way the predisposition to tonsillitis is incre
In general tonsillotomy is not a dangerous operation, but it is impo
to guarantee a prophylactic result, and since so little is known rega
the importance of the tonsil for the whole organism removal of this
should not be done without sufficient cause.

Tonsillotomy is performed with specially constructed tonsillotom
with knife and forceps, or hook-retractors. Some recommend the
vanocaustic loop or simple cold snare, but these latter methods hav
been generally accepted. For the removal of circumscribed hypert
of isolated portions, cutting forceps may be employed.

Tonsillotomes may be divided into two groups, those constructed
the old Fahnestock and those after the more recent Mackenzie pa

In the former instrument a ring provided with a cutting edge along its inner border slides between two bars, and at the moment that the tonsil is divided by the cutting ring it is drawn out by a projecting book. In the Mackenzie instrument a semicircular-shaped knife is pushed against a ring which surrounds the tonsil. The tonsil is not pulled out of its pocket, but the ring surrounding it is pressed down upon the pillars of the fauces. Hypertrophied tonsils can readily be removed with either form of tonsillotome, if the former projects from its pocket. Where the tonsil does not project, and there are the slightest adhesions, it is impossible to carry out the operation by this method. If adhesions are present and an instrument provided with a projecting hook is used, one of the pillars of the fauces may be drawn into the ring and be injured. In most cases, however, the operation cannot be performed at all and the instrument becomes caught in such a way as to be very annoying to the patient as well as to the physician. Under such conditions it is better to remove the tonsil with a knife. For this purpose it is best to employ a slightly curved probe-pointed scalpel, and either a two-pronged sharp retractor or a broad-bladed tooth-forceps. The tonsil is drawn inward with forceps or retractor; if any resistance is noted, due to adhesions, the latter can be divided by means of the probe-pointed scalpel. If the adhesions are very extensive, the tonsil must first be freed by means of a scalpel curved on the flat, or with Cowper's scissors. As much of the tonsil as projects beyond the pillars of the fauces is then cut off. This is best done in a direction from below upward, as otherwise the knife is liable to be deflected from the tonsil in the lower part of the incision, and the respective portion of the tonsil remains. Care should be taken not to injure the pillar of the fauces after the knife has traversed the tonsil. Such wounds are much more painful, especially afterward, than those of the tonsil itself, and unpleasant also for the reason that the purity of the *singing voice* may be permanently impaired thereby.

The danger of hemorrhage accompanying tonsillotomy has been much discussed. Hemorrhage is frequently very severe, and has repeatedly been fatal. It was formerly believed possible that the internal carotid might be injured during tonsillotomy, but modern anatomical investigations would show that this can be practically excluded. On the other hand, Merkel had drawn attention to the fact that an abnormal course of the external maxillary artery, when the latter projects toward the tonsil in a sharp curve, may under circumstances lead to severe arterial hemorrhage. More commonly the surgeon has to deal with secondary parenchymatous hemorrhage, which is frequently kept up through the fact of the patient's increasing blood-pressure, by hawking, coughing, and spitting, or by a tight collar causing congestion. One can never be sure that hemorrhage may not take place, even if the operation is performed with the galvanocautery; hemorrhage may at times follow the removal of the slough. To stop the bleeding, it frequently suffices to exclude the above-mentioned causes.

In case of arterial hemorrhage the bleeding vessel should if possible be caught with a long or preferably a curved clamp, and tied or twisted, or hemorrhage should be controlled by forcible compression. pression must occasionally be kept up for some time, a special sorium has been devised by v. Mikulicz, which can be allowed t in place. It has also been recommended in such cases to close th of the tonsil by closely suturing the pillars of the fauces. It is st hemorrhage is most liable to occur in dense fibrous tonsils. cases there was hæmophilia. Finally, it is possible that the exi acute angina with inflammatory paresis of the vessel-wall may closure of the latter.

Incision of the tonsil is another method frequently employed i hypertrophy of the tonsils, and one which is very useful when deep clefts in the tonsil filled with masses of detritus. This met gested by v. Hoffmann and especially recommended by Moritz produces evacuation of the clefts, and in this way removes chroni mation of the tonsillar tissue. Incision is made with a knife be to a right angle, on the flat or the edge, or with a slightly curve pointed bistoury. This operation can be performed without ar and is absolutely painless with cocaine, and causes very little hem The operation must occasionally be repeated when the clefts numerous, and particularly when incision was not carried su deep into the substance of the tonsil at the first operation.

SYPHILIS, TUBERCULOSIS, LEPROSY, RHINOSCLEROMA, GLANDERS OF THE PHARYNX.

Syphilis is the most common of specific inflammations of the Primary lesions frequently occur, especially on one tonsil, l mouly on both. They play an important part among ext lesions. According to Münchheimer's compilations, of 10,26 genital infections, 504 occurred on the tonsils. Infection may a result of unnatural intercourse, also through kissing, from instruments, etc. Especially to be noted is the infection of through spoons with which they have fed syphilitic children.

On the tonsil the primary lesion frequently, though not alway the cartilage-like, firm consistence of the initial lesion, but in of the cervical lymph-glands regularly occurs. This is fı marked. On account of the latter, confusion with malignan is very possible, particularly if, as is not infrequently the primary lesion pr s s a phagedenic character, with rapid necrosis. The diagnosis is frequently very difficult, but all d soon be dispelled, provided the possibility of primary lesion is co Frequently distinct secondary manifestations appear before the lesion has disappeared, thus rendering the diagnosis certain. N form of treatment is required in this stage; under circumstanc there is no tendency to heal, the latter may be combated by e curial treatment. Where the ulcers are phagedenic in character and other antiseptics should be applied.

Secondary manifestations, generally occurring in the form of typical mucous patches, have only a diagnostic significance, except in so far as their great infectiousness is concerned. It may be mentioned, however, that they frequently show a tendency to become eroded, and may possibly be confused with diphtheria or follicular tonsillitis.

Gummatous changes in the pharynx are very frequent, particularly in the posterior wall of the pharynx and on the soft palate, especially at the posterior surface of the latter. The ulcers themselves, when recognized, usually show the typical picture of gumma, but are frequently so covered by mucus of the pharynx that they are not easily recognized. Posterior rhinoscopy should never be omitted. Gummata are often present in large numbers, and by producing infiltration of the palatal muscles often cause functional disturbance of the latter—*i. e.*, difficulty in swallowing, the entrance of fluids into the nose, and their escape through the latter, and disturbances of speech possessing the character of rhinolalia aperta. These disturbances frequently precede the visible changes in the gumma when the process is principally located in the nasopharynx. As is well known, gummatous ulceration very frequently leads to perforation of the palate. If this perforation is situated at the base of the uvula, ulceration may completely destroy the latter. If the ulcers heal, there commonly occur marked scar formation and possibly adhesions, particularly if treatment was instituted late.

Treatment.—The general treatment is that of syphilis. Besides potassium iodide, mercury should be given; frequently a combination of both acts better.

Tuberculosis may occur in the pharynx, either in the lupous or the ordinary form of tuberculous infiltration and ulceration. This is almost always secondary.

In unquestionably primary cases lesions are found only on the tonsil. Orth in particular has confirmed the primary occurrence of tuberculosis in the tonsils. Schlenker and others have demonstrated that tuberculosis of the tonsils is not infrequently followed by tuberculous disease of the cervical lymphatic glands. Unfortunately no clinical distinction between ordinary hypertrophy of the tonsils and primary tuberculosis of the tonsils has been made. It is advisable, therefore, in cases in which enlarged tonsils are accompanied by obstinate recurring tuberculous lymphadenitis of the neck to remove the tonsils and make a histological examination of them. It might be possible in this way to prevent recurrences. Seifert found two apparently primary cases of tuberculous disease of the pharynx. Otherwise the disease occurs only in association with tuberculosis elsewhere.

Lupus.—The lupous form spreads by extension along the mucous membrane from the lips and skin of the face to the pharynx; very frequently also the larynx is invaded. The appearance of the infiltrated nodes, which become ulcerated and covered with a dirty grayish slough, not infrequently showing a tendency to bleed and become covered with brownish-red or yellowish-brown crusts, coincides with the description of lupus of the mucous membrane. The process shows a tendency here

also to undergo healing with marked scar formation, partic
young individuals.

SYMPTOMS.—In lupus of the pharynx the symptoms are f₁
insignificant. The author knows of patients who consulted th₁
cian only on account of the presence of lupus of the skin,
mentioning the disease of the pharynx, which was a great d
extensive (frequently the mucous membrane of the month an
was also involved). In general the most marked disturbances ₁
able to these complicating diseases. Those of the larynx pa:
may produce serious interference with swallowing, and 'm this
to impaired nutrition; there may also be respiratory difficulty.

PROGNOSIS.—The prognosis depends principally upon how ex
the larynx and lungs are involved and upon the terminatio
process in the latter. On the whole the prognosis is not so unt
as far as life is concerned, particularly in young individuals. Tl
cases in which in older individuals fresh processes occur ar₁
fatal as a result of further extension, though at first the typic₁
of lupus might lead to a wrong prognosis. In lupus of the pha
local lesions themselves frequently heal, but recurrences rarel
occur, and at the best the disease runs a very protracted cou
the same time lupus may be continuously progressing in oth
tions.

TREATMENT.—The treatment of lupus in these situations is ₁
as anywhere else. The foci can be completely removed surgic₁
scissors, sharp spoon, or galvanocautery.[1] Recurrence is, howe
prevented by the use of so-called selective substances, of whi
acid is the one principally employed. The latter must, how
used in sufficiently strong solutions (at least 50 per cent., be:
strength), and be thoroughly applied with a cotton swab, or b₁
with a stiff, short-haired brush. Where the parts are very
cocaine should first be applied. The posterior surface of the so
should not be forgotten (posterior rhinoscopy). The same t₁
should be applied to coexisting disease of the nose and lips, as c
new foci may originate from the latter. For foci which are a
from without, hot-air treatment, which was recently introduced
considered, and the author has occasionally seen very good resul
its employment in just such cases. Naturally care should be t₁
to burn the mucous membrane of the larynx, particularly if na:
ration is disturbed. Also by improving the arrangements for t:
with arc light and x-rays, it may be possible to obtain good r
the application of these measures in this situation.

In the medicinal treatment iodoform plays an important p
spite of the different opinions regarding this substance, the auth₁
not wish to do without it. It should not only be insufflated, l
oughly applied to the abraded or cauterized surface of the ulc
a brush or cotton swab. This is best accomplished if the iod

---

[1] In using the galvanocautery marked and annoying inflammatory œdema is liable

in the form of a paste. Submucous injections of iodoform-glycerin may be of advantage in case of marked infiltration of the mucous membrane.

Tuberculosis.—While the prognosis is fairly good in lupus, it is always worse in other forms of tuberculosis. Infiltration and resulting ulceration, besides disseminated tuberculous disease, are frequently but incorrectly described as miliary tuberculosis. *Infiltration* usually undergoes rapid ulceration; the latter attains considerable depth and shows all the characteristics described in connection with tuberculous disease of the mouth. It is most frequently found on both surfaces of the soft palate, and upon the posterior pharyngeal wall, where it occasionally attains considerable size and not infrequently involves the entire thickness of the soft palate, so that it is difficult to distinguish it from syphilitic ulceration.

DIAGNOSIS.—In most cases the diagnosis must depend upon histological examination of the secretion or scrapings or resected portions of tissue. Even if distinct pulmonary disease is present, it is not safe to be too positive of the tuberculous character of disease of the pharynx if the appearance is doubtful, as syphilis may occur at the same time as tuberculosis. Distinct disease of the lungs is rarely absent in these cases, and for this reason the prognosis is correspondingly grave. It is absolutely bad only in the *disseminated* form, in which all the soft parts of the pharynx are traversed by small confluent nodules, while at the same time the entire vicinity is found in a condition of inflammation, with marked redness and swelling. Frequently the structures involved are conspicuously livid and cyanotic in appearance. It is remarkable that in this form of disease the subjective symptoms are occasionally very mild. In most cases the general disturbances, high fever, and the signs of pulmonary disease occupy the prominent position in the clinical picture.

TREATMENT avails only in the forms with infiltration and ulceration, particularly if there ·is associated with the latter marked disturbance of swallowing. Cauterization with lactic acid may also be of advantage here, but should be employed with great care. This is true of all interfering measures, as otherwise the threatened disturbance of general nutrition will be actually produced. If there is inflammatory œdema of the surrounding tissues, it is advisable to employ iodoform or orthoform, and other local anæsthetics. Cocaine, which is used a great deal, is too transient in its action. The patient is very liable to become addicted to its use, so that it is better to reserve it for a time of necessity. Morphine has a certain field of usefulness, being the only remedy in disseminated tuberculosis where the latter causes much suffering. Otherwise in this obstinate form astringent lotions, aluminum acetate, etc., are indicated, beside the well-known general remedies.

The remaining specific inflammations of the pharynx are very rare.

Leprosy is being considered more as the number of cases observed is constantly being increased by fresh examples, and recently in Upper Silesia an autochthonous case of the disease was observed. In the pharynx there occur tuberous swellings, as described in Mikulicz's and

Michelson's *Atlas*, having the appearance of the intestine in typh
being very firm, with no tendency to ulcerate and undergoing ci
contraction. More rarely in the early stages are seen waxy 1
frequently occurring in large numbers in the substance of the sof
and on the posterior wall of the pharynx. This disease causes
ances only in the advanced forms, with marked mechanical inter

Rhinoscleroma.—In the early stages the infiltrations of rhinos
are similar to those of leprosy; they favor the middle line, and, ac
to the course of the disease, usually follow diseases of the month
by direct extension. In this situation the characteristic cup-shap
and later cicatricial contraction can be distinctly observed, and
them the diagnosis of rhinoscleroma positively made in later
There is usually extensive, if not complete, closure of the meso
from the epipharynx, and the soft palate is drawn upward and
the posterior pharyngeal wall in the form of a Gothic arch.
these cases disturbances are not severe provided the nodular, c
like infiltration does not lead to occlusion of the nose or the lower
of the pharynx.

Glanders.—In glanders the pharynx is not infrequently invol·
ulceration produced by this disease, and which is usually prec
a distinctly recognizable infiltration, is very similar in appeal
tuberculous ulceration. As a rule the question of diagnosis can
settled by bacteriological examination, inoculation into the pe
cavity of guinea-pigs, and the discovery of glanders nodule
testicles.

Diagnosis.—In all these diseases the diagnosis will be based
pally upon the observance of lesions located elsewhere, which ar
always present in glanders and leprosy; the integument is
affected, and in rhinoscleroma the nose or larynx is generally in
In rhinoscleroma, however, the disease in the pharynx is usu
most characteristic. In the other diseases the lesion of the ph
hardly recognizable without the disease of the skin or nose.

Treatment.—There is hardly any treatment for the last-nan
eases. If stenosis, caused by contraction of the infiltration, p
inconvenience, attempts may be made to dilate the former mecht
This treatment should, however, be commenced early. In these
little can be accomplished by attempts at dissection or destruc

STENOSIS AND ADHESIONS OF THE PHARYNX.

Congenital narrowing and atresia of the pharynx are extrem
and of little surgical importance. In regard to marked stenosi
deeper portions of the pharynx, the author refers to stenosis
œsophagus. Acquired atresia and stricture are more frequent,
quite rare. A small number of them are produced by caustics; t
majority result from syphilitic scars. Very rarely they are ca
leprosy or rhinoscleroma. Most cases of syphilitic stenosis res

the adhesion of opposite-lying portions of the pharynx, the seat of gummatous ulcers. Of the latter, three groups may be distinguished (P. Heymann): those situated between the soft palate and posterior pharyngeal wall, those between the soft palate and the root of the tongue, and those at the lower circumference of the mesopharynx and hypopharynx. These three groups, pure cases of which offer a great variety of findings and symptoms, are naturally combined in various ways owing to the well-known multiplicity of these ulcerations.

Adhesions at the Boundary between the Mesopharynx and Epipharynx.—These adhesions may cause relatively little disturbance and few manifestations provided there has been no serious loss of substance of the palatal arch and uvula. It might readily be assumed from the appearance that there was a simple posterior displacement of the soft palate. More frequently there are found, besides this retraction, defects of the uvula or the palatal arch; frequently the tonsil is embedded in the cicatricial bands or their surface is left so exposed by the latter that it appears as if lying unprotected in the cavity of the mouth. Complete closure of the nasopharynx as a result of such adhesions is rather rare. P. Heymann, however, found several hundred such cases in literature. More frequently adhesions are so extensive that there remains only a small opening leading to the nasopharynx. The latter is frequently difficult to find, particularly if, as is frequently the case, it presents a tortuous or crooked passage. In cases of total and also those of incomplete adhesions according to the size of the existing opening the greatest disturbance is difficulty of speech. Owing to closure of the nasopharynx the nasal sounds are imperfectly produced; moreover, the stiffness of the palatal structures prevents the formation of gutturals; and finally, if there is only a small opening left in the cicatricial tissue, it can only be imperfectly or not at all closed by the palatal muscles, and most vowels assume a nasal twang. Patients in whom there is complete or incomplete atresia infrequently are free from marked annoyance; naturally they may suffer inconvenience from being compelled to breathe through the mouth. The sense of smell is also entirely or almost entirely lost. It is annoying, finally, not to be able to snuff up the nasal secretions. In incomplete atresia the extent of the latter does not always determine the degree of disturbance. Moreover, where the existing opening cannot be closed by the palatal muscles, food, especially fluids, enter the nostrils. The latter accident is frequently the most annoying to the patients.

Atresia at the Boundary between Mesopharynx and Mouth and in the Hypopharynx.—These adhesions are almost always partial, otherwise the inability to take nourishment would render life impossible. But even considerable narrowing of the isthmus of the fauces may exist without serious disturbance. There are cases in which the opening was only the size of a lead-pencil, or would hardly admit the tip of a probe. In these cases of atresia disturbance of swallowing is naturally the most important feature. The patients are sometimes obliged to live on fluid or semifluid food. Speech is also considerably impaired if the move-

ments of the tongue are interfered with by fixation of the root
latter, or if at the same time, as is apparently true in most case:
tricial bands are developed at the entrance to the larynx.   Adl
of this border-zone are almost always combined with stricture
hypopharynx, consequently with closure of the latter from the
pharynx.   In this situation there may be present a number of
cicatricial trabeculæ or a complicated system of thin folds, b
which the passage follows its course.   Sometimes all parts of the er
to the larynx are adherent with the tongue and the arch of the
on the one hand, and to the posterior pharyngeal wall on the ot
that only a small passage remains for the entrance of food.   Tha
plete closure seldom occurs here might be referred to the fact t
account of the threatened danger of starvation patients continue (
nourishment in spite of the great difficulty, and in this way ke
passage open.

It is hardly possible to exhaust the variety of pictures which ma}
from a combination of the various forms of atresia, and for this
every case presents certain peculiarities.

Treatment.—The treatment of all these cases is extremely c
and tedious.   Even if the patient is seen before adhesions have f
it is hardly possible to prevent strictures; the mobility of the '
parts involved is so necessary for the continuance of life that it is
sible to keep the ulcerated surfaces separated for any length of
There does not seem to be any advantage therefore in torturi
patients in cases which come under observation during the early
of the disease by dilating with bougies, etc.   It is best to wait ur
process has terminated, efforts being made, however, to bring the |
to a termination as soon as possible.   In cases of syphilitic ulc
potassium iodide should be assiduously administered, at the sam
endeavoring to control the secondary infection usually present by
feeting the mouth with appropriate gargles, the application of iod
etc.   If cicatrization has been completed, the adhesions should l
separated provided the resulting disturbances render such m(
necessary.   That the extent of the anatomical changes does not i
furnish sufficient indication, and the functional disturbances mus
as a guide, is to be emphasized.

Gradual *dilatation* of existing openings should at first be atte
in all cases, owing to the difficulties surrounding operative trea
This is more apt to bring about good results in adhesions betw(
mesopharynx and the epipharynx; in deeper adhesions it is les:
ticable.   If it is to be employed here, it may be necessary on a
of the interference with respirations to perform tracheotomy.
the mesopharynx is closed from the cavity of the mouth, inter
is hardly ever necessary, as in this situation a sufficient opening
remains of itself.   On the other hand, in the hypopharynx sucl
ference has repeatedly been found necessary on account of the di
in swallowing.   In all cases in which there is stenosis in this si
swelling of the cicatricial tissue, and as a result of the latter as|

may occur, as was emphasized by P. Heymann, so that in the majority of cases these measures were preceded by tracheotomy. Gastrostomy has also been found necessary in a number of cases.

In all cases of stenosis in which treatment is not limited to dilatation with bougies the first problem is to divide the cicatricial bands. Owing to the peculiar localization of these bands the ordinary straight scalpels are frequently inadequate, and even Cooper's scissors are frequently not sufficiently curved. It is best for this purpose therefore to employ knives curved on the flat or short flat knives bent at sharp angles to the handles. Division is usually easy; occasionally considerable hemorrhage occurs, to control which the galvanocautery may be necessary, and in one case it was found necessary to ligate the carotid. In case of bands situated lower down, unless they can be made accessible by direct laryngoscopy, it is better to use the laryngeal mirror and instruments suitable for laryngeal operations.

In case of adhesions between the mesopharynx and the epipharynx division of the cicatricial bridges is almost certain to be followed by recurrence, and it is always necessary subsequently to dilate with bougies or to allow the patients themselves to use bivalve dilating instruments (Hajek). Continuous dilatation has been repeatedly effected by the use of a tube attached to a palate-plate which was passed through the stricture. Dieffenbach sutured the edges of the incision after division, but found that this was very difficult. For less skilful operators this suturing would hardly be possible, at least in those cases in which the line of incision runs transversely through the pharynx. Most authors have not found this method practicable. It might be possible to graft mucous membrane flaps over the surfaces of the wound possibly; even Thiersch skin-grafting might be employed. Experiences in this direction have not been reported in literature, and owing to the great difference in the course of the cicatricial bands it would be impossible to lay down any rule for such measures. In the hypopharynx there is apparently no or very little tendency to recurrence. In the case of adhesion of the soft palate recurrence has been observed even after years of dilatation with bougies.

TUMORS OF THE PHARYNX.

Benign Tumors of the Mesopharynx.—Benign tumors of the pharynx are not common. However, pedunculated fibromata (so-called polypi) do occur. Sometimes they are soft and œdematous, at other times firm. In most cases they originate in the soft palate. Some of these, the so-called lymphadenoid polypi, are characterized by a round-cell infiltration of their tissues. Occasionally also they contain true lymph-follicles, and under the latter circumstances are probably derived from rudimentary displaced tonsils. Other tumors of similar form, but covered with very thick, horny epidermis, occasionally also containing hair and other epidermal derivatives, may be considered *congenital dermoids*, even if they cannot always be discovered at the time of birth.

These tumors are sometimes thickly covered with hair; occasio only a few downy hairs are present, so that even after histolc examination it is not always easy to distinguish them from ord fibrous polypi.

Papillomata occur more frequently than polypi. They consist warty connective-tissue framework, covered by a thick layer of epide Sometimes they consist entirely of the latter. The pedicle is gen short and thin, more rarely very long. In most cases they are acc tally discovered on examination. Actual disturbance is only caus a very long pedicle, which may cause annoying tickling, or some

Fig. 356.

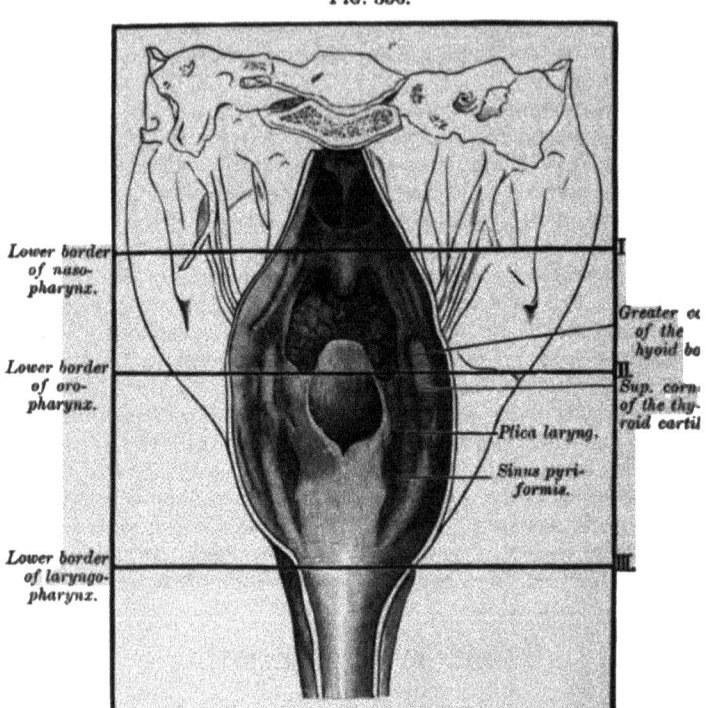

Lower border of naso-pharynx.

Lower border of oro-pharynx.

Lower border of laryngo-pharynx.

Greater o of the hyoid bo

Sup. corn of the thy-roid cartil

Plica laryng.

Sinus pyri-formis.

View of anterior wall of pharynx, seen by opening posterior wall in median line.

the tumor is swallowed by the patient and then regurgitated. But in such cases there are usually found other inflammatory manifesta in the pharynx, to which the complaints of the patient might properly be referred than to the tumors themselves.

The removal of these various tumors can readily be accomplished snare and forceps whenever occasion arises. The pedicle, though is usually tough. Dermoid tumors frequently have such a broad firm pedicle that it is impossible to grasp the latter with scissors. (

sionally also it is only apparently inserted into the arch of the palate, while actually attached high up in the nasopharynx.

Fig. 357.

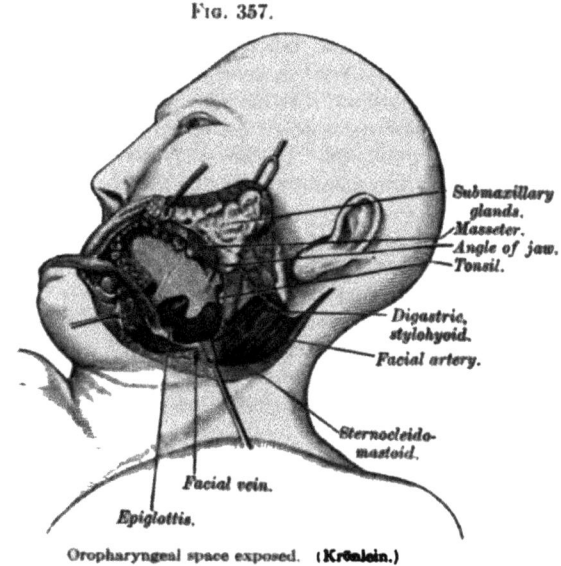

Oropharyngeal space exposed. (Krönlein.)

Fig. 358.

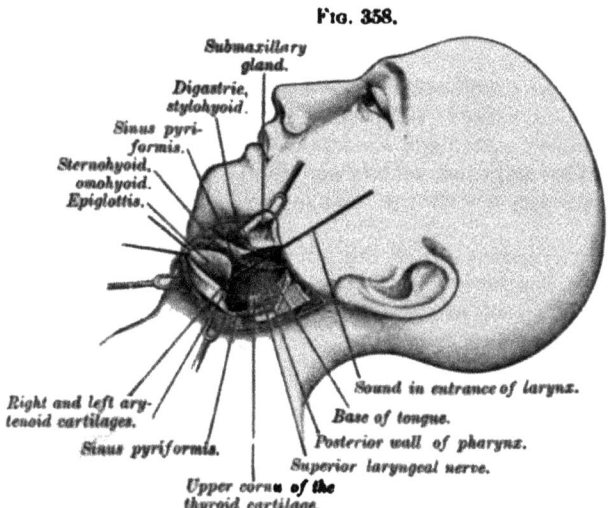

Laryngopharyngeal space exposed. (Krönlein.)

Vascular tumors not infrequently occur in this region; they are more commonly composed of bloodvessels than of lymphatics. Of the latter, cavernous angioma is the most frequent. The edge of the palate and

...nite sites; but they may extend far bey...
...Such large tumors frequently endan...
...hemorrhage; most of them, however, are...
Pedunculated tumors of this kind ha...
...readily removed, but removal of th...
...more difficult if an operation b...
...advisable to use multiple galvan...
...a dull-red heat should be employ...
...while still hot. In this way hem...
...sittings are required this meth...

...are usually combined with hæmang...
...manifestation like those in the tong...
...annoying that operative inter...
...circumstances it is better t...
...on the part of the larynx or...
...otherwise inflammatory symptor...
...these tumors also galvanopunctur...

...as far as the soft palate, but thi...
...hemorrhage from other part...
...part. True aneurysms occasionall...
...originate either from the i...
...arteries. In cases in which pu...
...mistaken for solid tumors, even f...
...has occasionally been followed by...

...on the posterior pharyngeal w...
...patients suffering from chronic puln...
...particularly in old alcoholi...
...They may cause hemorrhage which...
...pulmonary hemorrhage. They are...

...retention-cysts of the soft pala...
...significance. Very rarely larg...
...folds of the soft palate and lined with...
...considered congenital inclusions, bu...

...between the folds of the soft pala...
...fibroma, or true fibroma. As a rule these...
...and belong more properly among the...
...discussed later. Clinically they are very...
...but rarely there are found on the...
...they may have broad pedicles or n...
...tissues. They can usually be readily enu...

...of the **Mesopharynx.**—Mixed tumors occ...
...between benign and malignant tumors. The...

situated between the layers of the soft palate; occasionally they send a relatively thin process through the fascia of the pharynx, which is immediately connected with a larger tumor of the parotid (hour-glass shaped tumor of the parotid). The majority of them are benign in their early stages; they may attain large size, but only cause disturbance through their encroachment on space. As, on account of their situation and size, they are always exposed to mechanical irritation, they may suffer ulceration. The ulcers are usually crater-like, frequently very deep, reminding one of gummatous ulceration or actual malignant tumor. Such ulcerating tumors, on account of their decomposition, frequently produce an extremely unpleasant odor from the month. They frequently cause pain which may be very severe, radiating toward the ear. If they are not ulcerated, the surface is usually rounded, covered by smooth and movable mucous membrane.

It is a peculiarity of these tumors that, after having existed for years or decades, sometimes they suddenly begin to grow rapidly and to assume a very malignant character. In such cases they frequently show the histological structure of round-cell sarcoma, sometimes only at certain portions.

Regarding the position of these tumors among tumors in general, opinions differ widely. The subject has been more fully discussed in the chapter on similar mixed tumors of the salivary glands.

Unless these tumors have assumed a malignant character they can be readily enucleated, as they are completely encapsulated. Those of smaller size, situated only in the pharynx, can therefore be easily removed through the month without preliminary operation. Those of larger size, particularly the parotid-palatal tumors, must be attacked from without, and the same route is to be recommended if the tumor is not movable, as under such circumstances it may rightly be suspected of having undergone a malignant change. If the malignant character is pronounced, it is sometimes surprisingly easy to remove even very large tumors by the external route.

Benign Tumors of the Hypopharynx.—The lower portion of the pharynx is on the whole rarely the seat of tumors. Particularly, benign tumors have only been observed in isolated cases. *Lipoma* is occasionally found near the entrance to the larynx and generally shows an arborescent structure. The finger-like processes may hang into the larynx or into the cavity of the mouth and the œsophagus. In this way they may produce a great variety of symptoms, and these may change in the individual case owing to the fact that these tumors are freely movable and may be swallowed, aspirated, regurgitated, or coughed up. Other tumors similarly constructed are composed of pure connective tissue. These may also attain an enormous size. Tumors have been described that were 20 cm. in length and from 2 to 4 cm. in diameter, which, if situated in the pharynx and œsophagus or upon the larynx, naturally cause considerable suffering. Their point of insertion is usually situated further down in the pharynx, or even in the œsophagus.

the palatal arch are favorite si
boundaries of the pharynx.   S
on account of severe hemorrh
noticed by the patients.   Pedi
observed. The latter can be re
common diffuse forms may be
necessary.   In most cases it i
ture, instead of dissection; onl
instrument being withdrawn v
will be slight, and though seve
accomplish the purpose.

Lymphatic vascular tumors a
and may cause inflammatory n
These attacks may become
becomes necessary.   Under s
however, unless severe complie
septic manifestations set in, a
be considerably increased.   In
best form of treatment.

Racemose aneurysm may exte
causes serious disturbance   A
tumor plays a more important
on the soft palate. The latter
maxillary or the external care
was not noted, and they wer
tonsillar abscess, their incisio
hemorrhage.

Varices not infrequently
at the base of the tongue in
disease and circulatory di
also without apparent ca
be mistaken for gastric o
dangerous.

Cystic tumors, such
quently occur, but are
occur situated between tl
epithelium. They have
is no proof of this the

Other tumors occu
myxoma, chondroma,
contain other kinds of
tumors, which will l
to the latter.   Occas
smaller or larger lip
situated in the deep
through the mouth.

Mixed Tumors
special position l

suggest **the idea that the removal of retrovisceral struma** in
of a normal thyroid might bring about cachexia strumipriva,
observed several times in cases of struma of the tongue.

lly there **must** be mentioned *retropharyngeal tumors*, to which
specially has called attention. In the majority of cases they are
but **enchondroma** and mixed tumors do occur; in only a few
were they **malignant** in character. They belong to the connective-
group of tumors, and originate in the connective tissue of the retro-
space or the periosteum of the vertebral column. Most of these
tumors are **as** well encapsulated as the above-mentioned mixed tumors
of the soft palate. The pharyngeal mucous membrane is freely movable
over the tumors, and the latter are freely movable over the subjacent
structures. If they are not freely movable, this is due either to processes
which may develop in the direction of the sheath of the carotid or to a
malignant character of the tumor.

Symptoms.—The symptoms produced by these tumors vary considerably according to their situation and extent: they may interfere with
swallowing or with breathing, not only with breathing through the nose,
but with breathing through the mouth as well. Owing to the great
size they sometimes attain they considerably distend and displace the
structures of the pharynx.

Treatment.—Owing to the fact that they are so well circumscribed
all of these forms of tumors cannot infrequently be readily enucleated
through the mouth after dividing the mucous membrane covering them
or splitting the edge of the palate (Busch). But such an attempt is not
advisable unless they are freely movable. Under such circumstances it
will be better to employ the external route by the methods to be described
in the following pages, as in this way opening the pharynx can be
avoided. B. O. Chiari witnessed death from incomplete operation
through the mouth as a result of septic infection in a case of retrovisceral
struma.

Malignant Tumors of the Pharynx.—As the rare malignant tumors
of the epipharynx have been sufficiently discussed, the author will discuss here only the most frequent malignant tumors of the pharynx, those
of the tonsillar region. *Lymphosarcoma* occasionally originates in the
faucial tonsils as well as in the pharyngeal tonsil. In this situation a very
peculiar clinical picture is produced (Störk). At first they have the
appearance of a simple hypertrophy of the tonsil, which is conspicuous
only on account of the white color and nodular character of the surface.
Associated with this there is a firm, pale, œdematous thickening of the
neighboring palatal mucous membrane; subsequently the enlargement
of neighboring and distant lymphatic organs, the spleen, etc., produces
the picture of pseudoleukæmia. In the initial stages, however, the manifestations would render confusion with peritonsillar abscess very possible,
and this mistake has actually occurred before the advancement of the
process had pointed out the correct diagnosis. Later the disease affects
all the neighboring organs, larynx, etc., finally causing a painful death
through disturbance of nutrition and respiration.

en even then. The temptation is great in such cases to enter the pharynx with a bougie or œsophagoscopy tube: in no other disease is there so much nger of perforating the wall of the pharynx or œsophagus. It is still ore difficult to recognize these tumors if the posterior cricoarytenoid nscles are infiltrated and the picture f a double posticus paralysis is pro- uced, causing one to suspect some ervous disease or an aneurysm of the orta. If this condition is associated with œdematous infiltration of the mu- ous membrane covering the arytenoid cartilages, and if the difficulty in swal- lowing occurs suddenly for the first time during eating, there is great lia- bility of mistaking the condition for phlegmonous laryngitis caused by a foreign body, and this mistake has ac- tually occurred. As in these tumors

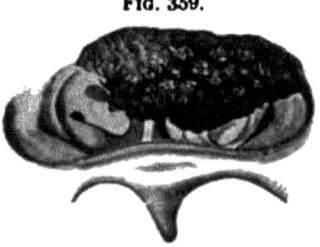

Fig. 359.

View of nasopharyngeal carcinoma in pharyngoscopic examination in a man aged fifty-four years.

the lymph-glands do not always become enlarged until later, and as, on the other hand, they become enlarged as a result of inflammatory process, the difficulties of diagnosis are numerous and frequently insurmountable.

Fig. 360.

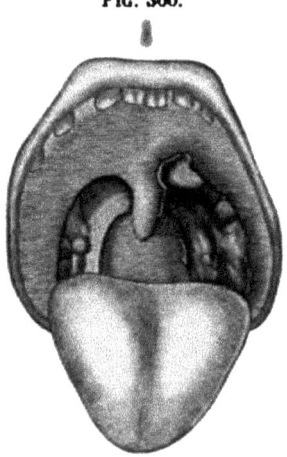

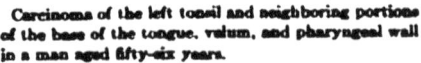

Carcinoma of the left tonsil and neighboring portions of the base of the tongue, velum, and pharyngeal wall in a man aged fifty-six years.

Fig. 361.

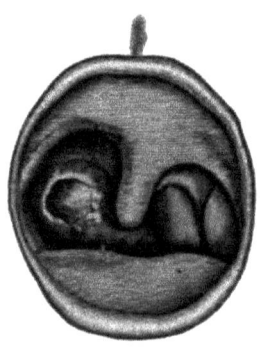

Carcinoma of both tonsils in a woman aged sixty-six years.

The prognosis in all these tumors is naturally worse the later they are recognized; it is better therefore in visible carcinoma of the tonsillar region than in deeply seated tumors of the hypopharynx; moreover, the former and tumors of the palate are more easily removed without severe impairment of nutrition and respiration, while after removal of larger

portions of the lower part of the pharynx the patients are depende
artificial nourishment unless it is possible to restore the alimenta
age by plastic operations similar to those of the œsophagus.   As
therefore it will be necessary to abstain from removing such deep
tumors, and to attempt alleviating the condition of the patient
trostomy or possibly tracheotomy.   Frequently this is more of a
than relief, and in such cases it is proper to employ morphine as
resort.

CHAPTER XXXII.

OPERATIONS ON THE PHARYNX.

THE indications for opening the pharynx are the presence of foreign bodies, stenosis, or new growths. The first two indications are at present hardly ever considered; though firmly embedded, and especially pointed foreign bodies cannot always be reached by means of the laryngoscope. Stenosis of benign character which is not amenable to dilatation with bougies is rare. Thus pharyngotomy is limited to tumors, and particularly to malignant tumors.

The pharynx is accessible by two routes: from in front and from the side. Otherwise the methods differ only as to the choice of a high or low incision or the combination of several incisions. The methods which follow the anterior route have fallen into bad repute on account of unfavorable immediate results. According to authors, the principal danger is the division of both superior laryngeal nerves; the latter injury is difficult to avoid, and causes complete anæsthesia of the entrance to the larynx, thus predisposing to aspiration pneumonia. Furthermore, the transverse incision is apparently liable to infection (subsequent phlegmon of the neck and inflammation of mediastinum). The danger of injury of the laryngeal nerve can be more readily avoided by suprahyoid pharyngotomy. By this method the muscles attached to the hyoid bone are divided immediately above the latter, and after dividing the mucous membrane one enters immediately in front of the epiglottis. In this way only the vicinity of the latter is made accessible. In subhyoid pharyngotomy the thyrohyoid ligament is divided between clamps. This ligament is inserted into the posterior border of the arch of the hyoid bone. It is thick in the median line, more delicate in its lateral portions. The epiglottis may be divided transversely. Thus the whole entrance to the larynx and pyriform sinuses are made accessible, but not the structures situated lower down. If the superior laryngeal nerves are to be avoided, the incision must stop about 1 to 1.5 cm. in front of the posterior extremity of the hyoid bone, or the latter may be divided at this site, so that the incision can be carried out alone as far as its posterior extremity.

The lateral incisions generally furnish more room and cause less danger. For small incision (as, for instance, in case of foreign bodies in the pyriform sinus) one may choose one side of the midhyoid or the suprahyoid portion of the pharynx. For tumors situated anteriorly and which are readily accessible, and in which regionary metastases are not to be expected, the transverse incision of the cheek according to Jäger may be indicated. Usually, however, longitudinal incisions are necessary. The latter possess the advantage also of permitting the easy removal of lymph-glands in cases of malignant tumors.

According to the investigations of Sappey, and recently those of
as well as the author's observations, in cases of malignant t
different groups of lymph-glands are affected according to the |
of the larynx involved. The lymph-vessels leading from the po
and lateral portions of all those parts enter the lymph-glands
retrovisceral connective tissue. In case of tumors originating
tonsils the first to be affected are the small glands situated at the su
pole in the peritonsillar tissue; later those glands situated alo
sternomastoid become involved. In case of tumor originating
pyriform sinuses, the arytenoepiglottidean fold, and the posterio
of the larynx, and consequently also anterior wall of the hypoph
the glands situated between the superior border of the thyroid ca
and the hyoid bone are first affected, later the above-mentione
glands of the neck. All these glands can be rendered accessi
lateral incisions, possibly also by adding a transverse incision just
or above the hyoid bone.

The region of the tonsil is best reached by placing a longit
incision further forward either from the angle of the mouth dow
with temporary division of the inferior maxilla (compare operati
the tongue), or in most cases, better still, according to the met
v. Mikulicz by making a *permanent resection of the ascending ra
the lower jaw.* An incision is made along the sternomastoid as fai
as the hyoid bone, the inferior maxilla is divided (wire saw) imme
above the insertion of the masseter, the resected portion enucleate
the tumor and any associated lymph-glands removed from withou
this way the entire diseased area is removed *in toto,* and last of
cavity of the mouth is opened. The author is able to state from po
experience that the motions of the jaw are completely restored, a
latter function remains normal even where there is recurrence.
slight deformity is produced by the displacement of the jaw. Ir
of smaller-sized tumors v. Langenbeck's temporary resection ful
same purpose and causes less destruction. If, however, as som
occurs, bony union of the fragments of the lower jaw is not effect
functional result is very bad.

In cases of tumors situated further back and lower down, resec
the lower jaw is generally not necessary; under such circums
lateral classical pharyngotomy of v. Langenbeck should be perfo
An incision is made along the anterior border of the sternomastoi
the mastoid process as far at least as the inferior border of the
cartilage, or even lower down. After dividing the fascia and pl
the lateral wall of the pharynx is forced into the wound by me
a catheter or similar instrument passed into the former. Durii
step the head should not be turned too far laterally in order
contract this space unnecessarily. The pharyngeal wall is then d
held with clamps, and turned outward. The finger can now
serted, and under guidance of the latter the incision prolon
far as the tumor and the latter removed. Below the angle of t
the visual field is extensive; close to the former, it is rather con

Frequently a transverse incision along the superior or inferior border of the hyoid may be useful (Krönlein, Bräm). In this way it is possible to turn the larynx out of the wound and thus render especially the pyriform sinuses accessible.

Whatever route is chosen in individual cases (numerous small modifications and combinations have been described as special methods), the principal problem is to expose thoroughly the tumor and the related glands; even the smallest of the latter should be removed. In most cases recurrence takes place in the glands, particularly at the base of the skull and in the retrovisceral space. Unless the defect is too large, the pharyngeal wall can be sutured. It is practicable, however, unless it is desirable to perform gastrostomy previously, to pass a Nélaton catheter through the nose to a point below the suture, for the purpose of subsequently feeding the patient. It can be fastened here with a piece of catgut in order to prevent its being vomited up after anæsthesia. The rest of the wound should be allowed to remain open and be packed with iodoform gauze; if the suture of the pharynx is exceptionally secure, the wound can be subsequently sutured; if this is not the case and the external wound is sutured, there is risk of causing a severe abscess. It is not advisable to insert a drainage-tube into the wound on account of the danger of erosion of the carotid. If the defect is so large that primary suture of the pharynx is impossible, the pharyngeal wound, provided the edges of the latter can be sufficiently retracted, may be sutured to the edges of the skin-wound according to v. Bergmann's suggestion. The secretion, which is usually abundant, can in this way freely escape externally. It is not necessary to insert a permanent catheter, as the sutured fistula readily allows the entrance of a tube for the purpose of feeding. If the pharyngeal wall were sutured, it is necessary for the purpose of maintaining the passage to begin dilatation with bougies through the mouth or the nose. If a fistula remains and is small, it may be closed by repeated cauterization, in other cases by resection, turning in the edges, and sewing up the edges of the fistula. If in case of extensive defects recurrence does not take place, attempts may be made to perform a plastic operation similar to those for defects of the œsophagus.

Prophylactic tracheotomy is unnecessary, and is best omitted if the tumor is situated sufficiently low down or is apparently sufficiently movable to assume that removal may be performed without the entrance of blood into the larynx. In opening the intact pharynx by means of a longitudinal incision this can always be avoided. In this situation transverse incisions are more dangerous. Prophylactic tracheotomy should always be performed if the wound for removal of the tumor is situated in the vicinity of the larynx. The tampon-cannula should be replaced by an ordinary cannula. The latter should remain in place sufficiently long. The author once saw a patient in whom tracheotomy had been omitted, and everything progressed well until the fourteenth day; then the patient died of inflammatory œdema of the arytenoepiglottidean folds before tracheotomy could be performed.

INDEX.

Lightning Source UK Ltd.
Milton Keynes UK
UKHW020623051218
333473UK00010B/280/P